FAMILY NURSING
Theory and Practice

THIRD EDITION

FAMILY NURSING

Theory and Practice

Marilyn M. Friedman, RN, MS, MA, PhD
Professor of Nursing
California State University, Los Angeles
Los Angeles, California

APPLETON & LANGE
Norwalk, Connecticut

0-8385-2543-1

93 94 95 96 / 10 9 8 7 6 5 4 3

Prentice Hall International (UK) Limited, *London*
Prentice Hall of Australia Pty. Limited, *Sydney*
Prentice Hall Canada, Inc., *Toronto*
Prentice Hall Hispanoamericana, S.A., *Mexico*
Prentice Hall of India Private Limited, *New Delhi*
Prentice Hall of Japan, Inc., *Tokyo*
Simon & Schuster Asia Pte. Ltd., *Singapore*
Editora Prentice Hall do Brasil Ltda., *Rio de Janeiro*
Prentice Hall, *Englewood Cliffs, New Jersey*

Library of Congress Cataloging-in-Publication Data

Friedman, Marilyn M.
Family nursing : theory and practice / Marilyn M. Friedman. — 3rd ed.
p. cm.
Includes bibliographical references and index.
ISBN 0-8385-2543-1
1. Family nursing. I. Title.
[DNLM: 1. Family—nurses' instruction. 2. Family Health. 3. Nursing Process—programmed instruction. WY 18 F911f]
RT120.F34F75 1992
610.73—dc20
DNLM/DLC 91-33191
for Library of Congress CIP

Senior Editor: Barbara Ellen Norwitz
Production Editor: Sheilah Holmes
Designer: Janice Barsevich

Cover Photo: Gustav Vigeland: The Family. (Granite)
Vigeland Sculpture Park, Oslo, Norway.

PRINTED IN THE UNITED STATES OF AMERICA

This Third Edition is dedicated
to my mother who left me with
the legacy of caring and commitment
to family.

Contributors

Kim Miller, RN, PhD
Assistant Professor
California State University
Los Angeles, California

Irene S. Morgan, RN, FNP, MS
Assistant Professor
California State University
Chico, California

Genevieve Monahan, RN, MS
Assistant Professor
California State University
Los Angeles, California

Reviewers

Noreen Meinhart, RN, MS
Formerly Clinical Nurse Specialist
UCLA Medical Center
Los Angeles, California

Judith E. Lausch, RN, MSN
Assistant Professor
Indiana University
Kokomo, Indiana

Martha A. From, EdD, RNC
Visiting Nurse Association
of Greater Philadelphia
Philadelphia, Pennsylvania

Sharon E. Beck, RN, EdM, MSN
Assistant Professor
LaSalle University
Philadelphia, Pennsylvania

Contents

Preface

It has been 14 years now since I completed the first edition of this text. At that time there were only three family-centered texts published. None of these texts, however, discussed family theory, assessment, or intervention in any depth. Now in 1992, there is a proliferation of texts in family-centered nursing that contain in-depth discussion of theories (family, family systems, and nursing) and their application to family nursing. The growth of publications about family nursing, the holding of family nursing conferences, the establishment of a family and health section of the National Council for Family Relations, and the increase in family nursing courses in undergraduate and graduate nursing programs presents strong evidence of the development of family nursing as both an integral part of generalist practice and a specialty area for those nurses engaged in advanced family nursing practice.

Moreover, there is a growing recognition that family nursing is conceptually and empirically distinct from nursing of family members. Due to the heavy influence of family therapy and application of systems theory, family nurses are increasingly "thinking interactionally" in their writings and discussions of families and family nursing practice.

I continue to be awed, however, by the contrast between what is promulgated in the nursing literature, and what actually exists in practice. A family-centered approach remains a stated ideal rather than a prevailing practice—not only in inpatient but also community and clinic settings. One literature review which surveyed published material detailing the extent to which family assessments were being completed by nurses from various areas in nursing confirmed that the focus is still on the individual (Temple, 1983). Nevertheless, in Temple's study (1983) where she sampled 99 nurses in community, school, inpatient and outpatient settings, she found that nurses who were more educated and who had completed family assesment courses, incorporated family assessment into their nursing practice to a greater extent.

My ardent belief is that health professionals, regardless of the setting, must broaden their commitment so that they serve families as units, as well as family subsystems (e.g., parental subsystems) and individual family members. One of the primary obstacles to providing family health care is a lack of substantive knowledge. Vast amounts of literature are available on the family—in the fields of sociology (family sociology), social psychology, anthropology (cross-cultural family studies), family therapy, social work, and nursing. But what do nurse educators teach in nursing that actually enables a nurse to work with families? Even though we see growing interest in family nursing, many schools of nursing do not include adequate family theory in their curriculum to provide the necessary foundation for family-centered practice. In health professional programs, there is typically an enormous concentration on the individual client or patient, with minimal focus on the family system. No one would negate the importance of studying the individual client comprehensively, but because the family is greater than and different from the sum of its parts, both the individual and group/family level of assessment and intervention must be nursing's focus. Sweeney (1970), two decades ago, expressed a similar conviction relative to public health nursing:

> The difference between philosophy and practice in public health nursing will be reconciled only when the public health nurse internalizes family concepts in relation to the needs of individuals and the needs of the family as a whole.

Several leaders in family nursing have recently acknowledged that systematic family assessment is emphasized in nursing curricula and publications, but that there is a lack of published writing about and emphasis on family nursing interventions (Gilliss, 1989a and Wright and Leahey, 1988). Based on my concern to extend this text to more adequately address the full practice of family nursing, rather than primarily theory and assessment, the text's focus in the Third Edition has been broadened to include family nursing diagnoses and family nursing interventions. One chapter (Chapter 18) has been added to cover general family nursing interventions. In addition, specific family practice areas, family nursing diagnoses, and family nursing intervention are addressed. Since there are so few published books on family nursing diagnoses and interventions, my discussion of these areas reflect the embryonic state of knowledge about family nursing interventions. Many of the suggestions made here were drawn from my own clinical experience or translated from individually-oriented nursing and mental health interventions.

This text is intended for undergraduate and graduate family nursing students and practitioners who are not involved in advanced family therapy or family systems nursing (Wright and Leahy, 1988a). Advanced family nursing practice requires the completion of a specialized program at the Masters level. Hence, I included family nursing interventions which are basic and straightforward; these suggest interventions, although certainly necessary within family nursing practice, are insufficient for working with the very complex family where more sophisticated, indirect interviewing and counseling skills are required.

In this edition, the same basic comprehensive family assessment tool, as in the first and second editions, is presented, with some modification. The family assessment model is based on three theoretical perspectives: a structural-functional perspective, a family developmental perspective and a systems perspective. Each chapter has been updated and contains both a theoretical and applied component that is related to each of the practice areas.

The family assessment process and much of the family theory presented in this textbook represent the product of my teaching of family and community health nursing as well as a graduate seminar in family nursing. I first started out with a very rudimentary tool. Gradually, as the result of insights gained from usage and student and faculty feedback, the family assessment tool grew into a series of self-learning modules which have been incorporated in much of the content within this book. The learning objectives and study questions were retained from the original modules to assist students with their own learning. The study questions (evaluation) at the end of the chapter test the objectives, and upon successful completion of the study questions the learner will have mastered the chapter objectives.

The assessment content and process presented in the following chapters has proved to be a valuable teaching-learning tool in both undergraduate and graduate courses. One obvious limitation to its usage in its pure form is that it is quite detailed and elaborate, precluding use in everyday practice. I believe, however, that a detailed approach is initially necessary to learn family nursing meaningfully. Once the content and skills are grasped, a more practical, attenuated assessment process may be initiated.

One way of using the comprehensive assessment tool with more clinical efficiency is to use the broad categories of assessment as *guides* to screen the family as to its basic strengths and problems. In comprehensively screening families, one or two presenting problem areas are usually identified. An in-depth assessment of these problem areas can then be accomplished, saving the practitioner considerable time and effort. Using interviewing skills to gain the family members' perceptions of experiences/events and observations of family interactions are important data collection methodologies to utilize in family nursing practice.

This book is subdivided into five broad areas. Part I includes three introductory chapters that discuss the family's importance and family definitions (Chapter 1), family nursing's evolution, focus and goals (Chapter 2), and the family nursing process (Chapter 3). The chapter on family nursing (Chapter 2) covers the gamut of goals and roles of the family nurse—from health promotion through rehabilitation. The rising costs of medical care, the implementation of DRG's, the rising proportion of older, chronically ill individuals, and the recognition that many chronic illnesses can be prevented or ameliorated with life-style changes are prominent trends which have greatly expanded the role of the family nurse in both health promotion and acute and long-term care in the home.

I have revised the chapters within Part II to expand the discussion of the basic theoretical approaches used in family nursing practice (Chapters 4–7). Chapter 4 includes the progress being made to reformulate family theories to fit a nursing perspective and to use nursing theories in family nursing practice. In the family development chapter (Chapter 6), family developmental theory is applied to single-parent and stepparent families. Greater depth of content is presented on the older family in this chapter also.

Part III introduces the reader to the actual family assessment model or tool, family nursing diagnoses (based primarily on NANDA), and family nursing interventions. I have integrated pertinent theory and content within each of these chapters. The specific topical areas where theory, assessment, nursing diagnoses and intervention are addressed are found in chapters focused on identifying family and sociocultural data, family structure, family functions, and family coping. Family structural dimensions are crucial to family nursing practice, since they cover family dynamics as seen in family communication patterns and processes (Chapter 10), the family power structure (Chapter 11), and the family role structure (Chapter 12). The affective function (Chapter 14), family socialization function (Chapter 15), and the health care function (Chapter 16), are the three most relevant family functions to assess in family nursing.

The sociocultural chapter in Part III is significantly expanded to cover the latest conceptual and research developments in the area. Social support research and theory is also now incorporated into this chapter.

Part IV addresses general family nursing interventions in Chapter 18. New intervention areas are highlighted under a discussion of nursing case management for the family who has a disabled or chronically ill/disabled family member or is experiencing the impact of the illness/disability on the family.

In Part V, cultural differences among families from the two largest minority groups in the United States, Mexican-Americans and Black Americans, are addressed in chapters 19 and 20. Current literature about the status of the Black American and Mexican-American family, coupled with an expanded description of family nursing interventions that are culturally sensitive and appropriate, make these chapters quite useful for working with culturally diverse clients.

The Appendices contain the complete family assessment tool (a shortened and a more detailed version), a family case description, and a case example of the use of the family nursing process. The family nursing example is included to give students a concrete model of family nursing practice and also an opportunity to retest themselves on the use of the Friedman Family Assessment Model and application of the family nursing process. Chapters in Part III describe the knowledge base needed to complete the family assessment and to develop family nursing diagnoses and intervention guidelines.

Acknowledgments

I particularly would like to thank the three contributors to the Third Edition: Dr. Kim Miller, a gerontology expert who revised the older family content in the family development chapter (Chapter 6), and Irene Morgan, who extensively updated and expanded Chapter 16, the Health Care Function, and Genevieve Monahan who expanded the case study and family nursing process application in Appendices C and D. I am also indebted to those family nursing leaders such as Dr. Lorrain Wright, Dr. Maureen Leahey, Dr. Wendy Watson, and Dr. Shirley Hanson who through their writings and professional friendship encouraged me to revise and expand this text. Noreen Meinhart, who carefully read the entire manuscript, corrected my English and typing errors, and questioned sentences that just didn't make sense, deserves a big round of applause. And lastly, a special thanks to my husband, Amnon and my dog, Tasha, who spent countless hours tolerating the noise from the computer and two years of having our bedroom filled with boxes and piles of books/papers/articles for the "revision in progress."

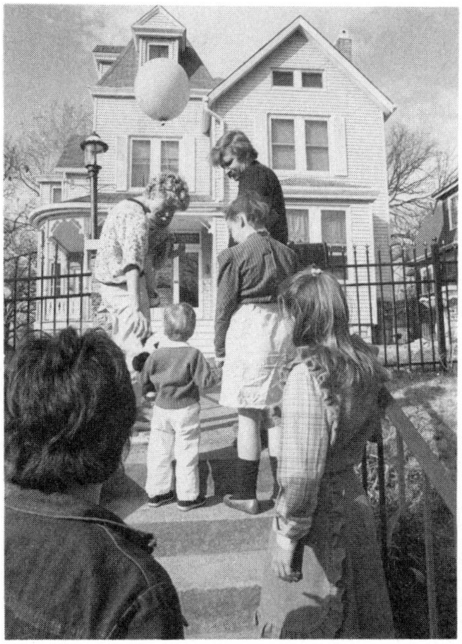

PART I

Introductory Concepts and Processes

Part I includes three foundational chapters for family nursing practice. Chapter 1 discusses the family's importance and family definitions. Chapter 2 covers family nursing's evolution, focus, and goals. In Chapter 3, the family nursing process is described and carefully applied to family nursing.

CHAPTER ONE

Introduction to the Family

Learning Objectives

1. Describe the basic purposes the family serves for society and the individual family members.
2. Explain why it is important for nurses to work with families.
3. Describe how family and society mutually affect each other.
4. Give examples of how the family influences the health status of its members, and of how the family is influenced by an illness of one or more of its members.
5. Define family, nuclear (conjugal) family, extended family, and family of orientation or origin.
6. Explain the difference between the meaning of health and family health.
7. Identify several demographic trends that have had major impact on the American family.
8. Discuss some of the factors associated with the growth of childless families, single-parent families, cohabiting families, and unmarried teenage mothers.
9. Define variant family forms and give examples of several types of traditional and nontraditional family forms.
10. Identify several stressors commonly found in single-parent and in step-parent families.

INTRODUCTION

One of the most important aspects of nursing is the emphasis placed on the family unit. The family—along with the individual, group, and community—is nursing's client or recipient of care.

Empirically we realize that the health of family members and the quality of family life is closely related. Until recently, however, remarkably little attention has been paid to the family as an object of systematic study in nursing. Apart from simple evaluative labeling of families with terms such as "good," "problem," "multiproblem," or "disorganized," nurses in the past were generally unable to objectively describe the families they were caring for. This situation is changing. Today the study of families in both undergraduate and graduate programs has grown significantly.

This chapter will set the stage for a systematic study of family theories and research (sometimes referred to as family science and family nursing science) and for family nursing practice by describing basic purposes of the family, the rationale for nurses working with families, how the society and family mutually influence each other, and most importantly, the salient interrelationship between the health status of family and the health status of its individual members. The chapter also discusses the state of the American family and its future, basic family definitions, and changing family forms.

Basic Purposes of the Family

Because the family forms the basic unit of our society, it is the social institution that has the most marked effect on its members. This basic unit so strongly influences the development of an individual that it may determine the success or failure of that person's life.

The family serves as the critical intervening variable (or as some authors term it, "buffer" or "bargaining agent") between society and the individual. In other words, the basic purpose of the family is *mediation*—taking the basic societal expectations and obligations and molding and modifying them to some extent to fit the needs and interests of its individual family members. At the same time the family provides new "recruits" for society, preparing children for assuming roles in society (Williams and Leaman, 1973).

Each family member has basic physical, personal, and social needs. The family must serve to mediate the demands and wishes of all the individuals within the unit. A family is expected to be concerned with the needs and demands of parent(s) as well as children, making it a difficult task to assign priorities to diverse individual needs at any particular time. On the other hand, society expects each member to fulfill certain obligations and demands. Hence, the family has to mediate the needs and demands of the family member with those of society.

Although a number of groups have a mediating function, the family is of central importance in that it is *the* primary group for the individual. Each family member belongs to a number of groups, but usually only the family is concerned with the total individual and all facets of his or her life. The highest priority of the family is usually the welfare of its family members. Other groups such as co-workers, church, school, and friends do not have concern for the whole individual, but usually limit themselves to one facet of an individual's life; for example, cooperation and friendliness at work, sincerity and involvement in church affairs, or productivity and achievement in school. This is not to say that other groups cannot serve as, or even replace, the family. In communes, monasteries, custodial hospitals, kibbutzim, or various rooming situations, nonfamily primary groups may provide this same critical mediating function.

A difference, however, that is not substitutable between these primary groups and the family is that the family still retains the replacement or reproduction responsibility. The other primary groups do not generate new members in order to guarantee the survival of the community.

To restate the family's role, the family unit occupies a position between the individual and society (Bronfenbrenner, 1979). Its functions here are twofold: (1) to meet the needs of the individuals in it and (2) to meet the needs of the society of which it is a part. These functions, which are fundamental to human adaptation, cannot be fulfilled separately. They must be joined in the family.

For society, the family, through its procreation and socialization of new members, functions to fill a vital need. It forms a grouping of individuals that society treats as an entity; it creates a network of kinship systems that help stabilize a society, even in its industrialized state; and it provides status, incentives, and roles for its members within the larger social system (Lidz, 1963).

The family also functions to meet the needs of its members. For the spouse or adult members it serves to stabilize their lives—meeting their affectional, socioeconomic, and sexual needs. For the children, the family provides physical and emotional care, and concomitantly directs their personality development. The family system is the main learning context for an individual's behavior, thoughts, and feelings. The family's mediating function also protects individuals from direct contact with society.

Parents are the primary "teachers," because parents interpret the world and society to children. The environment—outside forces—is important mainly as it affects parents, because parents are the ones who translate to the children the major meanings these outside forces have.*

The family has long been seen as the most vital context for healthy growth and development. It has a crucial influence on the formation of an individual's identity and feelings of self-esteem. Minuchin (1977), a noted family therapist, so beautifully summarizes the dual role that the family plays:

> The family, then, is the matrix of its members' sense of identity—of belonging and of being different. Its chief task is to foster their psychosocial growth and well-being throughout their life in common. . . . The family also forms the smallest social unit which transmits a society's demands and values, and thus, preserves them. The fam-

** The interpretation parents give of the world and society is naturally based on their experiences and their "reality." If they have been discriminated against or lived in a crime-ridden community, they may see the world as being dangerous, hostile, a place to avoid, and thereby impart these perceptions to their children. If, on the other hand, the world has provided stability and security for them, this perspective will be transmitted to their children.*

> ily must adapt to society's needs while it fosters it's members' growth, all the while maintaining enough continuity to fulfill its function as the individual's reference group. (p. 3)

An individual is the repository of group (especially primary group or family) experience. His or her identity is both individual (intrapersonal experiences) and social (interpersonal experiences). A person's intrapsychic experiences are largely developed from his or her interpersonal experiences, as through the parent–child relationship (Mead, 1934). A meaningful conception of an individual's mental health status can be achieved only when we relate the functioning of the individual to the human relation patterns of that person's primary group or family.

Why Work With the Family?

In the preface it was noted that family-centered practice has been promulgated by community health nursing since its inception. Why has there been the emphasis on working with families? Tinkham and Voorhies (1984) believe that the family provides the critical resource for delivering efficacious health services to people. They refer to the family as being the community health nurse's "patient," with the major focus being family health needs and their resolution.

The following summary highlights the most cogent reasons why the family unit must be a central focus of our care.

1. In a family unit, any dysfunction (illness, injury, separation) that affects one or more family members may, and frequently will, in some way affect other members as well as the unit as a whole. The family is a closely knit, interdependent network where the problems of an individual "seep in" and affect the other family members and the whole system. If a nurse assesses only the individual and not the family, he or she may be missing the gestalt needed to gain a holistic assessment. One of the important tenets of family therapy is that the symptoms of the identified patient (the family member with the overt behavioral problems or psychosomatic illness) are indices of the family's level of adaptation, or in this case, maladaptation.
2. There is such a strong interrelationship between family and health status of its members that the role of the family is crucial during every facet of health care of its individual family members—from preventive strategies through the rehabilitative phase. Assessing and rendering family health care is critical for assisting each family member to achieve an optimum level of wellness.
3. Through family health care that focuses on health promotion, "self-care," health education, and family counseling, significant inroads can be made to curtail risks that life-style and environmental hazards create. The goal is to raise the level of wellness of the whole family, which should then significantly raise the wellness level of each of its members.
4. Case finding is another good reason for providing family health care. The presence of health problems in one member may lead to discovery of disease or risk factors in other family members; this is often the case when visiting families with chronic health problems or communicable disease. The family-centered nurse works through the family to reach its members.
5. One can achieve a clearer understanding of the individuals and their functioning when they are viewed within their family context.
6. Inasmuch as the family is a vital support system for individuals, this resource needs to be assessed and incorporated into treatment plans for individuals.

THE FAMILY–SOCIETY INTERFACE

As the basic unit in society, the family shapes and is shaped by the external forces (community and larger social systems) surrounding it. Most sociologists would agree that the influence of society on the family is greater than that of the family on society, although the family exerts an effect on the society also. In spite of the greater impact society exerts on the family, the family should not be considered a passive, reactionary agent in the process of social change. Throughout history the family has demonstrated tremendous resiliency and adaptiveness, just as political, educational, and other societal institutions have shown their ability to change as need dictates. Moreover, the forces operating in society and in the family are continually intervening, interacting, and changing.

Society, with its beliefs, values, and customs, pervades every facet of family life, such as the age at which children may go to work and the age at which they are legally given adult status. Society also sanctions illness definitions, sick-role behaviors, and the appropriateness of treatments. The adulation of youth by society and the participation of women in the labor force has altered the functions of the family relative to its role in assisting parents and grandparents.

On the other hand, the family influences society, which in turn may alter social norms. For instance, the egalitarian roles that women have assumed in family life have made drastic changes in the way society now views women and their roles and capacities. The recent controversies over family planning services and abortion laws further exemplify the way in which the family exerts pressure on society to change. With rising expectations for accessibility to comprehensive health services, families continue to push for health legislation.

The great forces of a modern technological nation, with its emphasis on individual achievement and autonomy, have been effective in shaping family patterns in such a way that a more atomistic nuclear family has emerged (Goode, 1964). The nuclear family structure, however, is not unique to this postindustrial society; apparently the nuclear family was the predominant kinship structure in the past (Laslett, 1971). Despite the long-standing belief associated with a nostalgic view of the family in agrarian, preindustrial times, that many kinfolk lived together in extended families, the nuclear family—a group composed of parents and their children only—was the most common type of domestic unit. Given the high mortality characteristic of these societies, the number of persons that lived long enough to become grandparents and share a household with their married children and grandchildren was extremely limited. In addition, families were larger, so that there were not enough grandparents to spread around to the grandparents' offspring. The extended family households that did exist—those that included kin beyond the nuclear family—were likely to be among the rich, who had sufficient resources to support additional family members.

INTERACTION OF HEALTH/ILLNESS AND THE FAMILY

Family members' health/illness status and the family mutually influence each other. An illness within the family affects the whole family and its interactions, while the family in turn affects the course of an illness and members' health status. Hence, the impact of the health/illness status on the family and the family's impact on the health/illness status are reciprocal or highly interdependent (Gilliss et al., 1989; Wright and Leahey, 1984). Families tend to be both a reactor to health problems and an actor in determining members' health problems.

Turning to the interaction between the family and its members' health status, the family is the primary source for health and illness notions and health behavior. In one way or another, the family tends to be involved in the decision-making and therapeutic process at every stage of a family member's health and illness, from the state of being well (when promotion of health and preventive strategies are taught) to diagnosis, treatment, and recuperation. The process of becoming a "patient" and receiving health services encompasses a series of decisions and events involving the interaction of a number of persons, including family, friends, and professional providers of care. Generally speaking, the role the family plays in this process varies over time depending on an individual's health, the type of health problem (e.g., whether it is acute, chronic, severe), and the degree of familial concern and involvement.

Six stages of health/illness and family interaction will be presented to further illustrate the interdependency of the family and its members' health status.* These stages also present a temporal sequencing of a family's experience with illness.

Prevention of Illness and Risk Reduction Stage

The family can play a vital role in all forms of health promotion and risk reduction. Many forms of health promotion, prevention, and risk reduction exist. Many of these revolve around life-style issues such as the cessation of smoking and engaging in regular exercise. Whether a child gets a particular immunization, a father is encouraged to get more exercise and eat less, or a mother receives proper prenatal care, all involve, to a great degree, family decisions and participation. Health promotion begins in the family. Wellness strategies, to be successful, usually require improvements in the life-style of an entire family. Moreover, within a family, members learn about their own health status and body image—such as whether they are frail and sickly or healthy and resilient.

Family Symptom Experience Illness and Appraisal Stage

This stage begins when symptoms are (1) recognized; (2) interpreted as to their seriousness, possible cause, and importance or meaning; and (3) met with varying degrees of concern. The stage consists of the family's beliefs about the symptoms or illness of a family member and how to deal with the illness (Doherty and Campbell, 1988).

Because the family serves as the basic point of reference for assessing health behavior and provides basic definitions of health and illness, it influences the indi-

* *The following six stages represent an adaptation of Suchman's (1965) five stages of illness and medical care and Doherty and Campbell's (1988) five stages of the family health and illness cycle.*

vidual's perceptions. In the American family, the mother is frequently the major interpreter of the meaning of particular symptoms and what action should be taken. Litman (1974), in family studies he conducted, reported that the mother acted as health decision maker 67.7 percent of the time, while the father acted in this capacity only 15.7 percent of the time. This central family member (usually the mother) who influences health appraisal is called in some of the literature the "family health expert" (Doherty and Baird, 1987).

Families expose their members to health hazards and provide the basic interpretations of their symptoms. Families of lower-income groups are often slower to respond to initial symptoms or may not recognize symptoms as signs of disease (Koos, 1954).

Families not only influence recognition and interpretation of symptoms of illness, but they may be the *genesis* of illness among family members. Family social disorganization often has negative health consequences for family members. A variety of specific health problems have been found more frequently in stressed or disorganized families, among them tuberculosis (Holmes, 1956), arthritis (Scotch and Greiger, 1962), mental disorders (Leighton, et al, 1963), hypertension (Harburg et al, 1973), coronary heart disease (Syme et al, 1964), and stroke fatalities (Neser, 1975). Many studies, as illustrated in a decade literature review (Ross, Mirowsky and Goldsteen, 1990), demonstrate the pervasive influence of family on health. They found that four family factors provided explanations for this causal pattern, for example, marriage, parenthood, wife's employment and the family's social support system.

Care-seeking Stage

The care-seeking stage begins when the family decides that the ailing member is really sick and needs help. The ill person and family start to seek alleviation, information, advice, and professional validation from extended family, friends, neighbors, and other nonprofessionals (the lay referral structure). The decisions as to whether a member's illness should be treated at home or in a medical clinic or hospital tends to be negotiated within the family. For example, Richardson (1970), in a study of low-income, urban households, found that about one-half of those with illnesses reported consulting another family member concerning what they should do about the situation. Knapp and associates (1966) also found that the family was the most frequently mentioned source of information concerning home remedies and self-medication.

Not only does the family provide the basic definitions of health, but family members may press a family member into this stage if they believe he or she is failing to react favorably. This process may be extremely difficult for the family, particularly when a psychiatric disorder is the major problem. This is because the family may have to label the person as mentally ill and isolate him or her and/or acknowledge their own feelings of guilt and shame. The problem is compounded when the affected person denies the disorder or blames the family (Vincent, 1970).

Family's Contact With Health System Stage

This stage commences when contact is made with a health agency or professional or with an indigenous or folk practitioner. Studies have clearly shown that the family is again instrumental in deciding where the treatment is to be given and by whom (Pratt, 1976). The family health expert will refer a family member to whatever types of service or practitioner that is felt appropriate. The family, in serving to refer the family member, is called the primary health referral agent (Williams and Leaman, 1973). Of course, decisions about what services to use are also determined by the availability and accessibility of health care to the family.

Most health care utilization data show that while the more affluent families use primary care physicians and medical specialists for their care, the most common resource for initial medical care for poor families is the emergency room. Among working- and middle-class families, there has also been a growth in the use of prepaid group practice (health maintenance organization) systems.

The type of health care sought varies tremendously. The folk practitioner, the unorthodox "healer," the holistic health practitioner (using sometimes alternative modalities such as acupressure and acupuncture), the superspecialist (such as a neurosurgeon), the independent nurse practitioner, the primary care physician, and the family or individual therapist, should all be considered as possible sources of health care (thus broadening antiquated definitions of medical care).

How do families decide what clinic or health provider to contact? Although such variables as acceptability, appropriateness, perceived adequacy of service, and seriousness of condition are important, the accessibility and proximity to a primary care facility seems to also be a prime determinant of whom families contact (Abernathy and Schrems, 1971).

Acute Response of Patient and Family Stage

As the patient accepts care of health practitioners, he or she surrenders certain prerogatives and decisions, and is expected to assume the patient role, characterized by a dependence on the health professional's advice, the willingness to comply with medical advice, and a striving to recover. Parsons (1951) coined this social state, "the sick role." How this role is further defined and enacted at home will be influenced by the family's sociocultural and idiosyncratic background. Some families exclude the sick member from all responsibilities and "serve and assist" to the fullest extent. Other families expect little change in the ill member's behavior, hoping that he or she can carry on as usual; this way of handling is seen frequently when it is the mother who is sick. Litman (1974) explains the difficulty mothers often have when sick:

> In view of both her rather pervasive and pivotal role as an agent of cure and care within the family setting, the mother may find it not only extremely difficult to fulfill her obligations to all the members of the household when one or more is ill, but she may experience considerable difficulty in maintaining her normal role and responsibility when she herself is the one who is ill. (p. 505)

Hence, mothers generally have a great deal of reluctance in accepting a patient role.

Thus the family unit plays a pivotal role in determining the sick member's patient role behaviors. The family is also instrumental in deciding where the treatment should be given—hospital, home, or clinic. Efforts by health professionals to treat illness and promote good health may often conflict with family values and attitudinal patterns, making medical compliance problematic.

The acute response stage also concerns the immediate adjustment the family must make to the family member's illness, diagnosis, and treatment. For serious or life-threatening illness, a family crisis may ensue, wherein the family undergoes a period of disorganization in response to the powerful stressor event (Hill, 1949).

Adaptation to Illness and Recovery Stage

The presence of a serious, chronic illness in one family member usually has a profound impact on the family system, especially on its role structure and the carrying out of family functions. The disruptive effect may, in turn, negatively affect the outcome of rehabilitation efforts. Can the patient resume his or her prior (preillness) role responsibilities or is he or she able to establish a new, "workable" role in the family? The way in which this question is solved usually has to do with two factors: (1) the seriousness of the disability and (2) the "centrality" of the patient within the family unit (Sussman and Slater, 1963). When either the nature of the person's condition is serious (greatly disabling or progressively deteriorating) or the family member is a pivotal, crucial person to the family's functioning, the impact on family is much more pronounced.

Families play an important supportive role during the course of a client's convalescence or rehabilitation. In the absence of this support, the success of convalescence/rehabilitation decreases significantly.

In summary, within the six stages, the ways in which families influence the health of their members are: (1) as a cause or the source of illness, (2) as a factor affecting the trajectory and outcome of illness once present, (3) as a locus for spread of illness from one family member to another, (4) as a determinant of health care utilization, and (5) as a determinant of the extent to which the ill or disabled member adapts to his or her condition.

FAMILY DEFINITIONS

The family has been defined in various ways. Definitions of the family differ depending on the theoretical orientation of the "definer"—that is, by the kind of explanation the writer seeks to make concerning the family. For instance, writers who follow the interactionist theoretical orientation of the family see the family as an arena of interacting personalities, thus emphasizing the family's dynamic transactional characteristics. Writers who espouse a general systems perspective define the family as a small open social system composed of a set of highly interdependent parts and affected by both its internal structure and extreme systems.

A widely referenced, traditionally oriented definition of the family by Burgess and associates (1963) is as follows:

1. The family is composed of persons joined together by bonds of marriage, blood, or adoption.
2. The members of a family usually live together in a single household; or, if they live separately, consider the household their home.
3. Family members interact and communicate with each other in family social roles such as husband and wife, mother and father, son and daughter, brother and sister.
4. The family shares a common culture that is derived primarily from societal culture containing some unique features of its own.

Although this definition is commonly used, it is limited in terms of applicability and comprehensiveness. Any definition of the family must cover the wide array of family forms present today, and traditional definitions such as the above definition do not do this.

Whall (1986), in her concept analysis of the family as the unit of care in nursing, defines family as "a self-identified group of two or more individuals whose association is characterized by special terms, who may or may not be related by blood lines or law, but who function in such a way that they consider themselves to be a family" (p. 241). Taking into account who individuals identify as family members is a crucial component of this definition. Bozett (1987) incorporates the individual's definition by referring to family as "who the patient says it is" (p. 4). Family Service America (1984) also defines family in a comprehensive manner—as "two or more people joined together by bonds of sharing and intimacy" (p. 7).

Incorporating two central notions from the above definitions, family in this text refers to *two or more persons who are joined together by bonds of sharing and emotional closeness and who identify themselves as being part of the family.* Because this definition is purposefully broad, it then encompasses the variety of relationships formally excluded by traditional definitions. This includes extended family living in two or more households, cohabiting couples, childless families, gay and lesbian families, and single-parent families.

The following additional family definitions connoting general family types are presented to facilitate an understanding of family literature.

- *Nuclear (conjugal) family*—The family of marriage, parenthood, or procreation; it is composed of a husband, wife, and their immediate children—natural, adopted, or both.
- *Family of orientation (family of origin)*—The family unit into which a person is born.
- *Extended family*—The nuclear family and other related (by blood) persons, who are most commonly members of the family of orientation of one of the nuclear family mates. These are "kin"—grandparents, aunts, uncles, and cousins.

FAMILY HEALTH

Given that family nursing is ultimately concerned with the health of the family, the concept of family health—or as Dunn calls it, family wellness—needs to be clarified. In reviewing the literature in this area, it is clear that this concept is probably even less consistently and clearly defined than the concept of health. In both cases the concepts are defined so broadly and abstractly that to fully operationalize them becomes a most difficult task.

Stemming from systems theory, we first need to assume that family health is more than just a sum of its parts (the health status of each of the family members). It is greater than and different from its parts. In systems terms, this notion is called "nonsummativity." Yet, in the literature we see that the term "family health" or "familial health" is used ambiguously (Johnson, 1984), sometimes referring to the health of the individual family members and sometimes to the health of the family unit itself. Because only individuals can have medical diseases, it is obvious that the former usage of the term is flawed.

In family research, family health is most often conceptualized as family functioning or family adaptation (McCubbin and Patterson, 1983a), although variations within this broad definition exist. The World Health Organization (1974) proposes a similar definition of this latter definition. They state that familial health "connotes the relative functioning of the family as the primary social agent in the promotion of health and well-being" (p. 17).

The meaning of family health also differs depending on the discipline of the author or the theoretical perspective he or she adopts. For instance, in family mental health where an interactional perspective is taken, family health is referred to as the state of the family's internal processes or dynamics such as their interpersonal relationships. The focus is on relationships between the family and its subsystems, such as the parental or parent–child subsystem, or between the family and its members.

If a systems perspective is adopted, the outcome of internal interactions and exchange between the family and its environment are emphasized. One of the outcomes is a balance between growth or change and stability or equilibrium in the family (Wright and Leahey, 1984). Both tendencies are needed in the proper balance for a family to be functional or healthy.

Public health and community welfare authors use different indicators of family health. These address the relationships of family to the community and its stability as a unit. They include poverty and divorce rates among families, presence of criminal and juvenile problems, and high school dropout and unemployment rates as indicators of family health.

Family nursing authors tend to use a family mental health or systems perspective in defining family health. There is also growing interest in using nursing theories in family nursing. One example of the application of a nursing theory to working with families comes from Tadych (1985). Applying Orem's self-care theory, family health refers to the extent to which the family assists its members to meet their self-care requisites, as well as the extent to which it fulfills its family functions and accomplishes the tasks appropriate to the family's developmental level (p. 52).

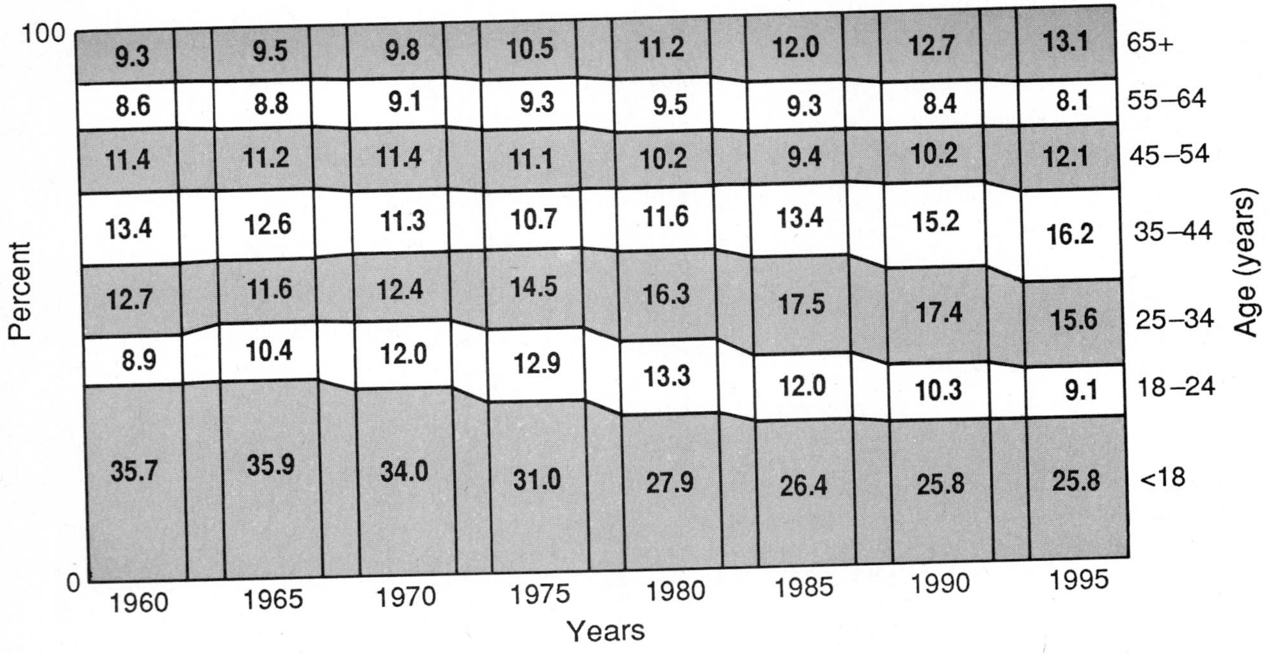

Figure 1–1
The U.S. population is getting older (age distribution of the U.S. population). (Source: U.S. Bureau of the Census, 1982.)

THE AMERICAN FAMILY

The pace of social change in recent decades has accelerated, with the family especially feeling its impact. In this process the family has demonstrated remarkable resiliency and ability to adapt to environmental flux. As the family interfaces with multiple institutions in society, it is in a perpetual state of evolution (Berardo, 1988). It mediates, translates, and incorporates social change within its structure (Goode, 1964). With the family evidencing increasing complexities in household and family patterns, family members now have more options to pursue life-styles that reflect their differences and preferences. Nevertheless, many family social scientists and family health professionals are concerned about the state of the American family and see many of the rapid family changes occurring as a result of adults pursuing their own goals of equality and individual freedom. Their concerns largely focus on the effects these various family changes have on the children.

Evidence of the profound changes and enormous diversity within American families comes from demographic data primarily compiled by the U.S. Bureau of the Census. Naisbitt in *Megatrends* (1984) colorfully describes these changes in the 1980s as a "decade of unprecedented diversity." He explains that there is no longer such a thing as the typical family:

> Instead, the diversity in American households of the 1980s has become a Rubik's cube of complexity. And like Rubik's cube, the chances of getting back to its original state are practically nil. (p. 261)

Demographic Trends

Aging of the Population. Probably the most important trend in demography is the increased general life expectancy and the fact that majority of the population now survives into old age. Because of this, the United States is in the midst of a demographic revolution, the inexorable aging of our population (Fig. 1–1). Senior citizen growth is particularly rapid in the group over 75 years of age (Fig. 1–2).

The aging population will have an enormous impact on the family and on health care. For instance, because women live 7 to 8 years longer than men, most older persons, especially over 75, are women who live alone and are poor. In terms of health care, with over 13 percent of the U. S. population in 1995 being over 65 years of age (and the proportion will steadily rise to 24 percent in 2050), the nation's health care will be crit-

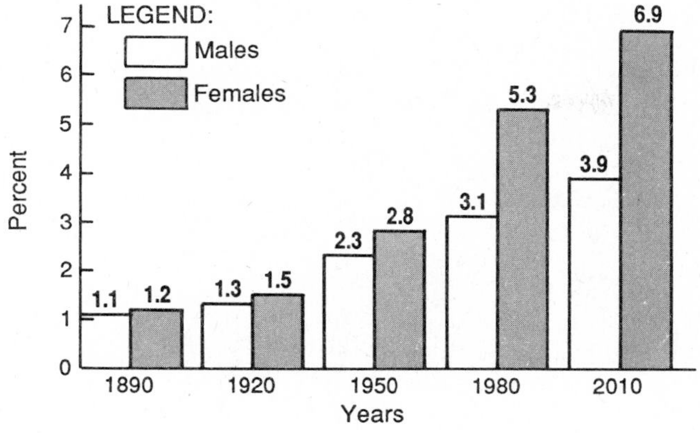

Figure 1–2
Increase in the very old population (percent of population 75 years and older, by sex). (Source: U.S. Bureau of the Census, 1978.)

ically strained. The rapid growth of the very old, who are the biggest users of health care services as well as caregiver assistance, will have a profound effect on family life (Pifer and Bronte, 1986).

Family or Household Size. The decrease in family and household size is a major long-term demographic trend. According to the U. S. Bureau of the Census (1988), the size of the American household was at a historic low of 2.66 persons in 1987. Concomitantly, women also have experienced a shortened childbearing period, this period referring to the years they have raising children, from the youngest to the oldest child. These recent decreases in family size reflect the cumulative impact of recent decline in fertility (down to 1.8 children per mother), and the increases in age of first marriage, rates of divorce, and rates of illegitimate births (Santi, 1987).

Marriage, Divorce, and Remarriage. The United States is found to have one of the highest marriage rates among developed counties. This is partly due to having one of the highest divorce and subsequent remarriage rates (Glick, 1988a). The divorce rate in the United States continues to climb. In 1988, White reported that estimates for recent marriages ending in divorce range from 40 to 50 percent. The long-term upward trend in marital disruption for the United States has nearly been matched by the upward trend in remarriages, reflecting an overall preference for marriage over single life (Teachman et al, 1987). Inasmuch as men remarry more than women, many divorced women live in a state of poverty or near poverty because of their disadvantaged economic position. The prominence of no-fault divorce has enhanced the disadvantageous economic position of the divorced woman by effectively removing legal support for the husband's long-term commitment to support the mother of his children (White, 1988).

Increase in First Births to Older Mothers. In a recent report from the National Center for Health Statistics (Ventura, 1989), national data were summarized that indicated there has been a significant increase in the numbers of first births to older mothers, ages 30 to 34 and particularly ages 35 to 39. These women tend to be better educated and during their pregnancy to receive prenatal care. Although the typical ages of childbearing continue to be 15 to 19 years, women in their early 30s accounted for 12 percent of all first births in 1986 compared with just three percent in 1970.

The dramatic rise in first births among older women is the result of several other demographic trends. First, marriage has been postponed by a sizable proportion of young people; second, there has been a sharp decline and then a leveling off of first births for women in their 20s, leaving large numbers of women still childless at age 30 and older. In addition, there was a substantial growth in the number of women age 25 to 39 from 1970 to 1986. These are the children born during the baby boom years following World War II. And lastly, national surveys show that most women intend to have at least one child, with only about 10 percent of women in their early 30s expecting to remain childless (Ventura, 1989).

Women's Employment. In the aftermath of World War II, the labor force participation of women rose steadily. Whereas single women's employment rates held constant after World War II, the employment rates of married women rose dramatically. Over 60 percent of married women with school-aged children were employed in the United States in 1981. Among mothers with preschoolers, the rates were somewhat lower (47 percent) (Moore et al, 1984).

Other family demographic trends are also significant to understanding the present state of the American family as well as its future. These are presented here under each of the varied family forms.

VARIED FAMILY FORMS

Never in recorded history has a society been composed of a greater multiplicity of attitudes, values, behaviors, and life-styles. These social, behavioral, and cultural differences are reflected in a variety of family forms. Hence, families using health services come from all walks of life and represent all types of life-styles. Many, if not most, of our clients are not part of the idealized traditional nuclear family. It is imperative for health care professionals to understand and appreciate the wide varieties of family forms, as well as some of the reasons for their existence.

One of the primary reasons for the growing array of heterogeneous family forms is our affluent, pluralistic society, which is highly differentiated, specialized, and values personal freedom, choice, and independence. In addition, the various family forms represent different adaptations to environmental demands placed on people and families. Each family form has its own particular strengths and vulnerabilities. Nonetheless, it is probably true that certain family arrangements are probably more suitable for fulfilling certain basic functions than other forms. However, in studies that compare different family forms with each other, it has been very difficult to sort out the effect of the family form from the many other variables, that also influence the outcomes being studied, such as socioeconomic factors, family developmental stage, and child care arrangements (Macklin, 1988).

In family sociology, the various family forms are classified as traditional and nontraditional, and as normative and nonnormative or variant family forms. Variant family forms refer to those family structures that are a variation from the norm. They include all deviations from the traditional nuclear family, which is characterized by households of husband, wife, and children living apart from both sets of parents with the male as the breadwinner and wife as the homemaker (Sussman et al, 1971). The term "variant" is used in an attempt to avoid negative connotations toward any ex-

TABLE 1–1. DIFFERENT FAMILY FORMS IN THE UNITED STATES

Traditional Variant Family Forms	Nontraditional Variant Family Forms
The most common traditional types of variant family forms now existing are: 1. Nuclear family—dual worker/dual career, husband, wife, and children living in same household. a. First marriage families b. Blended or step-parent families 2. Nuclear dyad—husband and wife alone; childless, or no children living at home. a. Single career b. Dual career 1. Wife's career continuous 2. Wife's career interrupted 3. Single-parent family—one head, as a consequence of divorce, abandonment, or separation. a. Working/career b. Unemployed 4. Single adult living alone. 5. Three-generation extended family—may characterize any variant of family forms (1, 2, or 3 above) living in a common household. 6. Middle-aged or elderly couple—husband as provider, wife at home (children have been launched into college, career, or marriage). 7. Extended kin network. Two or more nuclear households of primary kin or unmarried members living in close geographical proximity and operating within a reciprocal system of exchange of goods and services.	The most common nontraditional variant family forms are: 1. Unmarried parent and child family—usually mother and child. 2. Unmarried couple and child family—usually a common-law-type of marriage. 3. Cohabiting couple—unmarried couple living together. 4. Gay/lesbian family—persons of the same sex living together as "marital partners." 5. Commune family—household of more than one monogamous couple with children, sharing common facilities, resources, and experiences; socialization of the child is a group activity.

Adapted from Sussman (1974), Macklin (1988).

isting type of family and to recognize the diversity of options available to people and families.

As can be seen in Table 1–1, a multitude of different family forms exist. Because of their significance for family nursing, the major types of family forms will be described.

The Nuclear Family

The "vanishing" nuclear family constitutes one of the most significant demographic and social transformations in recent history. With the acceleration of the divorce rate, out-of-wedlock births, and cohabitation from 1965 to the present, family forms other than the nuclear family have rapidly proliferated. According to the 1990 U.S. Census the nuclear family consisting of a husband provider, a wife homemaker, and children, that was once the norm, accounts for 26 percent of all households (U.S. Bureau of the Census, February 1991). Hofferth (1985) estimated that 70 percent of all white children and 94 percent of all black children born in 1986 have spent or will spend part of their lives before age 18 in a nonnuclear family.

Although it is recognized that the traditional nuclear family is no longer modal, family scientists have asked "to what extent is the traditional family the norm?" This type of family appears to still be the "ideal" norm, but not the "real" norm. Surveys suggest the majority of Americans still wish for traditional family life. Although at any one point in time the majority of adults are not living in traditional nuclear households, over the course of their lives, most will do so. Yet increasing numbers, as previously described, are living in nontraditional family forms. Yankelovich (1981), reporting the findings of a large national survey of adults he conducted, noted that there is greater acceptance of egalitarianism, as seen in the growth of shared parenting and decision making, as well as a greater tolerance for nontraditional living arrangements.

Two growing variations within nuclear families are the dual-worker/dual-career and the childless family. Adoptive families are also another type of nuclear family noted in the literature as having special circumstances and needs.

The Dual-worker Family. With the striking increase in employment among married women, the great majority of families will have both spouses simultaneously employed for some period of the family's life cycle. In most dual-worker families, where both spouses are employed either part or full-time, the majority of women (and many men) have what might be called jobs—positions that are not a major life interest and are undertaken for economic reasons (Skinner, 1984). There is a growing minority of families, however, where both husband and wife pursue careers while maintaining a family. Career people tend to view their positions as a primary source of personal satisfaction and identity. Skinner (1984), in summarizing research of dual-career families, reported that a significant feature of the dual-career life-style is that it is associated with considerable stress and strain, with more stress and strain reported by the wife than her husband. The basis of this stress is primarily due to the competing demands of the occupational structure and those associated with the family—child care, homemaking, and marital responsibilities. Two-career couples tend to do more sharing of traditionally female tasks than do one-career or dual-worker families, particularly in the area of child care (Barnett and Baruch, 1987; Macklin, 1988). But it appears that in many families, the wife still assumes the major responsibility for domestic tasks (Spitze, 1988).

A crucial concern in the dual-worker literature is about the effects of both parents working on the children. "There is no evidence to date to suggest that the dual-career life-style, in and of itself, is stressful for the children" (Skinner, 1984).

There is also growing research interest in one form of the dual-career family—the commuter family, in which spouses voluntarily live in separate residences for at least a majority of each week because of geographically separated jobs. This is usually a temporary pattern. Research findings have pointed to the difficulties that this life-style imposes (Macklin, 1988).

The Childless Family. One type of traditional variant nuclear family is the family without children. An extensive number of recent research studies have been published on the correlates and consequences of childlessness as well as the reasons for not having children (Houseknecht, 1987). About 5 percent or more of all ever-married women in the United States are voluntarily childless. The rate is expected to go up to 10 percent in the near future not only because of delayed marriage and childbearing patterns but because of the many career and educational options now available to women (Macklin, 1988).

The Extended Family

The traditional extended family is one in which the couple shares household arrangements and expenses with parents, siblings, or other close relatives. The children are then reared by several generations and have a choice of models after which to pattern their behavior. This type of family is more frequent in working-class and recent immigrant families. As people live longer, and divorces, teenage pregnancies, and out-of-wedlock births increase, houses also have become home to several generations, usually on a temporary basis. Demographers also have found that because of increased longevity, four- and five-generation families are becoming commonplace among poor and working-class families (Otten, 1989).

There is also another form of extended family—the extended kin network family. Here two or more nuclear households of primary kin or unmarried kin live in close proximity and operate within a reciprocal system of social support, including the exchange of goods and services. This type of family form is modal in the Latino community (see Chap. 19 for greater detail).

Although the great majority of Americans do not live in the two types of extended families mentioned, greater extended family ties are possible and widespread today due to advances in transportation and communication. The nuclear American family is not as isolated as it superficially appears. The many ways in which families rely on one another create an extended family context that has been verified in several important studies. The frequently repeated myth that the nuclear family is isolated from family supports is not borne out by this research, the evidence showing that a modified extended family usually exists within a rich network of generational interaction (Hill, 1970; Kingson et al, 1986). Primary kin—parents and siblings of spouses—form the most important network of extended kinship relations. The common modified extended family of today differs from the isolated nuclear family in that it provides significant support and continuing assistance to other nuclear families within the extended-family network (Shanas et al, 1968). This type of extended family is typically set up on an egalitarian basis and is composed of a series of nuclear families that equally value these extended-family bonds (Litwak, 1972).

The Single-parent Family

The single-parent family is one in which there is one head of household, mother or father. The traditional variant single-parent family is one where the head is widowed, divorced, abandoned, or separated. The nontraditional variant single-parent family is one where the head—practically always the mother—has never been married (Table 1–1).

Demographic Trends. One of the most dramatic demographic changes taking place in the United States is the radical shift in the modal household from one headed by a marital pair rearing their dependent-age children to a household headed by a single adult (Rossi, 1986). Since 1940 the number of single-parent families has increased in the United States, from 12 percent in 1940 to 25.7 percent in 1986. Breaking these statistics

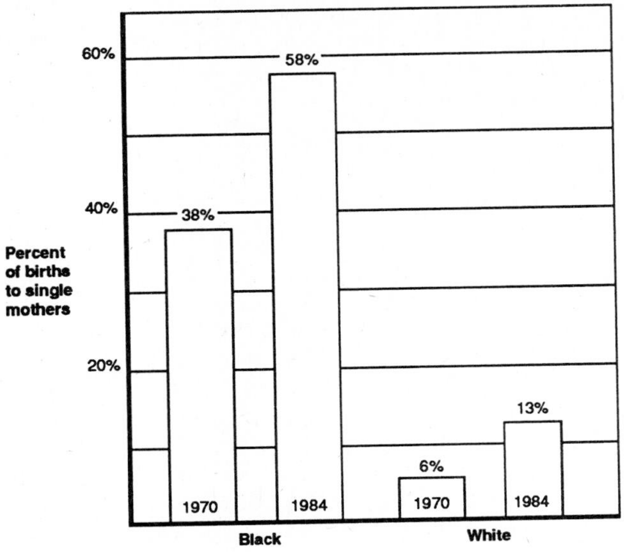

Figure 1–3
Rising proportion of births to unmarried women. (National Center for Health Statistics, 1986.)

down by black and white families, 50 percent of all black families were single-parent families, while 15 percent of all white families were single-parent families. There was a 69 percent increase in the number of single mothers from 1970 to 1985 (U.S. Bureau of the Census, 1985).

The proportion of children nationally who are under the age of 18 and are cared for by a single parent, however, has skyrocketed, from 9 percent of all children in 1960 to 24 percent of all children in 1986. Among black children the proportion is much greater, from 22 percent in 1960 to 53 percent in 1986 (Fig. 1–3). Sixty percent of all children will spend about a year or longer in a single-parent home before they reach the age of 18.

Factors associated with the rapid increase in the numbers of one-parent families are (1) the upsurge in divorce, (2) the large amount of financial aid to one-parent families with dependent children, and (3) the tremendous growth in the number and proportion of births that occurred to unmarried mothers—from 5 percent of all births in 1960 to 22 percent of all births in 1985. Within this group, the largest increase was in black births, which rose from 22 percent in 1960 to 60 percent in 1985 (Glick, 1988b).

Among unmarried mothers, the significant increase is within the teenage mother group. From 1970 to 1987 there was a 22 percent increase in births among unmarried women ages 15 to 17. Ninety percent of these teenage mothers had not completed high school and were on means-tested support programs (U.S. Bureau of the Census, 1985). About 88 percent of single parent families in 1986 were mother–child families (Chilman, 1988). Moreover, of all single-parent families, the largest group is headed by divorced and separated mothers (55 percent), followed by never-married mothers (24 percent) (U.S. Bureau of the Census, 1985).

Mendes (1988), in reviewing the research on single-parent families, emphasizes the fact that single-parent families are not homogeneous. They are, in fact, very diverse in terms of their resources, opportunities, and limitations. She identifies five common life-styles of the single parent:

1. Sole executive life-style. Here the single parent is the only parent actually involved in the lives and care of the children. In some cases, he or she attempts to fulfill both father and mother roles and is very much prone to stress, fatigue, and role overload. In other families, the sole executive handles what he or she can do without undue stress, and then coordinates the allocation of some of the other functions by assigning them to competent persons within or outside the family.
2. Auxiliary parent. In this life-style the custodial parent shares one or more of the parental responsibilities with an auxiliary parent, usually the father of one or more of the children.
3. Unrelated substitute. In this life-style the custodial parent shares one or more parental functions with a person who is not related to the family, such as a live-in housekeeper who is "like a mother" to the children.
4. Related substitute. Here the related substitute is a blood or legal relative who assumes a parental role. These persons are often grandmothers, but could also be aunts, uncles, cousins, or siblings of the children.
5. Titular parent. The titular parent lives with the children, but has, for all intents and purposes, abdicated the parental role. Teenage mothers or mothers who are alcoholics, drug addicts, or mentally disturbed are sometimes parents in name only. In these cases there may be a parental child acting as parent, or a parent of the titular parent who assumes the child care and domestic responsibilities.

Each of these types of single-parent families has its own set of problems and strengths. Crucial to the successful functioning of any of these types of families, however, is its integration into a viable psychosocial support system.

As a group, single-parent families are disadvantaged when compared to other forms of families. They are characterized as having a high rate of poverty, are disproportionately from disadvantaged minority backgrounds, are more mobile, and the single parents are relatively undereducated. This is more often the case in female-headed than in male-headed families.

Of the generic features of single-parent families, poverty is the most serious. Families headed by women (over 10 million in 1985) had a poverty rate of 34.5 percent and accounted for nearly half of all poor families. *Newsweek* (Gelman et al, 1985) calls these women a "new class of poor." Single parenthood appears to be a major factor in "the feminization of poverty." Several variables are cited as causative factors: the minimal to nonexistent child support from fathers, the inequities of the workplace for women, and cutbacks in social welfare programs during the tenure of the last two conservative presidents.

Role changes and role conflicts are other generic features of single parents. Role problems revolve around playing both mother and father roles; and the role overload of working, raising a family, domestic responsibilities, and of attempting to have a personal life. And lastly, since most single divorced parents will remarry, there is the necessity of making another major role change—relinquishing the other parent role and forming new marital and parental roles on remarriage (Hogan et al, 1984; LeMasters, 1974; Macklin, 1988).

About 12 percent of all single parents were men in 1985. Father-headed families have more than doubled since 1970 (U. S. Bureau of the Census, 1986). Although courts still favor mothers as custodial parents, men are making more vigorous claims to custody rights. Single fathers experience the same role change and role overload problems. They are on average, however, much better off financially.

The Unmarried Teenage Mother. As mentioned earlier, a very large increase of pregnancies is occurring within the unmarried teenage group, particularly among black adolescent girls. Births to unmarried teenagers are also high, and would be even higher if not for abortion. It is estimated that about half of teenage pregnancies are resolved by abortions (Chilman, 1988). The causes for the increase in unmarried teenage families are multiple. The major factors cited in the literature are early sexual activity, no use or ineffective use of contraceptives, poverty, failing to marry before the child's birth, and relatively greater acceptance of unwed adolescent motherhood among lower-class African-Americans (Chilman, 1988). The fact that over 50 percent of black urban male youths are unemployed is one reason for the low marriage rate in the black teenage group. The shortage of young black men as compared to young black women also explains why so many young black teenage mothers do not marry.

Services to adolescent single parents to date are sorely inadequate. A continuum of services is needed. They range from primary preventive services in sex education and birth control to outreach programs, support networks, counseling, and school-based clinics and parenting classes, as well as services to the extended families of unmarried teenage mothers.

Single parents as a whole also have special needs. In addition to providing parenting classes and peer support networks, social policy changes are required so that adequate child care facilities and institutional supports such as flexible working hours can be established.

The Single Adult Living Alone

The number of people living alone has also grown. In 1986, 24 percent of all households were made up of people living alone. A preponderance of elderly women live alone, but the large increase in lone living is among those adults in their 20s and 30s (Glick, 1988a).

Many home health clients, especially older chronically ill or disabled individuals, are single people living alone. Although these solitary people do not appear to fit into the text's definition of family, they probably have extended family members, siblings or children being the most common, which they identify as their family. Most solitary people are part of some loosely formed family network. If this network is not made up of relatives, then it may be composed of friends such as those residing in the same retirement home, nursing home, or neighborhood. Pets can also be important family members.

Then there are those individuals who are truly "loners." They have a greater need for health and psychosocial services, because they have no support system and sometimes aren't interested in developing one. Long-term and home care nurses can help these types of clients by developing a supportive relationship with them, and thereby can reduce the client's social isolation.

The Step-parent Family

Although divorce has been increasingly common, this trend has been accompanied by high rates of remarriage. This situation has produced a growing number of step-parent or blended families. It was estimated that in 1981 about one child in five was living with a step-parent (Pollack, 1981). Usually these types of families are comprised of a mother, her biological children, and a step-father.

This family form typically is one that initially is a complex and stressful merger. One of the primary reasons for this is the difficulty associated with integrating a step-father into an already established family and the mixed allegiance or divided loyalities that the wife-mother feels towards her husband and children (Visher and Visher, 1979).

McCubbin and Dahl (1985) summarized literature about parents in a remarriage. They state that the three most widely referenced problem areas are disciplining children, adjusting to children's personalities and habits, and winning acceptance. Macklin (1988) adds to this list of problem areas the role ambiguity of step-parents and step-kin, unrealistic expectations of family members, lack of time for step-parents to learn the new parental role, and conflict over finances and child rearing.

The Binuclear Family

The binuclear family refers to the postdivorced family in which the child is a member of a family system composed of two nuclear households, maternal and paternal, with varying degrees of cooperation between and time spent in each household (Ahrons and Perlmutter, 1982). With the movement toward sex-role equity, increased participation by some fathers in parenting, and the growing awareness of the loss of being a noncustodial parent and the negative consequences to children where there is no father contact, various ways of active coparenting have emerged. The most widely discussed form of active coparenting is joint custody, where both parents have equal legal rights and responsibilities to the minor child irrespective of residential arrangements.

There has been increased attention given to coparenting and joint custody. Nevertheless, these family arrangements are only seen among a small fraction of divorced families. A case in point: in a nationally representative sample of children in single-parent and step-parent families, almost half of the children had not seen their nonresidential parent in the past year. The residential parent assumed a disproportionately large amount of the child care (Furstenberg and Nord, 1985).

Nontraditional Variant Family Forms

Nontraditional variant family forms cover a wide gamut of family forms that are very different from one another in structure and dynamics, although probably more similar to one another in goals and values than to the traditional nuclear family. Specific family forms here include open marriages, communal families, cohabiting couples, group marriages, and gay and lesbian families (Cogswell, 1975; Macklin, 1988). Refer to Table 1–1.

Cogswell (1975) reports that one theme implicit in the literature relates to the nontraditional families' rejection of the myth of the idealized traditional nuclear family. Advocates of these types of families see the nuclear family as restrictive to one's personal preferences and goals. Those in nontraditional family arrangements often stress the value of self-actualization, independence, gender equality, intimacy in a variety of interpersonal relationships (not exclusively marital), and openness in communication. The delay of marriage and parenthood, the reduction of family size, and the high divorce rate are all evidence that other options besides marriage and family are present for both sexes.

The Nonmarital Heterosexual Cohabiting Family

There is a substantial growth in the number of U. S. couples living together unmarried (U. S. Bureau of the Census, 1985). This wave of cohabitation appeared in the 1960s and has continued, with over a 100 percent increase nationally in the number of cohabiting household units from 1977 to 1986 (from nearly 1 to 2.2 million households). This trend is expected to continue. In an earlier era, cohabitation was limited to the very rich, those in the theater, and the very poor, according to Weiss (1988). But today, cohabitation has become a much more acceptable nontraditional family form of young adults before and in between marriages.

LOOKING AT THE FUTURE OF THE AMERICAN FAMILY

The dramatic changes of recent years have led some alarmists to proclaim the demise of the family, while other positivists have seen the family as remarkably adaptive and resilient. It seems reasonable to conclude that the family is continuing its age-old process of gradual evolution, adapting to the changing economic and social realities of society. Nevertheless, many families are in trouble. It is only in recognizing the stressed state of these families that social action, broadened family-focused health services, and urgently needed domestic policy changes will occur.

FAMILY NURSING IMPLICATIONS

A description of the above family forms illustrates the broad array of structures prevalent in families today. There is no "right," "wrong," "proper," or "improper" form of family. Families must be understood within their own context. Labels and types serve only as a reference to the family's living arrangements and primary group network. Every effort must be made to understand the uniqueness of each particular family. Society places complex and often conflicting demands on people; hence, the need for a range of family forms to coexist. Health professionals serving families must be tolerant and sensitive to the diversity of family life-styles and should abandon the traditional model of the "ideal family."

☐ *STUDY QUESTIONS*

Choose all correct answers to the following questions.

1. Which of these characteristics belong in a broadened, nondiscriminatory definition of "family"?
   a. Composed of one or more persons.
   b. Geographic dispersion.
   c. Emotional involvement and commitment.
   d. Sense of identity as a family.

2. Which is correct?
   a. The family of parenthood/procreation is the family into which you were born.
   b. The family of orientation/origin is the family of marriage.
   c. The extended family includes the immediate community, including but not limited to the family plus relatives.
   d. None of the above.

3. The family functions to meet the *needs of society* by:
   a. Mediating between society's expectations and the needs of the individual.
   b. Providing recruits for society's needs.
   c. Reproduction and socialization.

4. The family functions to meet the *needs of its members* by:
   a. Providing recruits for society.
   b. Serving as a "buffer" between society and the individual.
   c. Facilitating the personality development of the individual.

5. Which of these is (are) the main reason(s) for community health nurses to work with the family?
   a. The entire family is affected by the health problem of a family member.
   b. Promotion of health functioning of the whole family will positively affect each family member and his or her health status.
   c. By working with the whole family, the nurse may be able to discover health problems that other family members are having.

6. Which of these is (are) example(s) of how the ill family member can adversely affect the family?
   a. Birth of handicapped child disrupts marital relationship.
   b. Emotional disturbance of husband disrupts the economic and emotional stability of the family.
   c. Family is brought together in common effort to help the ill member get well.

How does the family affect the health of its family members in each of the following six stages of health/illness?

7. Prevention of illness and risk reduction stage.

8. Family and symptom experience illness appraisal stage.

9. Care-seeking stage.

10. Family's contact with health system stage.

11. Acute response of patient and family stage.

12. Adaptation to illness and recovery stage.

13. Some ways in which society has been able to influence/change family values, attitudes, or sanctions are:
    a. Judicial rulings on constitutional rights of people.
    b. Postponement of marriage and childbearing.
    c. Health legislation.
    d. Advances in technology.

14. How does the meaning of family health differ from the meaning of health?

Fill in the correct answers to the following questions.

15. Variant family forms refer to:

16. Give three examples of traditional variant family forms.

17. Give three examples of nontraditional (experimental) family forms.

18. Name three stressors that commonly affect single-parent families.

19. List three major recent demographic trends that have helped shape the American family.

Choose the correct answer(s) to the following question.

20. What are the usual ties between nuclear and extended family (circle all accurate descriptions)?

a. A modified extended family exists within a network of generational interaction.

b. Parents and siblings of spouses form the most important network of extended kinship relations.

c. The extended family network provides significant support and continuing assistance to the nuclear families within the network.

21. Relative to the single-parent family, the cohabiting family, and the family with an unmarried teenage mother, which of the following factors are associated with *all three of these family forms?*

a. Birth control technology
b. Poverty
c. High divorce rates
d. Unavailability of males
e. Postponement of marriage
f. Early premarital coitus

CHAPTER TWO

Family Nursing: Focus, Evolution, and Goals

Learning Objectives

1. Explain the differences in how the family is conceptualized in the three levels of family nursing practice.
2. Describe how the family is incorporated into the American Nurses' Association's standards of practice in community health nursing, maternal–child nursing, psychiatric–mental health nursing, and rehabilitation nursing.
3. Differentiate between how goals and priorities are set by the family nurse versus how goals are set and prioritized by the family-centered community health nurse.
4. Identify the four specialty areas in nursing that historically have been most ardently involved in family health care.
5. Briefly describe the three levels of prevention.
6. Explain why health promotion is a primary thrust within family nursing.
7. Discuss the primary factors leading to increased interest in health promotion today.
8. Identify factors that have impeded the growth of health promotion, self-care, and family nursing.
9. Define high-level wellness (Dunn's definition) by explaining its major facets.
10. Identify the five key dimensions of wellness, as described by Ardell.
11. Explain the purpose and contents of the health hazard appraisal tool used in preventive medicine.
12. Identify a nursing theory that focuses specifically on self-care.
13. Describe the family nurse's role in primary, secondary, and tertiary prevention.

INTRODUCTION

This text is about family nursing and the basic knowledge base—consisting of theory, factual information, research, and clinical implications—needed to practice basic family nursing. The chapter begins the discussion of the family nursing area by addressing what family nursing encompasses, its evolution, and how several of the specialty areas incorporate family into their standards of care. Finally, the goal of family nursing, promotion and maintenance of family health, is analyzed by using Leavell and associates' (1965) levels-of-prevention framework as a vehicle for discussing the family nurse's role within the three levels of prevention. Particular emphasis is given to primary prevention and health promotion, because this focus is seen as the main thrust of family nursing. Discussions of family health, the wellness life-style, and risk appraisal and reduction are also elaborated upon as part of health promotion.

FAMILY NURSING: DEFINING THE SPECIALTY

Family nursing today is indeed becoming a specialty area that cuts across the various other specialty areas of nursing. Although as a distinct specialty it is still in its infancy (Hanson, 1987), there is strong evidence that family nursing is a growing, dynamic specialty area of focus in practice, education, and research. When the first edition of this text was written in 1979 to 1980, there were no definitions of family nursing. Several texts discussed family nursing (Ford, 1979; Sobol and Robischon, 1975); family-centered community nursing (Reinhardt and Quinn, 1973); family-focused nursing (Janosik and Miller, 1980); and family health care (Hymovich and Barnard, 1979); but notions about a specialty in family nursing were absent. Today, texts and articles in the area of family nursing are extensive.

There is, however, disagreement over what family nursing actually encompasses and how it differs from community health nursing (Friedman, 1986) and family therapy (Gilliss et al, 1989b). A review of the family nursing literature reveals that within the definition of family nursing three levels of family nursing practice or foci are evident. The level of family nursing that is practiced depends on how the family nurse conceptualizes the family and works with it. The degree of family-centeredness also is dependent on the philosophy of the system within which the nurse works. Work environments (what leadership rewards and negatively reinforces) are major determinants of behavior. Each of these three levels or foci of family nursing are components of family nursing.

Level I: Family As Context

In level I, family nursing is conceptualized as a field where the family is viewed as context to the patient or client (Bozett, 1987) (Fig. 2–1). The family, as typically the client's most important primary group, is visualized as a stressor of or resource to the client. The family is the background or secondary focus and the individual, the foreground or primary focus relative to assessment and intervention.

The nurse may involve the family to varying degrees. In some cases the nurse may assess the family as part of the client's social support system, but with little incorporation of the family into the client's plan of care. In other cases, the nurse may show extensive involvement of the family in the client's care. The family's potential or actual as well as tangible and socioemotional impact on the client, is assessed and integrated into the treatment plan.

Most nursing theories conceptualize the family's role in this light. Most specialty areas also view the family as a crucial social environment of the client and hence a primary social support resource. A case in point is the definition of family-centered care promulgated by the interdisciplinary Association for the Care of Children's Health (1989). They state that family-centered care is a philosophy of pediatric health care that considers and treats the child in the context of the family and recognizes the family as the primary and continuing provider of care for the child. Where the family is incorporated into the assessment and plan of care of the patient, some authors call this family-centered or family-focused care (Bozett, 1987).

Level II: Family As Sum of Its Members

In the second type of family nursing practice, the family is seen as an accumulation or sum of the individual family members. When care is made available to or provided for all the family members, family health care or family nursing is seen as being provided. This is a model that is implicit to much of practice within family primary care and community health nursing. No explicit model of this conceptualization of family nursing practice exists.

There is a growing effort in family primary care to see the family as a whole as the focus of care (Doherty and Campbell, 1988) rather than as a sum of its parts, but with cost-containment efforts and lack of reimbursement for family care, these efforts are not widespread. In this level, the foreground is each of the clients, seen as separate rather than interacting units.

Level III: Family As Client

In the third type of family nursing practice conceptualization, the family is viewed as client or as the primary focus of assessment and care. The family is now in the foreground, with the individual family members in the background or context. The family is viewed as an interactional system. The focus is on internal family dynamics and relationships, the family's structure and functions, as well as the interdependence of family subsystems with the whole and of the family with its outer environment. The connections between illness, the individuals in the family, and the family are analyzed and incorporated into the treatment plan (Wright and Leahey, 1988). It is in this latter type of conceptualization and care that the unique contributions of family nursing are evident. This type of practice involves using a different paradigm or epistemo-

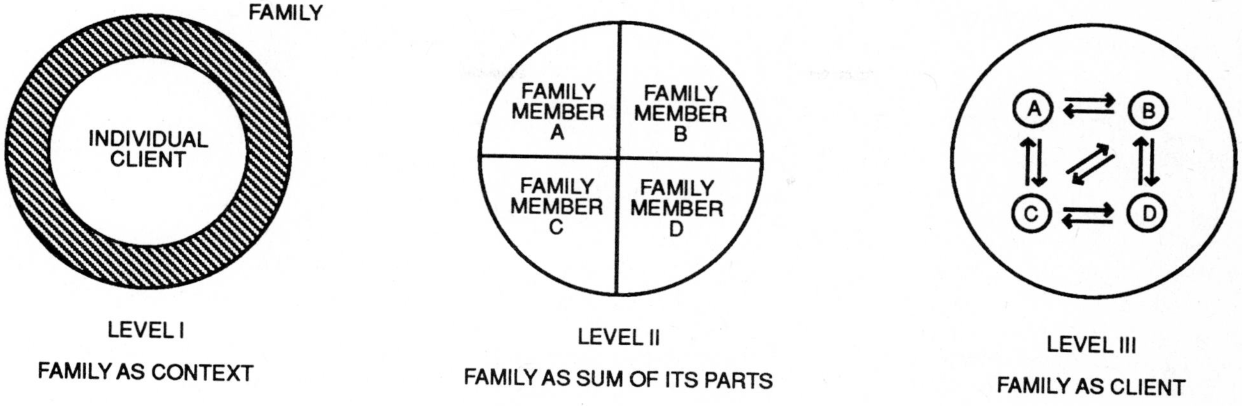

Figure 2–1
Levels of family nursing practice.

logical framework for assessment and care, involving holism, circular causality, and other general systems notions.

Wright and Leahey (1988) refer to advanced clinical assessment and intervention skills based on an integration of nursing, family therapy, and systems theory as "family systems nursing." This is a level-III focus, as it is on interaction or the reciprocity between family functioning and health/illness.

Although there is some dissent in the literature over what constitutes family nursing, it is seen in this text as consisting of the third level of conceptualization or practice. This is not to say that visualizing and working with the family as context is not important; in fact, working with families in this way is critical to providing comprehensive nursing care to individual clients. Focusing on family nursing as the third level of practice also does not preclude nurses from practicing at two or three levels simultaneously or over time. In order to define the knowledge base needed and the nursing processes involved, however, clarity as to the level of care is imperative. Therefore, the focus of family nursing in this text refers to nursing practice where the family is seen and treated as the client or recipient of care.

Distinguishing Family Nursing from Other Practice Areas

Because family nursing historically has been aligned primarily with community health nursing (Whall, 1986a), some confusion exists between what is community health or public health nursing and family nursing. Whereas family nursing focuses on the family as its target or recipient of care, community health nursing's target of service is the community (Kark, 1974). The health of the community rather than the health of the family is the ultimate goal of community health nursing. It is through families that community health nurses improve and preserve the health of communities. The difference here is a matter of ultimate goals and priorities. The implications of this difference are that in rendering personal health services to a family—for example, a single-parent family of mother and young children—the "noncommunity-oriented" family nurse would be concerned with the family's unique problems first, and second with the community health problems common to young families (the first commitment being a client and family). In a community health setting, the nurse would be cognizant of the pressing maternal–child health problems in the community that were relevant to the client family, such as immunizations and family planning, and prioritize these needs along with the unique health needs of the family.

Another point of confusion is the difference between family nursing and family therapy (Gilliss et al, 1989). In Wright and Leahey's text, *Nurses and Families* (1984), they distinguish family interviewing from family therapy. Family therapy that is systems-oriented and practiced within a nursing perspective, was in later writings called family systems nursing by Wright and Leahey (1988). These family nursing experts believe that advanced preparation is needed to practice as a family systems nursing clinician. However, family interviewing, consisting of basic family nursing assessment and intervention, should be part of baccalaureate preparation. The nurse here is able to complete family assessments of healthy/functional and dysfunctional families. The family nurse or interviewer intervenes using educative–supportive strategies that are direct and straightforward. In family systems nursing or family therapy versus family interviewing or basic family nursing, interventions particularly vary. In the former case, the nursing interventions include more complex and indirect psychosocial interventions (Wright and Leahey, 1984, 1988).

Family nurse researchers working as a special interest group under the auspices of the Family Nursing Continuing Education Project, Oregon Health Sciences University (Kirschling et al, 1989), were also interested in clarifying what family nurses actually do. To address this question they conducted a national survey of 263 nurses who identified themselves as being family nurses, asking them about their practice and interaction with their clients. From this data, the researchers identified unique characteristics of family nursing practice. The following four major themes emerged when participants were queried as to what they did differently when they cared for families rather than individuals:

- Recognition and integration of family concepts.
- Application of a broader perspective as identified in the nurses' approach to nursing care, primarily by assessing the family.
- A focus on family interaction and family dynamics.
- Involvement of family members in care, particularly in areas of decision making and caregiving.

THE INCORPORATION OF FAMILY INTO ANA'S STANDARDS OF CARE

Ideally, in all clinical areas of nursing practice, family nursing should be a reality. In some settings and specialty areas, however, family assessment and involvement are more difficult to achieve than in others. For instance, in the episodic settings—especially in intensive care units and emergency rooms, where immediate life-saving measures are needed—a predominant patient focus is understandable.

Evidence of what specialty areas believe to be the appropriate standards and scope of their practice are found in publications from the American Nurses' Association (ANA), which is responsible for defining and establishing the scope of nursing practice and standards in both the general field and in areas of specialization. A review of the ANA's *Social Policy Statement* (1980), the ANA's standards of care in psychiatric–mental health nursing practice (1982), community health nursing practice (1986), maternal and child health nursing practice (1983) and the scope of practice statement on rehabilitation nursing (1988), reveals a growing recognition of the family in health assessment and care. Highlights on how the family is incorporated in each of these documents provides some sense of what different specialties believe ought to be the nature and extent of professional involvement with families.

In the ANA's important *Social Policy Statement* (1980), the organization describes the family, along with the individual client and group, as nursing's focus of care. The family is also identified as a necessary unit of nursing services.

The psychiatric–mental health nursing standards (1982) are individually oriented, with only limited incorporation of the notion of family as client or family as context. The nursing process framework is used as the basis for the standards. Nursing assessment sources of health data, however, do include information about the family system. Only two of the 10 standards explicitly incorporate family into the actual standards of care. These two standards address intervention: health education and psychotherapy. Under psychotherapy, advanced clinical expertise is identified as being needed to intervene on the family level. Extensive family involvement appears to be seen as a specialty area in psychiatric–mental health nursing–that is, within family therapy and not as an integral part of psychiatric–mental health practice.

The *Standards of Community Health Nursing Practice* (1986) again are written in a nursing process framework. Community health nursing in this document is interpreted broadly to cover the subspecialty areas of public health, home health, occupational health, school nursing, and primary care nurse practitioners. The nursing process is utilized to assess, plan, diagnose, intervene, and evaluate individuals, *families*, and communities. Collaboration with families is stressed. Hence, community health nursing practice directs its services to individuals, families, and groups, although the dominant responsibility is to the population as a whole. Nevertheless, family nursing care is promulgated as a vital component within community health nursing practice.

The *Standards of Maternal and Child Health Nursing Practice* (1983) are not written according to a nursing process framework. They are content oriented. Family is heavily identified and integrated throughout these standards. For instance, the standards state that nurses assist families to achieve health promotion and to cope with health problems and role transitions. Another standard directs the nurse to intervene with families at risk to prevent health problems. Family is defined as both client and context in these standards.

The last standards that were reviewed were those in

rehabilitation nursing. Because rehabilitation nursing involves long-term care of clients and families with complex needs, this field should show a family-centered approach in its scope of practice documents. *The Standards for Rehabilitation Nursing: Scope of Practice* (1988) were developed jointly by the ANA and the Association of Rehabilitation Nurses and are organized by selected North American Nursing Diagnosis Association (NANDA) diagnoses. Unfortunately the standards are predominantly individually oriented, but families are definitely conceptualized as an important resource of the client. In a more limited way families are seen as clients. Nurses are directed to help families adjust to the impact of the disability and to educate families about the client's health problem and rehabilitation regime.

FAMILY NURSING'S HISTORICAL LEGACY

"The concept of family nursing has always been with us in nursing" (Ford, 1979, p. 4). It has, however, seen decline and regrowth.

In the preindustrialized, colonial era, when family members worked at home in cottage industries or farming, family care predominated. Then came industrialization, with family members moving into factories to work. Health care gradually moved from the home to the hospital.

In England, Florence Nightingale was aware of the importance of the family and home environment in the care of the sick. She mentions the needs of family members in military camps and the need "to keep whole families out of pauperism by nursing the breadwinner back to health" (Beard, 1915, as cited in Whall, 1986a, pp. 242–243).

During the 1800s and early 1900s in the United States, public health nurses and their equivalents in England served families in the home (initially the poor, but later also those with communicable diseases). With bureaucratization in society, specialization in medicine grew (obstetrics, pediatrics, surgery, and so forth). Nursing also became specialized, and family medicine and nursing practice fell into disuse. Insurance coverage limitations, private and public reimbursement policies and referrals, and lack of preventive funding also were policies that later mitigated against family-focused care (Ford, 1979).

Public health nursing, maternal–child health, and midwifery managed to bridge the gap in some instances and stand as examples of both family-centered and fractionalized care. For instance, obstetrics often ignores the baby and family, and communicable disease public health nursing services typically only include the family with regard to case finding. An example of where family nursing continued was in the Frontier Nursing Service. Here the Frontier Nursing Service provided both midwifery and public health nursing services to families.

The four specialty groups in nursing that have been the most ardent in focusing on the family have been community health nursing, which sees the family as client; parent–child nursing, which sees the family as context and client; psychiatric–mental health nursing, which sees extensive family involvement within the family therapy specialization; and the family primary care or nurse practitioner specialty, which often sees the family as a sum of its members. Each of these specialty groups has been informed by both specific developments in its own area of specialization and by more general developments within nursing, social science, and society. For instance, in community health nursing, the legacy was to consider the family as a focus of service. But not until the 1970s was there much substantive content within nursing programs that addressed family theory, assessment, and intervention. In the 1970s we saw texts focusing on family theory and its application to family-centered community health nursing. In community health nursing, sociological and cultural theories of family behavior (such as family socialization, poverty, roles, values, dynamics, and cultural diversity) were important in influencing the field.

Psychiatric–mental health nursing, in contrast, was more heavily influenced by the theories and clinical writings of the family therapy movement. Since these nurses work with troubled families, this knowledge base was more important to assist them in assessing and intervening with dysfunctional families. Family therapy theories and practice, however, are only one psychotherapeutic modality in mental health. Hence, family nursing assessment and intervention are not widespread throughout the whole specialty area.

Maternal or parent–child nursing has a long history of family involvement—beginning with the early days of midwifery and visiting of mothers and children in the home. It has long been recognized that when caring for mothers and children, the family is crucial. Family-centered texts in pediatrics and maternity are the norm. Most texts primarily see the family as context. Parent–child family-focused nursing has been particularly influenced by growth and development, mother–child bonding, role, and socialization theories.

Family nurse practitioners are the fourth specialty area identified as being family focused. In the 1960s it was recognized among health care planners and legislators that specialization in medicine was not meeting the primary health care needs of the whole population in the United States. Federal monies were granted to medical schools to open up family practice programs. The nurse-practitioner movement, particularly the family nurse-practitioner movement, grew on the coattails of this larger movement concerned with cost-effective, accessible care to all sectors of society. Nurse-practitioner programs have also been heavily federally funded. Family nurse practitioners care for the whole family, but their predominant focus is to see the family as a sum of its members (level II). Some family nurse-practitioner programs, however, are incorporating advanced family nursing content into their curricula to attempt to broaden services and to help students "think family" (Wright and Leahey, 1984).

In addition to the more specific influences each of these specialty areas experienced, certain more general factors enhanced the growth of family nursing. These include:

1. The increased recognition in nursing and society of the need for health promotion and a health focus, rather than the practically exclusive disease orientation.
2. Our aging population and the growth of chronic illness, which have brought self-care and the needs of family caregivers into prominence.
3. The enormous growth in family research and literature.
4. The widespread realization that there are many troubled families in our communities.
5. The promulgation and general acceptance of certain family-based theories, such as attachment and bonding theory and general systems theory.
6. The marriage and family therapy movements and the growth in child guidance, marriage, and family clinics and services.
7. The extensive and influential family communication research in the 1950s and 1960s which showed that troubled mothers and their communication patterns were associated with troubled children.

LEVELS OF PREVENTION

Leavell and associates (1965) developed a framework, referred to as levels of prevention, which is used here to explain the goals of family nursing. The levels of prevention cover the entire spectrum of health and illness, as well as the goals appropriate for each of the levels. The three levels are:

1. Primary prevention, which involves health promotion and specific preventive measures designed to keep people free of disease and injury.
2. Secondary prevention, consisting of early detection, diagnosis, and treatment.
3. Tertiary prevention, which covers the stage of recovery and rehabilitation, is designed to minimize the client's disability and maximize his or her level of functioning (Fig. 2–2).

The three levels of prevention constitute the major goals of family nursing. They consist of the promotion, maintenance, and restoration of health (Hanson, 1987). Health promotion is a major thrust of family nursing. Certainly, however, early detection, diagnosis, and treatment are also important goals. Tertiary prevention or rehabilitation and restoration of health are especially important goals in family nursing today, given the growth in home health care and the prevalence of chronic disease and disability among our rapidly increasing older population.

FAMILY HEALTH PROMOTION

A primary goal of family nursing is health promotion of the family as a whole and each of its members. Health behaviors, values, and attitudes are learned in the family (Crooks et al, 1987; Pender, 1987). One of the basic functions of the family is the health care function, the purpose of which is to meet family members' health needs. Because of its lasting effects, teaching of health behaviors is perhaps the most important of these health needs.

Health promotion is included under primary prevention by Leavell and associates (1965). However, a clear distinction needs to be made between health promotion and prevention or health-protective behaviors. Health promotion is not disease or health problem specific. It is designed to contribute to the growth, enlargement, or excellence of health. It is a positive, dynamic process that focuses on improving the quality of life and well-being, not merely avoiding disease. Health promotion involves "approach" behaviors consisting of a number of actions and activities whose end is high-level wellness (Dunn, 1961).

In contrast, prevention (of illness) is disease or health problem specific and involves "avoidance" behaviors. Primary prevention then also consists of activities that protect persons from specific diseases or decrease the likelihood that they will acquire diseases or health problems. Both prevention and health promotion are important goals, and are complementary to each other (Duncan and Gold, 1986; Pender, 1987).

Family health promotion involves both promoting family members' health and promoting family system health (Loveland-Cherry, 1988). In the former case the emphasis is on the individual family members in the

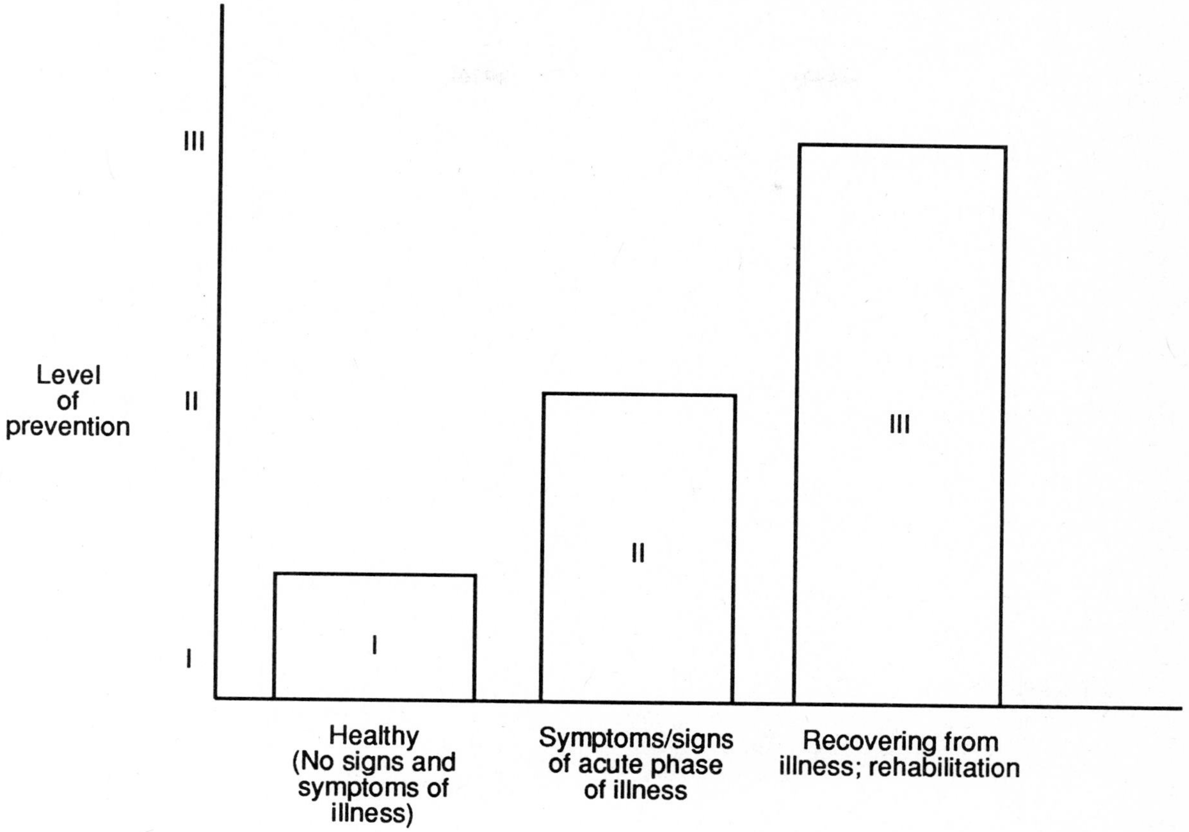

Figure 2–2
Relationship of levels of prevention to health–illness stages.

context of the family, while in the latter case the focus is health promotion of the family system both internally and in interaction with its external interacting systems, such as the social welfare or educational systems. Here the goals are the promotion of the health of the family unit. Inasmuch as practically all the health-promotion literature deals with the individual rather than the family unit, that emphasis is reflected here.

Nevertheless, the health-promotion concept can be easily applied to the family as a whole. Because the family is a small interactional system, it means, however, that different areas need to be assessed (such as communication patterns, parent–child relationships, and interaction with social support resources) and different strategies applied. In the family assessment and intervention chapters that follow, health promotion of the family system is incorporated.

Health promotion and primary prevention of acute and chronic health problems pose the greatest health challenge to our society. Perhaps our most important goal should be to assist people (individuals and families) to learn how to be healthy in a natural, enjoyable way, rather than focusing on assisting clients on how not to get sick, or worse yet, assisting clients only when they are sick.

Thus, primary prevention, including health promotion may be viewed as a most exciting and important role. This role has, however, largely been overlooked in practice, although much rhetoric about the significance of health teaching and prevention is heard. The adherence of health professionals to the medical model—in which health and illness are looked on as discrete, separate entities and the client is seen as a set of physiological systems—has led us and society (the consumers) to primarily view health care in terms of curative medical care. Individuals, when ill, "turn themselves over" to health providers. There has been little encouragement or reward from society or health care professionals for assuming self-responsibility for staying well or striving to improve one's total functioning (Bruhn and Cordova, 1978). Moreover, many health care professionals act as poor role models for their clients; they often smoke and are overweight, sedentary, and under apparent stress, and thus are not in a position to speak effectively about improvements in life-style.

Nurses and other health care professionals have been taught to respond to illness and crisis but not how to teach/counsel "symptom-free" individuals and families to enhance their level of wellness. Interestingly enough, the present health promotion movement commonly referred to as holistic health care, self-care, wellness training, or life-style modification, was for the most part not initiated and led by health care professionals but by laypersons and groups.

Recently these health promotion movements have become "respectable" in most health care professional circles; even the most esoteric modalities for stress reduction and pain control are being looked on as "helpful" by many health care practitioners. There is much more openness and acceptance of alternative modalities, including yoga, meditation, biofeedback, acupressure, acupuncture, guided imagery, visualization, and body therapies.

Wellness training, holistic health care, and self-care all share in the fundamental belief of taking responsibility for one's own health. The basic assumption underlying self-care is that people have self-directing and self-healing powers that can be consciously mobilized and applied. Inherent also is the belief that individuals and families should have control over their own actions. In addition, it is felt that the responsibility for one's health lies not with the health care professional but with the individual (Leonard, 1976).

Factors Leading to Renewed Interest in Health Promotion

Several of the important factors that have led to the renewed interest in health promotions are discussed below.

Need for a Change in Focus. Our present health care system is crisis oriented, with treatment being given in many cases too little, too late. In the case of chronic illness, our prevailing cause of morbidity and mortality, one is not treating and eradicating disease, but only minimizing its impact, repairing the damage as much as possible, and treating its complications. Some now recognize that we are spending most of our money treating the end result of self-destructive life-styles rather than focusing in on the causative factor of ill health, such as life-style and environmental hazards (Ardell and Newman, 1977; Pender, 1987).

The Surgeon General's landmark report, *Healthy People* (U.S. Public Health Service, 1979) and its companion report, *Promoting Health/Preventing Disease: Objectives for the Nation* (U.S. Public Health Service, 1980) emphasized the fact that life-style modifications were the most significant changes needed to achieve health gains in our nation. Six life-style changes were identified: cessation of smoking; reduction of alcohol misuse; dietary changes to reduce excess calories, fat, salt, and sugar; exercise; periodic screening procedures for major disorders such as high blood pressure and diabetes; and use of seatbelts and following speed limits on highways.

Rising Costs. There is a growing concern among laypersons, legislators, and some health-care professionals that the present system of health care is both costly and relatively ineffective, with no cost containment or conservation of health resources in sight. We spend enormous amounts of money for hospital and medical care with little improvement to show for it. Longevity has not significantly improved in recent years, even though we keep pumping more and more money into a leaky system. Compliance studies show that there is a widespread lack of medical compliance by patients, which naturally raises costs even more. Ardell (1977) reminds us that Americans spend vast amounts of money on the treatment of diseases that could be prevented for free.

Demystification of Primary Health Care. There have been unprecedented public disclosures of the inadequacies and inequities of professional service. For instance, the women's movement has focused national attention on the poor quality of care received by women in a male-dominated system. The downward transfer of functions (from physicians to nurse practitioners and physician assistants, and from registered nurses to vocational nurses, community workers, and nurse's aides) has helped with the demystification process.

Consumerism and Popular Demands for Increased Self-control. Consumers today expect to be informed about the findings of their medical services and to be given more self-control over their lives. This usually translates into being given sufficient information to be reasonably informed so that they can make their own choices and evaluate services. The need for greater self-control is related to present societal values and to antitechnology and antiauthority sentiments.

Changes in Life-style and Increased Educational Levels. A considerable number of educated, middle-class persons and families are placing a greater value on health, personal fulfillment, and the quality of their lives (Harris and Gurin, 1985). Although the general level of health knowledge in our society is relatively low, this group, through reading of a multitude of health-oriented articles and books and exposure to mass media, conferences, and so forth, has become quite informed about general health-promotional strategies and environmental hazards and risks. This shift in values and the improvement of education level has led to improved life-styles for many, albeit generally limited to the more affluent classes (Harris and Gurin, 1985).

Lack of Accessible and Available Professional Health Services. A major impetus to self-care may arise from situations where professional health services are not readily available or accessible (Levin et al, 1976). A shocking 37 million Americans in 1987 had no health insurance (U.S. Dept. of Health and Human Services, 1989b). The uninsured, however, may use self-care for treating common primary care problems rather than for learning health promotional strategies.

Growing Recognition of the Interrelationship Between Stress and Illness. It is estimated that 80 percent of all illnesses are stress induced, with stress being responsible for aggravating all illnesses and illnesses aggravating existing stress. Multiple studies have shown the negative role stress plays on an individual's or family's health status (Pelletier, 1979). Because of this, treatment of the problem alone is not adequate. In the case of the individual, the whole person must be considered, with an integration of body and mind being of prime importance for recovery and wellness. Stress reduction has become one of the five major dimensions of wellness training (Ardell, 1977) or a wellness or healthy life-style.

Impediments to Family Health Promotion

Although there has been a substantial growth in health promotion, self-care, and family nursing, certain factors have created major impediments or obstacles to the growth in these areas so that all sectors of society may benefit. The major impediment is money. Lack of third-party reimbursement for family assessments and interventions and for health promotion and preventive activities creates a situation whereby only the more affluent can afford the out-of-pocket expenses involved in health-care-professional-initiated activities or have access to the education needed for self-care. A second obstacle is the attitudes and socialization of physicians and nurses in the United States. We are still very illness oriented and pay lip service to the importance of health promotion. The medical model is still the dominant model for practice, policy-making, and funding. Little attention or value is placed on health and the psychological and social factors involved in health care (Doherty and Campbell, 1988). Other obstacles are our value system, where materialism and accumulation of goods are so important; the presence of social problems such as inadequate health care, employment, and educational opportunities for the stigmatized (the poor, minorities, senior citizens, and women); and widespread environmental hazards (air and water pollution and exposure to toxic substances).

What Does Health Promotion/Primary Prevention Involve?

The goal of health promotion or primary prevention is high-level wellness. In 1961, Halbert Dunn, the father of the wellness orientation, defined high-level wellness as "An integrated method of functioning which is oriented towards maximizing the potential of which the individual is capable within the environment where he is functioning." The key words are: (1) "integrated," meaning to function as a whole. This is in contrast to the situation where a person functions in a disjointed way—where various facets of an individual are in conflict with other aspects of that person. Ardell speaks of an "integrated" life-style, where each of the key dimensions of high-level wellness (self-responsibility, nutritional awareness, physical fitness, stress management, and environmental sensitivity) are balanced and consonant with each other, producing a synergistic effect. (2) "Maximizing potential" connotes a dynamic state where a person is continually striving to grow and improve his or her level of wellness. Abraham Maslow's hierarchy of needs (1954) has a similar connotation; here man is seen as striving to meet higher needs as the lower, more basic needs are met. And (3) "within his environment" suggests that we have to look at individuals within their psychosocial and physical environments when assessing their level of wellness. The primary group (family) is the central social environment of individuals. In spite of poor and deprived environments, some individuals (in some literature they are referred to as the "invulnerables") may achieve high-level wellness. Dunn calls this status "emergent wellness." According to him, families and communities can be similarly assessed using the same definition of high-level wellness. Travis (1976), a "wellness doctor," gives this explanation of the meaning of high-level wellness:

> The ideas of measuring wellness and helping people attain high levels of wellness are relatively new. Most of us think in terms of illness and assume that the absence of illness indicates wellness. This is not true. There are many degrees of wellness as there are many degrees of illness.

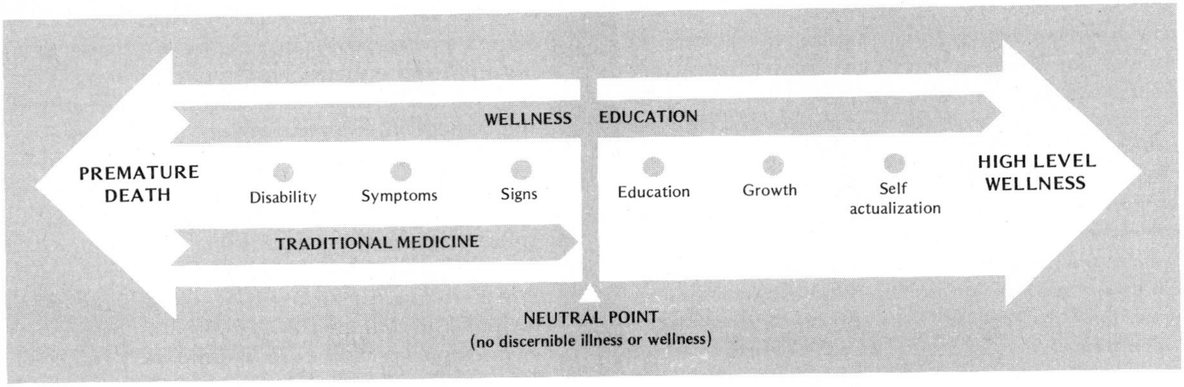

Figure 2–3
The health–illness continuum and its relationship to health care. (Travis, 1976.)

Travis explains his diagram (shown in Fig. 2–3) as follows:

> Moving from the center to the left shows a progressively worsening state of health. Moving to the right of center shows increasingly levels of health and well-being. Traditional medicine is oriented towards curing evidence of disease, but usually stops at the midpoint. Wellness education begins at any point on the scale with the goal of helping a person to move as far to the right as possible.

Health has an enriched and extended meaning for Travis (1976):

> Wellness is not a static state. It results when a person begins to see himself as a growing, changing person. High level wellness means giving good care to your physical self, using your mind constructively, expressing your emotions effectively, being creatively involved with those around you, being concerned about your physical and psychological environment and becoming aware of other levels of consciousness.

Wellness Life-Style

Ardell (1977) wrote a most interesting and enlightening book for laypersons and health professions alike, titled *High-Level Wellness—An Alternative to Doctors, Drugs, and Disease*. In his book he describes five key dimensions of a life-style philosophy he calls high-level wellness. Using Ardell's framework, but integrating more recent notions of Pender (1987), each of the five dimensions of a wellness life-style is described (Fig. 2–4).

Self-responsibility and Self-care. Self-responsibility and self-care are the foundations on which the other dimensions of the wellness life-style rest. Without a sense of active accountability for one's own health, the necessary motivation will be lacking to engage in a health-producing life-style. Families also need a strong sense of accountability to create a home environment where eustress (healthy stress) and self-actualizing health behaviors are promoted.

Families need to be given the feeling that their health lies primarily in their hands. They need to believe that a wellness life-style fueled by a strong sense of self and family responsibility can be more gratifying than living a life filled with high-risk behaviors.

A major factor accounting for insufficient self-responsibility is the unavailability of self-care-oriented health education. In fact, health professionals often discourage their clients from engaging in independent actions on their own behalf. Ardell (1977) and Vickory and Fries (1981) write that part of self-responsibility and self-care is knowing how to use the health care system effectively, coupled with creating a life-style that keeps individuals well and out of the medical system as much as possible.

Self-care covers the entire spectrum of health–illness, from primary prevention through tertiary prevention (Steiger and Lipson, 1985). The growing interest in health promotion today has gone hand-in-hand with the renewed interest in self-care. Goeppinger and Labuhn (1988) elaborate on the historical and political roots for self-health care. They point out that in the 1970s there was a resurgence of the "pioneering" value of being self-reliant and some influential anti-medical books appeared, such as Illich's *Medical Nemesis, the Expropriation of Health* (1976), which fostered the growth of self-care. In the 1980s the social climate has stressed egalitarianism, individualism, independence, and freedom of choice. These values also enhance the attractiveness of self-care.

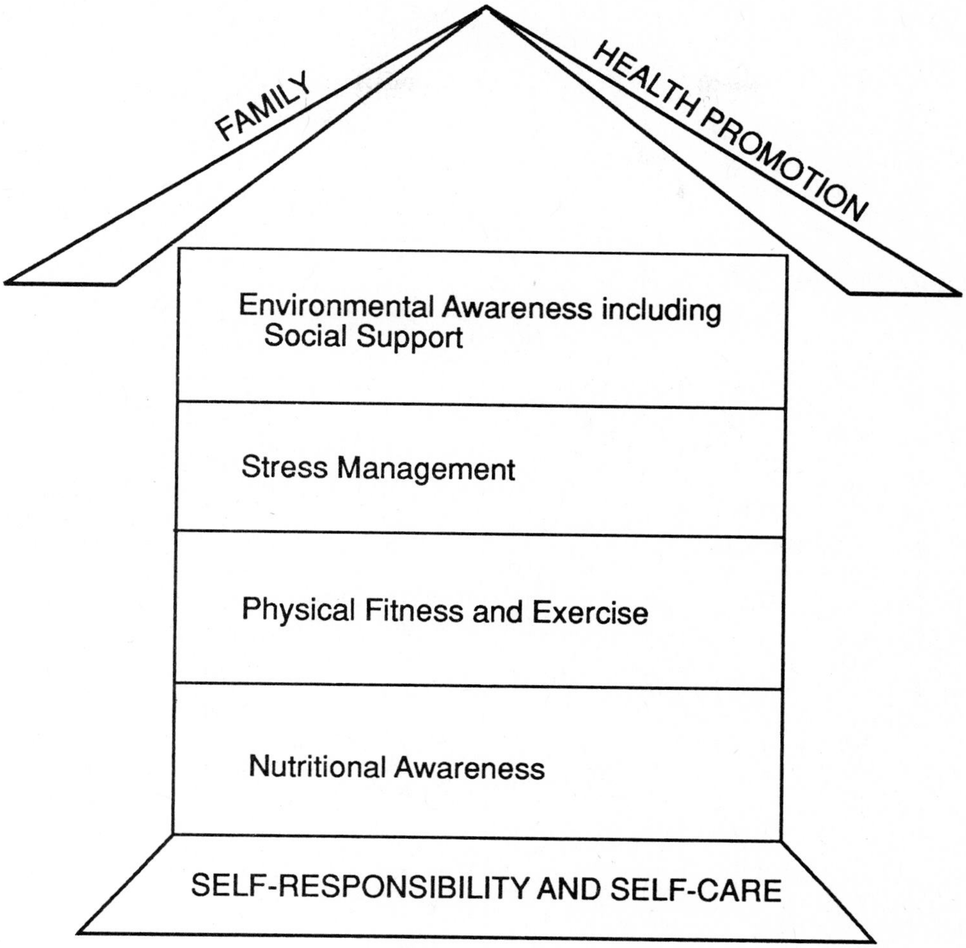

Figure 2–4
The wellness life-style.

Self-health care is typically viewed as lay-initiated (Levin et al, 1976) and is based on the assumption that laypersons are capable of carrying out their own health care. Orem (1980) is the primary nursing theorist who emphasizes people's natural self-care capabilities. She calls clients self-care agents and defines self-care as "the practice of activities that individuals personally initiate and perform on their own behalf in maintaining life, health, and well-being" (p. 35). Nursing, according to Orem, intercedes when a client has self-care deficits and requires professional nursing intervention.

A comprehensive definition of self-health care was developed by Goeppinger (1982). She describes self-health care as that which "encompasses those activities, continuous and episodic, volitional and unintentional, which people can do for themselves, individually or collectively, in a variety of health and illness matters" (p. 380).

The importance of self-care behavior has frequently been neglected in the health-promotion literature, which tends to emphasize the role of health care professionals in initiating health-promotion activities. Yet knowing what people and families do on their own behalf is one critical key to any health-promotion intervention. Several large epidemiological studies (Belloc, 1973; Harris and Gurin, 1985; Langlie, 1979; Prohaska et al, 1985) show that Americans engage in many self-initiated health-promotion activities. These need to be reinforced and supported by health care professionals.

Nutritional Awareness. Nutritional awareness connotes not only an awareness of the composition of a healthy diet but also good nutritional habits. Because adequate nutrition is a crucial component in the maintenance of health, it plays a major role in both a wellness life-style and in the prevention of the major chronic diseases. Many health leaders have voiced their concern over the poor state of the American people's nutrition. One such example is cited. As early as 1975, the United States Senate Select Committee, at the conclusion of years of fact-finding studies and testimony relative to our dietary habits and nutritional status reported:

> We have reached the point where nutrition, or the lack or the excess or the quality of it, may be the nation's number one public health problem. The threat is not beri beri, pellagra, or scurvy. Rather we face the more subtle, but more deadly, reality of millions of Americans loading their stomachs with food which is likely to make them obese, to give them high blood pressure, to induce heart disease, diabetes, and cancer—in short, to kill them over the long term. (p. 5)

Five of the 10 leading causes of death are related to faulty diets: heart disease, stroke, diabetes, arteriosclerosis, and cirrhosis of the liver (Ardell, 1977). Twenty-five health problems are associated with being overweight (including congestive heart failure; renal disease; breast, uterine, rectal, and colon cancer; osteoarthritis; and shortened life span). Because most adults and many children have a weight problem, this adds up to a mammoth number of at least partially preventable health problems (Spence, 1989).

Guidelines on nutrition have been disseminated by the U. S. Department of Agriculture (1985) and the American Heart Association (Barnett, 1986). Table 2–1 combines their recommendations about levels of sodium, cholesterol, fat, protein, and carbohydrates. It is within the context of the family that faulty dietary habits are learned, involving familial behavioral patterns that are central to daily life. Although difficult, it is within this same context that such patterns may be changed.

TABLE 2–1. RECOMMENDATIONS FOR A HEALTHY DIET

Recommendation	Method
1. Eat a variety of foods, with proper proportions of protein, carbohydrates, and fats.	• Protein should constitute 15% of total calories.
2. Maintain ideal weight.	• Use the 1959 leaner Metropolitan Life weight tables rather than the 1983 tables.
3. Avoid too much unsaturated fat, saturated fat, and cholesterol.	• Total (saturated and unsaturated) fat should be less than 30% of caloric intake. Saturated fat should be below 10% of all calories and as low as possible. Cholesterol should not exceed 100 mg per 1,000 calories.
4. Eat foods that provide an adequate amount of starch and fiber.	• Carbohydrates should account for 50 to 55% or more of total calories. Complex carbohydrates or starches are recommended.
5. Avoid too much sugar.	
6. Avoid too much sodium and salt.	• Sodium and salt should account for 1 g per 1000 calories and no more than 3 g per day.
7. If you drink alcohol, do so in moderation.	• Alcohol should not exceed 50 mL per day (the equivalent of two drinks).

From: U.S. Department of Agriculture (1985), American Heart Association (1986).

Stress Management. The 1980s are thought by many to be the age of stress—stressful personal lives, jobs, relationships, societal stress, and so forth. Nonetheless, it should be noted that it is not the stress we encounter that seems to make the big difference in outcomes, but the way in which we handle stress. If individuals try to master stress instead of feeling helpless and overwhelmed by it, then many times stress will not have negative consequences (Kobasa, 1984). Persons with "hardy personalities" seem particularly stress-resistant.

According to Brown (1974), 80 percent of our present illnesses are stress induced, and all of our health problems can be aggravated by stress. Hans Selye (1974), the father of the stress theory, points out that it is the effects of prolonged stress (or "distress") that are particularly deleterious on the body, causing such problems as migraine headaches, peptic ulcers, heart attacks, hypertension, mental illness, and suicide. Selye coined the word "eustress," referring to the positive aspects of stress. In the family context, eustress is used to refer to "a positive type of stress that takes place when families benefit from or enjoy facing the challenges of life" (McCubbin and Dahl, 1985, p. 374). Because of the ubiquity of stressors in our environment today, stress has to be managed so that eustress (an appropriate amount of stress for enjoying life and being stimulated and productive) can be maintained.

One component of stress management involves the use of techniques to gain mental relaxation in times of duress. A multiplicity of such strategies and techniques for stress reduction and relaxation is discussed in the literature.* Families need to be sensitive to the amount of stress within the home environment and how as a group to provide an eustressful environment. Effective ways of coping with stress should be taught and accessible to family members.

Stress reduction techniques are varied and range from common sense solutions, such as avoiding the stress producer (often an impossibility), to the more complex, such as biofeedback. Other stress reduction techniques include deep breathing and meditation, autogenic training, visualization, muscle relaxation exercises, cognitive reappraisal, hypnosis, developing goal alternatives, change avoidance, counterconditioning to avoid stress arousal, physical exercise, assertive communication, environmental modification, time blocking and time management, music therapy, diversion, and changing addictions to drugs/substances (Bulechek and McCloskey, 1985; Lachman, 1983; Pender, 1987; Steiger and Lipson, 1985).

Exercise and Physical Fitness. "Physical fitness is critical for dynamic, fulfilling and productive living" (Pender, 1987, p. 285). Unless individuals are reasonably fit, high-level wellness cannot be maintained. Yet our modern "comfortable" (as compared to previous eras) life-style has led most Americans to become sedentary and "physically disadvantaged" (Cantu, 1980). Current estimates from large surveys report that 40 to 64 percent of American adults get insufficient exercise to maintain healthy cardiovascular systems, 24 to 40 percent never exercise, and 12 to 20 percent exercise consistently enough to get cardiovascular benefits (Haydon, 1987; Rippe, 1989). Moreover, fitness levels of American children are on the decline. The large proportion of sedentary, inactive children in our nation are at greater risk for future coronary heart disease (Haydon, 1987).

Although there have been improvements made in the proportion of American adults who regularly exercise (Gurin and Harris, 1987), these gains are primarily limited to those in the upper middle classes (Haydon, 1987). Not all sectors of our society by any means have joined the so-called fitness revolution or boom.

The wide-ranging benefits of exercise have been convincingly shown in study after study (Rippe, 1989). Several significant studies have found substantial cardiovascular benefits, increased longevity, and better general health among those who exhibit a lifelong pattern of consistent exercise.

The benefits of regular exercise are many. Psychologically they consist of mood elevation and improved psychological well-being, self-concept, and body image. Most regular exercisers report a higher level of relaxed energy, reduction in feelings of tension and stress in their personal lives and on the job, and better eating habits and control of their weight. Physiological benefits include lowering the heart rate, blood pressure, percentage of body fat, and blood lipids and cholestrol levels. Also there are strength, flexibility, and coordination benefits as well as a slowing down of osteoporosis (Ardell, 1977; Hales and Hales, 1985; Pender, 1987; Rippe, 1989; Steiger and Lipson, 1985).

The family offers an excellent context for reducing the prevalence of overweight, sedentary, physically disadvantaged children and adults. Health behaviors, such as exercising and leading an active life-style, are heavily influenced by parental behaviors and attitudes. The value of consistent, natural, enjoyable exercising as part of one's life-style is translated to children primarily through parents' role modeling. Family recreational and leisure-time activities are excellent ways to promote the value of physical fitness as well as healthy, positive family relationships.

Environmental Awareness. Steiger and Lipson (1985) remind us that

> Health and illness are as inextricably connected with environmental factors as they are to social and cultural factors. It has become more and more apparent in recent years that health hazards in the home, on the road, in the workplace, and in the broader environment have striking, if sometimes subtle, effects on health. (p. 276)

Environmental awareness encompasses the physical and social environmental influences on the family and its members—that is, how the environment either enhances or diminishes health and well-being. The air we breathe, the community in which we reside, and the neighborhoods' characteristics are all examples of the physical and social environments that affect us. The smaller spatial circle surrounding individuals is their personal environment or space (such as a bedroom or office) as well as their primary group and network of friendships. Social support networks are crucial to health promotion and maintenance of both individuals and families. (See Chap. 8 for an elaboration of social support systems.)

In order to achieve the level of environmental sen-

** Lachman (1983) and McQuade and Aikman (1975) are two books that describe primary strategies used for stress reduction and management. The several health-promotion texts found in the References also have good descriptions of stress-management techniques.*

sitivity needed to enhance health, the effects the environment has on one's personal and family health and well-being need to be recognized (Ardell, 1977). Just as individuals need to be aware of their environment and its effects on them, so do parents need to look at their home, neighborhood, school, community, and sets of relationships to assess how these settings and groups collectively and individually are affecting them and their children.

Environments need to be suitable for the developmental stages of the children and the family as a whole. One of the most difficult problems poor and working-class families face is that their home, neighborhood, and community environments are not conducive to wellness, and yet they do not have the option to move.

Wellness Life-style Pays Off

A large-scale health survey conducted in the mid-1960s of 7000 adults in California who were later followed for 5.5 years demonstrates the values of a healthy life-style. Belloc (1973) demonstrated that (1) an individual's overall health status was improved, and (2) an 11.5-year greater life expectancy could be achieved for men age 45 whose life-style incorporated six or seven of the "old health habits" traditionally stressed versus men of the same age who followed only three or less "habits." These life-lengthening habits were: (1) no smoking, (2) no alcohol or only in moderation, (3) 7 or 8 hours of sleep nightly, (4) regular meals with no snacking in between, (5) daily breakfast, (6) normal weight, and (7) moderate, regular exercise. For women the same positive correlation between habits and longevity appeared, although only 7 years were gained by incorporating six or seven "habits" into their lives versus three or less (Belloc, 1973).

The clinical implications for promoting the health of the family as a whole and its members are consistently compelling throughout the entire life cycle of the family. Many of the life-style principles apply equally well to the family and individual. When the adult family members stress the values and habits inherent in healthy living, the children—through identification and imitative learning—also learn a more healthy life-style. In fact, role modeling by significant others (parents, important peers, teachers has been found to be the best learning device. As the old adage says, "actions speak louder than words." Parents also need to understand normal growth and developmental patterns, including the important developmental tasks their children are struggling to achieve, so that they, in turn, can encourage and foster health-promotion strategies that are developmentally appropriate.

Many strategies are available for helping individuals and families with life-style modification programs. Texts also cover screening or health promotion assessment methods and tools. Several excellent nursing texts are Edelman and Mandle (1986), Pender (1987), and Steiger and Lipson (1985).

PRIMARY PREVENTION: SPECIFIC PREVENTIVE MEASURES AND RISK APPRAISAL

Primary prevention, in addition to health promotion, involves maintaining and improving the level of individual and family resistance to particular diseases. It also covers risk appraisal and reduction methods.

Specific Preventive Measures

Increasing resistance to social, emotional, and biological forces that precipitate disease is a goal of primary prevention. A wellness life-style, as described previously, should accomplish this "resistance." Specific preventive measures also are needed. These encompass preventive measures such as immunizations and fluoride treatment.

Risk Appraisal and Reduction

In preventive medicine, the most common way in which primary prevention is practiced is by determining long-term risks to which a client is exposed and then by prescribing measures that will reduce the individual's risk factors. In many cases, a health-hazard appraisal method or tool is used. Here the total personal risks to a client are estimated by identifying the average risk for the major causes of death in the client's own age, sex, and racial group. From this, one can develop a prognosis for the well client. Using this appraisal method, the health care practitioner can make an estimation of those causes most likely to bring about disease and death in the client, and recommend life-style changes and medical treatment to reduce risk. Table 2–2 is an example of the use of the health hazard appraisal method.

The Family's Role in Primary Prevention

Families have been found to be the most important source of help for American adults who have changed their life-styles to a more wellness-oriented one. A Gallop national survey in 1985 confirmed that when it comes to health matters, most people get more help from their family than any other source, even their doctor (Gurin, 1985).

In summary, primary prevention—health promotion and disease prevention—is a primary thrust of family nursing. Family nurses should help families

TABLE 2–2. HEALTH HAZARD APPRAISAL TOOL

Name: John Doe
Age: 43
Race and Sex: White male
Occupation: Small businessman

Rank—Disease/Injury	Prognostic Criteria	Patient Findings	Treatment (Rx)
1. Arteriosclerotic heart disease	Blood pressure	120/70	
	Cholesterol level	280	Reduce saturated fats, calories, and red meats.
	Diabetes	No	
	Exercise	Sedentary—none	Initiate regular exercise program.
	Family history	None	
	Smoking	2 packs a day for 20 years	Referred to stop-smoking clinic.
	Weight	200 lb (5 ft 11 in)	Weight reduction diet. Reduce to 165 lb.
2. Auto accidents	Alcohol	Occasionally (socially)	Recommended to always use seatbelts in car.
	Drugs	None	
	Mileage	30,000/year	
	Seatbelts	Occasional use	
3. Suicide	Depression	None observed, patient denies	
	Family history	Negative	
4. Cirrhosis of liver	Alcohol use	Social occasions only	

Adapted from Edelman and Mandle (1986), Robbins and Hall (1970).

take responsibility for their own health and incorporate wellness life-style changes into both their family's life-style and their members' personal lives. The family continues to play a crucial role in helping its members learn new ways to live more healthy lives. By believing in families' abilities to provide their own self-health care and to act in their own best interests, we will provide positive support and more effectively become resource persons and facilitators to families.

SECONDARY PREVENTION

Case finding is the key to secondary prevention so that early diagnosis and prompt treatment can be instituted. If the nature of the disease precludes cure, then the goal is to control the progression of the disease and prevent disability.

The nurse's role here would be to refer all family members for screening, health histories, and physical examinations (or complete the screening and checkups himself or herself). Additionally, depending on the setting, initiation and follow-through of referrals for diagnosis and treatment tailor-made to suit the member's family needs may be indicated. Health teaching, along with careful referral and follow-up, are concomitant functions at this time.

The Issue of the Yearly Physical for Healthy Adults

How effective and necessary is the annual or periodic health examination of an ostensibly healthy adult patient? This continues to be an area of dispute, although the weight of the evidence now leans towards longer intervals between physicals than previously recommended, as well as much more selective testing for only certain major diseases. Annual physicals are losing favor with the health community. Several important health and medical associations (the American Medical Association, American Heart Association, Canadian Task Force on the Periodic Health Examination, and American College of Physicians) have promulgated new recommendations for health maintenance checkups (Oppenheim, 1984; Parachini, 1987).

Most health care professionals have been socialized to believe that the annual physical was a sacrosanct part of good health care, and that a host of hidden diseases can be detected before they become serious. But is this so? "Not really," states the American College of Physicians, which in 1980 proclaimed the annual physical unnecessary (Oppenheim, 1984). Spitzer and Brown (1975) found that only a relatively few diseases or risk factors could reasonably be found in a preclinical state such that the disease's natural outcome could be altered. It is also evident that there has been a proliferation of unvalidated procedures prescribed in physical examinations.

Several organizations have developed their own tables, according to age and gender, for when physicals should be completed on healthy persons and what exams and tests should be performed. For instance, the AMA now advises healthy adults until age 40 to have a checkup every 5 years, then every 1 to 3 years after that. Four diseases can be effectively and easily screened for in the physical: cervical cancer (Pap smear), hypertension (blood pressure readings), bowel cancer (stool blood test), and breast cancer (breast exam and mammogram). Blood cholesterol testing for atherosclerosis is also simple and effective (Oppenheim, 1984).

When clients come in for physicals, primary care practitioners are encouraged to ask more comprehensive questions about clients' health behaviors and using a family-centered approach follow up more concertedly on needed life-style modifications.

TERTIARY PREVENTION

Rehabilitation is the primary focus of tertiary prevention. Recovery and maintenance care for chronically ill people are also included under this rubric. Rehabilitation involves restoring individuals disabled by disease or injury to a level of functioning optimal for them—or to their greatest usefulness—physically, socially, emotionally, and vocationally. In learning to live with a permanent disability, the client and family need tremendous support and extensive teaching of self and dependent care. The nurse plays central roles in tertiary prevention, particularly in view of the growth of home health care. In addition to direct caregiving, the family nurse's most significant roles are that of coordinator or case manager, patient/family advocate, teacher, counsellor, and environmental modifier.

This chapter has defined the several levels of family nursing. The text will primarily address the third level of practice in which the family is considered the client. The historical legacy and growth of family nursing was presented as well as the extent to which specialty areas have incorporated family into their respective standards of practice. The goals of family nursing are described by using the levels of prevention as an organizing framework. Because of the pervasive health problems among American family members, family health promotion is an especially critical goal for family nurses today.

□ STUDY QUESTIONS

1. One major difference between the three levels of family nursing practice is:
   a. The setting in which family nursing is practiced.
   b. The conceptualization of the family.
   c. The specialty area of the nurse.
   d. None of the above.

2. What is the different mission of the family-centered community health nurse versus the family-centered nurse working in other settings?

3. Which of the following statements is/are true about the levels of prevention? The levels:
   a. Specifically identify the nurse's role in prevention of disease.
   b. Cover the entire spectrum of health and disease.
   c. Identify goals for each of the three levels of prevention.
   d. Are generally synonymous with preventive, curative, and rehabilitative phases of health care.

Match the correct level of prevention from the right-hand column (items 4–12) with the description in the left-hand column.

4. Case finding.	a. Primary prevention.
5. Health promotion.	b. Secondary prevention.
6. Specific preventive measures.	c. Tertiary prevention.

7. Early detection and treatment.
8. Convalescence.
9. Minimizing the complications of the disease.
10. Rehabilitation.
11. Health maintenance.
12. Risk avoidance and reduction.

13. The family as client is an integral part of the ANA standards of practice in two specialty areas in nursing. Which are these?
a. Rehabilitation nursing.
b. Medical-surgical nursing.
c. Psychiatric-mental health nursing.
d. Community health nursing.
e. Maternal-child nursing.
f. Family nurse practitioners.

Which of these above specialty areas have been most ardently involved in incorporating families into their practice?

14. Identify five factors that have led to increased interest and involvement in health promotion.

15. What are three important components of Dunn's definition of high-level wellness?

16. Discuss briefly each of the five key dimensions making up a wellness life style.

17. The health-hazard appraisal tool contains and asks for what kinds of information?

18. What nursing theorist discusses self-health care (or self care) as a central concept in her model?

19. How does the meaning of family health differ from the meaning of health?

20. Why is health promotion considered a primary thrust of family nursing?

21. Which of the following impeding factors with respect to family health promotion is said to be the most significant?
a. Health care professionals socialization and attitudes.
b. Third party reimbursement (funding).
c. The American value system.
d. Presence of societal social problems.

CHAPTER THREE

The Family Nursing Process

Learning Objectives

1. Explain the difference between using the nursing process in family nursing and using the nursing process in working with individuals.
2. Describe each of the five basic steps within the nursing process relative to its purpose and meaning.
3. Discuss the preparation needed to adequately visit a family.
4. Identify several sources of family assessment data.
5. Explain the advantages of using the problem, etiology or contributing factors, and defining characteristics when making a family nursing diagnosis.
6. Explain why family strengths are helpful to include as part of the family assessment.
7. Describe several variables that the family nurse would consider when determining priorities for nursing care.
8. Identify within what phases of the nursing process the identification of resources is included.
9. Apply the premise that "families have the right and responsibility to make their own health decisions" at each step of the nursing process.
10. Name the classification system of client problems used in community health nursing.
11. Identify strengths and limitations of the North American Nursing Diagnoses Association (NANDA) in terms of making family nursing diagnoses.
12. Describe several factors that influence the particular family nursing intervention selected.
13. Differentiate Freeman's from Wright and Leahey's types of family nursing interventions.
14. Select two concepts of change that are important to assist families in changing their behavior.
15. List two family problems that confront family nurses and interpret the meaning of these problematic behaviors.

INTRODUCTION

Comprehensive family nursing is a complex process, making it necessary to have a logical, systematic approach for working with families and individual family members. This approach is the nursing process. According to Yura and Walsh (1978), "The nursing process is the core and essence of nursing. It is central to all nursing actions, applicable in any setting, within any frame of reference, any concept, theory, or philosophy." "Process" refers to a deliberate and conscious act of moving from one point to another (in this case through a series of circular, dynamic steps or phases) toward goal fulfillment. It is basically a systematic problem-solving process that is utilized when working with individuals, families, groups, or communities.

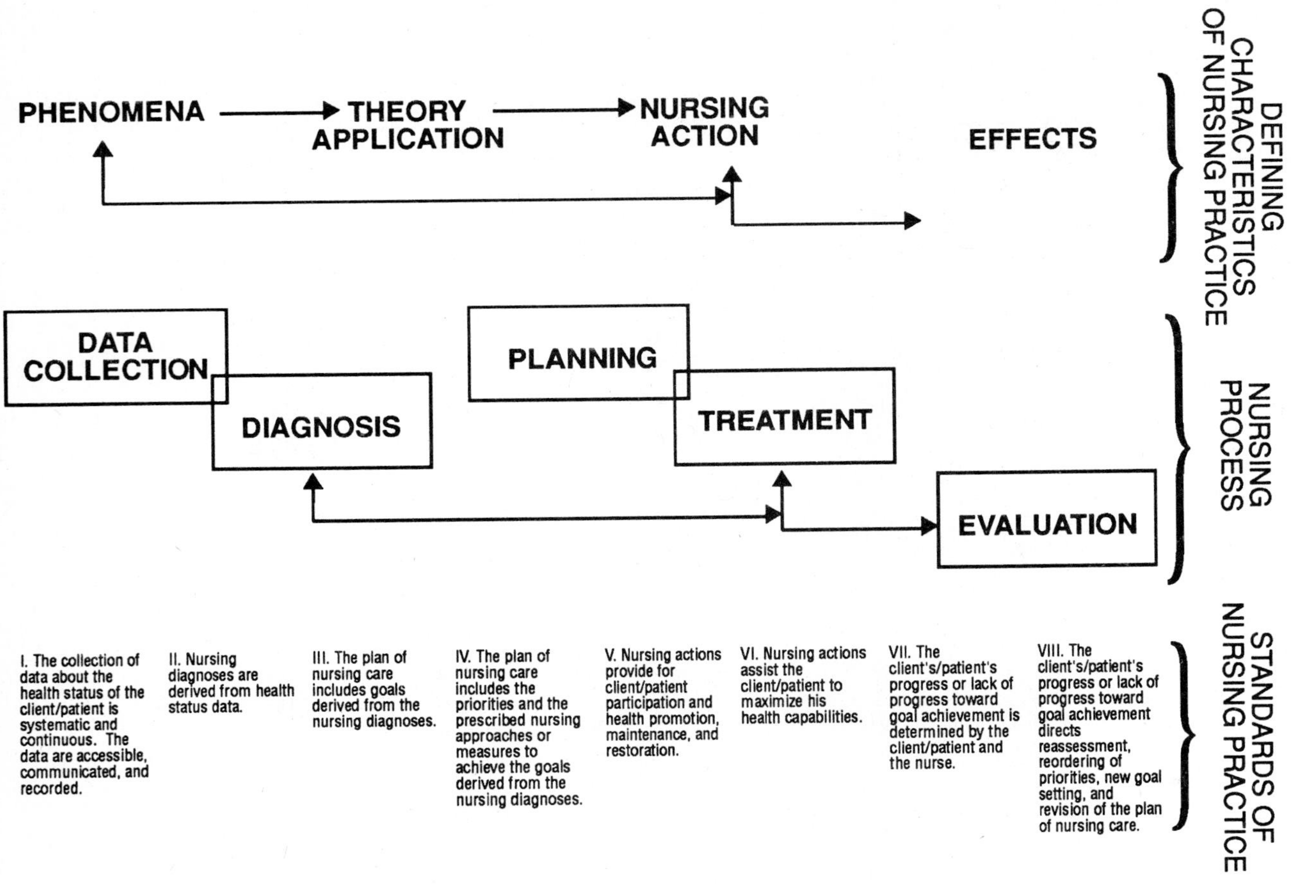

Figure 3–1
Relationship of the nursing process to the standards of nursing practice. (From: American Nurses' Association, 1980.)

The American Nurses' Association (ANA) description of the nursing process within *Social Policy Statement* (1980) is particularly informative because it links process to nursing standards of care (Fig. 3–1).

THE FAMILY NURSING PROCESS

The family nursing process will differ relative to who is the focus of care. This focus difference depends on the nurse's conceptualization of the family in his or her practice. If he or she sees the family as the background or context of the individual patient, then the individual family members are the focus and the nursing process is individually oriented, as is the traditional way of proceeding. If, however, the nurse conceptualizes the family as the unit of service, then, even though the process itself does not vary, the family as a unit or system is the focus.

Most family nurses in practice work simultaneously with both individual members and the family. This means the family nurse will utilize the nursing process on two levels—on the individual and the family level. In this case, assessment, diagnosis, planning, intervention, and evaluation will be more extensive and complex.

If feasible, it is important to assess and focus on both levels of analysis. Our nursing services are typically very specialized if we assess and work only with the family as a system. And conversely, an adequate understanding of each family member cannot be gained without viewing that member within the context of the primary group—the family.

This two-level approach to assessing and carrying

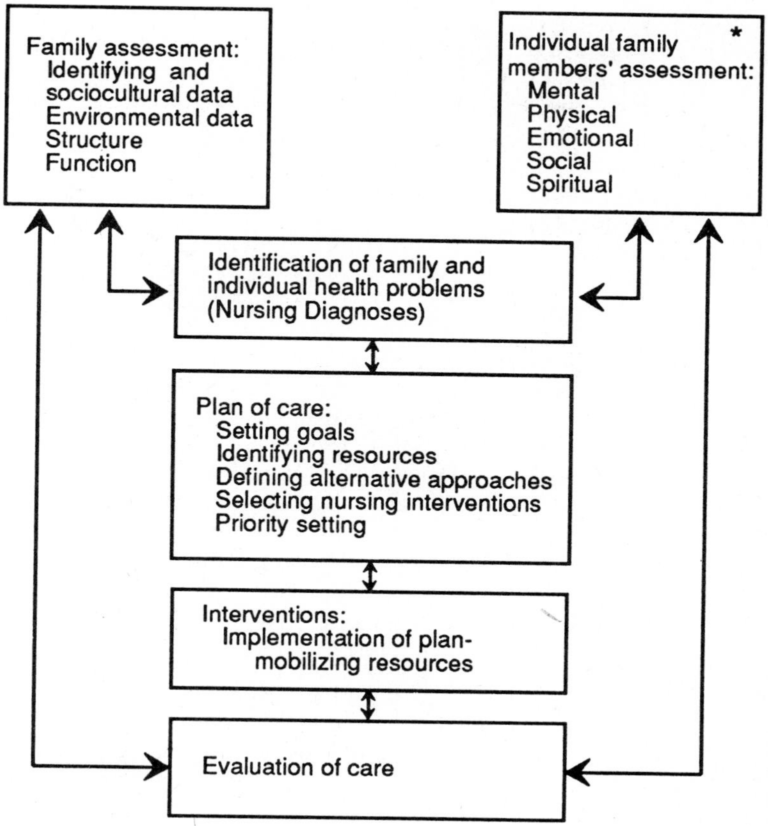

Figure 3–2
Steps in the individual and family nursing process. [a]Individual client nursing process is not covered in this text.

out family nursing care is illustrated in Figure 3–2. In reality, the steps in the diagram are interdependent and not strictly sequential or linear in organization. In practice, one or more steps or phases may overlap or take place simultaneously, with movement back and forth among the various steps.

FAMILY ASSESSMENT

Family Assessment: An Interactional Level of Analysis

Although in the above section I have stated that family nursing care often involves assessment and intervention at both the individual and family level, for purposes of this text and in this chapter, only family assessment, planning, and intervention is discussed. Many texts cover the nursing process used with individual clients.

In order to work effectively with family clients, conducting assessments and providing care, the family nurse must "think interactionally" (Wright and Leahey, 1984). Wright and Leahey (1984) explain that "perhaps the most significant variable that promotes or impedes family-centered care is how the nurse conceptualizes problems." Knowledge of family theory and research as well as a systematic framework for assessing and working with families greatly helps the nurse to make the transition from an individualistic to a familistic perspective. To this end, this text presents foundational family science knowledge, as well as a comprehensive family assessment tool.

The Assessment Process

The process of nursing assessment is highlighted by continuous information gathering and professional judgments that attach meaning to the information being gathered. In other words, data are collected in a systematic fashion (using a family assessment tool), classified, and analyzed as to their meaning. Often cursory data are collected on each of the major areas. When the assessor then finds significant probable or potential problems, he or she then probes those areas more deeply. The amount and type of information is also dependent on the client, who may wish to convey more information in one area than another. Data collection is the *sine qua non* of problem identification. Although assessment is the first step of the nursing process, data continues, however, to be gathered throughout the provision of services, showing the dynamic, interactive, and flexible nature of this process.

Sources of Assessment Data. Family data collection comes from many sources: client interviews relative to past and present events, objective findings (eg, observations of home and its facilities), subjective appraisals (eg, responses of individuals and family members), written and oral information from referrals, various agencies working with family, and other health team members.

The interview is a face-to-face meeting with one or more family members. It is desirable when possible to interview the whole family during the initial assessment phase. This minimizes the distortion of information, gives everyone a chance to share their perceptions, and gives the nurse an opportunity to see the interactions of family members (Holman, 1983). The interview should be focused, but, according to the purpose of the interview, varies in how structured it is.

One of the important roles of the family health nurse is that of a participant observer in the family. While the nurse is actively working with families, he or she must also have the ability to "stand back" and objectively observe the conditions and situations existing in the home.

Several family system tools are used to gather information during family interview. The genogram, ecomap, and family sculpture are commonly used for this purpose. They are discussed in subsequent chapters. The Friedman family assessment tool used in this text can be used to structure interview questions and foci.

More structured checklists, inventories, and questionnaires can be used in data collection (Holman, 1983). They may be especially useful when a great deal of information is needed to be gleaned or recorded. When a nurse is seeing a family over an extended period of time, or there is more than one nurse working with the family, checklists and other structured, easily completed tools may be useful. In home health care agencies, family assessment checklists are commonly used for this purpose. Home assessment inventories are also used by nurses in rehabilitation who visit families in the home to assess the home setting in terms of its suitability for the disabled client.

In addition, one of the most frequent uses of structured family assessment tools is in the area of family research. There are numerous good family assessment instruments. Most of these can be found in three family assessment instrument texts listed in the References: Filsinger (1983), Grotevant and Carlson (1989), and Jacob and Tennenbaum (1988).

Building a Trusting Relationship. The establishment of a trusting relationship in which there is mutual respect and open, honest communication goes hand in hand with the assessment process and orientation phase of working with a family. Trust and rapport building set the stage for and are the cornerstones of effective family nursing care.

Family nursing usually involves a continuing series of interactions with a family. The nurse's effectiveness in assisting the family to identify and meet its needs depends not only on the nurse's professional expertise, but also on how sensitive the nurse is to what the family is experiencing (Matteoli, 1974). A family in need of help will often open up rapidly if there is someone to whom the family members can freely express their concerns and problems. The family is then in a beginning position for helping itself. "The nurse's function is to create a trusting relationship within which this may occur" (Matteoli, 1974, p. 2). Trust is developed by the nurse conveying an acceptance of the family, and acknowledging the family's right to their own feelings and beliefs, irrespective of the nurse's goals, values, or expectations.

The orientation phase in working with families is seen as the time for assisting the family to begin to express its present concerns so that the nurse may more fully understand the family and the meaning of its experience; the family members may deepen their understanding of their own concerns during this phase; the family may begin to problem solve; and family members may feel some sense of relief from sharing their concerns.

Preparation for Family Visits. When visiting the family in the home, careful preparation must precede the actual visit. Because the nurse is often on her or his own in the family's home without immediate access to resources (except by phone), the preparatory aspect of the home visit is critical to success. Because home visits are quite costly in terms of both time and money, the most efficient and cost-effective method is to be as prepared as time constraints and other reality factors permit. This implies the reading of available records, discussing the family with health care team members who know the family well, and anticipating the types of needs that the family might have (both common developmental and unique situational needs). In this way the nurse can gather whatever teaching supplies, information, assessment, and intervention tools (e.g., tongue blades, developmental screening kit, dressings) are needed before leaving the agency. Flexibility, of course, is essential, because unanticipated or priority needs often become apparent, and part of the preparation may not be needed—or at least not on the particular visit. When the family has a telephone, calling to introduce oneself, stating the reason for the visit and making arrangements, is preferable (Leahy et al, 1977). Much wasted time and effort have been expended either by needless visits to families who are not home or due to the nurse being inadequately prepared.

The nurse's sensitivity will add to his or her observation. Sensitivity has to do with the ability to role take and empathize with others. Dyer (1973) points out that families operate on two levels of activity. The first level is the activity of work (what the family is overtly doing, who is doing what, and how they are doing it). The other level is the feeling level (how the family members feel about what they are doing). It is crucial to understand both levels.

After having collected the data on a systematic family assessment tool, the next step is analyzing the data. The data need to be summarized and collated, grouping similar data together and arranging them in orderly form so that accurate conclusions and problems can be identified. It is also at this time that gaps in information become obvious, indicating where further probing and detailing of information are needed.

Family Strengths. In analyzing the data, several family health care professionals are recommending that family strengths be identified (Clemen-Stone et al, 1987; Power and Dell Orto, 1988; Wright and Leahey, 1984). The strengths can be used as resources to draw upon when planning nursing interventions. Several authors have identified family strengths, most notably Otto (1973), Pratt (1976), Curran (1983), and most recently Beavers and Hampson (1990) and Power and coworkers (1988). They deal with the family atmosphere, flexibility and adaptibility, the extent of autonomy of members, as well as cohesiveness, the relationship of the family to the community, and communication skills. Table 3–1 gives the family strengths identified by Power and Dell Orto (1988).

TABLE 3–1. FAMILY STRENGTHS

Communication Skills
- The ability to listen.
- The ability of the family members to discuss their concerns (family expressiveness).

A Shared Family Paradigm
- Shared common perceptions of reality within the family.
- Family's willingness to have hope and appreciate that change is possible.

Intra-family Support
- The ability to provide reinforcements to each other.
- The ability of family members to provide an atmosphere of belonging.

Self-Care Abilities
- The ability of family members to take responsibility for health problems.
- Family members' willingness to take good care of themselves.

Problem-solving Skills
- The ability of family members to use negotiation in family problem-solving.
- The ability to focus on the present, rather than on past events or disappointments.
- Family members have the capacity to use everyday experiences as resources.

Adapted from Power et al (1988).

FAMILY NURSING DIAGNOSES

The family assessment culminates in an identification of family problems. Many family health problems are within the nurse's scope of practice, and are called **family nursing diagnoses.** Other family problems, however, fall under the scope of practice of other professions and fields, such as medicine, law, education, recreation, or social welfare. In these cases, the family's problems still need to be identified and discussed with the family, which serves to verify that the need or problem is mutually perceived. Often the nursing role here is to refer the family to appropriate resources and to provide the necessary coordination, teaching, and support related to the problem and referral. Other family problems are the concern of several health care professionals, with each having a different way of assessing and working with the family. In these instances, collaboration and coordination with the other team members is imperative to avoid unnecessary client confusion and lack of efficient, effective services. These problems are called **collaborative problems** (Carpenito, 1987).

Family nursing diagnoses are an extension of nursing diagnoses to the family system and are the outcome of the nursing assessment. Family nursing diagnoses include actual or potential health problems that nurses, by virtue of their education and experience, are capable and licensed to treat (Gordon, 1978 and 1982). They are used "as a basis for projecting outcomes, planning intervention, and evaluating outcome attainment" (Gordon, 1985, p. viii).

At the family level, the nursing diagnosis can be derived from using one of the family or nursing theories or from using North American Nursing Diagnosis Association (NANDA) diagnoses. For instance, if a structural-functional or interactional framework is utilized, family nursing diagnoses might include role conflicts or transitions, child-rearing problems, value conflicts, or communication problems. If a systems framework is utilized, then the family's closed boundaries relative to interactions with the community, lack of an intact parental subsystem, or excessive separateness of family members from each other are possible nursing diagnoses. In the discussions of each of the assessment and intervention areas that follow (Chaps. 8 to 17), the reader will be able to gain insight into the types of family nursing diagnoses and other family problems that may result from deficiencies in the family system, its structure or functions.

Nursing Diagnoses: The NANDA Classification

The nursing diagnosis movement represents a very significant effort on behalf of nurse leaders to systematize nursing practice and promote the use of a standardized list of diagnoses in practice. The North American Nursing Diagnosis Association (NANDA) includes, although secondarily, family problems when they define nursing diagnosis. For example, Carpenito (1987) defines nursing diagnosis as:

> A nursing diagnosis is a statement that describes the human responses (health state or actual/potential altered interaction pattern of an individual or group which the nurse can legally identify and for which the nurse can order the definitive interventions to maintain the health state or to reduce, eliminate, or prevent alterations. (p. 5)

In her definition the family is one type of group the nursing diagnoses may address. Yet in spite of this, nursing diagnoses at present remain heavily individually oriented. Family, again as discussed by Carpenito (1987), "is used to describe any person or persons who serve as support systems to the client" (p. 2). Hence, when families are the focus of nursing diagnoses, they tend primarily to be seen as context—as resources to the patient.

However, in examining a recent list of the 98 accepted NANDA nursing diagnoses, there are some diagnoses that can or do address family system and subsystem health problems. Table 3–2 lists these selected nursing diagnoses.

In addition to the NANDA nursing diagnoses being individually oriented, four other problems or limitations are apparent in the use of NANDA diagnoses in family nursing practice.

TABLE 3–2. SELECTED NANDA NURSING DIAGNOSES APPROPRIATE FOR FAMILY NURSING PRACTICE

NANDA Diagnostic Category	Nursing Diagnosis
Health perception–health management pattern	• Altered health management • Health-seeking behaviors
Activity–exercise pattern	• Impaired home maintenance management
Cognitive–perceptual pattern	• Knowledge deficit • Decisional conflict
Role–relationship pattern	• Anticipatory grieving • Dysfunctional grieving • Parental role conflict • Social isolation • Alteration in family processes • Altered role performance • Potential alteration in parenting • Altered parenting • Potential for violence
Coping–stress tolerance patterns	• Family coping: Potential for growth • Ineffective family coping: Compromised • Ineffective family coping: Disabling

Adapted from McFarland and McFarlane (1989).

1. They are atheoretical, which can be both a strength and a weakness, depending on one's viewpoint. This limitation is generally noted in the literature.
2. For the most part, the family-oriented nursing diagnoses are very broad and may not be sufficiently specific to guide nursing interventions. However, specifying the signs and symptoms of the problem and etiological or contributing factors can handle this limitation.
3. They are essentially illness oriented (Donnelly, 1990).
4. The present list is incomplete and does not cover the array of family nursing actual or potential problems/diagnoses that clinicians see.

It should be noted that nursing diagnoses are in the process of development and nurses are encouraged to submit refinements of accepted diagnoses to NANDA. Realizing these gaps, a special interest group of family nurses is engaged in describing the diagnosis "Impaired family caregiver." They plan to submit this important nursing diagnosis to NANDA to extend the list of accepted nursing diagnoses.

Donnelly (1990) describes another large gap in the NANDA accepted list. She notes with concern the essential absence of standardized diagnostic categories that address family and health promotion. She identifies only one NANDA diagnosis that "hints" at family health promotion concepts: "Family coping: Potential for growth."

Until the NANDA-approved nursing diagnosis list is expanded and refined, NANDA diagnoses offer partial assistance to the family nurse. Efforts are urgently needed to broaden the accepted list of diagnoses to adequately cover family-as-client throughout the broad spectrum of health–illness concerns (Donnelly, 1990).

Gordon's (1978 and 1985) and the NANDA format for stating nursing diagnoses consists of the statement of the diagnosis, signs and symptoms (defining characteristics) and etiologic or contributing factors. This formatting provides a rich and broadened resource for goal setting and formulating treatment plans. An example of a common family health problem is "Impaired verbal communication (NANDA diagnosis) between mother and daughter characterized by mutual hostility; related to (contributing factors) values, control, and limit-setting conflicts and mother's low self-esteem." In this case the diagnosis from NANDA was used but the signs and symptoms and contributing factors were not identified by NANDA and thus were generated by the author. Another common family nursing diagnosis from NANDA is an alteration in parenting. Here there is an array of defining characteristics that may help the clinician in identifying the signs and symptoms. This diagnosis appears to be more broadly described. For example, the alteration in parenting could be characterized by inadequate child care provision and multiple parental surrogates with etiological factors being economic, knowledge deficit (mother), and social isolation (family). The nursing care plan shown in Table 3–3 illustrates how this aspect is schematically handled in a nursing care plan tool.

Nursing Diagnosis: The Omaha System

Another classification system of client problems that has received favorable evaluation from agencies who have used the system is the Omaha system, developed

TABLE 3–3. STUDENT TOOL USED TO ASSESS, PLAN, AND IMPLEMENT NURSING CARE

I. Assessment
   A. Assessment of individual family members
   B. Assessment of family[a]
      1. Identifying and sociocultural data
      2. Environmental data
      3. Family structure
      4. Family functions
      5. Family coping
II. Nursing care plan (family)

Family Nursing Diagnosis Including Etiological or Contributing Factors	Signs and Symptoms of Problem (Defining Characteristics)	Goals	Intervention	Evaluation
Family overprotection of son, Bobby, due to parental: 1. Guilt about unwanted pregnancy. 2. Anxiety about child's health condition: asthma.	Mother dresses Bobby even though at age 4, he is able to do this himself. Mother wouldn't let Bobby play outside for fear of his hurting himself. Child is clinging to mother when strangers present. Parents view Bobby as a special, "fragile" child.	Mother will let Bobby dress himself, with help only in realistically difficult tasks. Mother will let Bobby play with brother and friends outside in the afternoon.	***Modifying Behavior*** Explored parents' feelings and behavior toward child. Discussed with the parents their child's developmental needs. Discussed with sibling activities they might enjoy playing together. ***Manipulation of Contributing Factors*** Advised mother to discuss with her doctor child's health condition and prognosis.	Mother is letting Bobby dress himself when there is time. Bobby enjoys doing so. Under mother's supervision, Bobby is playing in the outside garden of house. Father is beginning to play ball at the park with both of the boys.

[a]To be discussed in later chapters.

by the Visiting Nurse Association of Omaha (VNA of Omaha, 1986). As part of a larger operationalization of the nursing process, an orderly, comprehensive list of client problems has been generated and tested. Client problems are grouped under four major domains: environmental, psychosocial, physiological, and health behaviors. These problems are also individually oriented, but include some family-as-client problems within the listing. An implementation manual is available (VNA of Omaha, 1986) and the system has been well operationalized for use in home health agencies.

Specifying the Level of the Problem

In terms of family problem identification, the nurse needs to indicate at what family system level the problem lies—at the family unit level or at the level of one of the family subsystems or sets of relationships such as the marital dyad, the parent–child subsystem, or the sibling subsystem.

Importance of Family Participation

Active family participation through the nursing process should be of central concern. In terms of identifying problems and strengths, the family nurse and the family are jointly responsible for this part of the process.

Diagnosis involves the process of putting information together with the family to formulate the problem(s) and to explore a possible course of action. A case in point: It is not enough for the nurse working with a family to observe that the family is under stress and is not following its plan for bringing in family or friends to help. Together with the family, the nurse needs to generate a diagnosis as to what is happening and why the family is not able to follow through with its intended action. If the nurse has collected adequate information and verified it with the family, the diagnosis will be reasonably correct. His or her diagnosis should then lead to goals and intervention aimed at assisting the family to cope more effectively.

Interrelationship of Data and Problems

One of the problems in determining health needs or problems of families is that all the information gathered is interrelated, and there are almost insurmountable difficulties involved in sorting out the cause-and-effect relationships. This is because, according to systems theory, there is circular causality. Feedback loops exist (which will be discussed in Chapter 6) wherein one person's behavior (A) sets off another person's behavior (B) causing A to act in response to his or her (A's) previous behavior plus B's response. Also, there is an overlapping of family problems such as role and power conflicts, and certain problems are not of the same type or level of generality or specificity as others. Pulling out the cardinal health problems and showing other related problem areas (economic, housing, community, education) as variables has often assisted in the listing of discrete problems (they are discrete for purposes of planning, but in real life never are).

Potential Problems. The problems identified in family nursing often focus on the family's ability to cope with a health or environmental problem. In many situations there will be no present medical illness or disability. In these cases the most frequent diagnoses are preventive or health promotional, such as reduction of risks (nutritional modification—salt, caloric, sugar, and fat reduction; lowering stress levels) and life-style improvements (regular exercise, more rest and relaxation, better communication).

By definition, a nursing diagnosis may involve potential health problems that originate from existing or anticipated conditions. Freeman (1970, p. 58) calls these "foreseeable crisis or stress points." Because of anticipated periods of unusual demand on the family and its members, anticipatory guidance or health teaching, health counseling, and the initiation of referrals to community resources are often indicated. Examples of foreseeable stressors are pregnancy, movement into a new community, retirement, adolescence, wife beginning full-time employment, and the progressive deterioration of an aging parent.

Triage Process and Priority Setting

One word of caution is necessary concerning the problems identified by a referring agency. The presenting problem, or reason for referral to the agency, is rarely the only problem. In fact, it may be the least serious problem the family faces. Archer and Fleshman (1975) recommend that family-centered community health nurses use a sorting or triage process when working with families, because there is always too much to do and a scarcity of resources. The triage process they recommend is based on a hierarchy of needs, as described below.

Of low priority and hierarchy relative to providing services are those needs that are impossible to do anything about, because of either client or agency constraints. Thus it is fruitless for individual nurses to "spin their wheels." Other needs or problems will resolve themselves or can be handled by the family's support system or someone less costly and more available, such as the homemaker-home health aide. Again, valuable professional health services should not be committed to these problems. Some needs require more resources than the agency or community can commit, and if a nurse attempts to meet these needs, other families will probably suffer from neglect. Thus realistic priorities, given limited resources, must be established.

There are also needs and problems that are beyond the control of the client or the control and/or level of expertise of the nurse. These limitations must be recognized. If the problem is not within our area of expertise, it needs to be referred. The needs for which family health nurses can affect change or on which he or she can make a discernible, positive health impact in an efficient manner are the problems we should be assisting families to alleviate or ameliorate.

Archer and Fleshman (1975) point out that community nurses have long been considered "generalists," engaging in all sorts of problem areas. But this characterization has resulted in frustration, case overload, and cost ineffectiveness.

Once family and individual health problems have been identified, they should be listed in order of priority, according to their importance to the client. There is often a disjuncture between how the professional views client needs and how the client (or members within the family) view their own problems. Only by ranking needs and priorities from the client's perspective can plans for intervention have any chance of success. The widespread use of problem-oriented records provides a ready vehicle for listing problems. These identified problems will then form the basis for setting goals and planning intervention.

PLANNING

Goal Setting

Planning first involves joint formulation of client-centered goals. The mutual setting of goals consists of identifying possible resources, delineating alternative approaches to meeting goals, selecting specific nursing interventions, mobilizing resources (including the family's own self-care capacities), and operationalizing the plan (setting of priorities and spelling out how the plan will be phased in). The nursing care plan serves as a blueprint for action.

Mutual goal setting with families is the cornerstone of effective planning. One of the basic premises of family nursing is that clients have the ultimate responsibility for managing their own lives (the principle of self-determination) and that we respect others' beliefs (Carey, 1989). Tinkham and Voorhies (1977) help families determine their own-health goals by providing them with all the relevant information about themselves. This allows them to make sounder decisions about what goals and services they wish to plan. Thus the main determinant of what goals are set is the family, not the nurse and what he or she hopes to achieve (Otto, 1973).

Mutual goal setting with family members is consistently superior to unilateral goal setting for several reasons: (1) the process of mutual goal setting has a positive effect on interactions with families; (2) people tend to resist being told what to do, but are likely to work toward goals that they themselves choose and support; and (3) people who make decisions tend to feel accountable for them (Carey, 1989).

Goal setting has been increasingly recognized as a highly important component in planning. The development of clear-cut, specific, and acceptable goals is crucial. If the nursing goals are not clear, it does not make much difference what activities are carried out because the end point is not known. To the extent that the stated objectives are defined and accepted as valid by the family, the desired action is likely to follow. In addition to the acceptability, clarity, and specificity of goals, they also need to be stated in behavioral terms so that they can be measured (evaluated).

There are several levels of goals. The first level includes the specific, immediate, and measurable short-term goals; in the middle of the continuum are intermediate-level goals; and at the other end of the continuum are the long-term, more general, ultimate goals that indicate the broad purposes the nurse and family hope to achieve. Short-term goals are necessary to motivate and give confidence to the family and individuals that progress is being made, as well as to guide the family toward the larger, more comprehensive goal.

In goal setting it is desirable to work with the family in differentiating those problems that need to be resolved by nursing intervention, those problems the family as the self-care agent can handle by itself, and those problems that need to be referred to other members of the health care team or handled on a collective basis. A case in point is an elderly couple that needs (1) assistance in obtaining Medicaid, (2) diet counseling, and (3) basic nursing care for the nonambulatory husband. The nurse may decide to handle diet counseling herself, refer the couple to a social worker for Medicaid assistance, and suggest a home health aide to provide the routine nursing care needed for the husband. As a member of the health care team serving families, the family-centered nurse must also be continually alert to situations where team conferences (formal or informal) might be beneficial to the clients. Collaborative planning with other team members helps foster a better understanding of client's needs, in addition to mapping out who will do what.

Generating Alternative Approaches and Identifying Resources

After setting goals, the health care professional and family need to generate alternative ways for reaching the stated goals. As these are delineated, possible resources for handling needs are identified. Such resources include use of family inner strengths, including their self-care resources, the family's support system, and physical and community sources of assistance.

Family strengths, as discussed previously, are useful in assisting nurse and family in resolving family health problems. Otto (1973) reports that he has successfully used a family-strength method in counseling of families. He explains that family strengths are first identified and then progressively shared with family members so as to increase their awareness of their resources and to take inventory of further potentials or strengths they have. Members are encouraged to discover latent strengths and unfulfilled potentials as part of their problem-solving efforts.

Specific actions or approaches facilitated by the nurse are selected from the available alternatives and resources. These are approaches that both family and nurse feel are appropriate and, hopefully, have a high probability of success. Some of the strategies may involve some or all family members, other health care team members, or extended family and friends, as well as the nurse.

In thinking through the planning of nursing approaches, the nurse needs to ask the following questions:

- Will the proposed approaches result in increased dependence or increased independence on the part of the family?
- Is this action within the information and skill level of the family members or their own resources?
- Will this action diminish or strengthen the coping abilities of the family (Dyer, 1973)?
- Does the family and/or its members have sufficient commitment and motivation to adhere to the plan?
- Are there adequate resources available to carry out the plan?

Families have the right and responsibility to make their own health decisions. Because of this premise of family nursing, there will be certain actions that fully informed families choose that we may personally and professionally disagree with. So important is the issue of client information and understanding of possible consequences of action (so that he or she can make a reasonable decision), that we now have informed consent laws in most states. Archer and Fleshman (1985) cite the example of a client who was exposed to rubella during the first trimester of pregnancy, with tests showing no immunity to the rubella virus. The nurse's responsibility in such an instance would be to discuss with the parents the risk of having an infant who is deformed and to inform them of possible alternatives (obtain abortion, continue pregnancy, seek further consultation). The parents need time and an opportunity to discuss their feelings and thoughts, as well as assistance with problem solving. However, we cannot make decisions for them. We may draw on professional judgment and knowledge to recommend a particular course of action after hearing their concerns, but we should in no way reject or withdraw our support if the client makes a decision counter to our advice.

Some of the approaches we plan with families are less than ideal, but are hopefully realistic and an improvement to the client's (family's) present situation. Seeking obtainable ways to reach goals is both realistic and pragmatic.

Priority Setting

The operationalization of the nursing care plan follows the mutual selection of approaches designed to reach each of the stated goals. Priority setting of interventions and a phasing in and coordinating of the plan leads to its implementation.

Organizing nursing interventions by priority will provide a more efficient, effective, and safe means for reaching goals and differentiating between short- and long-term goals.

The family's ranking of priorities is paramount in the joint setting of priorities. Some nurses assign planned intervention low-, medium-, and high-priority ratings, with high-priority actions being those that must be carried out immediately or very soon. Reality factors such as agency policies, time and money constraints, and availability of personnel and other resources also influence priorities. In addition to client safety or life-threatening situations, two important factors to consider in assigning priorities are (1) the client's sense of urgency (this is important in building of rapport) and (2) actions that will, or might have, therapeutic effects on future actions. Some actions are prerequisite to others.

FAMILY NURSING INTERVENTION

The intervention phase begins with the completion of the nursing care plan. Implementation may be carried out by a number of people: the client (individual or family), the nurse(s), other health care team members, the extended family, and other persons in the family's social network.

Subsequent to the family assessment and a joint discussion of family concerns and problems, the family nurse and family need to decide whether family intervention is indicated. Criteria for making this decision includes the family's interest and motivation in receiving help and working on its problems, the family's level of functioning, the nurse's own skill level, and the resources available (Wright and Leahey, 1984). In addition to routine health promotional and preventive care, Wright and Leahey (1984) suggest that families normally need help in the following circumstances:

1. A family presents with a problem(s) in which the relationships between family members are affected.
2. A family member presents with an illness that is having an obvious detrimental impact upon the other family members.
3. The family members are contributing to the symptoms or problems of an individual.
4. One family member's improvement leads to symptoms or deterioration in another family member.

During the execution of nursing interventions, new data will be continually coming in. As this information (client's responses, changes in situation, and so on) is collected, the nurse needs to be sufficiently flexible and adaptable to reassess the situation with the family and extemporaneously make modifications to the plan.

Levels of Family Nursing Intervention

There are different levels of family nursing interventions with respect to the complexity of the interventions themselves. Wright and Leahey (1984) divide these into two levels of family intervention—beginning and advanced. In the basic level of family nursing practice, interventions are generally supportive and educative, as well as direct and straightforward. At the advanced level of family nursing practice, interventions include some of the more complex and indirect psychosocial family therapy interventions.

Nursing Intervention Typologies

Freeman's Classification. Freeman (1970), in her classic community health nursing text, classifies nursing intervention as being:

TABLE 3–4. WRIGHT AND LEAHEY'S CLASSIFICATION OF INTERVENTIONS DIRECTED AT THREE LEVELS OF FAMILY FUNCTIONING

1. **Cognitive.** Interventions directed at the cognitive level of family functioning consist of those nursing actions where new information or ideas on a situation or experience are presented. Teaching and reframing strategies fall under this category.
2. **Affective.** Nursing actions directed at the affective aspects of family functioning are those designed to alter family members' emotions so that they can problem-solve more effectively. Helping parents reduce their anxiety about the care of their sick child is an example of this type of intervention.
3. **Behavioral.** Nursing strategies directed at assisting family members to interact/behave differently with each other and with those outside of the family are included here. Teaching family members to communicate more functionally, such as listening to each other without interrupting, is an example of a strategy that fits this category.

Adapted from Wright and Leahey (1984).

1. Supplemental. Here the nurse acts as a direct provider of nursing services by intervening in areas where the family is unable to do so.
2. Facilitative. In this case the family nurse removes barriers to needed services, such as medical, social welfare, transportation, or home health care services.
3. Developmental. Nursing goals are aimed at improving the capacity of the recipient of care to act on his or her own behalf (eg, promoting of family group self-care and self-responsibility). Assisting families to utilize their own self-health care resources, such as their internal and external social support systems, is one such intervention (Milardo, 1988). Chapter 8 discusses social support in more detail.

Wright and Leahey's Classification. Wright and Leahey (1984) have detailed the process of implementing psychosocially oriented family nursing interventions. They classify family nursing interventions as being directed at three levels of family functioning: cognitive, affective, and behavioral (Table 3–4).

Interventions Aimed at Changing Family Behavior

When nurses are working with families, interventions are typically aimed at helping the family members change their behavior, with the ultimate goal being the enhancement of family system functioning or high-level family wellness. For the nurse working with families over a period of time, it must be remembered that change in families comes about "over time through a sequence of interventive moves, each one growing out of information gained, in part, through observing the outcomes of the previous interventions" (Hartman and Laird, 1983, p. 306).

Concepts of change are helpful in thinking about ways of helping families to change. Wright and Leahey (1984) have highlighted some important concepts of change that they have found critical in assisting them to work with families with health problems:

- Change depends upon context.
- Change depends upon the (client's) perception of the problem.
- Change depends upon realistic goals.
- Understanding alone does not lead to change.
- Change does not necessarily occur equally in all family members.
- Change can have myriad causes. (p. 68)

Specific Family Nursing Interventions

A myriad of family nursing interventions exist that may be used in working with families. Which interventions are selected are often the result of the theoretical model the family nurse utilizes in the care of a particular family, as well as the family nursing diagnosis made and the goals formulated. For example, anticipatory guidance (a type of teaching strategy) is emphasized in the developmental model, while crisis intervention strategies are used frequently when a family stress and coping model is applied in practice.

Moreover, the specific intervention strategies health care professionals utilize with families may depend on the level of functioning of the family. Leavitt (1982) classifies families into highly functional, moderately dysfunctional, highly dysfunctional, acute and highly dysfunctional, and chronic. Depending on the family's degree of functionality, nursing interventions vary. For instance, with the highly functional family, the family nursing actions are largely preventive and health promotive (teaching, information providing). In contrast, with the highly dysfunctional, acute family, short-term and long-term therapeutic, supportive, and preventive actions are advised (Leavitt, 1982).

The particular interventions implemented also depend on the families, as they are active participants in goal setting and selection of interventions. In any case, educative (teaching) and supportive strategies are core intervention strategies regardless of all the other factors involved.

In each of the assessment and intervention chapters, specific interventions stressed in that particular area are identified. Further discussion of the specific family nursing interventions is presented in Chapter 18. A listing of the family nursing interventions cited in the literature appears in Table 3–5.

TABLE 3–5. FAMILY NURSING INTERVENTIONS

Behavior modification
Contracting
Case management/coordination
Collaborative strategies
Counseling, including support, cognitive reappraisal, and reframing
Empowering families through active participation
Environmental modification
Family advocacy
Family crisis intervention
Networking, including use of self-help groups and social support
Providing information and technical expertise
Role modeling
Role supplementation
Teaching strategies, including stress management, life-style modifications, and anticipatory guidance

Barriers to Implementing Interventions

Apathy and Value Differences. In reporting his work with culturally diverse and poor families in the community, Dyer (1973) mentions two related problems with which family nurses are confronted—family apathy and indecision. The first of these problematic behaviors must not only be recognized as a major problem, but more importantly, must be interpreted as to its possible meaning.

The first of these problematic behaviors is apathy. Behavioral manifestations of apathy are apparent. When the nurse finds health problems that he or she feels vitally affect the family and discusses these problems and recommendations, the family responds with a "so what" attitude and gives no signs of action or concern. Does the family really not care? Not usually. It is often the case that there are differences in values, especially if the family is of a different socioeconomic or ethnic background. Whereas the nurse feels health should be a top priority, the more basic physiological and safety needs for economic security, livable housing, and adequate food may have a greater urgency for such families. Many health practices (eg, carefully planned nutrition, cleanliness, preventive health care) are not part of the general life experiences of the poor. Thus, what the nurse may perceive as apathy is really just a continuation of the family's life experience and differences in values. The nurse is often faced with the task of trying to help families obtain their more basic needs so that they can work at improving their own health.

The educational task is even more difficult if the

family's social network or social system (relatives, friends, and neighbors) does not support needed health actions. Some research shows that if members of a group adopting new practices support each other, the possibility of changing behavior is greater. Based on this understanding, many therapeutic self-help groups have been formed to assist group members to adopt new behavioral patterns (eg, Alcoholics Anonymous, Parents Anonymous, Weight Watchers, Colostomy Club, Reach for Recovery, psychotherapy groups).

Apathy, Hopelessness, and Futility. In addition to value differences, apathy may also be the outcome of a sense of hopelessness—the belief that "whatever the family does, it won't matter anyway" or fatalism—the feeling that "what will be, will be." Fatalism is a central theme among the poor and powerless. Certain problems may be just too overwhelming for individuals to know where to begin. Breaking a task up into small, sequential steps may help a family proceed successfully toward a goal that at first seems insurmountable. It must be remembered, though, that not trying to accomplish a goal is a common way of coping to "save face," since it avoids the embarrassment of being found inadequate or of failing.

Apathy and Futility. The second explanation for apathetic behavior on the part of a family is that family members may have a sense of futility about the effectiveness or availability of services: "So I have cancer? There is nothing that can be done if they do find it!" Without a perception that effective and accessible treatment exists, clients are not going to seek health care services (Becker, 1972). The family-centered nurse will need to probe a situation where apathy exists to attempt to determine what is going on. Is faulty information the problem, or finances, or management of family resources, or excessive fear (and thus avoidance)?

Indecision. Dyer (1973) describes indecision as the third behavioral area nurses in the community find problematic. In this case the family does not appear completely apathetic, but it cannot seem to make a decision. What are the causes of this type of behavior? Dyer identifies several. First, indecision often results from the inability to see the advantage of one action over another. Whatever is done, the advantages or disadvantages seem to be equal. In this case the nurse needs to help the family to problem solve, exploring both the pros and cons of different actions, in addition to the family members' feelings. It is hoped that this process results in one approach gaining superiority in family members' minds so they can take action. Some clients desperately want direct advice on what to do. Very careful consideration should be given to their requests. Temporary dependence is sometimes the best avenue, but generally this approach only solves a particular problem, and in the meantime the family has not learned how to cope independently with the next problem. Being a supportive resource person is the preferable role.

Indecision may also be the result of unexpressed fears and concerns. Marked anxiety and fear immobilize problem-solving abilities.

De-facto decision making (letting things just happen) may also be a part of the family's life-style. This type of decision making has been found to be predominant in disorganized families and in many poor families.

EVALUATION

The fifth component of the nursing process is evaluation. The evaluation is based on how effective the interventions were that the family, nurse, and others instituted. Effectiveness is determined by looking at family responses and outcomes (how the family responded), rather than the interventions implemented. The evaluation, again, is a joint endeavor between the nurse and the family.

Although a client-centered approach to evaluation is most relevant, it is often frustrating because of the difficulties in establishing objective criteria for desired outcomes and because of factors other than planned interventions that intervene and affect family/client outcomes. Because of such factors, one never gets a clear-cut, "pure" look at the efficacy of nursing intervention.

The nursing care plan contains the framework for evaluation. If clear, specific behavioral goals have been delineated, these can then serve as the criteria for evaluating the degree of effectiveness achieved. In some instances there may be a need to develop even more specific criteria for evaluation of goals. For example, the goal, "The family will seek medical services for their sick baby," may need more specific criteria to judge whether the goal has been attained. Criteria for evaluation might include the fact that the family has been seen by a pediatrician and has received treatment for the baby's illness. In many cases, however, the goal is written in more specific terms to avoid further criteria development, such as, "The child will obtain diagnostic and treatment services from pediatrician within 1 to 3 days."

Evaluation is an ongoing process that occurs each time a nurse updates the nursing care plan. Before care plans are expanded or modified, certain nursing actions will need to be looked at jointly by the nurse and family to see if they are really helpful. Unless family responses to nursing intervention are jointly evaluated, ineffective nursing action may persist.

The following questions should be contemplated when evaluating:

1. Is there a consensus between the family and other health care team members on the evaluation?
2. What additional data need to be collected to evaluate progress?
3. Were there any unforeseen outcomes that need to be considered?
4. If the family's behavior and perceptions indicate that the problem has not been satisfactorily resolved, what are the reasons?
5. Were the nursing diagnoses, goals, and approaches realistic and accurate?

There are various methods of evaluation used in nursing; the most important factor is that the method needs to be tailored to the goals and interventions being evaluated.

MODIFICATION

Modification follows the evaluation plan and begins the cyclical process of returning to the assessment and reassessing—feeding in the new information obtained from previous encounters, and then continuing to revise each phase in the cycle as needed.

Modification is often difficult to do, as it can be frustrating and ego deflating to admit our plan and implementation were ineffective. So often in working with families on a long-term basis we see only very slow results or perhaps no movement of a family at all—at least not when we are working with them. At this point we need to make sure that if we continue our search for a more accurate diagnosis or a more effective plan, our efforts have some chance of success and the resources to be expended will be commensurate with the gain achieved. It is most important, however, to keep foremost in our minds the principle of self-determination—that families have a right to decide what is best for them and to make their own health decisions.

Table 3–3 presents a family nursing care plan example, using the process outlined in this chapter.

□ *STUDY QUESTIONS*

Choose the correct answer(s) to the following question.

1. The primary difference between the nursing process when working with families versus working solely with individual clients is (select the best answer):
   a. The community setting must be assessed.
   b. The level of assessment, diagnosis, planning, implementation, and evaluation is broadened to include both the family and its members.
   c. The level of assessment, diagnosis, planning, implementation, and evaluation is the family system.
   d. Prevention and health promotion are the aim versus cure and rehabilitation when working with individuals.

2. Match the correct process characteristics in the left-hand column with the nursing phase/component on the right.

PROCESS CHARACTERISTICS	PHASE/COMPONENTS OF NURSING PROCESS
a. Continuous data collection	1. Assessment
b. Approaches based on identified goals	2. Diagnosis
c. Client outcome appraisal	3. Goal setting
d. Anticipated behaviorally stated client responses	4. Plan of care
e. Setting of priorities	5. Intervention
f. Nursing action, therapy, or approaches	6. Evaluation
g. Execution of the nursing care plan	7. Modification

h. Existing or potential family and individual health problem
i. Mobilizing community resources
j. Identification of resources
k. Refinement and revision efforts
l. Defining alternative approaches

3. The nursing assessment is (choose the best answer):
   a. Based on initial gathering of data.
   b. Done by all persons involved in providing client care.
   c. A sensitive and continuing process conducted by all involved health providers.

4. One objective in terms of completing a family assessment process is the setting up of priorities for intervention.
   a. True.
   b. False.
   c. Uncertain.

Match the nurse's statements with the appropriate step in the nursing process.

a. Establishing a relationship.
b. Obtaining information.
c. Clarification of focal problem.
d. Assessment of strengths and resources.
e. Formulation of a therapeutic plan and mobilization of client's and others' resources.

5. "How have things been with your family?"

6. "I'm concerned about your problem and would like to know more."

7. "Can you tell me about the fight with your wife?"

8. "Tell me how I can help you."

9. "Do you feel you can talk easily with your sister about your worries?"

10. List the three activities the family health nurse should carry out in preparation for a home visit.

Fill in the spaces in the following question.

11. NANDA recommends that a nursing diagnosis contain the statement of the problem, its etiology or contributing factors and defining characteristics. Explain one advantage to using this method for diagnosing client problems.
____
____

Choose the correct answer(s) to the following question.

12. In planning nursing intervention, priorities need to be established. These variables are significant when establishing priorities:
    a. Family/individual interests and perceptions.
    b. Degree of urgency or acuteness of problem.

c. Availability of resources.
d. Agency policies.
e. Actions that are prerequisite to other actions.

Fill in the space in the following question.

13. Active family involvement in the nursing process should occur during ______
____
______________________ phase(s) of the nursing process.

After reading the vignettes, answer the following questions.

14. Mr. and Mrs. Wade's daughter, age 5, has been observed several times by kindergarten teachers in grand mal seizures. The school nurse, while visiting family, discusses the convulsions and need for medical follow-up at a special clinic in a nearby community. She notes that the parents change the subject, brushing off observed seizures as temper tantrums. They state that the family does not have time to take her to a doctor.
a. What type of problem does the school nurse have in working with this family?
b. What may be the basis for this problem?

15. Mrs. J., a single parent with limited income, is having difficulty raising her only son, age 10. She describes him as rebellious, disobedient, and irresponsible. Because of this parenting difficulty, she feels that she is a failure in the mothering role. The community health nurse, who is visiting because Mrs. J. is pregnant, listens to her concerns regarding her son. For several years, teachers and a church minister have encouraged her to take the child for counseling, but she could never decide whether this would be helpful or more damaging.
a. This type of behavior problem is called ______________.
b. What may be the basis for the problem?

Select one answer to the following questions.

16. A widely used (in community health nursing) classification scheme for client problems is the:
a. NANDA system of nursing diagnosis.
b. Freeman classification.
c. Omaha system.
d. None of the above.

17. In the list below select two *major* concepts of change that are important to consider when assisting families to make changes.
a. Change depends on the nature of the stressors families face.
b. Change only occurs if both parents are in agreement.
c. Gaining the right information leads to change.
d. Change is situationally determined.
e. The client's perception of the problem is critical in considering change.

Provide the short answers indicated.

18. What are three sources of data for family assessment? ______________
____

19. Which family intervention is selected depends on multiple factors. Three considerations are (a) ____________, (b) ____________, and (c) ____________.

20. Which classification of interventions contains "supplemental," "facilitative," and "developmental" categories? ____________

21. What is a basic difference between Freeman's and Wright and Leahey's classification relative to nursing interventions? ______________________________
____

22. Relative to family nursing practice, indicate whether the following about NANDA nursing diagnoses classification is a strength, a limitation, or neither in the list below (s = strength, 1= limitation, and n = neither).
   ______a. Diagnoses are individually oriented.
   ______b. Diagnoses are illness-oriented.
   ______c. Diagnoses cuts across all nursing settings.
   ______d. Diagnoses are each generated by a group of experts, submitted to NANDA and carefully considered.
   ______e. NANDA nursing diagnoses are in state of expansion and refinement.
   ______ f. Statements of family problems are broad.

PART II

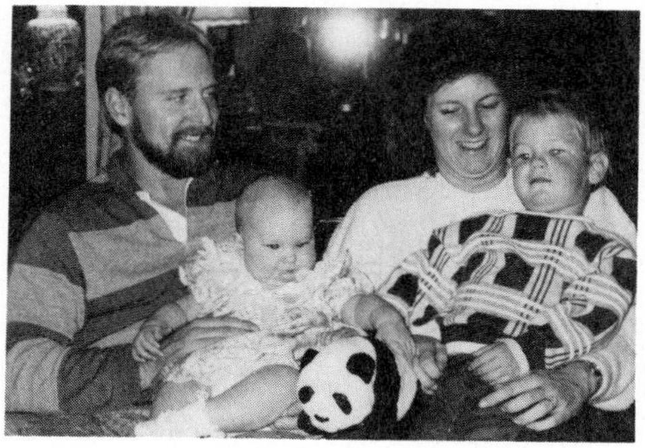

Theoretical Foundations

The theoretical foundations for family nursing practice are described in Part II. Theoretical perspectives used in family nursing are reviewed in Chapter 4. Although family social science and family therapy theories still form the basis for most of family nursing practice to date, notable progress is being made to reformulate family theories to fit a nursing perspective and to use nursing theories in family nursing practice. Chapters 5 to 7 present the three theories that are the primary basis for the Friedman Family Assessment Model (see Appendices A and B for the complete model). These three theoretical perspectives are structural–functional theory (Chap. 5), family developmental theory (Chap. 6), and systems theory (Chap. 7).

CHAPTER FOUR

Theoretical Approaches Used in Family Nursing

Learning Objectives

1. Explain the advantages inherent in deriving family nursing practice from a theoretical framework, a nursing model or theory, a family therapy theory, and family social science theories.
2. In each of the five nursing models described, identify the model's orientation or level of analysis.
3. Describe the five major theories utilized in the family social sciences for analyzing families.
4. Define family interactional theory.
5. Trace major alterations that occurred in family functions during the change from an agrarian, nonindustrialized society to present society.
6. Identify the grand theory under which the family ecological theory fits.

THEORETICAL FRAMEWORKS

A theoretical framework is needed to guide clinical practice in all areas of nursing. Theory-based nursing practice is probably even more important in family nursing practice, since to "think interactionally" with respect to family phenomena and problems is counter to our previous education in nursing, and hence more challenging.

A theoretical framework or perspective provides the mechanism by which we can organize our observations, focus our inquiries, and communicate our findings (Meleis, 1985). Theories describe, explain, and predict social phenomena such as family behavior. For the applied sciences such as nursing, using a theoretical perspective for assessment assists the nurse to sort out and organize a large amount of disparate data about the family, give meaning to the data in terms of problems and strengths identification, and provide guidance for goal setting and interventions.

Theories vary tremendously in their level of abstraction or generality, as well as in their scope of applicability and the number of phenomena they address. Theories are generally classified as grand, middle range, or low level (also called single domain), based on the above criteria.

In family nursing practice we basically use theories from three disciplines or specialty areas. These are theories from nursing, family social sciences, and family therapy. These theories range from the more abstract of the family theories (eg, family systems theory) to more focused middle-level theories such as family stress theory. Within the various theories, theoretical perspectives, conceptual models, or "streams of influence," much overlap of concepts and ideas can be seen. There has been a substantial amount of cross-fertilization between theorists, whereby concepts originating in one theory have been translated into similar concepts in another. Many of the notions within nursing theories incorporate concepts borrowed from earlier grand and middle-range theories of sociology, anthropology, and psychology. Concepts of interaction, stressors, environment, self-concept, or self-esteem are examples of nursing theories' borrowed concepts from the behavioral and social sciences. Likewise the family theories have used the earlier grand theories and concepts of developmental theory, symbolic interactionism, structural–functional theory, social exchange theory, and general systems theory, and applied them to the family.

A good grounding in the major theoretical approaches used in working with families is needed, since no *one* theory adequately addresses the behaviors and problems of all families. The theory or perspective the family nurse applies depends on the family's situation, the family nurse's skills and knowledge, the family's goals, and the nurse's position or role with the agency. Table 4–1 lists theories used in family nursing practice.

TABLE 4–1. THEORETICAL APPROACHES USED IN FAMILY NURSING PRACTICE

Nursing Theories/Conceptual Models
Systems orientation
Johnson's behavioral systems
Neuman's systems conceptual model
Developmental orientation
Orem's self-care conceptual model
Systems and interactional orientations
Roy's adaptation model
King's open systems model
Systems and developmental orientations
Roger's life process model
Family Social Science Theories
Developmental
Sociologically oriented: Duvall
Psychologically oriented: McGoldrick and Carter
Systems
Mainstream
Ecological model
Structural–functional
Interactional
Role theory
Family stress and coping theory
Institutional–historical
Other
Conflict theory
Social exchange theory
Social learning theory
Family Therapy Theories
Family systems (mainstream theoretical orientation)
Bowenian family systems theory
Structural (Minuchin) family theory
Interactional or family communications theory
Behavioral
Psychodynamic
Experiential–humanistic
Family crisis intervention

NURSING THEORIES

Nursing has moved from a technically based vocation to a discipline with competing paradigms or schools of theories (Meleis, 1985). According to Fawcett (1984), conceptual models or theories in nursing can be classified into three types, which vary according to their world view and their theoretical orientation (the type of earlier sociological or psychological grand theory upon which the model is based). These three types of theory are (1) developmental, stressing change and growth; (2) interactional, stressing roles, communication, and self-concept; and (3) systems, stressing the interdependency between parts and wholes and circular causality. It should be noted that these same three types of theories are also found within the family social science theories. Fawcett (1984) has classified six of the widely referenced theories or conceptual models into the following typology.

- Systems: Johnson's behavioral systems model, Neuman's systems model.
- Developmental: Orem's self-care model.
- Interactional: No major theorist noted.
- Systems and interactional models (characteristics of both): King's open systems model, Roy's adaptation model.
- Systems and developmental models (characteristics of both): Roger's life process model.

Although all the nursing theories began as individually oriented theories and considered the family only as part of the patient's context, as the theorists and others have elaborated on and refined the major nursing theories, they have tended to increase their focus on the family (Whall, 1986a). Most have significantly broadened their focus so as to view the family as a client, along with the individual person and the community.

Five of the leading nursing theories or models are briefly described with respect to how the family is incorporated into the model and the model's relevancy for family nursing.

Neuman's Systems Model

In Neuman's publications in the 1970s about her systems model, she did not discuss the family as such. In a later compilation of chapters about the Neuman model, edited by Neuman (1982), the model was expanded relative to family so that the recipient of nursing care included families. Two chapters from this latter text applied Neuman's model to a family system (Reed, 1982) and family therapy (Goldblum-Graff and Graff, 1982). In these chapters the family is described as an appropriate target for both assessment and primary, secondary, and tertiary interventions. The nursing process is used as the link between family theory and nursing practice (Fawcett, 1984). Recently Mischke-Berkey and associates (1989) have assiduously adapted the Neuman model for use in family assessment and intervention. Neuman's model, because family concepts have been identified and applied, appears to be quite useful for guiding family nursing practice.

Orem's Self-care Model

Orem's theories of self-care, self-care deficit, and nursing system are individually oriented. Individuals (clients) are considered the primary recipient of nursing care. The family is seen as a basic conditioning factor for the family members (the clients), or as the primary context within which the individual functions. The nurse also assists dependent-care agents (those adult members who care for dependent individuals) and in doing so relates to them as individuals rather than families or family subsystems (Orem, 1983).

Orem has not articulated how family theory concepts could be incorporated into her model of nursing practice (Tadych, 1985). Tadych (1985), however, takes on the task of describing how family structure, functions, and development could be articulated with Orem's model. Because the unit of analysis differs between the two theories, the articulation that Tadych describes is complementary. Although the self-care philosophy is quite relevant for family nursing, Orem's present concepts do not provide the foundational concepts for working with families as clients. Chin (1985) has suggested that one reason why there is a lack of applicability of Orem's model to the family as a unit is that self-care requisites for families are not the same as for individuals. She suggests that universal functions of the family become the basis for self-care requisites of the family. This is certainly an improvement over attempting to use Orem's individually oriented self-care requisites to assess a family. Further efforts such as this are needed so that Orem's theory will be more useful for working with the family as client.

King's Open Systems Model

In King's 1981 text, the family was indexed extensively (Whall, 1986a). King viewed the family as a social system and a major concept within her model. The family is treated as both context and client. King explains that "a theory of goal attainment is useful for nurses when called to assist families to maintain their health or cope with problems or illness" (1983, p. 182). King continues to describe her model as assisting nurses to help family members set goals to resolve problems and make decisions. Because the model is systems and interactionally oriented, with further elaboration of family content, it should be quite useful in family nursing.

Roy's Adaptation Model

Describing her adaptation model and how family is incorporated, Roy explained that the family as well as the individual, group, social organization, and community may be the unit of analysis and a focus of nursing practice. Just as nurses assess the person as an adaptive system, so they need to assess the family when a family is the focus of care. "Nursing interventions are the enhancing of stimuli [focal, contextual, and residual] to promote adaptation of the family system" (Roy, 1983, p. 275). Further refinement and elaboration of family concepts are needed, but basic congruency and applicability of the model to family nursing practice exists. Hence, Roy's theory of adaptation also seems to hold promise in terms of describing/explaining family nursing phenomena. Whereas Roy suggests that nursing problems involve ineffective coping mechanisms, which cause ineffective responses, disrupting the integrity of the person, this notion could easily be broadened to the family unit, where ineffective family coping patterns lead to family functioning problems (McCubbin and Figley, 1983). Moreover, this theory stresses health promotion and the importance of assisting clients in manipulating their environment; both notions are also significant in family nursing.

Roger's Life Process Model

In the case of Roger's theory, the focus of nursing is on the life processes of human beings. The goal of nursing is to promote symphonic interaction between human beings and their environment (Meleis, 1985). In earlier writings from 1970 to 1980, Rogers did not discuss the family. But in 1983 she asserted that her conceptual model was as applicable to families as it was to individuals. For Rogers the family was conceptualized as an irreducible, four-dimensional, negentropic family energy field that has become a focus of study in nursing. Whall (1981) clearly shows the congruency and applicability of Roger's theory to family assessment, illustrating this by using Roger's concepts of complementarity, resonancy, and helicy to describe the family system. Rogers' legacy is clearly associated with general systems theory, and because of this orientation there is a good fit between Rogerian nursing theory and family nursing.

Summary

As yet, application of nursing theory to family nursing practice is incomplete, but growing impressively (Clements and Roberts, 1983; Whall, 1983; Whall and Fawcett, 1991). Nursing theories hold great promise in that when applied to the family, they will hopefully describe and explain not only the family in the context of health and illness but will delineate the nurse's role in assessment and intervention. Unfortunately, at this point in time, nursing theories are still in beginning stages of application to family nursing. Family theories are much more complete in their description and more powerful in their explanation of family behavior (family social science theories) and family intervention (family therapy theories), but need to be reformulated or adapted so that they fit the perspective of nursing (Whall, 1986b).

FAMILY SOCIAL SCIENCE THEORIES

An Eclectic Approach

At present no one theory from nursing, family therapy, or the family social sciences fully describes the relationships and dynamics of family life among the diverse variety of families with which we work. Nor does one theoretical perspective give us a sufficiently broad knowledge base upon which to assess and intervene. Hence, we are forced to draw upon multiple theories to work effectively with families. Some theories, however, are much broader in scope, such as Roger's life process theory or general systems theory applied to the family, while other theories are clearly middle range (more limited in scope and the phenomena they describe). Examples of middle-range theories are family stress theory (Hill, 1949), family role theory (Rose, 1962), and family communication theory (Watzlawick et al, 1967).

Of the three genres of theory, the family social science theories are the most well developed and informative with respect to how families function, the environment–family interchange, interactions within the family, how the family changes over time, and the family's reactions to stress. One striking limitation in using these theories as a basis for assessment and intervention in family nursing is that their clinical application is lacking. The obvious reason is that these theories emanate from sociology and social psychology—academic disciplines, not professional disciplines. This text covers some of the major social science theories relevant to family nursing practice and makes clinical applications both to family assessment and family intervention.

Family therapy theories, in contrast, are practice theories, as are nursing theories. They describe family assessment and family intervention strategies for the professional discipline(s) involved. The major drawback in using these theories, however, is that they may not be congruent with the nursing perspective (Whall, 1986b) and, for the beginning family nurse particularly, may not be entirely appropriate. In addition, the family therapy theories are designed for working with families with identified mental health problems, and hence, may not be as germane in working with healthy families or families with other types of health–illness problems.

Whall (1986b) urges family nurse therapists to reformulate existing family therapy theories to fit the nursing perspective in accordance with the nursing theory the nurse is using. In this way, the modified family theory will more effectively guide family nurse practice.

Reviewing the literature on social science theoretical frameworks used to study families, it is clear that there is little consensus as to what theories constitute the major theoretical frameworks. For example, Nye and Berardo (1966) delineate the following theoretical–conceptual approaches utilized to study the family: anthropologic, structural, functional, situational, psychoanalytic, economic, institutional, interactional, social-psychological, developmental, Western Christian, and legal. Nevertheless, only eight frameworks that are directly relevant to understanding the family and to family-centered practice are described in this text. These are systems theory, structural–functional theory, family interactional theory, family developmental theory, the institutional–historical approach, conflict theory, social exchange theory, and social learning theory. The first five of these theories are the most salient in terms of family analysis.

Systems Theory

In general systems theory, the family is viewed as an open social system with boundaries, self-regulatory mechanisms, interacting and superordinate systems, and subcomponents. The family ecological framework, a framework adopted by family-centered social workers, is viewed as fitting within the systems framework. Bronfenbrenner (1979), a renowned psychologist, has proposed that we study the family as part of its "ecological environment"—or within the family's larger network of social institutions. For Bronfenbrenner, the family is pictured as part of nested structures, with the individual family members nested within the immediate setting that includes the family. This setting is known as the microsystem. The individual and family are situated within and affected by a mesosystem (the immediate larger environment) and an even larger environment—a macrosystem, a social setting that includes a community's ideology, values, and social institutions (McCubbin and Dahl, 1985). Chapter 7 is devoted to an in-depth discussion of the systems framework.

Structural–Functional Theory

Using this framework, the family is also viewed as a social system, but with more of an outcome rather than a process orientation, which is more characteristic of systems theory. The analysis of the family's functional and structural dimensions, as the name implies, receives primary attention. This approach has been selected as one of the text's prime organizing and theoretical framework and, as such, will be discussed in Chapter 5. In addition, Part III (Chaps. 8 to 17)) elaborates on and describes the operation of the structural–functional framework. Within this framework, content germane to family nursing is covered.

Family Developmental Theory

Developmental theories explain how and what changes occur to human organisms or groups over time. Family developmental theory is a reformulation of earlier theories of development of the individual, as described by Freud, Erikson, and Havighurst, plus the incorporation of concepts of role and interpersonal interactions.

The developmental framework provides a unique perspective for assessing and intervening with families (Reed, 1986). It focuses on an analysis of the family as it progresses and changes throughout its life cycle—from inception through old age and dissolution. Chapter 6 describes this approach in detail.

The Institutional–Historical Approach

The 5th framework for analyzing the family is the institutional or historical approach. The institutional framework, later broadened to include a more general historical or cross-cultural approach, was one of the first approaches used in analyzing families in sociology and anthropology (Leslie and Korman, 1989). The institutional approach examines a society at some point in history and analyzes how the family institution performs specialized functions for its members; how it interacts with other societal institutions, including religious, educational, governmental, and economic systems; and how it is affected by and affects social change within society.

Historical analysis of families (theory generation and research) is relatively recent and has considerably increased our understanding of the family's response to changing social and economic conditions, how people react to social change and what change means in their family life. The cumulative impact of historical studies about the family has been to revise the simplistic view of social change and family behavior over time (Hareven, 1987).

Many historical studies of the family have been influenced by the "new social history perspective" of the 1960s, which stimulated an interest in reconstructing the life patterns of ordinary people rather than the elite or celebrated, a commitment to linking individuals and family behavior to larger social structures and processes, and a view of families and their members as active agents confronting historical forces rather than passive victims. Relative to the latter trend, the most important development in family historical research is the focus on family strategies (Hareven, 1987). Here "the emphasis has shifted to the ways in which families take charge of their lives and allocate their resources in the struggle to survive and to secure their own and their children's future (Hareven, 1987, p. 49). This focus is closely linked to a life cycle and life course perspective whereby individuals and families are viewed as changing their individual and family strategies throughout their family life cycle and individual life course.

A central concept within this approach is social change. Family historians focus on change in families over time and see change as more omnipresent in the family than stability (Gordon, 1978). By understanding the long-term changes that have occurred in families, we are better able to understand the contemporary American family.

The concept of modernization is also a major theme or concept in much historical literature. Modernization is actually a process, not an event that simply happened. It began well before the Industrial and French Revolutions, but certainly these "dual revolutions" contributed heavily to the cultural, societal, and family changes that followed. Social change among families does not, however, follow a simple linear trend as postulated in modernization theory. Although cultural lag has occurred, native white middle-class families have more uniformly changed and fit the "modal patterns" that modernization theory describes. Many immigrant families, minority families, rural families, and poor families have, however, displayed a diversity of family life patterns unlike those described about the modern American family. To complicate matters further, many immigrant and minority families retain characteristics of both "the old and the new" simultaneously.

Societal Changes Affecting Families. Recent and ongoing societal changes have influenced family life, and hence should briefly be mentioned before discussing the changes in the family over time. We assume a reciprocal relationship exists between families and society, with society, however, exerting a more sustained impact on families. Economic trends and changes are believed to have exerted the greatest impact on the family, but in addition to this factor, technological advances, demographic trends, sociocultural trends, and political trends are important factors that have influenced the family (Clark, 1984; Toffler, 1990).

The most obvious economic trend today is the rising costs in all areas of family life. This is particularly true in terms of the cost of health care (Nelson and Roark, 1985), particularly burdensome for poor families, older families (who are living on preinflationary dollars), and beginning families. Under the rubric of technological advances is included the knowledge explosion (Toffler, 1970); the increased ability to prolong life (Clark, 1984); environmental pollution (air, water, food, and noise); the use of nuclear energy and automation (Clark, 1984); and birth control advances. Automation has made a great difference in the home. The majority of women are now working and have had to reallocate their time; automation has allowed working wives to spend less time working in the home. Birth control advances are the last major technological advance to be mentioned here. Having better control over reproduction has literally transformed the family, in particular the life cycles of families. Women are no longer having as many children and, equally important, are having their children in a shorter period of time, making the child-rearing period of the family's life shorter. Couples now have more time alone—before the advent of children and after they have been launched (Duvall, 1977).

The two most obvious demographic trends are that our population has increased significantly, and that our country has aged (the proportion of those over 65 continues to grow each year). In addition, our country is more urbanized and more recently, suburbanized. Increased social mobility of families and the growing numbers of culturally diverse peoples are other trends that have had a great impact on families—who they are and where they live.

Changes in Family Functions. Using an institutional approach, the functions that the family carries out for society and its members, how these dovetail with the functions that other institutions provide for the family, and how the family's functions have changed over time are examined in Table 4–2. Certain functions have changed, primarily in response to societal and economic changes. If one examines the American family as it existed before industrialization—when an agrarian life-style and culture predominated—and compares the family during that period with today, profound changes in family functions become apparent.

It is clear that industrialization and urbanization have intruded forcefully on the family, and its institutions have assumed many functions that were once the family's domain. In addition to changes in family func-

TABLE 4–2. CHANGES IN FAMILY FUNCTIONS: PRE- AND POSTINDUSTRIALIZATION PERIODS

Family Function	Family Functions Before Industrialization (Agrarian Setting)	Present-day Family Function (Urban Setting)
1. Economic	Work and family were not separate spheres. Family served as sole economic unit. It was a self-contained, self-sufficient unit: home and business were combined; all family members helped. Family both produced and consumed its products. Family was supported by strong kinship associations (the extended family).	The family's economic function is much more limited. Food and clothes are bought outside of the home. Children are no longer economic assets. Single individuals survive well on their own. Family providers, who in many cases are both spouses, work outside of home, bringing home money to buy outside products and services.
2. Status conferring	Family conferred privilege, honor, and status on people. Family affiliation was crucial in locating and placing someone in society.	Function is still present but much decreased in importance except among upper class families. People are seen primarily as individuals, not as family members.

TABLE 4–2. (*Continued*)

Family Function	Family Functions Before Industrialization (Agrarian Setting)	Present-day Family Function (Urban Setting)
3. Education	Education ("schooling") was done primarily in home. Father taught son vocation. Mother taught daughter homemaking and child-rearing skills.	Education is carried on outside of home to great extent; very formalized and institutionalized, which has a pervasive influence on children, in both school and extracurricular activities (eg, sports, music, school clubs). Economic activities need specialized training. Occupational skills and knowledge are learned outside of home.
4. Socialization of children	Child rearing occurred in the home and was the responsibility of mothers, grandmothers, aunts, and older female children. Parents were fully "in charge" of child rearing.	Socialization function remains as a major function, but is shared with outside institutions (eg, nursery schools, baby sitters, child-care centers, teachers, counselors). Parents' authority and control is diminished, especially after preschool period.
5. Health care function (care of ill/older family members)	Protection, supervision, and care of family members, especially of dependent, disabled, or aged individuals, was entirely family's responsibility. The aged, dependent, and infirm were cared for at home.	This function has decreased greatly, although still present. The family's ethnic background and degree of acculturation to white, middle-class culture influences the family functioning in this area. With older or disabled persons, society takes responsibility when family cannot or will not care for these dependent members. The high proportion of working women and the larger number of elderly in our society has also made home care by family members more difficult.
6. Religious	Religious training and practices were carried out in both the home and in religious institutions.	There is increasing secularization within society and religion has a declining influence on everyday behavior. Family religious involvement also declined. Religion is primarily taught in outside agencies.
7. Recreational	Because family was without commercial recreation, family-centered activities predominated.	Commercialization of recreation is ubiquitous. Family-centered activities are greatly curtailed.
8. Reproduction (procreation)	Marriage and family were necessary for survival.	Having a child creates a family, but marriage or having a family is not necessary. Nevertheless, reproduction remians the one *universal* family function.
9. Affective	Primary group relationships were not as strong; extended family was more important affectively.	This function not only remains, but has increased in importance. The usual American family has weakened extended family ties, whereas emotional relationships between the mates and parent–child are very intense. The result is a great emotional strain in relationships. Historically there existed an economic basis for marriage, which now is usually an affective basis, making divorce more of an acceptable alternative if the affective basis for the marriage fails.

tions, family values and the timing of family transitions have been markedly altered. Demos (1970), in describing the transfer of functions from the family to other social institutions, points out that the preindustrial family served as a workshop, church, reformatory, school, and asylum. Today, the old live apart in old-age homes, in housing projects for senior citizens, or in their own apartment or house separate from the family. Rather than having to depend on the family for assistance, economic support is now provided to the old, unemployed, disabled, and dependent through Social Security or welfare programs. The young are no longer trained at home, but are educated in schools, and by the mass media, peers, and various other associations and groups.

Activities that traditionally took place within the home or involved the entire family now take place elsewhere and engage only certain family members. For instance, economic activity, which traditionally the family engaged in at home as a whole, has until recently been the father's responsibility—one that took him out of the home and away from family life. Today, with the growing number of dual-career/worker families both spouses are engaged in economic activities. One of the most interesting books in this area is by Christopher Lasch, a social historian. His brilliant book, *Haven in a Heartless World* (1977) expounds on the erosion of family in terms of the loss or partial loss of important family functions.

The affective function of the family is a central family function today. And kinship ties, thought at one time to be "weakened" or "practically absent" because of the demands created by industrialization and urbanization, continue to be "alive and well." Given the bureaucratized, impersonal character of public life, people may increasingly look to their families for more emotional solace and support than in earlier times.

Comparative Analyses. The institutional framework also includes comparisons between different cultures (comparative studies) and different settings, especially of urban and rural environments and their effects on the family. Some of the significant forces facing families of rural and urban environments are outlined in Table 4–3. Each of the characteristics listed should be understood as representing one end of a continuum describing the differences between rural and urban life. Obviously, no single community fully conforms in all respects to the somewhat exaggerated characteristics outlined here.

It is assumed that more disruptive forces are part of city living, although this assumption is now being questioned, as more recent literature has pointed out the unique set of stresses and strains that rural families in America face (Bushy, 1990).

TABLE 4–3. COMPARISON OF URBAN AND RURAL COMMUNITY CHARACTERISTICS

Rural Setting	Urban Setting
1. Geographic and social isolation	1. Geographic and social proximity
2. Homogeneity of community residents	2. Heterogeneity of community residents
3. Agricultural employment	3. Industrial employment
4. Sparsely populated	4. Densely populated
5. A subsistence economy	5. A consumer economy
6. Personal relationships	6. Impersonal relationships
7. More traditional/ conservative values and behavior	7. Less traditional/ conservative values and behavior

Limitations of the Institutional–Historical Approach. This approach explains broad patterns of family life occurring over time. Nevertheless, it is not concerned with individual family members or with single family units and their individual differences (Rodgers, 1973). Nor do many of the historical and institutional writings adequately describe the complexity of the contemporary American family. Hence, this approach provides a broad, macroscopic understanding of the family, but does not serve as a useful family nursing practice model.

Family Interactional Theory

The family interactional approach stems from symbolic interaction as applied to the family by Hill and Hansen (1960), Turner (1970), Rose (1962), and others. The writings of Mead (1934), Cooley (1909), Thomas (1923) and Blumer (1962) largely form the original conceptual legacy for the grand sociological theory of symbolic interaction.

In the family interactional approach the general focus is on the ways in which family members relate to one another. Thus the family is viewed as a set of interacting personalities, and internal family dynamics and the relation between the individual and the family group is addressed in detail (Stryker, 1964). Schraneveldt (1973) explains that

> within the family, each member occupies position(s) where a number of roles are assigned. The individual perceives norms or role expectations held individually or collectively by other family members for his attributes and

behaviors. . . . It is this tendency to shape the phenomenal world into roles which is the key to role-taking as a core process in interaction. An individual defines his role expectations in a given situation in terms of a reference group and by his own self-conception. Individual family members role-play. The family and its individual members are studied through the analysis of overt interactions. Each family is not only supported, but limited by family life pattern which has evolved in its interaction in society. Through this limitation or support, each family in interactional process achieves its own tempos or rhythms of family living. A unique, differentiating characteristic of the interactional approach is that it is based on the action of the family resulting from communication processes. It views family behavior as an adjustive process: cues are given, individual members respond to these stimuli.

In other words, the interactional approach strives to interpret family phenomena in terms of internal dynamics. These processes or dynamics consist of role playing, status relations, communication patterns, decision making, coping patterns, and socialization, with the assessment of roles and communication processes forming the core of the framework. Both personality and socialization are also viewed as central concerns of the interactional framework.

Advantages to Using an Interactional Perspective

When assessing the family from an interactional frame of reference, wherein families are seen as a unity of interacting personalities, a shift takes place from viewing the family broadly—as a social institution—to viewing the family more narrowly, as an internal network of family relationships. With this approach, the family nurse centers his or her attention on how family members interact with each other and with the family as a whole. Because of this focus, the approach is especially useful in assessing and explaining family communications, roles, decision making, and problem solving (McCubbin and Dahl, 1985). It is also helpful in isolating and specifying potential sources of difficulty as family members relate to one another.

Disadvantages to Using an Interactional Perspective. The disadvantage of using this approach in working with families is that the interactional perspective does not conceptualize the family within its external environment, and hence does not explain how the external social systems interface and interact with the family. This approach, then, is limited by the fact that the family is viewed as being self-contained and operating within a vacuum (Pasquali et al, 1985). Because the family actively and constantly interacts with its environment, the family–environmental interface must be included in an assessment if comprehensive family nursing care is to be provided.

The same concepts and processes that the interactional framework focuses on are also considered as part of family structure, family function, and family coping in this text. Therefore, this approach was not selected as one of the text's organizing frameworks. Yet the vital content and notions from the interactional approach are contained with the coverage of family role, power, communications, socialization, affective function, and coping processes.

Role and Family Stress Theory

Family stress theory and role theory are two middle-range theories which are largely based on a symbolic interactionism or the interactional framework. Family stress theory was originally developed by Hill in 1949. His model, called the ABCX theory, describes how families experiencing the same stressor event adapt differently to that event. He identified three factors that, interacting together, make a difference as to whether the family goes into crisis or not. The three explanatory factors are (1) the stressor itself, (2) the family's existing resources, and (3) the family's perception of the stressor. Hill's theory was later expanded by McCubbin and Patterson (1983) to cover the postcrisis period. Called the Double ABCX Model, each of Hill's explanatory factors in the model were modified, the notion of coping was inserted as a central predictor, and family adaptation (ranging from maladaptation to bonadaptation) became the outcome described, rather than crisis or noncrisis. This model has been tested among families with chronically ill children.

Role theory is a second more specific symbolic interaction-based theory. As the name implies, family role theory analyzes the interactions and roles (formal and informal) that family members play vis-à-vis each other and during various situations. The impact of illness has been extensively studied, using role theory as the basis for explanation as to how the family is affected (Turk and Kerns, 1985). More extensive discussions of both these theories are found in Chapters 12 and 17, respectively.

Conflict Theory

Conflict or social conflict theory, one of the grand sociological theories, has been used by family professionals to assess and treat families, particularly where interpersonal dynamics, instability, and conflicts are problematic, and where the teaching of conflict-management strategies is needed. The primary thrust of social conflict theory is to describe and explain social change, conflict, and constraint (Murphy, 1983). Or as Sprey (1979) points out, the aim of conflict theory applied to marriage and the family is "to answer how and why stability and instability occur, and under what conditions harmonious interpersonal bonds are possible" (p. 130).

Two basic assumptions of conflict theory are that the family is in a constant state of change (change and conflict are inevitable) and that conflict, as a form of social interaction, has positive and unifying effects (Simmel, 1955). Sprey sees the family as an arena in which conflicting interests and alliances of common purpose contend (Sprey, 1969). Murphy (1983) asserts that "the focus of the conflict framework is not on the differences between and among the various members of the family, but is on the process or processes whereby differences are managed or resolved" (p. 127). Social conflict theory deals with change, competition, conflict, consensus, negotiation and bargaining, power and influence, aggression, and threats (Sprey, 1979). Hence, this theory is useful in working with families where there are power conflicts, decision-making struggles, and family violence.

Social Exchange Theory

Social exchange theory—which evolved out of sociology, classical economics, and behavioristic psychology—is another theory found useful in explaining family interactions (Beutler et al, 1989; Nye, 1979). Social exchange theory (Homans, 1958) asserts that "interaction between persons is an exchange of goods, material and nonmaterial" (p. 597). In applying exchange theory to families, Nye states that the most general (and central) proposition of the theory is "that humans avoid costly behavior and seek rewarding statuses, relationships, interaction and feeling states to the end that their profits are maximized" (p. 2). Many more specific propositions are subsumed under this general statement having to do with rewards, costs, profits, the norm of reciprocity, choice, and exchange. One can readily see the economics legacy in this terminology.

Exchange theory has been minimally used by family nurses. No publications by family nursing authors were found that described the use of social exchange theory to guide practice or research (Mercer, 1989).

The theory has been criticized by family scholars as inaccurately describing much of family behavior. A case in point is that exchange theory assumes that humans are rational, hedonistic, and know the options available to them. But in the family realm, rationality and hedonism are often laced with emotionality and altruism, and it is often the case that family members do not understand the various options available to them. Hence, the basic assumptions of exchange theory do not fit family behavior very well (Beutler et al, 1989). In spite of this criticism, Nye (1979) and others have used social exchange theory successfully to describe many aspects of family behavior—from child-rearing patterns to mother's employment patterns.

Social Learning Theory

Another lesser-referenced middle-range theory from behavioral psychology that has been applied to the family is social learning theory (Jacob and Tennenbaum, 1988). The counterpart to this theory in family therapy is family behavioral theory (under family therapy theories). Bandura (1977) is credited for developing social learning theory by broadening previous learning models through a greater emphasis on the social aspects of learning and the mutual, interactive effects of behavior, person, and environment. Bandura pointed out the important role that cognitive aspects of learning play, as well as how central role modeling is in learning. He contended, "that learning through observing complex behaviors and then modeling such patterns is the source by which the most important learning of the social world takes place" (Jacob and Tennenbaum, 1988, p. 9).

Social learning theory applied to the family is very useful in considering how family members are socialized, how they communicate and function in their family roles, and how they cope as individuals and as a family. Practice implications of this academically oriented theory are spelled out by family therapist authors who ascribe to family behavioral therapy.

FAMILY THERAPY THEORIES

Family therapy theories, in contrast to family social science theories, are practice theories, have been developed to work with troubled families, and therefore are pathology-oriented for the most part (Table 4–4). Family therapy theorists in the last 30 years have generated extensive theoretical writings on the family. Because these theorists are concerned with what can be done to facilitate change in "dysfunctional" families (Whall, 1983), their theories are both descriptive of functional and dysfunctional families and prescriptive (suggesting treatment strategies). Most family therapy theories to varying degrees have been derived from or deeply influenced by general systems theory (to be discussed in Chapter 6). Thus certain basic similarities between the theoretical perspectives are apparent. Nevertheless, multiple theoretical perspectives are

TABLE 4–4. DIFFERENCES BETWEEN NURSING THEORIES, FAMILY SOCIAL SCIENCE THEORIES, AND FAMILY THERAPY THEORIES

Criteria	Nursing Theories	Family Social Science Theories	Family Therapy Theories
Purpose of theory	Descriptive and prescriptive (practice models); guide nursing assessment and intervention efforts.	Descriptive and explanatory (academic models); explain family functioning and dynamics.	Descriptive and prescriptive (practice models); explain family dysfunction and guide therapeutic actions.
Discipline focus	Nursing focus.	Interdisciplinary (although primarily sociological).	Marriage and family therapy, and family mental health.
Target populations	Primarily those families with health and illness problems.	Primarily "normal" families (normality-oriented).	Primarily "troubled" families (pathology-oriented).

Adapted from Jones and Dimond (1982).

evident in the literature. Goldenberg and Goldenberg (1985) classify these approaches to family theory and clinical practice into those that (1) are psychodynamic in orientation, (2) are experiential or humanistic in emphasis, (3) are behavior in approach, and (4) conceptualize the family as a system, including the Bowenian, structural, and communication models.

Family crisis interventions or crisis theory is another theoretical perspective that is a type of family therapy model. It is a short-term, more focused practice model, in comparison to the other family therapy models. This theoretical approach has been found to be very useful in family nursing for working with families in crisis or under acute stress. Family crisis intervention, as an expansion of Gerald Caplan's crisis model, is elaborated on in Chapter 17.

The theorists who view the family as a system (Satir and other interactionists, Bowen, and Minuchin) because their observations and theories are so pertinent to family nursing, are mentioned at various points within this text.

As previously mentioned, Whall (1986b) and others have advocated the reformulation or adaptation of family therapy models so that they are congruent with nursing's perspective (its philosophy and practice perspectives). Several authors have shown how this reformulation is done. Jones (1986), for example, reformulated family interactional theory to be appropriate for nursing practice. In doing so she used the nursing process, formulated nursing diagnoses, and specified health promotion as the family nursing goal. McFarland (1988) has also effectively reformulated Bowen's family systems theory. Nursing concepts of health, environment, family, and nursing are defined within the context of Bowen's family systems theoretical perspective.

SUMMARY

In summary, a discussion of nursing theories that appear to have a good fit with family nursing were presented, as well as a brief explanation of the family therapy theoretical perspectives. Five conceptual frameworks used to explain family dynamics were also discussed. Two frameworks, the interactional and the historic frameworks, were briefly described in this chapter. Chapters 5 to 7 will elaborate on the remaining three frameworks. The systems, structural–functional, and developmental frameworks are particularly important in that they provide the broader perspective for the text's assessment and intervention guidelines.

☐ STUDY QUESTIONS

1. Match approaches used in studying family on the left with best descriptions in column on the right.

APPROACHES	DESCRIPTIONS
a. Systems approach b. Interactional approach c. Developmental approach d. Institutional approach e. Structural–functional approach	1. Studies family related to present situation—that is, behavior vis-à-vis "triggering" event. 2. Studies family progressing through life cycle. 3. Family viewed as an open social system and has a process orientation. 4. Deals with internal family dynamics. 5. Studies family functions in society as they change over time. 6. Describes family as having predictable natural history common to families and associated with changing ages and member composition. 7. Family viewed as social system with emphasis on purposes family achieves, its internal organization, and its relationship to the wider society.

Fill in the correct answer to the following question.

2. The interactional approach analyzes the family in respect to ___________.

3. Give three important areas the interactionist would assess using the above framework.

4. Match each family function from the left column with the appropriate description of it on the right column showing how the function has changed (as society changed from an agrarian to industrialized state);

FUNCTION	DESCRIPTION
a. Affective b. Socializing c. Economic d. Religious e. Care of disabled family members f. Educational g. Status conferring h. Reproduction	1. Continues to be crucial. 2. Decreased in importance or limited. 3. Increased in importance. 4. Function important; function shared with other institutions in society.

5. What advantages do the following genres of theoretical frameworks have?
   a. Nursing theories
   b. Family therapy theories
   c. Social science theories
   d. Theoretical frameworks in general

6. The family ecological theory can be most logically subsumed under:
   a. Roy's adaptation theory.
   b. Structural–functional theory.
   c. Family systems theory (in family therapy).
   d. General systems theory.
   e. Historical–institutional theory.

7. Match the five nursing models with their respective orientations or level of analysis.

NURSING MODEL	ORIENTATION
a. Roy's model	1. Individually oriented
b. Roger's model	
c. Neuman's model	2. Family oriented
d. Orem's model	
e. King's model	3. Individually and family oriented

C H A P T E R   F I V E

Structural–Functional Theory

Learning Objectives

1. Identify the three primary theoretical perspectives used in this text for completing a family assessment.
2. Define the components and basic characteristics of the structural–functional approach as applied to the family.
3. Explain the usefulness of the structural–functional approach to family nursing.
4. Analyze the relationship of family structure to family functions and the system's theory approach to the structural–functional approach.
5. List and briefly describe the five basic family functions.

A central assumption of this text is that clinical practice should be guided by theory. I also believe that the decision regarding what theory or theories to use in one's practice—that is, in assessing, planning, intervening, and evaluating—should be based on practical grounds. In other words, what theory(ies) best/most powerfully explains a situation and suggests meaningful and effective nursing goals and actions. I agree with Blau (1977), a noted sociologist and theoretician, who advises us, "a choice between [theoretical] perspectives can only be made on pragmatic grounds: which theory is more useful for clarifying given problems" (p. 3).

Looking at the potpourri of theories presented in Chapter 4 (nursing theories, family therapy theories, and family social science theories), several family social science theories appear at this time, because of the state of theory development among the nursing theories, to be the best, most powerful theoretical perspectives to use in family nursing. These, I believe, are structural–functional theory, developmental theory, and general systems theory. Applying three general theoretical models in addition to some less general theories encourages family nursing practice to be more holistic and comprehensive.

The structural–functional perspective applied to the family is comprehensive and recognizes the important interaction between the family and its internal and external environment. The developmental approach is needed to provide the information of family development and life cycle tasks, to examine changes in a family's life over time, and to assess how a family is handling its developmental tasks. A general systems approach applied to the family is also needed to look at adaptational and communications processes within the family. The structural–functional analysis tends to present a static view of the family, while both developmental and general systems theory handle change over time better. In addition, a structural–functional perspective minimizes the importance of growth, change and disequilibrium in a family, while a general systems theory explains these processes more fully and convincingly.

THE STRUCTURAL–FUNCTIONAL APPROACH

The structural–functional framework is a major theoretical frame of reference in sociology (Leslie and Korman, 1989), particularly in the areas of family and medical sociology. Applied to the family, the scope of the framework is very broad. The family is viewed as an open social system. Relationships between the family and other social systems (eg, the health care system, educational system) are examined. A description of the family's structural (organizational dimensions) and family functions are at the core of this approach.

According to Eshleman, the structural–functional approach has its origin in the functionalist branch of psychology (particularly Gestalt psychology), in social anthropology (as exhibited in the writings of Malinowski and Radcliffe-Brown), and in sociology (particularly as described by social systems theorists such as Parsons). The Gestalt position emphasizes that one must view the whole and its parts, exploring the interrelationship between the whole and its parts. Along the same line of thinking, social anthropologists have concluded that one cannot understand a particular aspect of social life detached from its general environment (Eshleman, 1974). Hence, structural–functionalists see the family, one of the social institutions of a society, as being "functional" for or congruent with the society. In the 1950s, theorists (Parsons and Bales, 1955; Parsons, 1951) envisioned a good fit between society and the family, a basic institution functioning to meet society's needs. Today, with such a changing heterogeneous society, this harmonious, stable picture of the relationship between society and the family has changed.

Most of the sociological literature applying the structural–functional approach to the family makes use of a more macroscopic approach, looking at the family as a subsystem of the wider society. The general assumptions made include the following (Leslie and Korman, 1989; Parsons and Bales, 1955):

1. A family is a social system with functional requirements.
2. A family is a small group possessing certain generic features common to all small groups.
3. The family as a social system accomplishes functions that serve the individual in addition to the society.
4. Individuals act in accordance with a set of internalized norms and values that are learned primarily in the family through socialization.

The structural–functional perspective is a very useful framework for assessing family life because it enables the family system to be examined holistically (as a unit), in parts (as subsystems or dimensions), and interactionally (as a system interacting with other institutions, such as the educational and health systems, the family's reference group(s), and the wider society). Mancini and Orthner (1988), family educators, remind family professionals that both a micro and macroscopic perspective is needed when working with families. They explain that "to understand families is to know about those internal dynamics, but also to know something about the common habitat, whether it be the values of society, current economic conditions, or governmental support for families" (p. 363). Structural–functional theory provides these two perspectives.

Structural–functional theory, then, has been selected, along with general systems theory and developmental theory, as the organizing framework for the text, because its use provides a comprehensive and holistic perspective for assessment purposes. The essence of family-centered nursing involves understanding the dynamics of the family and all the forces, both internal and external, that affect it. For this understanding, structural–functional theory serves as a suitable umbrella under which more specific theories can be placed and areas assessed.

CONCEPT OF STRUCTURE

The structural–functional approach primarily analyzes the family's structural characteristics—the arrangement of the parts that form the whole, and the functions it performs for both society and its subsystems. The structure of the family refers to how the family is organized, the manner in which units are arranged, and how these units relate to each other. The dimensions, or definitions, of this concept of family structure vary considerably. Some theorists base structure on the type of family form (eg, nuclear versus extended); type of power structure (eg, matriarchal versus patriarchal); or marital patterns (eg, exogamy versus endogamy) (Eshleman, 1974). Another way of looking at the family structure is by describing the subsystems as the structural dimension (Minuchin, 1974). Assuming that the family is a special kind of small group, the structural dimensions identified by small-group theory as being relevant for assessing such groups are used in this text. Parad and Caplan, in analyzing a family under stress, have used very similar structural dimensions, which they call the family life-style. Family life-style refers to "the reasonably stable patterning of family organization, subdivided into three interdependent elements of value system, communication network and role systems" (Parad and Caplan, 1965, p. 55). In this text a fourth element of structural dimension has been added to Parad and Caplan's structural elements—the power structure. To repeat, then, the four basic structural dimensions that are subsumed under structure, and that will be elaborated on in separate chapters, are (1) role structure, (2) value systems, (3) communication processes, and (4) power structure.

These elements are all intimately interrelated and interacting. When one aspect of the internal structure of the family is affected by input from the external environment, the processing of this input within the family system will also affect the other structural dimensions. The family's high degree of interrelatedness and interdependency is seen when a family health care professional observes how certain family behaviors often become indicators of several or all of the major organizing elements within the family. For instance, a husband, in an authoritarian way, is observed ordering his wife and children on when and what will be served for dinner. The mother is then seen directing the children to each prepare certain assigned parts of the meal. Mother and children carry out father's wishes with no comments or sign of feelings. No other communications are noted. We can see from this one vignette (and this would have to be verified by further observation of the family) that the power figure in this situation is the father; his role is one of a stern, commanding leader of the family, who probably needs and has much control over his family (because even details are controlled). The communication patterns here are one-way (father to mother and children, mother to children) and completely task centered. No feelings or sharing of thoughts are observed. Again speculating on this situation, the events are more likely congruent with the family's value system. One of the values central to this family probably would be male dominance, while another related value might be respect for and obedience to elders.

Family structure, or organization, is ultimately evaluated by how well the family is able to fulfill its family functions—the goals important to its members and society. The family's structure serves to facilitate the achievement of family functions, because the conservation and allocation of resources is a prime task for the family structure. Because of this important relationship, functions should be viewed in tandem with family structures.

CONCEPT OF FUNCTION

Family functions are commonly defined as outcomes or consequences of the family structure. Although some authors use "function" to mean "consequences of or results of," it is a little easier to think of family functions as being what the family does. Why does it exist? What purposes does it serve? As described in detail in Chapter 1, the family's basic functions meet the needs of both individual family members and wider society. Five family functions are most germane when assessing and intervening with families.

1. Affective function (personality maintenance function): for stabilization of adult personalities, meeting the psychological needs of family members.
2. Socialization and social placement function: for the primary socialization of children aimed at making them productive members of their society, as well as the conferring of status on family members.
3. Reproductive function: for maintenance of family continuity over the generations as well as for societal survival.
4. Economic function: for the provision of sufficient economic resources and their effective allocation.
5. Health care function: for the provision of physical necessities—food, clothing, shelter, health care (Fig. 5–1).*

Affective Function

The affective function is a central basis for both the formation and the continuation of the individual family unit, and it thus constitutes one of the most vital functions of families.† Today, when many societal tasks are performed outside the family unit, much of the family's effort is focused on meeting the needs of family members for affection and understanding. The ability to

* *These functions represent an adaptation or modification of several theorists' descriptions of family functions, including those of Murdock (1949), Ogburn (1933), Parsons and Bales (1955), and Hill (1965).*

† *See Chapter 14 for a detailed discussion of the affective function.*

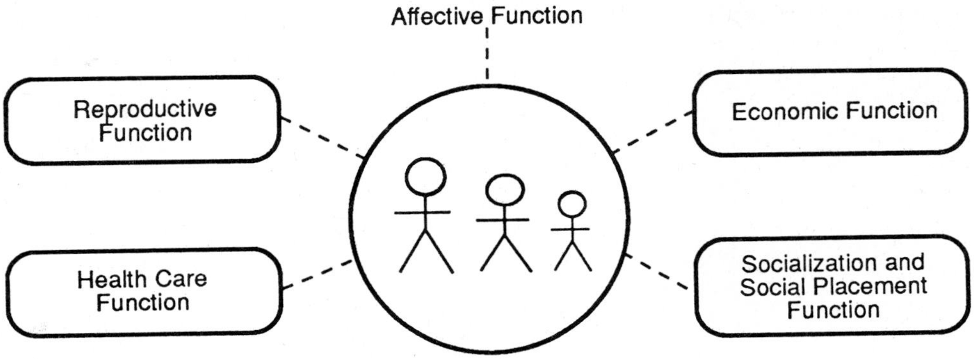

Figure 5–1
The five basic family functions.

provide for these needs is a key determinant of whether a given family will persist or dissolve. As Duvall (1977) says, "Family, happiness is gauged by the strength of family love." The family must meet the affectional needs of its members because the affectional responses of one family member to another provide the basic rewards of family life.

Primarily a parental role, this function deals with the family's perception and care of the socioemotional needs of all its members; it involves tension reduction and morale maintenance. The elevation of this function to a high level of importance within the family is a relatively new notion and found most strongly among middle class and affluent families, where choice is more feasible. In the middle and upper classes, personal happiness in the marital relationship based on companionship and love is critical. The importance of this function has a decreased emphasis in many working-class and lower-class families, largely because more basic functions such as providing the physical necessities of life predominate.

Socialization and Social Placement Function

Socialization of family members is an universal, crosscultural functional requisite for societal survival (Leslie and Korman, 1989). It refers to the myriad of learning experiences provided within the family aimed at teaching children how to function and assume adult social roles such as those of husband–father and wife–mother. The family has the primary responsibility of transforming an infant in a score of years into a social person capable of full participation in society. Furthermore, socialization should not be thought of as pertaining only to infant and child-rearing patterns, but rather as a lifelong process that includes internalizing the appropriate sets of norms and values for being a teenager, a bride, a parent, an employee on a new job, a grandparent, and a retired person (Eshleman, 1974). In short, socialization involves learning the culture.

Because this function is increasingly shared with schools, recreational, and child-care facilities, and other extrafamilial institutions, the family plays a reduced, yet critical, role in socialization. Parents still transmit their cultural heritage to their children.

An integral part of socialization in the family involves the inculcation of controls and values—giving the growing child (and adult) a sense of what is right and wrong. Kohlberg (1970) describes the process of moral development as having its foundations in the family. Moral development is seen as a process similar to the stages of emotional and cognitive development à la Erikson and Piaget, respectively. By identifying with parental figures and being consistently reinforced negatively and positively for their behavior, children develop a personal value system that is greatly influenced by the family's value system.

Social placement or status conferring is the other aspect of the socialization function. Conferring of status on children refers to passing on of the traditions, values, and privileges of the family, although today tradition no longer dictates life patterns of most adult Americans. At birth, a child automatically inherits his or her family's status—ethnic, racial, national, religious, economic, political, and educational. The family socializes the child into its social class, instilling in him or her all the relevant aspirations. Additionally, the family has the responsibility of providing necessary socialization and educational experiences that enable an individual to assume a vocation and roles in groups that are consistent with status expectations.

Educating parents about child-rearing patterns and ways they may cope with family problems are major components of family health care, beginning with genetic and reproductive counseling, continuing through prenatal and child care, and extending throughout the life cycle of the family. The common health concerns and family problems with which the family nurse can assist families are described within the various stages of the family's life cycle in Chapter 6. Chapter 15 describes the family socialization function more extensively.

Health Care Function: Providing Physical Necessities and Health Care

The physical functions of the family are met by the parents providing food, clothing, shelter, and protection against danger. Health care and health practices (which influence the individual family members' health status) are the most relevant part of this family function for the family nurse. Chapter 16 is devoted entirely to an exploration of this significant aspect.

Reproductive Function

One of the basic functions of the family is to insure continuity of the intergenerational family and of society—that is, provide recruits for society (Leslie and Korman, 1989). In the past, marriage and the family were designed to regulate and control sexual behavior as well as reproduction. Both these aspects, control of sexual behavior and birth control, are now less important functions of the family; it is not required in this society to limit sexual activity to those who are married or to have children within the confines of the traditional family. Once a child is born, a new family is born—with single-parent families becoming increasingly common. The number of births to unmarried mothers, for example, has continued to rise in the United States as greater acceptability and loosening of sexual mores has occurred (see Chap. 1 for demographic changes in the family).

Along with having children outside of the confines of the traditional family, greater use of birth control measures is another important trend, either within or outside the family context. Moreover, the move toward population control and family planning is affecting the importance of parenthood for both women and men. A shift of cultural priorities and personal values continues to deflate motherhood as a woman's central purpose in life and fatherhood as a man's chief reason to work. Increasingly, public expressions are heard against the bearing of more than two children per couple (as the couple's replacement quota), particularly in developing countries.

Economic Function

The economic function involves the family's provision of sufficient resources—financial, space, and material—and their appropriate allocation by decision-making processes.

An assessment of the family's economic resources provides the nurse with data relevant to the family's ability to allocate resources appropriately to meet family needs such as adequate clothing, food, shelter, and health care. By gaining an understanding of how a family distributes its resources, the family-centered nurse can also obtain a clearer perspective about the family's value system (what is important to the family) and what resources can be accessed to help it meet its needs.

Because this function is difficult for most poor families to fulfill satisfactorily, family nurses must accept the responsibility of assisting families to obtain appropriate community resources where they can secure needed information, employment, vocational counseling, and financial assistance.

☐ STUDY QUESTIONS

1. The text's family assessment tool is based upon three theoretical perspectives. These are:
   a. Orem's, Roy's, and Roger's nursing theories.
   b. Interactional, structural–functional, and institutional theories.
   c. Structural—functional, developmental, and general systems theories.
   d. Family coping, affective, and economic theories.
   e. Role, communications, and power theories.

2. The interactionist approach analyzes internal family dynamics. The structural–functional approach, which is broader in focus, analyzes what?

3. The following are reasons for using a structural–functional approach for assessing and working with families. Select the most accurate and inclusive reason:
   a. Because it is a microscopic approach, it centers on inner dynamics and provides information for transactional-based diagnoses.
   b. It consists of a comprehensive, holistic perspective by which not only the family can be assessed, but also the family's universe (its inner and outer environments).
   c. It provides the family health worker with an understanding of the forces from within and without that impinge on the family.
   d. Using this framework the common health problems are recognized as the family progresses through the life cycle.

4. The relationship of the family structure to family function is that (select one answer):
   a. The structure provides the organization for family functions to be accomplished.
   b. The functions mandate the family structure.
   c. Structure and function are separate entities and have no direct relationship to each other.

5. The structural–functional approach differs from the systems approach in what way? (Select the best, most inclusive answer.)
   a. They are two separate frameworks.
   b. The structural–functional approach is in opposition to the systems approach.
   c. The systems theory approach handles change over time better.
   d. The structural–functional approach emanated from theories in psychology (Gestalt), social anthropology (Malinowski), and social systems theory (Parsons).

6. Indicate whether the four descriptions in the left-hand column are structural dimensions or family functions.

a. Roles of two adult family members	1. Structure
b. Reproduction	2. Function
c. Communication patterns	
d. The provision of adequate economic support	

Family Case Study

7. *Using the following case study for data, list and then describe how this family is fulfilling each of the five basic family functions.*

Family Composition:

NAME	RELATIONSHIP	AGE
Emma	Wife	40
Arthur	Husband	44
Danny	Son	17
Ronny	Son	14
Leonard	Son	11
Sammy	Son	7
Cindy	Daughter	5
Arlie	Son	4
Iris	Daughter	2

All the children appeared in good health and were dressed adequately. Arthur and Emma were rather short and obese.

The house was located in a suburban area, in a neighborhood full of children and pets. The house has three bedrooms, one-and-a-half bathrooms, attached garage, with small front and backyards. The interior is reasonably clean and orderly with bare floors and sparse furniture. The TV is in the living room where there are no pictures, books, or decorations.

This is a Mexican-American family. All the members are bilingual. Arthur completed the 10th grade and served in the Army. He has since worked as a maintenance man on refrigeration units of food trucks. He has medical insurance through his company.

Emma has been a housewife since her marriage at 19. She has devoted most of her energies to the family and their care. She spends time cooking and provides hearty, nutritious meals, although overabundant in carbohydrates.

The children are in school with the exception of Iris. They do passable work. The older two boys are involved in athletics, which is a source of pride for the parents.

This is the only marriage for Arthur and Emma, who have been married for 21 years. There has been significant marital discord during the past 11 years.

From Emma's description of home life, she "wears the pants in the family." She describes her husband as a meek, passive man who takes no responsibility in the household. He brings home the check, eats and sleeps there. She states she finds him "sexually unattractive," and difficult to be "close" to. Emma says she wants to be with her children but that she has no love for her husband.

Arthur says he works and makes a living. "The house is a woman's responsibility," which he has left to his wife.

Emma does all of the disciplining and is the parent children go to for permissions. Emma states that when Arthur tells the children to do something and they disobey, their excuse is they didn't think that he really meant it. The children verified that Emma does the greater part of the disciplining and that when she is home, they really watch their behavior.

Emma prefers her children to her husband. They are the apparent reason the marriage holds together. She seems very fond of all her children, but she mentions Leonard and Iris the most. She seems to favor Leonard because other children tease him for being fat. She tries to give him special attention. She talks about Iris as being her baby.

Arthur appears to love all the children, but makes extra comments about the oldest sons. Arthur says his wife is a wonderful mother and good housekeeper but makes no comments about their personal relationship.

Danny and Ronny seem to pair off because of their ages. Leonard and Iris prefer mother's company, while Sammy cares for and plays with Arlie. Cindy, age 5, appears withdrawn and a loner.

CHAPTER SIX

Family Developmental Theory

Marilyn M. Friedman and Kim Miller

Learning Objectives

1. With respect to family developmental theory, discuss four basic assumptions.
2. Discuss the usefulness of the family developmental approach in assessing and working with families.
3. Define the meaning of family developmental tasks and the family life cycle.
4. Identify and describe each of the developmental stages within the life cycles of the two-parent nuclear family.
5. Identify three health promotion needs or health concerns that families commonly experience within each of the two-parent nuclear family's stages of development.
6. Describe developmental tasks of parents and how they relate to the nuclear family's stages of development.
7. Discuss adolescence and its impact on family.
8. Relative to the single-parent and/or divorced family, describe the family life cycle stages.
9. Relative to the step-parent family, describe the family life cycles stages.
10. Identify the primary assessment areas relative to family development and history, as well as two general family nursing interventions appropriate for assisting families developmentally.

One of the more recent frameworks generated for studying and working with families is that of family development. This theoretical approach attempts to account for change over time in the family system, including changes in interactions and relationships among family members over time. The family developmental approach is based on the observation that families are long-lived groups with a natural history, or life cycle, that must be assessed if the dynamics of the group are to be fully and accurately interpreted (Duvall and Miller, 1985). Although each family goes through each stage of development in its own unique way, all families are considered as examples of an overall normative pattern (Rodgers, 1973) and to follow a universal sequence of development (Goode, 1959).

Family development theory then describes family life over time as divided into a series of discrete stages. Stages are thought of as periods of relative stability that are qualitatively and quantitatively distinct from adjacent stages (Mederer and Hill, 1983).

The notion of life cycle stages rests on the assumption that in families there is high family member interdependence: families are forced to change each time members are added to or subtracted from the family, or each time the oldest child changes his or her developmental stage. For instance, changes in roles, marital adjustment, child rearing, and discipline have been found to change from stage to stage (Mederer and Hill, 1983). The family takes one kind of structure when children are infants of preschool age; another structure when the parents enter into the prime of life and the children reach adolescence; and finally another when the children mature, marry, and go their own ways. Rodgers (1973) describes these changes further:

> The structure of the group changes during its history. . . . As members interact with one another over a variety of matters happening in the group, a whole set of learned and shared experiences develop which become precedents for further interactions. Although many of these experiences are unique, a great many are related to the normal and inevitable issues that arise in living together. Recently married couples must work out a set of relationships which are mutually satisfactory concerning many matters. Once established, however, the relationships do not remain constant, but change subtly or perhaps dramatically because of later events, which may occur in the family or outside of it. . . . Many happenings are anticipated and prepared for, whereas many are unexpected—though not peculiar to that family alone. Thus, though each family's history is unique, it is also common. Furthermore, it has a certain quality of inevitability though not necessarily of predictability as to exact time or circumstance. The developmental approach does not seek to explain family dynamics in terms of its unique elements, but in terms of the common quality of its experience over its history. There exist many more events that are common than are unique. (p. 13)

The historical roots of family developmental theory can be traced to five theoretical legacies. Family developmental framework is eclectic, because it acquired concepts from different approaches to the study of the family. Contributions to family development theory were drawn from symbolic interactionism, structural functionalism, the sociology of work and professions, systems theory, and more recently from family life stress and crisis theory (Mattessich and Hill, 1987).

Four basic assumptions of family developmental theory, as outlined by Aldous (1978), are:

1. Families develop and change over time in similar, predictable ways.
2. As people mature and interact with others, they initiate actions as well as reactions to environmental demands.
3. Families and their members perform certain time-specific tasks that are set by themselves and by the cultural and societal context.
4. There is a tendency for families to have a discernible beginning and end.

Although family developmental theory is based on the common, general features of family life, it does not address situational or nonnormative stressors (unusual events), and can be criticized for its assumption of homogeneity (its lack of adequate attention to family diversity), its middle-class bias, its assumption of stability within each stage, and its lack of explaining the processes that occur between stages that allow families to change. Yet the use of this framework for assessment and intervention is exceedingly helpful, because it provides family care health professionals with ways of anticipating what to expect and hence what kinds of teaching and counseling services may be needed. Family developmental theory increases our understanding of families at different points in their life cycle and generates "typical" or "modal" descriptions of family life during the various stages (Duvall and Miller, 1985). Moreover, by assessing the family's developmental stage and its performance of the tasks appropriate to that stage, family health care professionals are provided with guidelines for analyzing family growth and health-promotion needs. The family nurse is better able to provide the support needed for smooth progression from one stage to another.

THE FAMILY LIFE CYCLE

There are predictable stages within the life cycle of every family. Just as individuals go through successive stages of growth and development, so do families as a unit go through successive stages of development. The most widely used formulation of the developmental stages of family life for the two-parent nuclear family is the eight-stage family life cycle of Duvall (1977); see Table 6–1. In addition, Carter and McGoldrick (1988) have more recently generated a similar six-stage model for family therapists. Table 6–2 compares Duvall's stages with the Carter and McGoldrick family life cycle stages.

In Duvall's paradigm, she uses the age and school placement of the oldest child as a guidepost for the life cycle intervals, with the exception of the two last stages of family life, when children are no longer present in the family. When there are several children in the family, some overlapping of different stages occur. Carter and McGoldrick (1988), in contrast, formulated family life cycle stages that focus on the major points at which family members enter or exit the family, thus upsetting the family's equilibrium. Emphasis here is placed on the altered relationships that are requisite so that the family can move from one life cycle stage to the next.

TABLE 6–1. THE EIGHT-STAGE FAMILY LIFE CYCLE

Stage I	Beginning families (also referred to as married couples or the stage of marriage)
Stage II	Childbearing families (the oldest child is an infant through 30 months)
Stage III	Families with preschool children (oldest child is 2½ to 6 years of age)
Stage IV	Families with school children (oldest child is 6 to 13 years of age)
Stage V	Families with teenagers (oldest child is 13 to 20 years of age)
Stage VI	Families launching young adults (covering the first child who has left through the last child leaving home)
Stage VII	Middle-aged parents (empty nest through retirement)
Stage VIII	Family in retirement and old age (also referred to as aging family members or retirement to death of both spouses)

Adapted from Duvall (1977), Duvall and Miller (1985).

Family Life Cycle Variations

Families vary, as do the family life cycle stages. Stages of the family life cycle follow no rigid pattern (Duvall, 1977). It then goes without saying that many families today do not fit into the traditional two-parent nuclear family life cycle stages of Duvall or Carter and McGoldrick. Variations in the traditional family life cycle are seen among families where couples do not marry, couples remain childless, and where there are homosexual unions and single-parent and step-parent families. More people are choosing various family forms and hence the original concept of the family life cycle, covering the two-parent nuclear family, is obviously limited in applicability. For nontraditional families or families that are poor or from minorities, variations in the timing and sequencing of family events exists (Teachman et al, 1987). Because of the preponderance of single-parent and step-parent families today, the life cycle stages of these two common forms of families are described later in the chapter.

Even within the traditional two-parent nuclear family there have been changes in the timing of life cycle stages. Increasingly young adults are living with parents, alone, or with other young adults (the "between family life cycle stage" of Carter and McGoldrick). Couples are postponing marriage, shortening the childrearing period (the result largely of birth control and work), and having fewer children. With these changes and people living longer, there is a corresponding greater number of years within the last two stages of the family life cycle—the middle years and retirement and old age stages.

TABLE 6–2. COMPARISON OF FAMILY LIFE CYCLE STAGES OF DUVALL, MILLER AND CARTER AND McGOLDRICK

Carter and McGoldrick (Family Therapy Perspective)	Duvall and Miller (Sociological Perspective)
1. Between families: the unattached young adult	No stage identified here, although Duvall considers young adult to be in process of "being launched." Because there is often a considerable time period between adolescence and marriage, addition of this "between stage" is indicated.
2. The joining of families through marriage: the newly married couple	1. Beginning families or the stage of marriage.
3. Families with young children (infancy through school age)	2. Childbearing families (oldest child up to 30 months of age).
	3. Families with preschool children (oldest child, 2½ to 5 years of age).
	4. Families with school-aged children (oldest child, 6 to 12 years of age).
4. Families with adolescents	5. Families with teenagers (oldest child, 13 to 20 years of age).
5. Launching children and moving on	6. Families launching young adults (all children leaving home).
	7. Middle-aged parents (empty nest, up to retirement).
6. Families in later life	8. Families in retirement and old age (retirement to death of both spouses).

Adapted from Carter and McGoldrick (1988), Duvall and Miller (1985).

Family Developmental Tasks

Just as individuals have developmental tasks* that they must achieve in order to feel satisfied during a stage of development and to be able to proceed successfully to the following stage, each stage of family development has its specific developmental tasks. Family develop-

* *Examples are the developmental tasks that are inherent within the following frames of reference: (1) Erikson's stages of psychosocial development, (2) Piaget's stages of cognitive development, (3) Kohlberg's stages of moral development, and (4) Freud's stages of psychosexual development.*

mental tasks refer to growth responsibilities that must be achieved by a family during each stage of its development so as to meet (1) its biological requirements, (2) its cultural imperatives, and (3) its own aspirations and values (Duvall, 1977).

How do the developmental tasks of the family differ from those of the individual family member? Although in reality many of them dovetail, family developmental tasks are generated when the family strives as a unit to meet the demands and needs of family members who in turn are striving to meet their individual developmental requisites. Family tasks are also created by community pressures for the family and its members to conform to the expectations of the family's reference group and the wider society.

In addition, family developmental tasks also include the tasks specific to each stage inherent in accomplishing the five basic functions of the family, consisting of (1) affective function (personality maintenance function); (2) socialization and social placement function; (3) health care function—provision and allocation of physical necessities and health care; (4) reproductive function; and (5) economic function (see Chap. 5 for a complete discussion of these functions).

The real challenge for families is to meet each of the members' needs, as well as to meet the general family functions. The meshing of individual developmental needs and family tasks is not always possible. For instance, the toddler's tasks involving the exploration of the environment are often in opposition to the mother's tasks of maintaining an orderly home.

TWO-PARENT NUCLEAR FAMILY LIFE CYCLE STAGES

The following family life cycle stages have been described by Duvall and Miller (1985) and Carter and McGoldrick (1988). They include nine stages of the family life cycle (Table 6–2). The "between stage" from the Carter and McGoldrick typology is added to Duvall and Miller's eight-stage model to give a more comprehensive depiction of changes in family life. These family life cycle stages portray the intact nuclear American family, but are limited in their applicability to single, divorced, and step-parent families. Common health concerns and health-promotion needs are also discussed within each of the respective family life cycle stages.

Transitional Stage: Between Families (the Unattached Young Adult)

This stage refers to the period of time when individuals are in their 20s, are financially independent, and have physically left their family of origin but have not begun their own family of marriage. The between-family stage is not considered a family life cycle stage by Duvall and other sociologists. Yet, because this period is such a commonly experienced one (adolescents do not go directly from their family of origin to a family of marriage, as was more frequently seen in the past), and because this period is such a pivotal transition, the stage was added in this text. This stage has also been largely ignored by family health care professionals and family therapists (Aylmer, 1988).

Demographic data support the importance of this stage. Today in the United States more young adults delay marriage while they live in bachelor quarters or cohabitate outside of marriage. First marriage in the United States occurs generally 3 years later than a generation ago. Five times as many young adults cohabitate outside of marriage today than in 1960 (Glick, 1989).

The between-family stage is considered by Aylmer (1988) and other family therapists to be the cornerstone for all the successive stages to follow; how the young adult goes through this stage profoundly affects who he or she marries as well as when and how marriage occurs. To complete this stage successfully the young adult must separate from the family of origin without cutting off or attaching reactively to an emotional surrogate.

Developmental Tasks. This stage is "between families," the development tasks are individual in nature rather than family-oriented. Carter and McGoldrick (1980) explain that the primary developmental task of the unattached young adult is "coming to terms with his or her family of origin" (p. 13). Three developmental tasks are listed by Carter and McGoldrick (1988, p. 15):

1. Differentiation of self in relation to family of origin.
2. Development of intimate peer relationships.
3. Establishment of self relative to work and financial independence.

It is a time for the young adult to form personal life goals and one's own sense of self before joining with another in marriage (Table 6–3). This is generally a difficult transitional stage, inasmuch as individuating from one's family of origin physically, financially, and emotionally is generally delayed in many families today.

This stage is typically experienced differently depending on one's gender. Carol Gilligan's seminal work, *In a Different Voice* (1982), describes the contrasting orientation of males and females through their socialization. Men generally are taught to pursue iden-

TABLE 6–3. THE TRANSITION STAGE: BETWEEN FAMILIES AND CONCOMITANT FAMILY DEVELOPMENTAL TASKS

Family Life Cycle Stage	Family Developmental Tasks
Transition stage: between families	1. Separating from family of origin. 2. Developing intimate peer relationships. 3. Establishing work and financial independence.

Adapted from Carter and McGoldrick (1988), Duvall and Miller (1985).

tity in self-expression; women, in self-sacrifice. As young men and women go through the unattached young adult period they have different identity issues to resolve. A balance of both autonomy and attachment is needed in relationships and work, but men generally struggle with issues of attachment and relationships, while women struggle with issues of autonomy.

Most of the above issues involve relationships between the young adult and his or her parents (Aylmer, 1988) and creating a new balance between separatedness and connectedness. How the parents of the young adult interact with their young adult child during this period is therefore vitally important. From a family systems perspective, there are reciprocal or circular effects taking place between the parents and young adults (each mutually influence each other's actions), which enhance or inhibit the process of separation and individuation of the young adult. If parents have an unsatisfying marriage and need the young adult to stay connected to meet their needs, this hinders the young adult's efforts at separating; in turn, if the young adult feels anxious and incompetent about managing independently, he or she will delay separation and attempt to keep the parents involved.

Health Concerns. Health concerns are both personal and familial during this transitional stage. Family planning and birth control use is a major concern and need. Sexually transmitted diseases are more frequently seen in this group (venereal disease, AIDS, etc). Accidents and suicides are leading causes of mortality. Mental health problems are also common, and as explained above, deal primarily with the issue of separating in a functional way from one's family of origin so that healthy, intimate heterosexual relationships can be formed.

Health promotion needs are similar to subsequent stages. Because young adults are now on their own, typically their life-styles do not incorporate the recommended health-protective practices such as avoidance of drugs, alcohol, and tobacco; as well as obtaining adequate sleep, nutrition, exercise, and preventive dental and medical examinations and care.

Stage I: Beginning Families

The marriage of a couple marks the beginning of a new family—the family of marriage or procreation—and the movement from the former family of origin or unattached single status to this new intimate relationship. The stage of marriage or married couples, as this stage is also called, today begins later. For example, according to 1985 U.S. Census data, 75 percent of men and 57 percent of women in the United States were still unmarried at age 21, a remarkable shift from 55 and 36 percent, respectively, in 1970.

Family Developmental Tasks. Establishing a mutually satisfying marriage, relating harmoniously to the kin network, and family planning constitute the three critical tasks of this period (Table 6–4).

Establishing a Mutually Satisfying Marriage. When two people become united in marriage, their initial concerns are preparing for a new type of life together. The resources of the two people are combined, their roles altered, and new functions assumed. Learning to live together while providing for each other's basic personality needs becomes a crucial developmental task. The couple has to mutually accommodate to each other in many small routines. For example, they must develop routines for eating, sleeping, getting up in the morning, cleaning house, sharing the bathroom, recreational pursuits, and going places they both enjoy. In this process of mutual accommodation, a set of patterned transactions are formed and then maintained by the couple, with each spouse triggering and monitoring the behavior of the other.

The success of the evolving relationship depends on the mutual accommodation just discussed and on a complementarity, or the fitting together of the needs and interests of the mates. Just as important, individ-

TABLE 6–4. TWO-PARENT NUCLEAR FAMILY LIFE CYCLE STAGE I AND CONCOMITANT FAMILY DEVELOPMENTAL TASKS

Family Life Cycle Stage	Family Developmental Tasks
Beginning families	1. Establishing a mutually satisfying marriage. 2. Relating harmoniously to the kin network. 3. Planning family (decisions about parenthood).

Adapted from Carter and McGoldrick (1988), Duvall and Miller (1985).

ual differences need to be acknowledged. In healthy relationships differences are seen to enrich the marital relationship. Achieving a satisfying relationship is dependent on the development of satisfactory ways to handle "differentness" (Satir, 1983) and conflicts. A healthy way of resolving problems is related to the mates' ability to empathize, be mutually supportive, be able to communicate openly and honestly (Raush et al, 1969), and approach a conflict with feelings of mutual respect (Jackson and Lederer, 1969).

Moreover, how successful the evolving marital relationship will be depends on how well each of the partners has differentiated or separated from their respective families of origin (the previous developmental task). A mature person must separate/differentiate from his or her own parents in order to form his or her own self-identity and healthy intimate relationships. An excellent description of this process and psychosocial problems during this period is presented by McGoldrick (1988).

Many couples experience problems in sexual adjustment, often because of ignorance and misinformation leading to unrealistic expectations and disappointment. Moreover, many couples bring their own unresolved needs and desires into the relationship, and these can adversely affect the sexual relationship (Goldenberg and Goldenberg, 1985).

Relating Harmoniously to Kin Network. A basic role shift occurs in the first marriage of a couple, as they move from their parental homes to their new setting. Concomitantly, they become members of three families—those of their respective families of origin in addition to the one they have recently created. The couple faces the tasks of separating themselves as a newly formed family from each of their families of origin and working out different relationships with parents, siblings, and in-laws, since their primary loyalty must shift to their marital relationship. For the couple this entails forming a new relationship with each set of parents, one that allows not only for mutual support and enjoyment but also for an autonomy that protects the newly formed family from outside intrusion that might undermine the building of a satisfying marriage.

Family Planning. Whether or not to have children and the timing of pregnancies becomes a significant family decision. Littlefield (1977) underscores the importance of considering the whole family pregnant when one is working in maternity care. The type of health care the family as a unit receives during the prenatal period greatly influences the family's ability to cope effectively with the tremendous changes after the baby's birth.

Health Concerns. The primary areas of concern are sexual and marital role adjustment, family planning education and counseling, prenatal education and counseling, and communication. It becomes increasingly apparent that counseling should be provided premaritally. Lack of information often results in sexual and emotional problems, fear, guilt feelings, unplanned pregnancies, and venereal disease either before or after marriage. These unfortunate events do not allow the couple to plan their lives and begin their relationship with a stable foundation.

Traditional marriage concepts are being challenged by love relationships, common-law marriages, and homosexual unions. People entering into nonmarriage unions often need as much if not more counsel from health care workers who may be called on to assist such couples. It is perhaps at this point that family nurses may be caught between two "families," the family of orientation and the forming union. In such a situation, family health professionals need not make value judgments but attempt to help each of the two groups to understand themselves and each other (Williams and Leaman, 1973).

Family Planning. Because family planning is such a cardinal responsibility for the nurse working with families, a more detailed discussion of this area follows. The absence of informed, effective family planning affects family health in many ways: maternal–infant morbidity and mortality; child neglect; ill health of parents; child development problems, including intelligence and learning ability; and marital discord. Informed and intentional family formation involves making decisions regarding the circumstances and timing of marriage, first pregnancy, birth spacing, and family size. Nevertheless, people have the right to make personal decisions about when and/or whether to have children, even aside from any family health considerations.

The number of births in the United States is on the rise, dipping to a low in 1975 and rising steadily thereafter through 1990, as projected from 1984 to 1990 (Family Service America, 1984). The rise in teenage pregnancies, particularly among black unmarried women, is much greater, and is seen as particularly problematic because of the vulnerability and lack of resources of this disadvantaged group of young adolescents (Chilman, 1988). Pregnancy is, not surprisingly, the chief cause of girls leaving school, as well as a frequent cause of premature marriage. Within marriage, early pregnancy (before 2 years) detracts from marital adjustment. All of these are important mental health factors for children and parents (Cohn and Lieberman, 1974).

The physical health of mother and child is a major

issue, documented in obstetrical and perinatal studies. Birth intervals of between 2 and 4 years and a maternal age in the 20s are the most favorable factors for reducing maternal and infant mortality and morbidity. Optimal family size, spacing, and timing of births reduces infant mortality (Cohn and Lieberman, 1974).

The rate of planned pregnancies is growing, as is the number of women or couples who are using contraceptives. Forty-five states, as well as the District of Columbia, have enacted legislation allowing teenage girls under the age of 18 to obtain contraceptives without parental consent. Yet a large proportion of sexually active adolescents and young adult women are not receiving family planning services (Chilman, 1988).

The disparity between the poor and more advantaged groups in their use of effective contraception is related to accessibility of services (Manisoff, 1977) and widespread ignorance about pregnancy and contraception among adolescents (Weatherley and Cartoof, 1988). Religious and sociopolitical factors have interceded to reduce women's and couple's reproductive rights. As of the early 1990s, due to pro-life opposition, the struggle to keep present services available is of growing concern. Public funding for birth control, particularly for abortions, has been cut and services gravely curtailed for the poor and young.

In addition to the need for more medical clinics and permissive legislation for teenagers to receive care, effective sex and family planning health education programs need to be devised and implemented in schools, churches, and health agencies. Such services should be focused not on the general premise that family planning is an end in itself, but on the health benefits of family planning to the individual and to the growth and development of the family.

Forcing birth control on families, however, is not ethical, because doing so destroys the sense of initiative, integrity, and competence. Teenage girls who want babies need to be counseled on physical and emotional readiness for parenthood and realistic protection from pregnancy along with good health supervision. Little has been done to balance the societal pressures toward sex and marriage with realistic contraception education.

Stage II: Childbearing Families

Stage II begins with the birth of the first child and continues through the infant's 30th month. Usually the parents are thrilled about their firstborn, but also quite apprehensive. This apprehensiveness about the baby usually decreases after several days, as the mother and baby begin to get to know each other. This unadulterated elation ends, however, when a new mother arrives home with baby after generally a very short stay at the hospital. She and the father are suddenly confronted with the all-engrossing roles that have been thrust upon them. It is especially difficult in the beginning because of the feelings of inadequacy of new parents; the lack of help from family and friends; the conflicting advice of helpful friends, family, and health care professionals; and the frequent waking up of the baby at night—which usually continues for about 3 to 4 weeks. Also, the mother is fatigued psychologically and physiologically. She often feels the burdens of household duties and perhaps work, in addition to caring for the baby. It is especially difficult if the new mother has been ill or has had a long, difficult labor and delivery or a cesarean section.

The arrival of a new baby into the home creates changes for every member of the family and for every set of relationships. A stranger has been admitted into a close-knit group, and suddenly the balance of the family shifts—each member takes on new roles and begins new relationships. In addition to a baby being born, a mother, father, and grandparents are born. The wife must now relate to the husband as both a spouse and a father and vice versa. And in families with previous children, the impact of the new baby is as significant on the siblings as on the married couple. Telling a child to adjust to a new brother or sister may be equivalent to a husband telling his wife that he is bringing home a mistress whom she is to love and accept as an equal (Williams and Leaman, 1973)! It is truly a time of developmental crisis for all involved.

Hence, although parenthood represents an extremely important goal for most couples, most find it a very difficult life change. The adjustment to marriage is usually not as hard as the adjustment to parenthood. Although a very meaningful and gratifying experience to most parents, the advent of the baby calls for a sudden change to an incessantly demanding role. Two important factors complicating the difficulty of assuming the parental role are that most persons today are not prepared to be parents and that many deleterious, unrealistic myths romanticizing rearing of children are current in our society (Fulcomer, 1977). Parenthood is the only major role for which little preparation is given, and difficulties in role transition adversely affect the quality of the marital and the parent–infant relationships.

Dramatic social changes in American society have also had a marked effect on new parents. The large proportion of women working outside the home and having careers, the rise in divorce and marital instability, the common use of contraception and abortion, and the large increase in costs of having and caring for children are all factors complicating the passage through the early childbearing life cycle stage (Bradt, 1988; Miller and Myers-Walls, 1983).

The Transition to Parenthood. The coming of the firstborn is a critical family experience and often a family crisis, as studies of families during this stage of the life cycle consistently illustrate (Clark, 1966; Hobbs and Cole, 1976; LeMasters, 1957).

To discover how the introduction of new children affected families, LeMasters (1957), in a classic study of family adjustment to the birth of the first child, interviewed 46 urban middle-class parents (ages 25 to 35) and estimated the extent to which they were in crisis. He found that 17 percent of the couples experienced no or only moderate problems, but that the remaining 83 percent experienced extensive and/or severe problems. The common problems parents reported were:

1. Husbands felt neglected (this was mentioned most frequently by the husbands).
2. There was an increased number of mate quarrels and arguments.
3. Interruptions in schedules were continual ("so tired all the time" was a typical comment).
4. Social and sexual life were disrupted and diminished.

Later studies (Hobbs and Cole, 1976) did not find as many couples reporting extensive crisis as LeMasters did, however. These "families in crisis" studies also suggested that families have an idealized, erroneous notion of parenting prior to the birth of the first child and that marital satisfaction drops sharply with the coming of the first baby (Miller and Sollie, 1980).

Clark (1966) conducted a study of families after the birth of a new baby that underscored both the difficulty in adjusting to parenting and the critical need after delivery for continuity of nursing services in the home and clinic.

Another important study dealing with couples' transition to parenthood was conducted by La Rossa and La Rossa (1981). The researchers conceptualized the transition process as best explained by a conflict model, in which scarcity of free time, conflicts of interest among the parents, and legitimacy of division of labor issues led to conflict between parental caretakers.

Miller and Myers-Walls (1983), based on their review of studies of new parents, summarized the specific parenting stressors identified in the research. The most commonly mentioned stressor appeared to be the loss of personal freedom due to parenting responsibilities; in addition, less time and companionship in marriage were frequently identified. Even more marital strain was reported in couples who have difficult children or children with serious health problems or handicaps.

TABLE 6–5. TWO-PARENT NUCLEAR FAMILY LIFE CYCLE STAGE II AND CONCOMITANT FAMILY DEVELOPMENTAL TASKS

Family Life Cycle Stage	Family Developmental Tasks
Childbearing families	1. Setting up the young family as a stable unit (integrating of new baby into family). 2. Reconciling conflicting developmental tasks and needs of various family members. 3. Maintaining a satisfying marital relationship. 4. Expanding relationships with extended family by adding parenting and grandparenting roles.

Adapted from Carter and McGoldrick (1988), Duvall and Miller (1985).

Family Developmental Tasks. After the coming of the firstborn, the family has several important developmental tasks. (Table 6–5). Husband, wife, and baby must all learn new roles, while the nuclear family unit expands in functions and responsibilities. This involves the simultaneous meshing of the developmental tasks of each family member and the family as a whole (Duvall, 1977).

The birth of a child makes radical changes in family organization. The functions of the couple must differentiate to meet the new demands of the infant for care and nurturance. And while the fulfilling of these responsibilities varies tremendously with the sociocultural position of the couple, a common pattern is for the parents to assume more traditional roles or division of responsibilities (La Rossa and La Rossa, 1981).

Relationships with the paternal and maternal extended family must also be realigned during this stage. New roles need to be established with respect to grandparenting and relationships between parents and grandparents (Bradt, 1988).

The most important role for family nurses to assess when working with the childbearing family is the parental role—how both parents interact with and care for the new infant, and how the infant responds. Klaus and Kendall (1976), Kendall (1974), Rubin (1967), and others verify the critical impact of early attachment and a beginning warm, positive parent–child relationship on the future parental relationship with the child. The parents' attitude about themselves as parents, their attitudes about the baby, and the characteristics of parental communication and stimulation of the infant (Davis, 1978) are related areas that need to be assessed.

Role changes and adaptation to new parental responsibilities often are more rapidly learned by the mother than by the father. The child is a reality to the expectant mother much earlier than for the father, who usually begins to feel like a father at the birth, but sometimes even later than that (Minuchin, 1974). The father often remains initially uncommitted while the woman is rapidly adjusting to a new family structure.

The way in which most fathers have traditionally been left out of the perinatal process has certainly delayed men from taking on this important role change and thereby hindered their emotional involvement. Fortunately, increased awareness of the important role fathers play in child care and the child's development has led to greater involvement of fathers in infant care among the middle-class (Hanson and Bozett, 1985).

The mother and father grow and develop their parental roles in response to the continually changing demands and developmental tasks of the growing youngster, the family as a whole, and themselves. According to Friedman (1957), parents go through five successive stages of development. The first two stages fall into this phase of family life. First, during the child's infancy, parents learn the meaning of cues their baby expresses in making his or her needs known. With each successive child, parents will go through this same stage as they adjust to each infant's unique cues.

The second stage of parental development, learning to accept child's growth and development, occurs in the toddler years. Just prior to and during this stage, parents—particularly parents with their first child—need guidance and support. Parents need to understand tasks the child is attempting to master and the child's needs for safety, limits, and toilet training. They need to understand the concept of developmental readiness, or "the teachable moment." At the same time, parents need guidance in understanding the tasks they themselves are mastering during this stage.

New marital communication patterns evolve with the coming of a child, with mates relating to each other both as mates and as parents. Spouse transactional patterns have been found to change drastically. Feldman (1961) observed that parents of infants talked less with each other and had less fun, less stimulating conversation, and a diminished quality of marital interaction. Some parents feel overwhelmed with the added responsibilities, particularly those in dual-worker families where both parents work full-time.

The reestablishment of satisfying communication patterns—including personal, marital, and parental feelings and concerns—is critical. Mates must continue to meet each other's personal adult psychological and sexual needs as well as share and interact with each other about parental responsibilities.

The sexual relationship of the mates generally declines during pregnancy and through the 6-week postpartum period. Sexual difficulties during the later period are common, arising from such factors as the mother's absorption in her new role, fatigue, and feelings of loss of sexual attractiveness, as well as the husband's feeling of being "left or pushed out" by the new baby.

Family communications now include a third member, making for a triad. Parents must learn to perceive and discern the communication cries of the infant. For instance, the baby's cries need to be differentiated into expressions of discomfort, hunger, overstimulation, sickness, or fatigue. And the baby begins responding to cuddles, fondling, and talking, which then are received and reinforced by the parents.

Family planning counseling usually occurs at the 6-week postpartum examination. Parents should then be encouraged to openly discuss family spacing and planning. Due to the increased personal and family demands new babies bring, parents need to realize that frequent, closely spaced pregnancies can be harmful to the mother, as well as to the father, siblings, and the family unit.

This life cycle stage requires an adjustment of relationships within the extended family and with friends. When other family members try to support and assist the new parents, tensions may result. Although grandparents, for instance, can be of great help to the new family, the potential for conflict exists because of differences in values and expectations existing between the generations.

Despite the importance of having a social network or social support system for achieving satisfaction with and positive feelings about family life, the young family needs to know when it needs help and from whom to accept it as well as when to depend on its own inner resources and strengths (Duvall, 1977).

A strong, viable marital relationship is essential to the stability and morale of the family. A satisfying husband–wife relationship will give the mates the strength and energy to "give" to the infant and to each other. Conflicting pressures and demands, such as between the mother's loyalty to infant and to husband, are problematic and can be agonizing. This type of conflict can become the central source of unhappiness during this life cycle stage.

Health Concerns. The main concerns of families in this stage are family-centered maternity education, well-baby care, early recognition and appropriate handling of physical health problems, immunizations, child development counseling, family planning, family interaction, and general health promotion (life-style) areas.

Other health concerns during this period of a family's life are inaccessibility and inadequacy of child-care facilities for working mothers, parent–child relationships, parenting including child abuse and neglect, and parent role transition problems.

Stage III: Families With Preschool Children

The third stage of the family life cycle commences when the firstborn child is about 2½ years old and terminates when he or she is 5. The family now may consist of three to five persons, with the paired positions of husband-father, wife-mother, son-brother, and daughter-sister. The family is becoming more complex and differentiated (Duvall and Miller, 1985).

Family life during this stage is busy and demanding for parents. Both parents have greater demands on their time, as it is probable that the mother is working also, part or full-time. Nevertheless, realizing that parents are the "architects of the family," designing and directing family development (Satir, 1983), it is critical for them to strengthen their partnership—in short, to keep the marriage alive and well.

Preschool children have much to learn at this stage, especially in the area of independence. They must achieve enough autonomy and self-sufficiency to be able to handle themselves without their parents in a variety of places. Experience in nursery school, kindergarten, Project Head Start, a day-care center, or similar programs is a good way to foster this kind of development. Structured preschool program are especially helpful in assisting parents with preschool children from inner-city, low-income families. A considerable rise in both IQ and social skills has been reported to occur after children have completed a 2-year nursery school experience (Kraft et al, 1968).

Many single-parent families exist within this particular life cycle stage. In 1984, 50 percent of black families and 15 percent of white families in the United States were headed by one parent, and in 88 percent of these families mothers were the head of household (Nortan and Glick, 1986). Among single-parent families, the role strain of parenting the preschooler, coupled with other roles, is great. Infant and preschool day care centers that are reasonable and of good quality are difficult if not impossible to locate in most communities. Mothers with careers and adolescent mothers are particularly in need of better child care facilities and programs (Adams and Adams, 1990).

Family Developmental Tasks. The family is now growing in both numbers and complexity. The need of preschoolers and other young children to explore the world around them, and parents' needs for their own privacy, makes housing and adequate space become major problems. Equipment and facilities also need to be childproofed, for it is at this stage that accidents become the most common causes of both mortality and disability. Assessing the home for safety hazards is of prime importance for the community health nurse, and health education must then be included so that the parents and children are cognizant of the risks involved and of ways of preventing accidents (Table 6–6).

TABLE 6–6. TWO-PARENT NUCLEAR FAMILY LIFE CYCLE STAGE III AND CONCOMITANT FAMILY DEVELOPMENTAL TASKS

Family Life Cycle Stage	Family Developmental Tasks
Families with preschool children	1. Meeting family members' needs for adequate housing, space, privacy, and safety. 2. Socializing the children. 3. Integrating new child members while still meeting needs of other children. 4. Maintaining healthy relationships within the family (marital and parent–child) and outside the family (extended family and community).

Adapted from Carter and McGoldrick (1988), Duvall and Miller (1985).

Due to both lack of specific resistance to the many bacterial and viral diseases and increased exposure, preschoolers are frequently sick with one minor infectious illness after another. Infectious diseases often "ping-pong" throughout the family. Frequent visits to the doctor, caring for sick kids, and running home from work to pick up an ill child from the nursery school are common weekly crises. Thus children's contacts with infectious and communicable diseases and their general susceptibility to disease are prime health concerns.

Accidents, falls, burns, and lacerations are also quite common occurrences. These are even more frequently seen where there are large families, families where an adult caretaker is not present (latchkey children), and in low-income families. Environmental safety and adequate child supervision are the keys to reducing accidents.

The husband–father assumes more involvement in the household responsibilities during this stage of family development than during any other stage, the largest percentage of this being spent in child-care activities. The father's involvement with child care at this time is especially important, as this relationship with the preschooler assists the child with his or her sexual identification. It is particularly critical for boys in the first 5 years of life to associate closely with a strong, limit-setting, warm father or father substitute so that their masculine role identity can be established (Walters, 1976).

A more mature role is also assumed by the preschooler, who gradually takes on more responsibility for his or her own care, plus helping the mother or father with household jobs. It is not the productivity of the child that is important here, but the learning that occurs.

Contrary to expectations, research has shown that the advent of the second child into the family has an even more deleterious effect on the marital relationship than does the first birth. Feldman (1961) reports that parental roles make the marital roles difficult, as exhibited by the following observations: couples perceive negative personality changes in each other; they are less satisfied with the home; there is more task-oriented interaction; fewer personal conversations and more child-centered conversations take place; more warmth is exhibited toward the children and less toward each other; and there is a lower level of sexual satisfaction (Feldman, 1969).

This well-recognized study parallels reports and observations of family counselors—that the marital relationship is often troubled at this phase of the cycle. In fact, many divorces occur within these years due to weak or unsatisfactory marital ties. Privacy and time together are prime necessities. Marriage counseling and marriage encounter groups have become important resources among the middle class. For the family without economic resources, however, limited assistance is available for strengthening a salvageable marriage. There is a trend for priests and ministers to become trained as marriage and family counselors and counsel couples who cannot afford private therapy.

A major task of the family is socializing the children. Preschoolers are developing critical self-attitudes (self-concepts) and rapidly learning to express themselves, as seen in their rapid grasp of language.

Another task during this period deals with how to integrate a new family member (second or third child) while still meeting the needs of older child(ren). The displacement of a child by a newborn is psychologically a very traumatic event. Preparation of children for the arrival of a new baby helps ameliorate the situation, especially if the parents are sensitive to the older child's feelings and behavior. Sibling rivalry is often expressed by hitting or negatively relating to new baby, regressive behaviors, and attention-getting activity. The best way to handle sibling rivalry is for the parents to spend a certain amount of time each day exclusively relating to the older child to give him or her the assurance that he or she is still loved and wanted.

About the time children become preschoolers, parents enter their third parenting stage, one of learning to separate from the children as they toddle off to nursery school, a day-care center, or kindergarten. This stage continues during the preschool and early school years. Separation is often difficult for parents and they need support and an explanation of how the preschoolers' mastery of developmental tasks contributes to their increasing autonomy.

Separation from parents is also difficult for preschool children. Separation may occur as parents go to work, to the hospital, or on trips or vacations. Family preparation for separation is important in helping the children adjust to change.

Assisting parents to obtain family planning services after the arrival of a new baby, or to continue with contraception if there has been no intervening pregnancy, is also indicated. It is, for instance, not unusual for a woman to have stopped using contraceptives because of a missed period with the belief that she was pregnant, only to find out later that her eventual pregnancy resulted from sexual intercourse without contraceptive protection.

Both parents need to have some outside interests and contacts to rejuvenate themselves to carry on the multitude of home tasks and responsibilities. The lower-class and single parent often does not have the opportunity to do this, and these families have the least satisfactory associations with the wider community due to their alienated position and the paucity of resources available to them.

Health Concerns. Numerous health concerns have been identified throughout our discussion of the preschool family. As indicated earlier, the major physical health problems concern the frequent communicable diseases of the children and the common falls, burns, poisonings, and other accidents that occur during the preschool age.

The prime psychosocial family health concern is the marital relationship. Studies verify the diminished satisfaction many couples experience during these years and the need for working to strengthen and reinvigorate this vital unit. Other important health concerns involve sibling rivalry, family planning, growth and developmental needs, parenting problems like setting limits (disciplining), child abuse and neglect, home safety, and family communication problems.

General health-promotion strategies continue to be germane during this stage, as life-style behaviors learned during childhood can have both short- and long-term consequences. Family health education directed at prevention of major health problems is indicated in the areas of smoking, alcohol and drug misuse, human sexuality, safety, diet and nutrition, exercise, and social support/stress management. "The chief goals for nurses working with the school age child and family are to assist them in establishing healthy lifestyles and in facilitating the child's optimal physical, intellectual, emotional, and social growth" (Wilson, 1988, p. 177).

Stage IV: Families With School-age Children

This stage commences when the firstborn is 6 years old and begins elementary school and ends at 13, the beginning of adolescence. Families usually reach their maximum number of members, and family relationships at the end of this stage (Duvall, 1977). Again these are busy years. Now children have their own activities and interests, in addition to the mandatory activities of life and school, and the parents' own activities. Each person is working on his or her own developmental tasks, just as the family attempts to fulfill its tasks (Table 6–7). According to Erikson (1950), parents are struggling with twin demands of finding fulfillment in rearing the next generation (the developmental task of generativity) and being concerned in their own growth; while school-age children are working at developing a sense of industry—the capacity for work enjoyment—and trying to eliminate or ward off a sense of inferiority.

The parental task at this time is that of learning to deal with the child's separation or, more simply, letting the child go. More and more, peer relationships and outside activities play larger roles in the life of the school-age child. These years are filled with family activities, but there are also forces gradually pushing the child to separate from the family in preparation for adolescence. Parents who have interests outside of their children will find it much easier to make the gradual separation. In instances where the mothering role is the central and only significant role in a woman's life, however, this separation process may be a very painful one and one that is strongly resisted.

TABLE 6–7. TWO-PARENT NUCLEAR FAMILY LIFE CYCLE STAGE IV AND CONCOMITANT FAMILY DEVELOPMENTAL TASKS

Family Life Cycle Stage	Family Developmental Tasks
Families with school-aged children	1. Socializing the children, including promoting school achievement and fostering of healthy peer relations of children. 2. Maintaining a satisfying marital relationship. 3. Meeting the physical health needs of family members.

Adapted from Carter and McGoldrick (1988), Duvall and Miller (1985).

During this stage parents feel intense pressure from the outside community via the school system and other extrafamilial associations to have their children conform to the community's standards for children. This tends to influence the middle-class family to stress more traditional values of achievement and productivity, and to cause some working-class families and many poor families to feel alienated from and at conflict with school and/or community values.

Children's handicaps may come to light during this period of a child's life. school nurses and teachers will detect many visual, hearing, and speech defects, in addition to learning problems, behavior disturbances, inadequate dental care, child abuse, substance abuse, and communicable diseases (Edelman and Mandle, 1986). Working with the family in the role of health educator and counselor, in addition to initiating appropriate referrals for follow-up screening, assumes much of a school nurse's energies. He or she also acts as a resource person to the school teacher, enabling the teacher to handle the common and more individualized health needs of her or his pupils more effectively.

There are a number of other handicapping conditions occasionally detected during the school years, including epilepsy, cerebral palsy, mental retardation, cancer, and orthopedic conditions. The family health nurse's primary function here—in addition to referral, teaching, and counseling parents regarding these conditions—would be to assist the family in coping so that any adverse impact of the handicap on the family will be minimized.

For children with behavior problems, family nurses in schools, clinics, doctor's offices, and community agencies should seek active parental involvement. Initiating a referral for family counseling/therapy is often very helpful in assisting the family to be aware of some of the family problems that may be adversely affecting the school-age child. When parents are able to reframe the child's behavior problem as a family problem and work toward its resolution with that new focus, many times more healthy family functioning results as well as more healthy child behaviors (Bradt, 1988).

Family Developmental Tasks. One of the critical tasks of parents in socializing their children at this time involves promoting school achievement. Another significant family task is maintaining a satisfying marital relationship. Again it has been reported that marital satisfaction is diminished during this stage. Two large studies reinforced these observations (Burr, 1970; Rollins and Feldman, 1970). Promoting open communication and supporting the spousal relationship is vital in working with the school-age family.

Stage V: Families With Teenagers

When the firstborn turns 13 years of age, the fifth stage of the family's life cycle commences. It usually lasts about 6 or 7 years, although it can be shorter if the child leaves the family early or longer if the child remains home later than 19 or 20 years of age. Other children in the home are usually of school age. The overarching family goal at the teenage stage is that of loosening family ties to allow greater responsibility and freedom for the teenager in preparation for becoming a young adult (Duvall, 1977).

Preto (1988), in discussing the transformation of the family system in adolescence, describes the family metamorphosis that takes place. It involves "profound shifts in relationship patterns across the generations, and while it may be signaled initially by the adolescent's physical maturity, it often parallels and coincides with changes in parents as they enter midlife and with major transformations faced by grandparents in old age" (p. 255).

This stage of the family's life is probably the most difficult, or certainly the most discussed and written about (Kidwell et al, 1983). The American family is affected by the tremendous developmental tasks of both the adolescent and parents and the inevitable conflicts and turmoil these create. The developmental tasks of adolescence demand a movement from dependence on and control by the parents and other adults, through a period of intense peer group activity and influence, to the assumption of adult roles (Adams, 1971).

The major challenges in working with a family with teenagers revolve around the developmental changes adolescents undergo in terms of cognitive changes, identity formation, and biological growth (Kidwell et al, 1983) and developmentally based conflicts and crises. Adams (1971) delineates three aspects of the adolescent process upon which much attention has been focused, namely, emancipation (increased autonomy), youth culture (development of peer relationships), and the generation gap (disparity of values and norms between parents and teenagers).

Parental Roles, Responsibilities, and Problems. Needless to say, parents find it a most difficult task to raise teenagers today. Nonetheless, parents need to stand firm against unreasonable testing of the limits that have been set in the family as they go through the process of gradually "letting go." Duvall (1977) also identifies the critical developmental task of this period to be the balancing of freedom with responsibility as teenagers mature and emancipate themselves. Friedman (1957) similarly defines the parental task during this stage as learning to accept rejection without deserting the child.

When the parents accept themselves as they are, with all their own weaknesses and strengths, and when they accept their several roles at this stage of development without undue conflict or sensitivity, they set the pattern for a similar sort of self-acceptance in their children. Relationships between parents and adolescents should be smoother when parents feel productive, satisfied, and in control of their own lives (Kidwell et al, 1983) and parents/families function flexibly (Preto, 1988).

Schultz (1972) and others have expressed the view that the increasing complexity of American life has made the role of parents unclear. Parents may feel in competition with a variety of social forces and institutions—from school authorities and counselors to birth control and premarital sex and cohabitation options. Other factors add to their considerably diminished influence. Because of specialization of occupations and professions, parents are no longer able to help children with their vocational plans. The residential mobility and lack of continuing trustworthy adult relationships for both adolescents and parents, in addition to the inability of many parents to discuss personal, sexual, and drug-related concerns openly and nonjudgmentally with their children, has also contributed to parent–adolescent problems.

Family Developmental Tasks. The first and central family developmental task is the balancing of freedom with responsibility as teenagers mature and become increasingly autonomous (Table 6–8). The parents must progressively change their relationship with their teenage son or daughter from the previously established dependent relationship to an increasingly independent one. This evolving shift in the parent–child

TABLE 6–8. TWO-PARENT NUCLEAR FAMILY LIFE CYCLE STAGE V AND CONCOMITANT FAMILY DEVELOPMENTAL TASKS

Family Life Cycle Stage	Family Developmental Tasks
Family with teenagers	1. Balancing of freedom with responsibility as teenagers mature and become increasingly autonomous. 2. Refocusing the marital relationship. 3. Communicating openly between parents and children.

Adapted from Carter and McGoldrick (1988), Duvall and Miller (1985).

relationship is typically one fraught with conflicts along the way.

In order for the family to adapt successfully during this stage, the family members, especially the parents, have to make a major "system change"—that is, set up new roles and norms and "let go" of the adolescent. Kidwell and associates (1983) summarize this needed change. "Paradoxically, the [family] system which can let go of its members is the system which will endure and reproduce itself effectively in later generations" (p. 88).

Parents who, in order to meet their own needs, do not let go, often find a major "revolution" by the teenager when separation occurs later. Parents may also thrust forth the adolescent into independence prematurely, ignoring his or her dependency needs. In this case the teenager may fail in attempts to achieve independence (Wright and Leahey, 1984).

As with the last three stages, the marital relationship is also a focus of concern. The second family developmental task is for couples to refocus their marital relationship (Wilson, 1988). Many couples have become so preoccupied with their parental responsibilities that their marriage no longer plays a central role in their lives. The husband usually spends much time away from home working and furthering his career, while the wife is probably also working while trying to keep up with housework and parental responsibilities. Under these conditions little time or energy is left for the marital relationship.

The other side of the coin, however, is that since the children are more responsible for themselves, the couple can more easily leave home to engage in their careers or establish individual and marital postparental interests. They can begin to build a foundation for the future stages of the family life cycle.

A third pressing family developmental task is for family members, particularly the parents and teenager, to openly communicate with each other. Because of the generation gap, open communication is often an ideal rather than a reality. There is often mutual rejection by parents and adolescents of each other's values and life-styles. Parents in multiproblem families have been found to frequently reject and then to disengage from their older children, thereby reducing whatever open communication channels there might have been.

Maintaining the family's ethical and moral standards is another family developmental task (Duvall and Miller, 1985). Although family rules need to change, family ethical and moral standards need to be maintained by parents. While adolescents are searching for their own beliefs and values, it is of paramount importance for parents to defend and adhere firmly to their own sound principles and standards. Adolescents are very sensitive to incongruities between what is "preached and practiced." Nonetheless, parents and children can learn from each other in the fast-changing and pluralistic society of today. Value transformations of youth are also transforming families. The adoption of a freer and more casual life-style symbolizes a value transformation affecting every phase of family life (Yankelowich, 1975).

Health Concerns. At this stage the physical health of the family members is usually good, but health promotion remains an important concern. Risk factors should be identified and discussed with families, as should the importance of a health life-style. From age 35 on, the risk of coronary heart disease rises appreciably in males, and at this point both adult members are beginning to feel more vulnerable to ill health as part of their developmental changes and are usually more receptive to health-promotion strategies. With teenagers, accidents—particularly automobile accidents—are a great hazard, and broken bones and athletic injuries are also common.

Drug and alcohol misuse, birth control, unwanted pregnancies, and sex education and counseling are relevant areas of concern. In discussing these topics with families, the nurse may get caught squarely in the middle of a parent–youth dispute or problem. Adolescents often seek health services for pregnancy testing, drug use, AIDS screening, birth control and abortion, and venereal disease diagnosis and care. There has been a legal trend to allow adolescents to receive health care without parental consent. Where parents are involved, separate interviews with the teenager and parents prior to bringing them together are often indicated.

Another health need is again in the area of support and assistance in strengthening the marital relationship and the adolescent–parent relationship. Direct supportive counseling or initiation of referral to community resources for counseling, as well as recreational, educational, and other services, may be needed. General health promotion education is also indicated.

Stage VI: Families Launching Young Adults

The beginning of this phase of family life is characterized by the first child leaving the parental home and ends with "the empty nest," when the last child has left home. This stage could be quite short or fairly long, depending on how many children are in the family or if any unmarried children remain at home after termination of high school or college. Although the usual length of this stage is 6 or 7 years, in recent years the stage is longer in some two-parent families due to more older children living at home after they have finished school and begun working. The motive is often economics—the high cost of living independently. The more widespread trend, however, has been for young adults, who generally delay marriage, to have a period of being unattached and live independently in their own living arrangements. From a large Canadian survey it was found that children who grow up in stepfamilies and single-parent families leave home earlier than those raised in families with two biological parents. This difference was not seen to be influenced by economic factors, but as due to parent differences and family milieu (Mitchell et al, 1989).

This phase is marked by the culmination of years of preparation of and by the children for an independent adult life. Parents, as they let their children go, are relinquishing 20 years or so of the parenting role and returning to their original marital dyad. Family developmental tasks are critical while the family is shifting from a household with children to a husband–wife pair. The major family goal is the reorganization of the family into a continuing unit while releasing matured young people into lives of their own (Duvall, 1977). During this stage the marital pair take on grandparent roles—another change in both roles and their self-image.

Early middle age, which is about the average age of parents during the launching of their oldest child, has been characterized as a "caught" period of life: caught between the demands of youth and the expectations of the elderly and caught between the world of work and the competing demands and involvement of the family, with the often seeming impossibility of meeting the demands of both realms. Studies indicate, however, that while the middle-aged may feel squeezed or "sandwiched" between the poles of youth and aging, at least for middle- and upper-class individuals, they can often appreciate their own importance and achievements: "They often know that they are the nation's decision-makers; they set the tone for life in this society. Society depends on middle-aged people's leadership and productivity" (Kerckhoff, 1976).

Family Developmental Tasks. As the family assists the oldest child in his or her launching, the parents are also involved with their younger children, helping them to become independent. And when the "released" son or daughter marries, the family task involves expanding the family circle to include new members by marriage and becoming accepting of the couple's own life-style and values (Table 6–9).

With the emptying of the nest, parents have more time to devote to other activities and relationships. Hopefully, they have not grown so far apart from each other that they cannot reinstitute or reestablish the wife and husband roles to the place of primary importance these roles once held. LeShan (1973) views this stage as a challenge to the marital relationship. When the children leave, marriage faces a moment of truth; is there strength enough to sustain it without the excuse of parenthood?

TABLE 6–9. TWO-PARENT NUCLEAR FAMILY LIFE CYCLE STAGE VI AND CONCOMITANT FAMILY DEVELOPMENTAL TASKS

Family Life Cycle Stage	Family Developmental Tasks
Families launching young adults	1. Expanding the family circle to include new family members acquired by marriage of children. 2. Continuing to renew and readjust in the marital relationship. 3. Assisting aging and ill parents of the husband and wife.

Adapted from Carter and McGoldrick (1988), Duvall and Miller (1985).

This period is usually much more difficult for the woman than for the man. In most families the central and enduring role—enduring in the sense that the role has existed 20 some years—for the woman has been the role of mother. Although less prevalent today because more women have returned to school or are involved with careers, the woman's identity and feelings of competency have been based on being a good mother. Despite the years of gradual separation of children preceding this stage, the launching often comes psychologically quite suddenly to her. With the children gone or going, the mother who does not work now finds herself with a clean house (not much work there anymore) and no place to go or purpose for her existence. Typically, middle-class husbands are at the peak of their careers and are spending long hours away from home, putting in a concentrated period of years to attempt to succeed occupationally, financially, or professionally, to fulfill their aspirations before it is too late. Many women have been so absorbed in their children that they have not prepared for this phase of their life and do not have other equally fulfilling commitments in which to invest their energies and talents. The middle-age crisis is more severe for women not only because of the children leaving home and the unavailability of their husbands, but also due to feelings of loss of femininity with the beginning of menopause (usually between 45 and 55) and loss of beauty when discernible signs of aging appear. If a woman has commitments outside of home (eg, work, and avocation), she usually has fewer problems than if she has remained home in the traditional role of housewife and full-time mother.

Men in middlescence (the name for middle age in the developmental literature) also face potential developmental crises. One potential crisis is the drive to get "ahead" in their careers with the realization that they have not succeeded or have not reached their aspirations. Also, signs of diminished masculinity, such as lower energy levels and lessened potency and sexual excitation, as well as figure, hair, and skin aging signs; and financial worries; are stressors for men during this family life cycle stage. The frequency of extramarital affairs, divorces, mental illness, alcoholism, and suicide all rise among adults of these age groups, underscoring the middle-age developmental crises that occur.

Friedman (1957) reiterates the significance of the marital relationship by characterizing the parental developmental stage at this point in the family life cycle as the building of a new life together.

Another important developmental task of the middle-years family is that of assisting aging and ill parents of the husband and wife. Even though the actual care of aging and/or dependent parents is not an expected function of the American family with the exception of certain ethnic groups, the husband and wife are expected to assist and support elderly family members as much as they feel is feasible. Such activity takes all forms—from frequent telephoning and supportive calls to assisting financially, providing transportation, and visiting and caring for their parent(s) in the home. In America the family is seen as primarily responsible for the succeeding generation, the offspring, and only secondarily for the previous generation, the parents (Kalish, 1975).

Three-generation families, although not the usual pattern, are not uncommon, particularly in "traditional" Asian, Hispanic, Greek, Italian, and Jewish families. Most often in the United States the multigenerational family seems to develop primarily when the nuclear family is disrupted by death or divorce, but financial expediency or child-care needs may also encourage such living arrangements. In fact, older parents typically desire to live independently so as not to impinge on their children's lives and, more importantly, to retain their own feelings of competence, independence, and privacy (Bengtson et al, 1987; Troll, 1971). Parents may also have to wrestle with the decision to place their parents in a nursing home or retirement or board-and-care facility during these years.

In summary it can be seen that as children disperse, parents must again learn independence. In readjusting, the marriage must be viable if parents' needs are to continue to be fulfilled. Parents have to readjust their relationship—to relate to each other as marital partners rather than primarily as parents. For this stage to be complete, children must be independent while maintaining ties and bonds with parents.

Health Concerns. The primary health concerns involve communication problems between young adults and their parents; role-transitional problems for wife and husband; caretaker concerns (for aging parents); and the emergence of chronic health conditions or predisposing factors such as high cholesterol levels, obesity, or high blood pressure. Family planning for the adolescent and young adult members remains important. Menopausal problems among women are common. The effects associated with prolonged drinking, smoking, and dietary practices become more obvious. Finally, the need for health-promotion strategies and a "wellness life-style" become more pressing for the adult members of the launching center family.

Stage VII: Middle-aged Parents

The seventh stage of the family life cycle, the stage of the middle years for parents, begins when the last child departs from the home and ends with retirement or death of one of the spouses. This stage usually starts when parents are about 45 to 55 years of age and ends with the retirement of a spouse, usually 16 to 18 years later. Typically, the marital couple in their middle years constitutes a nuclear family, although still interacting with their aging parent(s) and other members of their own family of origin, as well as with the new families of marriage of their offspring. The postparental couple is not usually isolated today; more middle-age couples are living out their full life span and spending a greater portion of it in a postparental phase, with extended kin relationships between four generations not being unusual (Troll, 1971).

The middle years include changes in marital adjustment (often better), in the distribution of power between husband and wife (more shared), and in roles (increased marital role differentiation) (Leslie and Korman, 1989). To many families with increased satisfaction and economic status (Rollins and Feldman, 1970), these years are seen as the prime of life. For example, Olson, McCubbin and associates (1983), in a large, cross-sectional, national survey of predominantly white middle class, intact families, found that marital and family satisfaction and quality of life increased and peaked during the postparental phase. Middle-aged families, in general, are also better off economically than at other stages of the family life cycle (McCullough and Rutenberg, 1988). Increased labor force participation by women and higher earning power than in previous periods by men account for the greater economic security experienced by most middle-aged families. Mutually enjoyable leisure activities and companionship is mentioned as the prime factor leading to marital happiness. Sexual satisfaction is also positively correlated with both good communication and marital satisfaction (Levin and Levin, 1975), even though middle-age husbands may experience a decline in sexual adequacy. Intimate husband-wife communication is essential for maintaining understanding and interest in each other throughout these years.

For some couples, however, these years are generally difficult and onerous ones, because of problems of aging, the loss of children, and a sense of themselves as failures in parenting and work efforts. Furthermore, it is not clear as to what happens with marital and family satisfaction across the family life cycle. Some marital satisfaction studies show that marital satisfaction drops soon after marriage and continues to decline through the middle years (Leslie and Korman, 1989).

Family Developmental Tasks. By the time the last child leaves home, many women have rechanneled their energies and lives in preparation for the empty nest. For some women, a middle-age crisis (discussed in previous stage) is experienced during the early period of this life cycle. Women work at encouraging their grown children to be independent by redefining their relationship with them (not intruding on their personal and family life). In order to maintain a sense of well-being and health, more women begin to live a healthier life-style of weight control, balanced diet, regular exercise program, and adequate rest, as well as to attain and enjoy a career, work, or creative accomplishments.

Occupationally, men may find the same frustrations and disappointments that were present in the previous stage. On the one hand, they may be at the peak of their career and not have to work as hard as previously; or on the other hand, may find their job monotonous after 20 to 30 years at the same type of work. Many middle-class workers suffer from the "plateau phenomenon"—where increased salaries and promotions are no longer available—leaving them to feel in a rut. Career discontent is said to reach alarming proportions under these conditions, with many persons making midlife job changes due to the feelings of discontentment, boredom, and stagnation. Because work has traditionally been a man's central role in life, this common experience of work discontentment greatly influences men's stress level and general health status.

The cultivation of leisure-time activities and interests is significant during this stage, since more time is now available and preparation for retirement must take place in a more planned fashion.

TABLE 6–10. TWO-PARENT NUCLEAR FAMILY LIFE CYCLE STAGE VII AND CONCOMITANT FAMILY DEVELOPMENTAL TASKS

Family Life Cycle Stage	Family Developmental Tasks
Middle-aged parents	1. Providing a health-promoting environment. 2. Sustaining satisfying and meaningful relationships with aging parents and children. 3. Strengthening the marital relationship.

Adapted from Carter and McGoldrick (1988), Duvall and Miller (1985).

An important developmental task for this stage is the provision of a healthy environment. (Table 6–10). It is in this period when taking on a healthier life-style becomes more prevalent for couples, despite the fact that they have probably been engaging in self-destructive habits for 45 to 65 years. Although not inadvisable to start now, since "better now than never" is always true, it is largely too late to reverse many of the physiological changes that have already taken place, such as arthritic changes due to inactivity; high blood pressure due to lack of exercise, prolonged stress, or poor dietary habits; and vital capacity diminution due to smoking.

The primary motivation of middle-aged persons to improve their life-style appears to be a feeling of susceptibility or vulnerability to illness and disease generated when a friend or family member of the same age group has a heart attack, stroke, or cancer. In addition to fear, a belief that regular checkups and healthful living habits are effective ways of reducing susceptibility to various diseases are also powerful motivating forces. Heart disease, cancer, and stroke account for two thirds of all causes of mortality between the ages of 46 and 64 years of age, with accidents the fourth cause of death (National Center for Health Statistics, 1989).

A second developmental task relates to sustaining satisfying and meaningful relationships with aging parents and children. By accepting and welcoming grandchildren into the family and promoting satisfying intergenerational relationships, this developmental task can be highly rewarding (Duvall, 1977). It allows the middle-age couple to continue feeling like a family and bring the joys of grandparenthood without the 24-hour responsibilities of parenthood. With increased life expectancy, being a grandparent typically occurs during this life cycle stage (Sprey and Matthews, 1982). Grandparents provide a wide range of support to their children and grandchildren in times of crisis and assist their children in the parent role through their encouragement and support (Bengtson and Robertson, 1985).

The more problematic role is that of relating to and assisting the aging parents and sometimes other older extended family members. Eighty-six percent of middle-aged couples have at least one parent each still alive (Hagestad, 1988). Thus, caregiving responsibilities for aging parents who are frail or ill is a frequent experience. More women find themselves in a "generational squeeze" in their attempt to balance the needs of their aging parents, their children, and grandchildren. Multiple intergenerational roles and relationships are likely to be more extensive among certain minorities, such as Asian and Latino families.

The third developmental task to be discussed here is that of strengthening the marital relationship. Now the couple is really alone after many years of being surrounded with other family members and relationships. Although appearing as a welcome relief, for many mates it is a difficult experience to have to relate to each other as marital partners rather than as parents. Wright and Leahey (1984) describe this family developmental task as being "reinvestment in couple identity with concurrent development of independent interests" (p. 49). The balance of dependency–independency between couples needs to be reexamined. Often couples develop different arrangements in marriage, such as having greater independent interests, as well as meaningful mutual interests.

For couples who experience problems, the reduced pressure of life in postparental years may lead not to marital bliss, but to marital "blahs." According to Kerckhoff (1976), marriage counselors have long observed that when trouble arises in the marriage during the middle years, it is often related to boredom of the union, not to its traumatic qualities. A common characteristic of this period relative to marriage is "smug complacency" and being in a "comfortable rut" (p. 9).

Health Concerns. The health concerns mentioned throughout the description of the life cycle stage include the following:

1. Health-promotion needs: adequate rest, leisure activities, and sleep; good nutrition; regular exercise program; reduction of weight down to optimum weight; cessation of smoking; reduction or cessation in use of alcohol; and preventive-health screening examination.
2. Marital relationship concerns.
3. Communication with and relating to children, in-laws, grandchildren, and aging parents.
4. Caretaker concerns: assisting in care of aging or disabled parents.

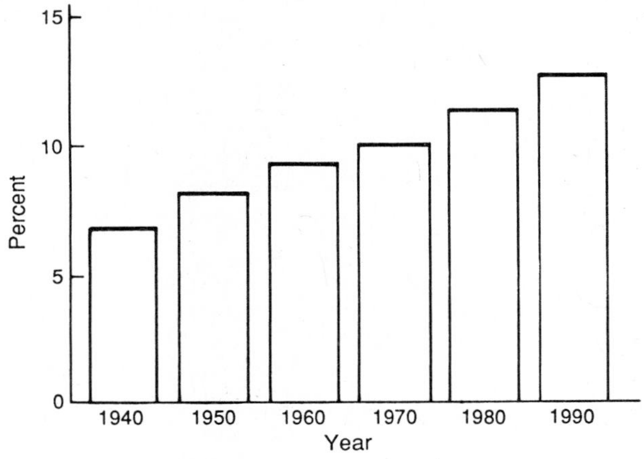

Figure 6–1
Growth of elderly population in the United States, percentage of population over 65. (U.S. Bureau of the Census, 1991).

Stage VIII: Families in Retirement and Old Age

The last stage of the life cycle of the family begins with the retirement of one or both spouses, continues through the loss of one spouse, and ends with the death of the other spouse (Duvall and Miller, 1985). The number of aging individuals—people 65 and older—in our country has rapidly increased during the last two decades, twice as fast as the rest of the population. In 1970, there were some 19.9 million people age 65 and older, representing about 9.8 percent of the total population. By 1990, according to Census Bureau figures, the elderly population had grown to some 31.7 million (12.7 percent of the total population). By the year 2020, 17.3 percent of the nation's population will be age 65 and older (Fig. 6–1). Information on population aging suggest that the "oldest old"—the 85-plus population—is growing especially rapidly. The 85-plus population grew to 2.2 million in 1980. It is projected that in year 2020 this population will increase to 7.1 million (2.7 percent of the population). As the result of improved disease prevention and health care, more people are also expected to survive into their 10th decade. Because of the increase in the very old population, it is increasingly possible that older people will themselves have at least one surviving parent (U.S. Bureau of the Census, 1984).

Perceptions of this stage of the life cycle differ significantly among aging families. Some persons are miserable, while others feel these are the best years of their lives. Much is dependent on the adequacy of financial resources, the ability to maintain a satisfactory home, and the individual's health status. Those who have lost their independence due to ill health generally have low morale; and poor physical health is often an antecedent to mental illness among the elderly (Lowenthal, 1972). Conversely, those elders who have maintained their health, have kept active, and have adequate economic resources represent a substantial proportion of older people and usually feel positive about this stage of life.

Society's Attitude Toward the Elderly. Our society emphasizes the achievements of those in the young adult years, glorifying the period of youth. Therefore, adults, through grooming, dress, and styles, try to maintain their youthful appearance as long as possible. Aging has always meant losing hair, friends, aspirations, and strength. For both the community at large and individual families, dealing with the aged has had a negative connotation, one loaded with feelings of being burdened down with imposing problems. Additionally, society has not allowed most aged people to remain productive. Hence, society's negative appraisal of older people has negatively affected their self-image.

Yet today many associations and much of the literature advocate and illustrate the strengths, resources, and other positive aspects of aging. This has begun to diminish the negativism and stereotypic thinking about the aged and help us recognize the assets of the older person and the great diversity of life-styles among members of this age group.

Our attitudes towards aging and the aged, albeit still negative, appear to be changing. Recent studies conducted on society's attitude toward the elderly have validated that the elderly are being viewed more positively (Austin, 1985; Schonfield, 1982). McCubbin and Dahl (1985) report that "many observers believe that age is regaining respect in the United States. A new generation of old people—better educated, more affluent, healthier and more active than previous elderly generations—is redefining the notion of 'being old'" (p. 276). This change in attitude will, in turn, enhance the elderly's image of themselves.

Losses Common to Aging People and Families. As aging progresses and retirement becomes a reality, there is a variety of stressors or losses experienced by the majority of older people and couples that confounds their role transition. These include the following:

- Economic—Adjusting to a substantially reduced income; later perhaps adjusting to economic dependency (depending on family or government for subsidy).
- Housing—Often moving to smaller quarters and later perhaps forced to move to an institutional setting.
- Social—Loss (death) of siblings, friends, and spouse.
- Work—Mandatory retirement and loss of the work role and a sense of productivity.
- Health—Declining physical, mental, and cognitive functions; caregiving for the less healthy spouse.

Retirement. With the loss of both the parental and the occupational roles, a substantial reorientation on the part of older individuals and couples becomes necessary. Retirement requires a resocialization to new roles and a new life-style. What such changes entail, however, is not entirely clear, because the roles and norms for the older person are ambiguous. Women who have been completely engrossed in their mothering role and husbands and/or wives who have been completely involved in their work, predictably, will have the greatest degree of difficulty adjusting. To fill the work vacuum, many men increasingly engage in domestic activities and assume a more expressive role, a change demanding a role shift on the part of the wife as well. The retired husband's adjustment to the sharing of household tasks depends on his value system. If he sees this type of activity as "woman's work" and considers it demeaning to him, he will feel devalued in such an activity. Troll (1971) found this attitude more true of the working-class man, who values the traditional breadwinner role more than the middle-class man. Retirement for women tends to be less difficult to adapt to as they still have their domestic roles to fall back on. Furthermore, women are more likely to retire by choice.

In any case, retirement necessitates role modification and is a time when, at least temporarily, declines in self-esteem, income, status, and health are frequently seen. But in spite of these new demands and losses, most older people report positive attitudes toward retirement (Kell and Patton, 1978).

Family Developmental Tasks. Maintaining satisfying living arrangements is a most important task of aging families (Table 6–11). Housing after retirement often becomes problematic. In the years immediately following retirement, the couple usually remains in its home until property taxes, neighborhood conditions, size or condition of house, or health forces it to find more modest accommodations. Although a majority of older people own their own homes, a substantial proportion of these are old and often rundown, and many are located in high-crime areas where older people are

TABLE 6–11. TWO-PARENT NUCLEAR FAMILY LIFE CYCLE STAGE VIII AND CONCOMITANT FAMILY DEVELOPMENTAL TASKS

Family Life Cycle Stage	Family Developmental Tasks
Families in the later years	1. Maintaining a satisfying living arrangement. 2. Adjusting to a reduced income. 3. Maintaining marital relationships. 4. Adjusting to loss of spouse. 5. Maintaining intergenerational family ties. 6. Continuing to make sense out of one's existence (life review and integration).

Adapted from Carter and McGoldrick (1988), Duvall and Miller (1985).

likely to be victims. Often, the elderly remain in these homes because no suitable options exist (Kalish, 1975). Nonetheless, older persons living in their own homes are generally better adjusted than those who live in their children's homes. Older people usually move in with one of their children because of a decline in health or economic status, not by choice, and this has proven to be a less satisfying arrangement for the elderly (Lopata, 1973).

One's living arrangements is a powerful predictor of well-being among the elderly (Berresi et al, 1984). Relocation is a traumatic experience for the elderly, whether it is a voluntary or involuntary move. It means leaving behind neighborhood ties and friendships that have provided the elderly with a sense of security and stability. Relocation means separation from one's heritage and the cues that bolster old memories (Lawton, 1980). Relocation does not affect all of the elderly in the same way. Given adequate preparation and careful planning of the change, the new environment may have positive impact on the elderly. Nevertheless, some research findings suggest that when older people move, some deterioration of their health often results (Lawton, 1985).

Only about 5 percent of older people live in institutions. The infirm are often forced to enter board-and-care, retirement, or nursing homes because of the lack of assistance in the home. The provision of full-time help in the home or, more feasibly, part-time health and homemaker services through a home health agency or homemaker agency, is more humane and protective of the older person's need to remain in his or her own home and retain his or her independence as long as possible, as well as less costly than institutionalization. Albeit difficult, one of the mates and/or grown children of the couple (or the remaining parent) often have to decide what is the best path to take—home health services, retirement home, nursing home, or living with grown children.

Adjusting to a reduced income is a second developmental task for the aging family. When men retire, there is an immediate drop in income, and usually as the years pass by, this income becomes less and less adequate because of the steady rise in cost of living and the depletion of savings. In 1989 one fifth of the older U.S. population was poor or near poor (AARP, 1990).

Older people have substantially less cash income than those under 65. The elderly rely heavily on Social Security benefits and asset income. More older women tend to be poor; nearly 71.8 percent of the elderly population are women. Black and Hispanic elderly have substantially lower money incomes as well as lower median incomes than their white counterparts (U.S. Senate Special Committee on Aging, 1987–1988).

Because of the frequency of long-term health problems, health expenses are a major financial concern. The elderly spend more on health care—both in actual dollars and as a percentage of total expenditure—than the nonelderly. Medicare has certainly alleviated part of this problem, but there are still unpredictable, and many times substantial, out-of-pocket expenses to be paid. For instance, Part B of Medicare covers only 80 percent of "reasonable" costs for medical services. And because of a fee-for-service type of payment system, some physicians will also have the patient return many more times for office visits than is absolutely necessary to provide safe and effective medical care. Medicaid is also available to those who are medically indigent and qualify for Supplementary Security Income (SSI). This health insurance program then supplements Medicare coverage.

As average life expectancy increases, more older people will spend more years with severely limiting medical problems. Even though women outlive men, and the gap in life expectancies between men and women is increasing, more married couples are surviving longer. Problems of caring for an elderly couple are often more difficult than providing for a widowed pensioner. Little consideration has been given to providing for the family unit in this phase of the life cycle, during which people have an increased likelihood of living in poverty as a result of the increased costs of health and social problems.

Maintaining marital relationships, a third developmental task, continues to be paramount to the family's happiness. Marriages perceived as satisfying in the later years usually have a long positive history, and vice versa. Research has also shown that marriage contributes greatly to both morale and continued activity of both older spouses (Lee, 1978).

One of the myths of old age is that sex drives and sexual activities are no longer possible (or should not exist). Considerable research has shown just the reverse, however. Such studies have found that although there is a slowing down of sexual capacity, the pleasure in sexual activity continues and may even increase (Lobsenz, 1975). Ill health sometimes diminishes the sex drive, but usually the lack of sexual activity is due to socio-emotional problems.

Adjusting to the loss of spouse, the fourth developmental task, is in general, the most traumatic developmental task. As the following statistics demonstrate, older women suffer the loss of spouse more than men do. According to statistics for 1986, three fourths of all older men were living with their spouses while only 38 percent of older women were living with their spouses. 51 percent were widowed (U.S. Senate Special Committee on Aging, 1987–1988).

In comparison with young groups, the aged are aware of dying as part of the normal process of living. One study reported that only 3 out of 80 dying elderly patients found it hard to discuss death (Duvall, 1977). The awareness of death does not, however, mean that the spouse left behind will find adjustment to loss easier. Loss of spouse takes its toll—the widowed die earlier than their married counterparts, and the living are more likely to have a serious health problem (social isolation, being suicidal or mentally ill). In addition, the loss of a spouse demands a total reorganization of family functions. This is especially difficult to achieve satisfactorily, since the loss has depleted the emotional and economic resources needed to deal with the change. For women this means a shift from mutual dependency and sharing activities of family living to being alone or associating with a group of unattached older women. For men the loss of spouse means the loss of a companion, as well as linkage to kin, family, and the social world in general. The aged widower does not have the same interest in or the ability to perform the homemaker-housekeeper roles and is often likely to need assistance in meal preparation, homemaking, and general care.

The extent of the difficult adjustment can be seen by the increase in suicides within the group of individuals over 65. Even though there is some increase in suicides among women over 65, the preponderance of suicides is found within the older male population. A review of suicide studies among this group showed that attempted and completed suicides often followed the loss of the mate (Rushing, 1968).

Studies of the widowed have consistently verified the difficult living conditions and life of the widowed. The widowed have lower morale and fewer social roles and ties than the married of the same age group. They have significantly less money to live on and are found to take poor care of themselves in terms of diet, exercise, alcohol, and tobacco consumption (Hutchison, 1975). Bild and Havighurst (1976), in a large study of the elderly in Chicago, reported that the loss of a spouse removed the strongest support of the elderly person, although children, when available, usually stepped in to fill the vacuum somewhat. Much more isolated still were the "never marrieds" and the childless widowed.

A fifth developmental task deals with the maintenance of intergenerational family ties. Although there is a tendency for the older person to disengage from social relationships, the family remains the focus of the aging person's social interactions and the primary source of social support. As the older person withdraws from activities in the surrounding world, relationships with spouse, children, grandchildren, and siblings become more important. The majority of older Americans live close by extended family members and have frequent contact with them (Harris et al, 1975; Shanas, 1968, 1980). Hence, family members are an important source of direct assistance and social interaction. Older families are found generally to reciprocate in the giving of help to the extent to which they are capable.

As people age they must continue to make sense out of their existence. Reminiscing about one's past life, called life review, is a common and vital activity, because it represents a search for the central meaning of life. It is viewed as a sixth "cognitive type" developmental task. Its importance lies in the fact that life review eases the adjustment to difficult situations and provides insight into past events. The elderly are concerned with the quality of their life and being able to live with respect, meaning, and dignity (Duvall, 1977).

Health Concerns. According to the 1987 to 1988 report prepared by the U.S. Senate Special Committee on Aging, the elderly are the heaviest users of health services. More than four out of five elderly have at least one chronic condition, and multiple conditions are commonplace among the elderly. The elderly made up 12 percent of the total population, but they use 33 percent of health care expenditures in the United States.

Factors such as diminishing physical vigor and function, inadequate financial resources, social isolation, loneliness, and the many other losses that the older person experiences demonstrate some of the psychophysiological vulnerabilities of human aging (Kelley et al, 1977). Therefore, multiple health concerns exist. Assisting the aging couple or individual with all phases of a chronic illness, from the acute phase through the rehabilitation phase, is needed. Both medically related functions (physical assessment, reporting untoward reactions) and nursing functions (assessing the client's response to illness and treatment and his or her coping abilities) are relevant here. Health promotion continues to be of critical importance, especially in areas of nutrition, exercise, injury prevention, safe use of medicines, use of preventive services, and smoking cessation.

Social isolation, depression, cognitive impairment (which may be related to a number of sources including Alzheimer's disease), and other psychological problems are serious health concerns, particularly when combined with physical ill health. Assessment and use of the family's or individual social support system should be an integral part of family health care.

The process of aging and declining health makes it necessary for marital partners to help each other. Because women live longer than men, on the average, they are usually the ones to take care of their ailing or disabled husbands. In most cases the illnesses are chronic and progressively disabling, so that there is time to adjust to the eventuality of the situation. Husbands find the task of caring for a wife more difficult, because the caretaker, nurturant, and homemaker roles are still seen largely as female roles.

Nutritional deficiencies are extensive among the elderly and contribute to many problems associated with aging (fatigue, confusion, depression, and constipation, to name a few).

Related problems of housing, a suitable income, adequate recreational and health care facilities adversely affect the elderly's health status. The incidence of falls and other accidents in the home is great, so that environmental safety measures are an important need. Government programs do not adequately provide secure retirement, as clearly demonstrated in problems concerned with the use of nursing homes, long-term board-and-care facilities, and mental hospitals as dumping grounds for the aged.

Family-centered health professionals can provide much indirect help by referring the older couple or individual to appropriate community resources to ameliorate their problems. Some of these community resources are:

> (1) senior centers that offer recreation, continuing-education programs, some health and (occasionally) legal services. . . ; (2) information and referral services that give relevant information in response to a telephone call or visit; (3) homemakers' services, including cooking and cleaning and providing social relationships—services that enable some elderly people to remain in their own homes rather than be relocated in institutions. . . ; (4) geriatric day-care facilities, in which older persons receive supervision and a variety of services during the day—usually restricted to individuals who are not capable of using senior centers; (5) nutritional programs, some of which transport recipients to a central location to eat and some of which, like the Meals-on-Wheels program, transport food to people who are not ambulatory; (6) the Foster Grandparent program, a federally subsidized program that pays low-income elderly people a small amount to care for, tutor, or play with institutionalized children; (7) the Retired Senior Volunteer Program, also federally subsidized, helping elderly persons to provide community services (Kalish, 1975, p. 117); and (8) case management services.

FAMILY LIFE CYCLE STAGES IN DIVORCED FAMILIES

One of the major variations in the family life cycle is seen when parents divorce. Although the great majority of families still consist of married couples, one of the most profound changes taking place over the past two decades has been the rise in divorces and female-headed households (88 percent of single-parent families are mother–child(ren) families). From 1970 to 1984 the number of one-parent families doubled (from 3.2 million in 1970 to 6.7 million in 1984) while the number of divorced couples increased by almost 300 percent (U. S. Bureau of the Census, 1986). Divorces are so common today (almost 50 percent of all marriages end in divorce) that the event is being viewed as a normative transition.

The single-parent, divorced family passes through the same life cycle stages, with most of the same responsibilities, as the two-parent nuclear family. The basic difference is the absence of the second parent to carry his or her (mostly his) share of the family tasks with respect to support, child rearing, companionship, and gender role modeling for the children. Hill (1986) explains that "the differences in paths of development of single-parent and two-parent families are seen primarily, not in stages encountered, but in the number, timing and length of the critical transitions experienced" (p. 28).

Carter and McGoldrick (1988) conceptualize divorce as an interruption or dislocation of the traditional family life cycle. Divorce, with its losses and shifts in family membership, creates major family destabilization and disequilibrium. Peck and Manocharian (1988) underscore the emotional and physical impact of divorce on the family. "Divorce affects family members at every generational level throughout the nuclear and extended family, thus producing a crisis for the family as a whole as well as for each individual within the family" (p. 335).

As with the two-parent nuclear family, there are crucial changes in roles and relationships and important family developmental tasks to be completed in order for the divorced family to move forward developmentally (Carter and McGoldrick, 1988). As a major disruptive force, divorce compounds the complexity of the developmental tasks the family is experiencing. Each subsequent life cycle stage is also affected, so that each postdivorce stage must be viewed within the context of both the stage itself and the consequences of the divorce.

After the divorce, family systems research has found that it takes about 1 to 3 years for the family to restabilize itself. "If a family can negotiate the crisis and the accompanying transitions that must be experienced in order to restabilize, it will have established a more fluid system that will allow a continuation of the normal family developmental process" (Peck and Manocharian, 1988, p. 335). Carter and McGoldrick have summarized the research and writings of Ahrons (1980) on the process of adjustment that divorced families go through. Table 6–12 outlines the pre- and postdivorce adjustment process, including concomitant emotional processes and family developmental issues.

To describe the impact of the divorce on the family life cycle stages, it first should be said that the impact varies depending on what stage the family is in when the divorce occurs. Other factors also make a difference in impact, such as ethnic, social, and economic factors. Divorce is the least disruptive during the first stage of marriage as there are fewer people involved, fewer traditions established, and fewer couple-based social ties (Peck and Manocharian, 1988). The impact is much greater during the third and fourth stages in those families with preschool and school-aged children. Moreover, the family is most at risk for divorce during these periods.

Young children are initially most affected by parents' divorce. Children may regress developmentally, making child rearing and separation of parents and children difficult. Single parenthood is often very onerous for the mother, who usually struggles both emotionally and economically. (Economic status of female-headed divorced families declines considerably following divorce.) A major and frequently seen problem is that the father loses his sense of connection to his children and/or the mother's attachment to the children and anger at the father leaves no room for the father. Yet maintaining both the mother–child and father–child relationships is very important for both parents and children. Unfortunately, for both father and children, a large proportion of children virtually lose contact with the father after the divorce (Hagestad, 1988).

When divorce occurs among families with school-aged children, the long-term impact of the divorce is even more profound on the school-aged child. Six to eight years of age was the age group that had the hardest time adjusting to divorce in one study (Wallerstein and Kelly, 1980). Children are old enough at that time to realize what is happening, but not to deal effectively with the divorce.

Families with adolescents are often already in turmoil, and divorce compounds the problem. For the single parent, raising the adolescent alone is difficult. Coparenting is also problematic when the adolescent is having behavior problems. Progressing through the developmental tasks of adolescence and the family life cycle is initially delayed.

In later stages of the family life cycle, children are likely to be affected less profoundly than in the previous family life cycle stages because they are older and better able to cope and function more autonomously. In the case of midlife divorce, older children may, however, be propelled into filial maturity, accepting of the dependency of a parent, particularly the mother, when a parent turns to a child for support during the divorce crisis.

During these later family life cycle stages, divorce is typically profoundly traumatizing to the divorced partners. Years of shared possessions, memories, and habits have created "a couple identity." Divorce during later years is likened to a death of a partner in some of the divorce literature.

LIFE CYCLE STAGES IN STEP-PARENT FAMILIES

Divorce is commonly a transitional state, followed by remarriage. Remarriage was so prevalent in the mid-1980s that nearly one half of all marriages were remarriages (U.S. Bureau of the Census, 1986). Before age 40 both men and women are remarrying fairly equally, but after age 40 remarriage is disproportionately a male transition (Hagestad, 1988).

In Table 6–13 Carter and McGoldrick (1988) present a developmental outline of the remarried family formation—the steps involved in the remarriage process, the prerequisite attitudes, and the developmental issues. The family's emotional process at the transition to remarriage is typically one that involves struggling with fears about investment in a new marriage and a new family; dealing with hostile or upset reactions of the children, extended families, and the

TABLE 6–12. DISLOCATIONS OF THE FAMILY LIFE CYCLE BY DIVORCE, REQUIRING ADDITIONAL STEPS TO RESTABILIZE AND PROCEED DEVELOPMENTALLY

	Phase	Emotional Process of Transition—Prerequisite Attitude	Developmental Issues
Divorce			
1.	The decision to divorce	Acceptance of inability to resolve marital tensions sufficiently to continue relationship.	Acceptance of one's own part in the failure of the marriage.
2.	Planning the breakup of the system	Supporting viable arrangements for all parts of the system.	a. Working cooperatively on problems of custody, visitation, and finances. b. Dealing with extended family about the divorce.
3.	Separation	a. Willingness to continue cooperative coparental relationship and joint financial support of children. b. Work on resolution of attachment to spouse.	a. Mourning loss of intact family. b. Restructuring marital and parent–child relationships and finances; adaptation to living apart. c. Realignment of relationships with extended family; staying connected with spouse's extended family.
4.	The divorce	More work on emotional divorce: Overcoming hurt, anger, guilt, etc.	a. Mourning loss of intact family: giving up fantasies of reunion. b. Retrieval of hopes, dreams, expectations from the marriage. c. Staying connected with extended families.
Postdivorce family			
1.	Single-parent (custodial household or primary residence)	Willingness to maintain financial responsibilities, continue parental contact with exspouse, and support contact of children with exspouse and his or her family.	a. Making flexible visitation arrangements with exspouse and his or her family. b. Rebuilding own financial resources. c. Rebuilding own social network.
2.	Single-parent (noncustodial)	Willingness to maintain parental contact with exspouse and support custodial parent's relationship with children.	a. Finding ways to continue effective parenting relationship with children. b. Maintaining financial responsibilities to exspouse and children. c. Rebuilding own social network.

(From: Carter B and McGoldrick M, eds. *The Changing Family Life Cycle, 2nd ed.* New York: Gardner Press, 1988, p 22.)

ex-spouse; worrying about the ambiguous new family situation; feeling guilty and concerned over the welfare of the children; and renewing of attachments (negative or positive) to the exspouse. Remarriage, again because it is a disruptive transitional process, impedes the family's movement through and completion of family developmental tasks. Step-parent adjustment and integration, as with divorce adjustment, seems to take a minimum of 2 to 3 years before a new structure allows the family to move on developmentally (Carter and McGoldrick, 1988).

IMPACT OF ILLNESS AND DISABILITY ON FAMILY DEVELOPMENTAL STAGES

Serious illness or long-term disability of a family member significantly affects the family and its functioning,

TABLE 6–13. REMARRIED FAMILY FORMATION: A DEVELOPMENTAL OUTLINE

Steps	Prerequisite Attitude	Developmental Issues
1. Entering the new relationship	Recovery from loss of first marriage (adequate "emotional divorce").	Recommitment to marriage and to forming a family with readiness to deal with the complexity and ambiguity.
2. Conceptualizing and planning new marriage and family	Accepting one's own fears and those of new spouse and children about remarriage and forming a stepfamily. Accepting need for time and patience for adjustment to complexity and ambiguity of: 1. Multiple new roles. 2. Boundaries: space, time, membership, and authority. 3. Affective Issues: guilt, loyalty conflicts, desire for mutuality, unresolvable past hurts.	a. Work on openness in the new relationships to avoid pseudomutuality. b. Plan for maintenance of cooperative financial and coparental relationships with ex-spouses. c. Plan to help children deal with fears, loyalty conflicts, and membership in two systems. d. Realignment of relationships with extended family to include new spouse and children. e. Plan maintenance of connections for children with extended family of ex-spouses(s).
3. Remarriage and reconstitution of family	Final resolution of attachment to previous spouse and ideal of "intact" family; acceptance of a different model of family with permeable boundaries.	a. Restructuring family boundaries to allow for inclusion of new spouse/step-parent. b. Realignment of relationships and financial arrangements throughout subsystems to permit interweaving of several systems. c. Making room for relationships of all children with biological (noncustodial) parents, grandparents, and other extended family. d. Sharing memories and histories to enhance stepfamily integration.

(From: Carter B and McGoldrick M, eds. *The Changing Family Life Cycle, 2nd ed.* New York: Gardner Press, 1988, p 24.)

just as the behavior of the family and its members significantly affects the course and characteristics of the illness or disability (Bahnson, 1987). Given this widely accepted assumption, it is clear that serious illness or disability profoundly influences family development, as well as individual family member development, especially of the sick or disabled member. Often when a family is delayed in meeting its family developmental tasks, it is the interaction of the developmental demands/stressors and a situational demand/stressor that compounds and overloads the family. The added family stress created by the presence of both types of stressors often results in lowered family functioning, whereby mastering of family developmental tasks becomes impeded or retarded.

The extent to which family developmental tasks are affected depends on several factors. One is certainly the family life cycle stage that the family is in; secondly, which family member becomes seriously ill or disabled makes a difference. Some particular life cycle stages are already developmentally hazardous, and certain individuals in the family are more central in terms of completing family developmental tasks of a particular stage. For instance, in a family with a teenager, if the adolescent sustains a serious injury and is left in a dependent state, this will greatly impede the adolescent's own mastery of the developmental task of becoming more independent from the family. Likewise the family developmental task dealing with balancing freedom with responsibility so as to assist the teenager to become increasingly autonomous will also be impeded. The challenge for the family is to attempt to resume working on normal developmental family tasks as soon as possible.

Another major factor that makes a difference in regards to the impact of illness or disability on family development is the formal and informal resources the family is utilizing. A good social support system of extended family and friends, as well as competent, helpful health and psychosocial supports, will augment the family's ability to more quickly get back on track developmentally.

When working with a family with a serious illness or disability, it is useful to compare the "ideal" family developmental tasks within the appropriate family life cycle stage with the family's actual behavior (Friedman, 1987). This type of comparison is useful in evaluating the probable impact of the illness or disability on the family.

ASSESSMENT AREAS: DEVELOPMENTAL STAGE AND HISTORY OF THE FAMILY

Throughout the assessment process, a focus on the family life cycle enhances the family health professional's understanding of the stresses that are impinging on the family and the actual or potential problems of the family. In completing the developmental part of a family assessment, the following areas are suggested:

1. The family's present developmental stage.
2. The extent to which the family is fulfilling the developmental tasks appropriate for the present developmental stage. It is important to note any significant deviations from the norm, as this may serve as an indication of impending or present problems.
3. The family's history from inception through present day, including developmental history and unique health and health-related events and experiences (eg, divorce, deaths, losses) that happened in the family's life. Some of this information (divorces, marriages, deaths) can be included on the family genogram (see Chap. 8 for the family genogram).
4. Both parents' families of origin (what life in family of origin was like; present and past relations with parents of parents).

As mentioned, both the family's common and unique experiences and perceptions as they progress through the family life cycle should be assessed to make the developmental history more comprehensive. A history of the family should also include a description of each parent's family of origin, because it is clear that the intergenerational influences on family life are crucial.

It may be more significant to elicit the developmental history from some families than others. It is important to make sure the family you are working with is open to exploring their past and that your collection of historic data in any of the suggested areas is relevant for understanding and working with the family.

To reiterate, developmental or historic data on a family can be gleaned by (1) asking about common experiences and tasks and how these were accomplished and perceived and (2) asking about special or unique family problems or experiences. The latter include divorces, deaths in nuclear or extended family, separations due to illness or military service, unemployment, and so forth. Asking parents about their present and past relationships with their family of orientation and what life in the original family was like gives the family-centered nurse a better appreciation and understanding of the parents during their formative years.

In order to elicit a family history, Satir (1983), begins by having parents first talk about their own marital relationship, focusing on this relationship because the parents are the family architects. Satir and the parents with the children present when appropriate, discuss the following areas:

- First meeting of the couple, their relationship prior to marriage, and how they decided to get married.
- Any obstacles to their marriage. Their responses to getting married.
- Marriage without the children; how they established tasks and roles.
- What life was like in both original family environments, including both parents' families of orientation.
- Any other people who live or have lived with the family.
- Relationships with in-laws.
- Description of each mate's parents and their relationship with them.
- Plans for and arrival of each new child. Were children planned? What was the impact of the arrival of each child?
- How much time does family spend together?
- Daily routine of family life.

Smoyak (1975), in her nursing practice as a family therapist, stresses the significance of assessing the parents' respective families of orientation:

> It is important to know how each present parent was reared and what lessons in childrearing were learned. How the two present parents put together their different backgrounds in childrearing is easier to understand when the background of each has been described. For instance, a German-Jew married to an English Protestant who live as a nuclear unit produce a very different set of mutual expectations than do two Catholic . . . Mexican-Americans living in an extended family. (p. 8)

She also inquires into each parent's ordinal position among their siblings, quoting Toman's (1961) work on family constellation, which showed that this position greatly influences the type of interactions and relationships one is likely to have with others, as well as one's personality development. For instance, Toman found that first-born children were more apt to be leaders than followers, while the reverse was more common among the last-born child. Another point of inquiry related to the couple's families of origin involves the state of health and marriage of the mates' own parents. Are they still alive, well, married, living together, residing nearby, or geographically distant? (Smoyak, 1975)

One of the ways family nurses obtain a better idea of the process of the family system over time, as well as assess the intergenerational family system is to construct a genogram. The genogram is a type of genealogical chart that traces the kinship history of families. It is widely used by family therapists, the advantage being that one can organize a large, unwieldy amount of data in a way that makes it comprehensible and helps reveal important patterns and themes in families (Hartman and Laird, 1983; McGoldrick and Gerson, 1985). Chapter 8 contains both a genogram and instructions for completing this type of family tree.

FAMILY NURSING INTERVENTIONS

One important goal of family nursing is to help families and their members move toward completion of individual and family developmental tasks (Friedman, 1987). Mastery of one set of family developmental tasks allows the family to progress developmentally to the next stage of family development. Family developmental tasks, if unfulfilled, produce dysfunctional families (Mattessich and Hill, 1987).

To accomplish this goal, the family nurse "assists families to achieve and maintain a balance between the personal growth needs of individual family members and optimum family functioning" (family developmental needs) (American Nurses' Association Division on Maternal and Child Health Nursing Practice, 1983). The balance between individual and group developmental needs is not easily achieved, particularly during certain stages, creating dissonance when an imbalance occurs.

When working with troubled families and individuals, family developmental theory helps family health professionals think about life cycle events that have established the context within which family and individual problems occur. Hence, it is important during both the diagnostic and planning phases that a developmental perspective be incorporated into family nursing practice.

It is also significant to incorporate a family developmental perspective into one's family nursing practice when working with healthy families. With healthy families, anticipatory guidance and teaching is often indicated in order to fulfill primary prevention goals (Bobak et al, 1989). Family nursing diagnoses, plans, and interventions should cover potential problems families may encounter because of the need to transform family structures so that family developmental tasks be accomplished. Helping families anticipate and go through different normative transitions in family life is a most germane family nursing goal.

The family nurse and other family clinicians assist families by teaching and counseling modalities. Referral to social support groups, such as a group for parents of infants or older ill parents, is also very helpful. Chapter 18 discusses general family nursing interventions in detail.

☐ STUDY QUESTIONS

1. Family developmental theory is built on some basic assumptions. What are these? (List at least three.)

Choose the correct answer(s) to the following questions.

2. Usually reliable predictions can be made regarding the common health concerns and forces that are at play within a family if the family nurse knows (select one answer):
   a. The developmental tasks of each member.
   b. The family life cycle stage.
   c. Where the family lives and their social class.
   d. The composition of the family

3. Which of the following illustrate the value of the developmental approach when assessing and working with families? (Choose all correct responses.)
   a. Gives cues as to the family's past problems and progress.
   b. Forecasts a given family's future needs.
   c. Views the common experiences of families during each of the life cycle stages.
   d. Highlights critical periods of family and individual growth and development.
   e. Helps to anticipate what to expect in terms of health concerns.
   f. Better able to evaluate the family normatively.

4. The best definition for the family life cycle is:
   a. Predictable stages within the history of the family.
   b. The growth and developmental stages of each family member as he or she progresses throughout life.
   c. Successive phases of growth and development of the family as a unit through its existence.

5. Family developmental tasks have these characteristics (choose all correct answers):
   a. They change in response to cultural imperatives and the family's unique aspirations and values.
   b. They change in response to the developmental needs of its members.
   c. They remain constant throughout the family's existence.
   d. They adapt the family's broad functions to meet the specific tasks of each stage.
   e. They satisfy the biological requirements of the family as a whole.
   f. They avoid clashing with individual needs.
   g. They are growth requirements that must be achieved by the family during each life cycle stage.
   h. Failure to achieve developmental tasks leads to difficulty in achieving later developmental tasks.
   i. Developmental tasks cover only aspects that directly influence psychosocial (interactional) components of family functioning.

6. The developmental approach seeks to explain family dynamics in terms of its:
   a. Unique elements.
   b. Common elements in its history as a family.
   c. Both common and unique elements of family history.

7. The developmental tasks of the family result from a combination of (more than one answer):
   a. Individual developmental tasks of family members.
   b. Sexual norms.
   c. Chronological ages and school placement.
   d. Community pressures for family to conform to societal norms.
   e. General family functions adapted to specific life cycle stages.

8. The stage of the family life cycles are defined by Duvall in terms of (select one answer):
   a. The age and school placement of the oldest child.
   b. The ages of the parents.
   c. The age of the middle child, if present.
   d. Years of marriage.

Complete the following outlines.

9. In the outline below, list the following:
—The eight phases in the family life cycle for the two-parent nuclear family (excluding the transition stage).
—A definition for each phase.
—Three basic health concerns (biopsychosocial and health concerns) Frequently present and appropriate for intervention by family nurse.

FAMILY LIFE CYCLE STAGE	DEFINITION OF PHASE	HEALTH CONCERNS OR NEEDS
I.		1.
		2.
		3.
II.		1.
		2.
		3.
III.		1.
		2.
		3.
IV.		1.
		2.
		3.
V.		1.
		2.
		3.
VI.		1.
		2.
		3.
VII.		1.
		2.
		3.
VIII.		1.
		2.
		3.

10. Within each of the eight life cycle stages of the family, identify the developmental tasks of parents as described by Friedman.

LIFE CYCLE STAGE	DEVELOPMENTAL TASK(S) OF PARENT
I.	1.
II.	1.
	2.
III.	1.
IV.	1.
V.	1.
	2.
VI.	1.
VII.	1.
VIII.	1.

Chose the correct answer(s) to the following question.

11. When does the marriage relationship, according to studies, appear to be the strongest and most satisfying?
a. Stage of preschool children.

b. Stage of childbearing families.
c. Stage of marriage.
d. The postparental period (middle-aged parents).
e. Stage of the contracting family (aging family).
f. Stage of families launching young adults.

12. Give the three aspects of the adolescent process that explain the developmental tasks and problems faced in this stage.

13. What is usual impact of adolescent family members on family as a whole?

*For each question from 14 to 21, select the lettered choice that applies to it.**

a. Beginning families
b. Childbearing families
c. Families with preschool children
d. Families with school-age children
e. Families with teenagers
f. Families as launching centers
g. Families in the middle years
h. Aging families

14. Beginning of loosening of family ties.

15. Reaching maximum size in number of members and of interrelationships.

16. Being totally responsible for the first time for another human being.

17. Establishing a home base.

18. Releasing members into lives of their own.

19. Rediscovery of couple as husband and wife.

20. Learning to supply adequate space, facilities, and equipment for a rapidly expanding family.

21. Dealing with death of spouse.

22. Which of the following descriptions apply to the single-parent or divorced family with respect to its development?
a. The single-parent or divorced family passes through the same family life cycle stages.
b. The characteristics of the family life cycle—after the divorce—differs because of the absence of a second parent in the family.
c. The single-parent or divorced family skips one or two of the family life cycle stages, depending on when the divorce occurred.
d. The timing of the family life cycle transitions will probably be delayed in the immediate postdivorce period.

23. In the step-parent family, remarriage creates initial crisis and destabilization. How generally does remarriage affect the family life cycle stages?

* *These questions are from Borlick M, et al.* Nursing Examination Review Book, *Vol 9:* Community Health Nursing. *2nd ed. Flushing, NY: Medical Examination Publishing Company; 1974.*

24. What general areas (name three) would you assess to gather information about family development and the family's history?

25. What broad family nursing interventions are appropriate for families having actual or potential developmental problems?

(An assessment question dealing with the developmental stage and history of the family is included in Chapter 9—the case study).

CHAPTER SEVEN

Systems Theory

Learning Objectives

1. Describe the characteristics of the paradigm associated with systems theory.
2. Define the following general systems theory terms: systems, social systems, open versus closed systems, differentiation, wholeness or nonsummativity, and feedback.
3. Relative to the family system, explain verbally or diagrammatically the family and its internal and external environment (the hierarchy of systems).
4. Apply the exchange and processing model (input-flow-output and feedback components) to the family system.
5. Compare the terms self-regulation, steady state, homeostasis, equilibrium, and adaptation.
6. Identify four prime characteristics of a family system.
7. Explain the significance of the family system and family subsystem boundaries.
8. Identify the three family interpersonal subsystems and explain their function.
9. Explain the term differentiation as it applies to the family system.
10. Name four characteristics of a successfully functioning, healthy family.

Three grand theories—developmental theory, structural–functional theory, and general systems theory—are used in this text to formulate the family assessment areas and questions. These theories also suggest how family problems may be labeled, and goals and implementation strategies. Of the three selected theories, systems theory is clearly the most inclusive and powerful, as is so convincingly demonstrated by the wide number of fields and substantive areas that have adapted this model as their organizing framework.

Systems theory has received wide usage in such diverse areas as educational systems, game theory, computer science, systems engineering, cybernetics, and information and communication areas. Growth in the use of systems theory in the health care fields has been especially impressive within the last 25 years, as evidenced by the proliferation of books using this approach to study individuals, the family, nursing and other health care professionals, the health care delivery system, and the community.

Systems theory form the conceptual basis for "thinking systems" or for working with family systems as client rather than the individual client. The influence of systems theory has probably stimulated most of the attempts to achieve a systematic understanding of the normal and troubled family.

SYSTEMS CONCEPTS AND PROPOSITIONS

Von Bertalanffy (1950), a biologist, is credited with first delineating general systems theory in biology and physics, although sociologists prior to and concurrent with Von Bertalanffy's early publications were also describing systems—social systems (Parsons, 1951). In looking at human behavior, be it of an individual, a family, or a whole community, the systems approach is a valuable "umbrella" under which various more middle-range theoretical perspectives may be subsumed (such as the ecological perspective, family communication theory, information processing theory, and adaptation theory). Systems theory constitutes a way of explaining a unit—the family—as it relates and interacts with other systems. It is an organizational theory that is more concerned with studying and describing the way things interrelate together than with analyzing the things themselves (Braden, 1984). It explains how each discrete variable affects the whole and how the whole affects each part. Furthermore, systems theory can be applied across disciplines so that universal laws are useful in working with various types of systems (Lee and Lancaster, 1988).

A Holistic Paradigm

In recent years within the physical, social, and applied human sciences, we have witnessed a "systems" revolution (Hartman and Laird, 1983), a shift in thinking from mechanistic, outcome-oriented theories to holistic, process-oriented theories. General systems theory has allowed health care professionals to do this. Systems theories provide us with the concepts and framework to think in terms of facts and events in the *context* of wholes, rather than as being created and sustained in a vacuum: "Looking at the world in terms of sets of integrated relations constitutes the systems view" (Lazlo, 1972, p. 19 as cited in Hartman and Laird, 1983, p. 59).

Previous to this theoretical framework, the tendency was towards reduction and "parts analysis," which Young (1982) and those in the holistic health movement labeled "the mechanistic paradigm."

The mechanistic model, in seeking to analyze and explain phenomena, reduces them to their parts—in many cases to their smallest parts, to find cause-and-effect relationships. Medical science and most of the sciences tend to operate within this linear (straight-line cause-and-effect or "A leads to B"), atomistic, reductionistic, and highly analytic paradigm. For example, using the mechanistic paradigm and linear thinking, infections in humans are explained in terms of bacterial invasions of certain cells and organs.

In contrast to this traditional paradigm is the systems paradigm, which is holistic (looks at whole systems like individuals or families, with regard to their interconnectedness rather than separateness), and posits circular causality. From a systems perspective, infections in humans would be conceptualized as an imbalance in man's interaction with his environment—where factors in the host (the person) influence the infectious agent and the infectious agent likewise affects the host.

It was Bateson (1979), a cultural anthropologist who is considered to be the father of the family therapy movement, who stressed the limits of linear thinking with respect to living systems. He proposed that in order to understand human behavior a shift to looking at ongoing processes, interrelationships, and circular causality was needed. For instance, applying the systems paradigm to the family, there is no true victim and prosecutor in a troubled family. A particular entity (in this case a family member) is focused upon in relation to the things he or she affects and is affected by rather than in relation to his or her individual characteristics. Since both the "victim" and "prosecutor" in a family are serially and simultaneously affecting each other's roles and responses, only circular causality can adequately begin to explain the above situation (Fig. 7–1).

In the 1950s and 1960s, Parson's (1951) social systems theory was used by sociology, social work, and nursing (Johnson's nursing theory grew out of Parson's work) to explain personal and group behavior. General systems theory, à la Von Bertalanffy (1966), began to filter into nursing's thinking and literature (Rogers' and Roy's nursing models and the family therapy systems models are examples of this trend). The ecological systems perspective was derived from the general systems model. This perspective focuses primarily on the adaptive balance that exists between living systems and their environments (Hartman and Laird, 1983).

Two other systems-derived theories, again more middle-range in scope, also revolutionized family-centered practice. These were the theories of cybernetics and family communication processes. Cybernetics is a science that deals with communication and control theory. Both parts and wholes are examined in cybernetics relative to their patterns of organization (Keeney, 1982; Weiner, 1948). Cybernetics and general systems theory provided the legacy for family communication theories (Bateson, 1979; Jackson, 1969; Satir, 1983; Watzlawick, et al, 1967), the theory that modern-day family therapists most heavily rely on both in terms of assessment and intervention.

The basis for the system approach is the assumption that matter, in all its forms, living and nonliving, can be regarded as forming systems that have discrete properties capable of being studied. Using a systems theory

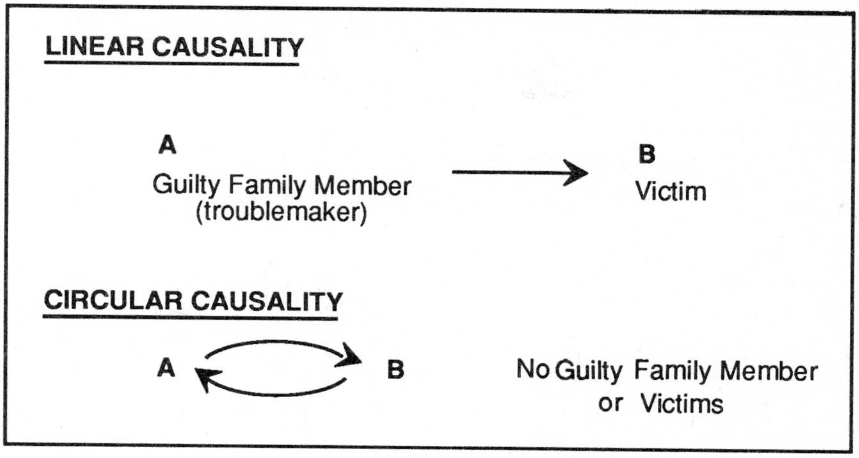

Figure 7–1
Comparison between linear and circular causality in a troubled family.

framework—namely, the organization of knowledge concerning the specific phenomena of interest as a complex system—one focuses on the *interaction among the various parts of the system* rather than on the function of the parts themselves (Buckley, 1967; Von Bertalanffy, 1966).

In the following discussion of systems theory, only the basic definitions and concepts used in a systems analysis of the family will be presented. Because these concepts are only briefly explained and systems theory is rather abstract, additional sources on this theory may be useful. The references in this chapter are suggested as supplementary reading to the discussion presented here.

DEFINITIONS OF CONCEPTS

Definitions of the following systems terms are eclectically derived. Three main sources were used: general systems theory, Parsons' (1951) social systems theory, and family systems theory from the family therapy field. Table 7–1 summarizes the main characteristics of system theory.

System. A system is defined as a goal-directed unit made up of interdependent, interacting parts that endure over a period of time. This system, together with its environment, make up a "universe," that is, the totality of what should be studied in a given situation. Systems and their parts have both functional and structural components. *Structure* pertains to the arrangement and organization among the parts of the system, whereas *function* refers to the purposes or goals of the system, such as activities necessary to assure the survival, continuity, and growth of the system. Function in systems analysis also is defined as the result or outcome of the structure.

Wholeness or Nonsummativity. A system is characterized by its property of wholeness or nonsummativity. The whole is greater than the sum of its parts, is the usual way that this concept is defined (Wright and Leahey, 1984; Young, 1982).

Social System. A social system is a model of social organization; it is a living system possessing a total unit distinctive from its component parts and distinguishable from its environment by a clearly defined boundary. Parsons and Bales (1955) define a social system as composed of two or more persons or social roles tied together by mutual interaction and interdependence (Anderson and Carter, 1974).

Open System. Systems are characterized on the basis of their degree of interaction with the surrounding environment. An open system exists in an environment

TABLE 7–1. KEY CHARACTERISTICS OF SYSTEMS THEORY

- Systems do not exist in a vacuum—the context in which systems function is critical.
- Interrelationships among parts of a system is the prime focus of a systems perspective.
- The whole is greater than the sum of its parts (nonsummativity).
- Whatever affects the system as a whole affects each of its parts.
- Causes and effects are interchangeable (circular causality notion).

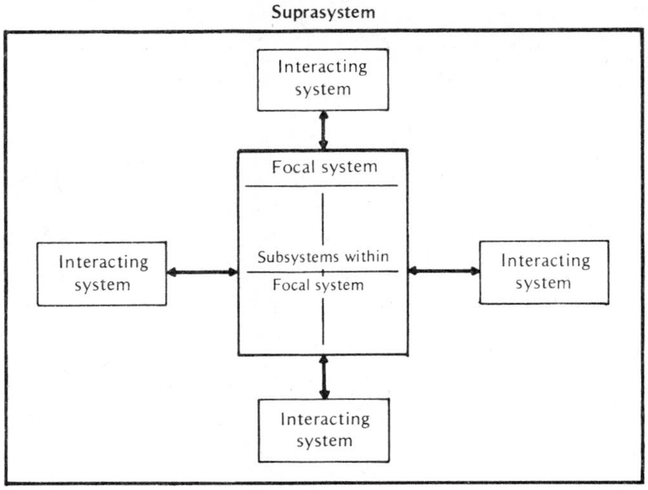

Figure 7–2
Schematic representation of the hierarchy of systems.

with which it interacts—from which it derives its inputs and to which it gives its outputs. This environmental interaction is necessary for its survival. (Buckley, 1967). By definition, all living systems are open systems.

Closed System. Theoretically, a closed system, in contrast to the open system, does not interact with the environment. A closed system would then be a self-contained unit, not dependent on continual environmental interchange for its survival. Because no totally closed system has yet been demonstrated in reality, "closed" denotes a relative lack of energy exchange across a system's boundaries (Parsons and Bales, 1955).

Hierarchy of Systems. No system functions in a vacuum. The system's universe, therefore, needs to be examined to determine its affect on the system under study. The universe—the system and its environment—contains a hierarchy of systems. Each higher-level unit contains lower-level systems. For instance, a hierarchy of systems from higher to lower levels might be as follows: community → family and other interacting systems → parental and other subsystems → individual organism → organ systems → tissues → cells. When using system theory as a working framework, one must be clear and specific about what system is being assessed. The system under study at a particular time is called the target or focal system. After specifying the target system, for example, the family, one would assess that system, and then the interacting systems within its environment, and finally its suprasystems and subsystems. In the case of the family focus, one would thus want to study the family *and* both its interacting, internal and external environments. The suprasystems are larger environmental systems of which the focal or target system is a part. The subsystems are smaller subunits or subcomponents of the focal system. For example, if the family is the focal system, then one suprasystem would be the family's cultural reference group and the subsystems would consist of the sets of family relationships (Fig. 7–2).

Boundaries. Each system has a boundary that demarcates the system from its environment. Auger (1976) explains that

> a boundary may be defined as a more or less open line forming a circle around the system where there is greater interchange of energy within the circle than on the outside. It is helpful to visualize a boundary as a "filter" which permits the constant exchange of elements, information, or energy between the system and its environment. . . . The more porous the filter, the greater the degree of interaction possible between the system and its environment. (p. 24)

In contrast, the less porous the boundary, the more isolated the system is from its environment. The ability of a boundary to control the degree of exchange is of great significance, because it regulates the amount and type of input from the environment at any time, enabling the system to maintain greater equilibrium (stability) or grow.

Input. As mentioned above, all open systems must receive input from their environment in order to survive. Input refers to such things as energy, matter, and information that the system receives and processes.

Flow and Transformation. Some input is immediately used by the system in its original state, while other forms of input must be transformed in order to be utilized by the system. In either case, the input must be processed. Whether unaltered or transformed, the processed input flows through the system and is released as output.

Output. The results of the system's processing of the input constitute the output. Output in the form of energy, matter, or information is released into the environment.

Feedback. Feedback refers to the process by which a system monitors the internal and environmental responses to its behavior (output) and accommodates or adjusts itself (Weiner, 1948). Feedback involves receiving and responding to the return of its own output. Information about how a system is functioning is looped back (feedback) from the output to the input, thus altering subsequent input (Goldenberg and Goldenberg, 1990). The system adjusts both internally by modification of subsystems and externally by controlling its boundaries. Thus it is able to control and modify inputs and outputs.

Feedback can be negative or positive feedback. *Positive feedback* refers to the system's output that is returned to the system as information that moves the system away from equilibrium and toward change. It involves amplifying feedback loops. Conversely *negative feedback* is informational output that is returned to the system, promoting equilibrium and stability of the system (Casey, 1989). The use of attenuating feedback loops maintain aspects of the system's functioning within prescribed limits (Goldenberg and Goldenberg, 1990). Figure 7–3 describes these last four terms diagrammatically.

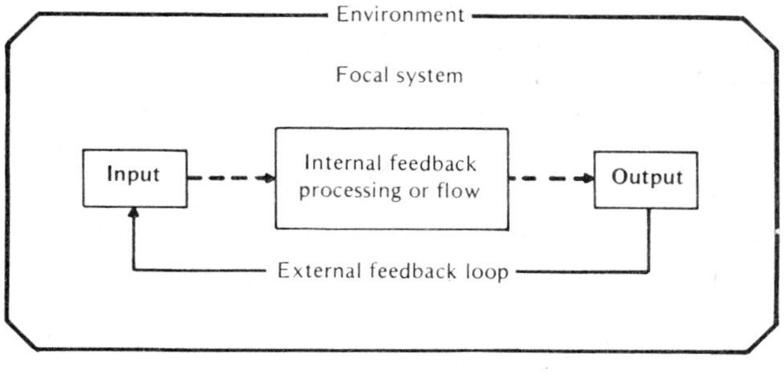

Figure 7–3
Energy, matter, and information exchange and processing model. (Adapted from Hazzard, 1971.)

Adaptation. A social, open system must continually adapt or adjust to demands and resources (inputs) from the outer environment and to its internal needs and changes. Adaptation is seen as the second component of feedback—that is, the system's adjustment to input. Adaptation can take two forms: (1) acceptance or rejection of incoming information or other input without change (assimilation is the acceptance of input without change) or (2) accommodation (modifying its structure in response to incoming information).

Self-regulation, Homeostasis, Steady State, and Equilibrium. All of these terms are used rather interchangeably in the literature, although there are fine distinctions between terms. Here only two distinctions will be pointed out. System self-regulation is a mechanism within systems that assists in balancing and controlling inputs and outputs, via feedback loops. When the system is in balance the result is homeostasis, a steady state, or equilibrium. This balance is not static, however, but dynamic and always changing within certain degrees of variation. Adaptation occurs through system self-regulatory mechanisms. The outcome of this regulation and adaptation is equilibrium, a steady state, or homeostasis (Hazzard, 1971).

Fishman (1985) asserts that when family members develop symptoms, these symptoms serve to maintain family homeostasis. For instance, if a child in a family "acts out" (consistently or over some time period), the focus of attention may shift from a conflictual marital relationship to how to manage the rebellious child.

Differentiation. General systems theory states that the growth and change toward a higher order of organization occur through differentiation. This term, then, denotes a living system's capability and propensity to progressively and serially advance to a higher order of complexity and organization. A social system, if acting normally, has a tendency to "grow" (called morphogenesis). The propensity to grow or change is counterbalanced by the tendency of a system to stabilize (return to a state of equilibrium or homeostasis). A balance between stability (called morphostasis) and change is needed for a system to grow or differentiate. Figure 7–4 illustrates the tendency for a system to have periods of both change and stability. Energy inputs flowing into the system are utilized for a system to grow in complexity and organization (Bowen, 1960).

Energy. "All dynamic, open systems require continuous supplies of energy in sufficient quantity so that demands for system integrity can be met." (Auger, 1976). The most important factor governing the amount of energy needed is the rate of utilization of

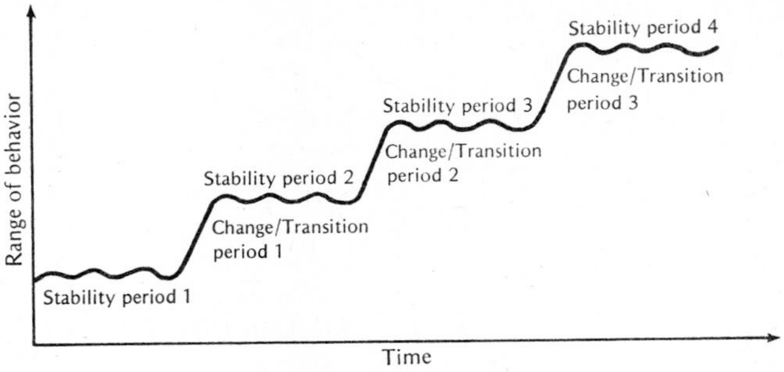

Figure 7–4
A system's tendency toward stability and change.

energy within the system itself. Systems with high levels of activity utilize large quantities of energy, and therefore must receive greater amounts of input from the environment in order to meet their energy demands. This, in turn, implies that the system's boundaries would have to be more open, or porous, to allow a greater input of energy.

FAMILY SYSTEMS DEFINITIONS

Family. The basic systems concepts and propositions will now be applied to the text's focal system, the family. The family is defined as a living social system. It is a small group of closely interrelated and interdependent individuals who are organized into a single unit so as to attain specific purposes, namely, family functions or goals. (See Chap. 5, where these functions are more fully discussed.)

Ripple Effect. The interrelationships found in a family system are so intricately tied together that a change in any one part inevitably results in changes in the entire system. Each family member and subsystem are affected by transitional and situational stressors, but the effects vary in intensity and quality. For example, family health professionals have observed a powerful collective quality when there is a sick or disabled child in the family. Boss (1988) explains that

> there is a ripple effect when a parent overfocuses on that child in the subsequent reaction of a sibling (or mate) who feels left out. The family member who feels neglected begins to distance himself or herself or to act out for attention. A sibling may run away; a mate may indulge in self-destructive behavior or have an affair. (p. 16)

Nonsummativity (Wholeness). One of the important properties of the family as an open system is called nonsummativity, which means that the family cannot be considered as merely the sum of its parts. The family viewed as a whole is greater than the sum of its parts. In other words, the assessment of the family *unit* cannot be based on knowledge about each of family members or sets of relationships (Wright and Leahey, 1984). "Family systems have emergent properties," state Hartman and Laird (1983, p. 62). By this they mean that the interrelatedness of components in the family system gives rise to new qualities and characteristics that are a function of that interrelatedness.

Hierarchy of Systems: Family as Focal System Figure 7–5 illustrates the relationship of the family to its subsystems, its interacting systems, such as the welfare and educational system, and its suprasystems, eg, the family's reference group(s), the community, and wider society.

Relative to the family system's environment, generally speaking, the more immediate the environment,

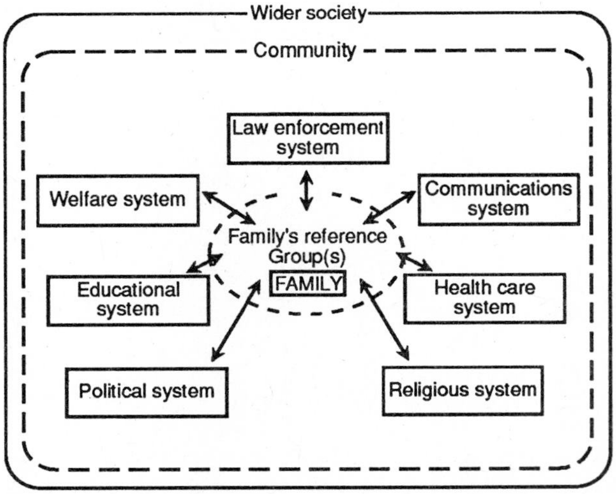

Figure 7–5
Schematic illustration of the family and its external environment.

the greater the influence on the system and the greater the input to the family. Conversely, more distant environments have less influence on the family. Thus systems with which the family continually interacts, such as the school system, generally have a more potent impact on the family than a remote suprasystem.

An example of a family suprasystem—its reference group—is described by Billingsley (1968). In the following quotation he explains how the black family is embedded within a whole network of mutually interdependent institutions and the wider black community:

> The Negro community includes within itself a number of institutions which are also viewed as subsystems. Prominent among these are: schools, churches, taverns, newspapers, neighborhood associations, lodges, fraternities, social clubs, age and sex peer groups, recreation associations and small businesses. (p. 5)

Open, Closed, and Random Family Systems. All families are, strictly speaking, open systems, because they exchange materials, energy, and information with their environment. Families are in constant interaction with their physical, social, and cultural environment. From a clinical perspective, it is possible, however, to identify degrees of openness, closedness, and/or randomness in a family and thus to evaluate a family's ability to change and to maintain stability. Kantor and Lehr (1975), in an in-depth qualitative study of families, described three types of families: open, closed, and random families.

In *open families* the exchange of information, friends, and activities is extensive. Open families welcome new ideas, information, techniques, opportunities, and resources. Moreover, open families take the initiative by actively seeking out new resources and using these resources to solve their problems. Creative and flexible solutions to problems are sought and are utilized in response to changing and unique needs (Satir, 1972).

Open families are those that perceive change as normal and desirable, and view people as inherently good and helpful and thus to be sought and needed. Open families reach out to the larger community and interact extensively with it. Family boundaries of the open family are much more permeable than in the closed family.

In contrast, *closed families* view change as threatening and are resistant to it. Strangers are perceived as being potentially harmful or at least not to be trusted. Closed families believe that man's negative qualities are a basic fact of life and that people must therefore be under strict control; thus, relationships have to be regulated by force and within the family there is extensive social control. These types of families are rigid; as a result, things and events in the closed family remain as constant and predictable as possible. Stability and tradition are core purposes of closed families. Kantor and Lehr (1975) describe the situation existing in the closed family:

> Locked doors, careful scrutiny of strangers in the neighborhood, parental control over the media, supervised excursions, and unlisted telephones are all features of a closed-type family. Closed bounding (boundary) goals include the preservation of territoriality, self-protection, privacy, and, in some families, secretiveness. Perimeter traffic control is never relinquished to outsiders or even to anyone within the family not specifically assigned bounding responsibilities. (p. 120)

The third type of family described by Kantor and Lehr is the *random family.* It is easy to think of this type of family as being the polar opposite of the closed family in terms of family social control and rigidity to change. Whereas time, activities, and family routines are closely regulated and controlled in the closed family, just the reverse is true in the random type family. Individual family members establish their own boundaries, values, activities, routines, and schedules. Traffic in and out of the family is loosely regulated even when strangers are involved. These are high-energy families that value spontaneity, free choice, very fluid norms, and challenge (Mercer, 1989). Here the core purpose of the family is exploration through use of members' sense of intuition (Kantor and Lehr, 1975). In the extreme, this type of family is chaotic and prone to dissolution.

Family Boundaries. Probably the most crucial means families have of facilitating adaptation to outside demands and internal needs is through their effective use of their semipermeable *family boundaries.* The function of metaphoric boundaries is to actively expand (or open) and retract (or close) according to need, thus regulating the amount of input from the environment and output to the environment (Reinhardt and Quinn, 1973). In other words, the key to successful family adaptation is selective permeability of family boundaries. In healthy family functioning, input is screened so that a family takes in what is needed from the environment and assimilates or modifies it to promote its own survival and growth.

When families have boundaries that are too rigid and impermeable, important resources are not forthcoming. These families are deprived of the necessary information and support, as well as, perhaps, the physical resources necessary for family wellness. Family boundary maintenance in information processing determines the openness of the system relative to exchanging information with the external environment. The amount of information a family can handle adequately is limited, and an excess of information or conflicting information from the outer environment amplifies and creates family disequilibrium. Conversely, too little information can also threaten family stability. In the healthy family, boundaries adequately screen information input and output. When an excessive amount of information flows into the family, the boundaries are closed, and when an underflow of information occurs, the boundaries are opened (Reinhardt and Quinn, 1973, pp. 90–91).

The family with an underflow of information from the environment creates a greater reliance upon inner familial resources. Relatively closed families may exhibit more energy than they can constructively discharge, with eventual disorganization the result.

The abused child is frequently found in families that are isolated and have closed boundaries with society. In healthier isolated families, the members tend to believe that all or most of the needs of the members can be met by the family itself or its reference group. Family self-sufficiency may be overemphasized, however, causing family members to view wider society in a distorted or negative way. The children of such families often experience great problems when they are required to interact with the wider society.

On the other hand, families that are indiscriminately open to information tend to become disorganized and chaotic. In this case, ineffective boundary regulation allows information to flow constantly into the family system, with resultant distortion and high levels of anxiety generated and manifested among family members. The children and adults of these families are forced into the extrafamilial environment of neighbors, community organizations, and state agencies in order to get their needs met. In these cases relationships within and outside of the family are generally shallow, nonrewarding, and frustrating to family members.

Family Adaptation. Family adaptation refers to the capacity of the family and its members to modify their behavior to each other and their outer world as the situation demands. In response to internal or external input, the family adapts by either accepting or rejecting incoming information, energy, or services, or by modifying the input to meet its needs.

In an open system the family balances inputs from the external and internal environments by the feedback process. Balanced adequately, this is called *family homeostasis, steady state,* or *equilibrium.* Homeostasis or its synonyms (steady state and equilibrium) should not imply stagnation, however, but the degree of balancing needed while continual change and growth are taking place. Healthy families are flexible, more spontaneous, open to growth and change, responsive to new stimulation, and not status-quo oriented (Lewis et al, 1976).

Because families must change in order to meet both internal and external demands, a sufficient range of behaviors and patterns, plus the flexibility to mobilize these when needed, is essential. Nevertheless, the family system has a tendency to offer resistance to change beyond a certain range and maintains preferred patterns as long as it possibly can. Although alternatives are feasible, the family's threshold of tolerance for change stimulates self-regulatory mechanisms that reestablish the accustomed range. An example of this phenomenon is that when a family member begins to distant himself or herself from the family, it is common for other family members to feel the distancing member is not doing his or her part. Guilt-producing techniques could then be used to return the family member to his or her usual family roles.

A steady state is achieved internally by balancing family members' roles. Family members help to maintain this internal balance either covertly or overtly. The family's repetitious, circular, and predictable communication patterns will reveal this balancing act.

Failure of Adaptive Strategies. As with individuals, the presence of stress in a family initially aids the family to mobilize its resources and work at solving its problems. Stress causes family homeostasis or its steady state to become precarious, in which case family members initially exert much effort to regain its balance. However, when initial attempts to resolve problems or to meet demands fail, stress increases. Often a stressor originally affects one individual, followed by one and then the other subsystems—until finally all family subsystems are involved (the ripple effect). For instance, problems in the spouse subsystem can be localized for a while. Then as they continue and intensify, other subsystems, especially the parent–child subsystem, becomes affected. Although stress is experienced by all the subsystems, each subsystem may tolerate and handle the stress differently, as discussed under the ripple effect earlier.

In time, if no solution is found to reduce the stress, the system eventually reaches its limits to respond adaptively, reaching a point of exhaustion. When important familial resources are depleted, family functioning deteriorates, and symptoms of family disorganization set in, such as overt symptoms of an individual family member's distress, economic difficulties, intrafamilial conflicts, or parenting problems. At this point a family crisis is present. If no outside assistance is received, the end result may be the family adapting at a lower level of functioning or perhaps the separation or loss of a family member. In contrast, a stable system under stress will move in the direction that tends to minimize the stress; for example, it will seek help from external sources when its internal resources are inadequate.

Family Subsystems. The family is a system of interacting personalities intricately organized into positions, roles, and norms, which are further organized into subsystems within the family. These subsystems become the basis for the family structure or organization. The family system differentiates and carries out its functions through personal and interpersonal subsystems (Kantor and Lehr, 1975). Interpersonal subsystems are made up of sets of relationships involving two or more family members. Each individual within the family is also a personal subsystem—the smallest of the subsystems in the family. Family subsystems, however, primarily refer to the interpersonal subsystems discussed here. Family members belong to different subsystems, where they have different levels of power and learn differentiated roles. An adult female, for example, can be a daughter, wife, or older sister. Each of these roles involves different complementary relationships and the use of a different cluster of behaviors (Minuchin, 1974).

The nuclear family has at least three interpersonal subsystems, each of which serves some unique function in addition to common objectives. These subsystems are listed in Table 7–2.

Minuchin (1974), a family therapist and the author of several important books in his field, has worked extensively with families using a systems-based approach in family counseling. He stresses the need to work with and through the several subsystems of the family to effect positive change within the whole family. His approach is to assist in the strengthening of the subsystems so that they function in an effective manner and do not lose their identity or unique contribution to the whole.

TABLE 7–2. FAMILY SUBSYSTEMS BASED ON SETS OF RELATIONSHIPS IN THE FAMILY

1. *The Spouse Subsystem.* Here two adult members relate to each other as (a) marital partners and (b) parents of their offspring.
2. *The Parent–Child Subsystem.* This subsystem is composed of the parents and their children. The subsystem has parenting functions (socialization) involving the mother–father roles and the children's roles.
3. *The Sibling Subsystem.* This subsystem is composed of the children and characterized by the children's relationships with each other.
4. *Other Subsystems.* There may also exist, for example, a grandparent–grandchild subsystem or uncle–nephew subsystems in an extended family.

Minuchin suggests that in the same way that the family system has a boundary, so does each subsystem, the purpose of which is to protect the differentiation of the system; that is, it is through the growth and evolution of subsystems that the whole family differentiates. Each subsystem has specific functions, which in turn lead to special demands on its members. Thus in the spouse system, the parent is given the child-rearing function. Clear and intact boundaries are required to deter any interference by other subsystems. For example, the spouse subsystem often becomes usurped by the parent–child subsystem because of the overwhelming demands on the adult members (parents) of the parenting role. In another case, the parent–child subsystem cannot function effectively if siblings interfere in the parent–child relationship and compromise the parents' capacity to parent one of their offspring. Minuchin calls this blurring of subsystem boundaries "diffuse" boundaries.

A brief explanation of each of the three subsystems will help illuminate their critical functions.

The Spouse Subsystem. The traditional spouse subsystem is formed when two adults of the opposite sex agree to join together for the primary purposes of mutual support and the meeting of each other's affectional and sexual needs. The couple needs to mutually accommodate, in addition to complementing, each other. The spouse subsystem is vital to the couple, because it acts as a refuge from external stresses and constitutes an avenue for contacting other social systems. It is also the most important subsystem of the family (Goldenberg and Goldenberg, 1985). Utilizing the systems framework, the spouse subsystem boundary needs to be intact and protected from the demands and needs of other systems. Children especially have a tendency to intrude on the spouse subsystem, creating a situation wherein husband and wife have a relationship based not on their own personal relationship with each other but on their parenting functions (Minuchin, 1974).

The Parent–Child Subsystem. With the birth or adoption of a child by the couple, the original dyadic family grows in complexity, because a new subsystem is created. The spouse subsystem now must differentiate itself to perform both mutual support (marital roles) and child-rearing (parental) functions. The parent–child subsystem involves parents and their relationship with each of their children (Minuchin, 1974).

The Sibling Subsystem. With the advent of additional children, the sibling subsystem comes into being. As only-children will attest, having a sister or brother is important. These relationships serve as the first social-skills laboratory for children. Here they learn to relate in the peer world. They learn to support, become, angry, negotiate, cooperate, and imitate each other. In their relating to siblings, children learn to play different roles, which then serve them when they go out into the extrafamilial world. Within these relationships there is an openness and honesty unmatched in outer society; that is, the child obtains constant feedback from siblings concerning his or her behavior.

The significance of the sibling subsystem is underscored by frequent observations made of only-children. Only-children accommodate in the adult world rather than their peer world, often exhibiting precocious development because of extensive parental exposure. Concurrently, they may have difficulty sharing, cooperating, and competing with children of their own age, and are usually more dependent in their behavior (Minuchin, 1974; Toman, 1961).

Differentiation. Differentiation refers to the family's propensity to evolve and grow so that as growth takes place the system becomes more complex, articulate, and discriminate. Developmental studies—studies of families throughout their life cycle—have demonstrated this tendency. Families are dynamic systems that are continually differentiating themselves both functionally and structurally. Because of the family's evolution and growth, there is also a concomitant need for increased numbers of specialized roles. This specialization and increased complexity are direct outcomes of differentiation (Minuchin, 1974).

CHARACTERISTICS OF HEALTHY FAMILIES

In concluding an exploration of the basic concepts and definition of systems theory and how these are applied and illustrated within the family system, it is fitting to draw a "composite picture" of the healthy family. According to Lewis and co-workers (1976), the healthy family is a maximally viable system characterized by complexity of structure; highly flexible organization capable and tolerant of internal changes; highly autonomous subsystems and considerable internal determination; and openness with the outer environment that results in a continual flow of a wide variety of information, experience, and input into the family. Pratt (1976) elaborates further by saying that healthy families are energized families in which people are developed in the matrix of the family through freedom and change. Rather than the holding back—conforming to prescribed social patterns through control and stability—the energized family is characterized as one in which there is:

1. Interaction by all members with each other regularly in a variety of contexts, (tasks or leisure-time activities).
2. Varied and active contacts with a wide range of other groups and organizations, including health, educational, political, recreational, and business associations in the community, so as to enhance and fulfill the interests of family members.
3. Active attempts to cope and master their lives by joining groups, seeking out information, discovering options, and making their own decisions.
4. A fluid internal organization, where role relationships are flexible and responsive to changing situations and needs, power is shared, each person participates in the decisions in which he or she is affected, and relationships support personal growth and autonomy (pp. 3–4).

THE RELATIONSHIP BETWEEN THE STRUCTURAL–FUNCTIONAL AND SYSTEMS THEORIES

With regard to the family, apparent similarities between structural–functional and systems theory include the notion that the family (the focal system) interacts with its inner and outer environments and must be examined in context. System theory characterizes the family and other systems as containing a structure and functions. In structural–functionalism, however, these two concepts represent the central thrust of the theory, certainly a much more important emphasis than found in systems theory. Both theories discuss adaptation, with structural–functionalism stressing the tendency toward equilibrium, while systems theory stressing the balance between equilibrium (stability) and change in its analysis.

System theory, as noted earlier, is derived from a holistic paradigm, where circular causation and feedback loops are essential elements. Structural–functionalism, counter to some of its assumptions, tends to resort to more "part analysis," linear notions of causation, and a more static view of the family.

Yet most of the more specific family theory has been generated within a structural–functional frame, and the structural and functional dimensions that are used in this text are most helpful for presenting the needed information, theory, and assessment guidelines. Hence, both theories converge and diverge at certain points. Nevertheless, both are useful in identifying and describing important content areas, explaining family behavior, and providing guidelines for family nursing practice.

☐ STUDY QUESTIONS

Are the following statements True or False?

1. A system is defined as a unit with distinct parts and boundaries, extending over a period of time and with some identified purpose.

2. A social system is either an animate or inanimate system.

3. Open systems depend on the environment for exchange of information, matter, and energy, whereas closed systems do not interact with the environment.

4. Family differentiation occurs when a system bifurcates or splits into smaller subunits or systems.

5. With greater energy use, system boundaries need to be more open.

6. Differentiation, particularly as it applies to families, describes the family's tendency to grow and evolve (as time progresses) into a more complex and specialized system.

7. Relative to the family system and its internal and external environments, supply the following information:
   a. Name a focal or target system.
   b. Name a suprasystem.
   c. Give three examples of interacting systems.
   d. Give three examples of family subsystems.

8. Draw a diagram of the energy, matter, and information exchange and process model and show a specific example of this energy exchange and processing pertinent to the family system.

9. Match the correct term from the left-hand column with characteristic from the right-hand column.

a. Equilibrium	1. Synonymous with balancing (used interchangeably)
b. Adaptation	2. The result of balancing
c. Homeostasis	3. A survival mechanism
d. Steady state	4. The whole is greater than its parts
e. Feedback loop	
f. Self-regulation	

10. Identify which of the following adjectives or terms accurately describe the paradigm used in systems theory.
    a. Reductionistic
    b. Objective
    c. Partial analysis

d. Atomistic
e. Linear causality
f. None of these

Choose the correct answer(s) to the following question.

11. The following elements and characteristics are true of the family system. It is a (an):
a. Open social system.
b. Highly organized system.
c. Highly interdependent system.
d. System with specified purposes.
e. System with necessary processes (eg, integration, adaptation, and decision making).
f. Independent system.
g. Undifferentiated system.
h. Suprasystem to the spouse, parent–child, and sibling systems.
i. Dynamic system but with little capacity for change.

12. What is the significance of the boundaries of the family system and subsystems?

13. Using the systems approach, explain how family boundaries function to maintain family homeostasis.

14. Match the proper function(s) on the left with each of the family subsystems on the right.

a. A social skills laboratory	1. Spouse subsystem
b. Mutual support	2. Parent–child subsystem
c. Meeting of adult affectional needs	3. Sibling subsystem
d. Learning to relate to peers	
e. Socialization function	
f. Disciplining—control and guidance function.	

15. Give four characteristics of a successfully functioning, healthy family.

16. Match the advantages/disadvantages and/or characteristics with "open," "closed," or random families.

a. Open families	1. Provide for change
b. Closed families	2. Are stagnated, rigid
c. Random families	3. Offers choices and flexibility
d. Does not apply to either	4. Change viewed as threatening
	5. Greater structuring and control mechanisms employed
	6. Privacy and territoriality stressed
	7. People seen as good, helpful, and needed
	8. Seek out new resources
	9. Family members set their own rules and schedules

17. Sequentially number the events below in terms of their sequencing when a family crisis occurs.

a. No solution is found to reduce stress—that is, failure of adaptive strategies exists.
b. Stress and strain are experienced.
c. A change occurs as stressor presents itself.
d. Family homeostasis or its steady state becomes precarious and family exerts additional efforts to maintain balance and reduce stress.
e. Stress spreads from one individual or subsystem to all subsystems of family.
f. System reaches point of exhaustion.
g. Family disorganization results.

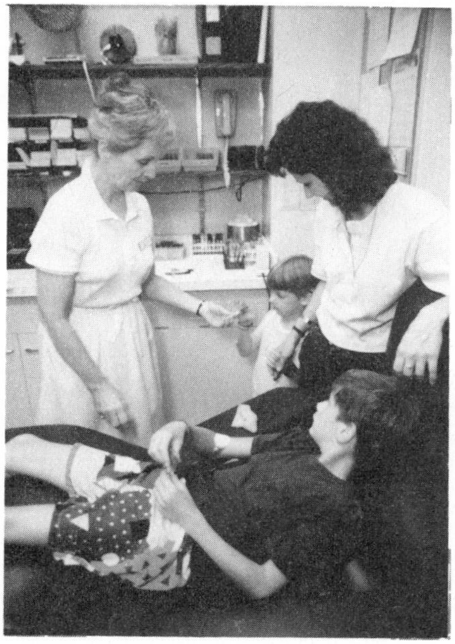

PART III

Family Nursing Practice: Theory, Assessment, Diagnosis, and Intervention

Part I dealt with the basic information on the family, the major approaches used to analyze families, and the prime goals and germane roles of the family nurse. The process of providing family nursing care and the developmental aspects of family life were also explored. From this broad perspective we now move into more specific applications for assessing families. The frameworks on which the assessment tool and the family nursing process are built are structural–functional theory, modified to meet the special needs of family health care; family developmental theory; and systems theory. There are five basic areas subsumed under this comprehensive approach: (1) identifying data, (2) environmental data, (3) family structural dimensions, (4) family functions, and (5) family coping strategies and processes.

Chapter 8 covers the identifying data and Chapter 9 the environmental data regarding the family. The four dimensions of family structure will be discussed in Chapters 10 through 13. Three of the most critical family functions (affective, socialization, and the health care function) are elaborated on in Chapters 14 through 16. Chapter 17 deals with family adaptation and family coping. In each of the chapters, assessment areas related to and part of the broad assessment topic give sufficient detail, in terms of both theory and application, for collecting and interpreting assessment data pertaining to families in a multitude of settings and throughout the family's life cycle. Family nursing interventions appropriate for the area being addressed are also presented. The actual family assessment tool, along with a suggested care plan form, is included as Appendices A and B. Appendix C presents a hypothetical family situation, which is followed by an analysis of the family in Appendix D.

CHAPTER EIGHT

Family Identifying Data: Sociocultural Assessment and Intervention

Learning Objectives

1. Define and describe the following family identifying data, applying content to a written case example:
   a. Family composition
   b. Type of family form
   c. Cultural (ethnic) and religious orientation
   d. Social class status including occupational, economic, and educational data
   e. Social class mobility
   f. Social supports/network
   g. Recreational activities
2. Diagram a family genogram and family ecomap.
3. Explain why an understanding of a family's cultural background is crucial for family health practice.
4. Discuss several of the major problems that result when cultural insensitivity and ignorance exist on the part of a health care professional.
5. Define these basic concepts: culture, ethnic groups, cultural pluralism, ethnic identity, stereotyping, acculturation, assimilation, cultural relativism, ethnocentrism, cultural imposition, cultural conflicts, cultural shock, indigenous health care system, and self-fulfilling prophecy.
6. Discuss the importance of the cross-cultural approach to family health care.
7. Identify some of the differences in values and norms among the social classes.
8. Describe family-oriented interventions appropriate for enhancing/maintaining social supports and financial and economic welfare and providing culturally sensitive services.
9. Differentiate between the concepts of social support, social networks, family social support, and family social networks.
10. Describe two nursing intervention strategies designed to maintain or promote family social support.
11. Summarize basic research findings relative to the impact of social support on health/illness.
12. Identify two strategies for assisting families with their health-related financial difficulties and two strategies for promoting family recreational activity.

Name (Last, First)	Sex	Relationship	Date/Place of Birth	Occupation	Education
1. (father)					
2. (mother)					
3. (oldest child)					
4.					
5.					
6.					
7.					
8.					

Figure 8–1
Family composition form.

IDENTIFYING DATA: GETTING TO KNOW THE FAMILY

As with all assessment tools, it is important to begin by obtaining broad identifying information about the family client. As discussed in Chapter 3, during the initial home visit (or client contact in another setting), the focus is typically on getting to know the family and all its members, as well as attempting to meet their immediate health needs. To learn about the family, a family composition roster and/or a family genogram afford(s) excellent assessment strategies. Duvall (1977) says that with information about who lives in the home and their relationships, along with knowledge of the time (family life cycle and season, day, and hour) and the family's social and cultural status, one can generally predict current family activities and issues.

Family Composition

Family composition refers to who the family members identify as being part of their family. This may include not only the household inhabitants, but also other extended family or fictive family members who are part of "the family," but do not live in the same household. Beginning with family composition also lets family members know of your interest in the whole family rather than just an interest in the individual for whom the visit or contact was ostensibly made. Completing a family composition roster involves collecting the following information:

- Family name
- Address
- Telephone number
- Family composition

In the family composition form given in Figure 8–1, the adult family members are recorded first, followed by the children in order of their birth beginning with the oldest. Include any other related or unrelated member(s) of the household next. If there are extended family members or friends who act as family members, although not living in the household, also include them at the end of the list. The relationship of each family member, as well as birthdate, birthplace, occupation, and education, are also identified.

The Family Genogram

The second assessment strategy for getting to know the family is the family genogram or family tree. The family genogram is a diagram that delineates the family constellation or family tree. It is an informative assessment tool used to get to know the family and the family's history and resources.

A genogram interview is seen as one part of a comprehensive clinical assessment of a family (McGoldrick and Gerson, 1985). The diagram maps relationships vertically (across generations) and horizontally (within the same generation) and often helps family nurses think systemically about how events and relationships in the nuclear family members' lives are related to family patterns of health and illness as well as to generate tentative hypotheses about what's going on in the family.

Based on the conventions used in diagraming family trees or genealogical charts and genetics, the family genogram incorporates information about three generations of the family (the nuclear family and the family of origin of each parent). Not only are the nuclear and extended family members included on the genogram, but also significant nonfamily members who have lived with or played a major role in the family's life. This visual representation of the family consists of information about members' age; gender; significant life events (eg, birth, marriage, divorce); health/illness status; death; and selected identifying features such as race, social class, ethnicity, religion, occupation, and place of residence.

There has been widespread use of family genograms

by family health practitioners and therapists, and much variety in the way genograms are diagrammed. McGoldrick and Gerson have written an entire book on genograms, *Genograms in Family Assessment* (1985). If a more thorough description of genograms and their application is needed, this excellent reference is suggested.

Constructing Genograms. Figure 8–2 shows an example of how a genogram is constructed. Symbols used in diagramming are also presented. The example given is relatively uncomplicated, given the number of families that have experienced multiple significant family transitions and events. Wright and Leahey (1984) explain the basic method involved in recording family data on the family genogram.

> Family members are placed on horizontal rows that signify generational lines. For example, a marriage or common-law relationship is denoted by a horizontal line. Children are denoted by vertical lines. Children are rank-ordered from left to right beginning with the eldest child. Each individual is represented. (p. 30)

Males are designated by squares, females by circles. Horizontal lines that are broken denote a separation or divorce. Household members are identified by encircling all the members of the household with a broken line.

Usually the family genogram is completed on the first visit and revised later as new information becomes available. Letting the family know that background information is needed to more fully understand the specific problems the family is experiencing, coupled with an explanation of the family tree method, usually suffice as explanations to gain family members' participation. It is suggested that questions about the immediate family are asked first (names, ages, sex of household members). Recent life cycle transitions as well as changes in the family situation (additions or deletions of members) may also be inquired about at this time (McGoldrick and Gerson, 1985).

After addressing the immediate family, asking about the parents' families of origin is recommended. Inquiring about the two extended families brings to focus the wider family context. Querying the mother about her side of the family and the father about his side of the family is a way to obtain this information. Moreover, questions should be asked about friends, clergy, caregivers, health care professionals, and others important to the family's functioning; this information may be included on the genogram or used to assess the family's social support system/network. At this point, non-family members may also be added as either household members or "family."

Difficult questions about family members' functioning are often saved to later in the interview, when greater trust and rapport is present. Areas family nurses should ask about include serious medical or psychological problems, work or school changes/problems, drug and alcohol problems, and trouble with the law (McGoldrick and Gerson, 1985).

THE FAMILY'S CULTURAL ORIENTATION

A family's cultural orientation or background may well be the most pertinent variable in understanding the family's behavior, value system, and functions. Because culture permeates and circumscribes our individual, familial, and social actions, its consequences are pervasive and its implication for practice broad.

Because understanding the family's cultural background is so critical in working with families, familial differences among the two largest ethnic groups in the United States are explored in Chapters 19 and 20. Chapter 13 on the family's value system will also help the family nurse look at cultural patterns, because family values are often a reflection of the value system of the family's reference groups, a major one being the ethnic subculture with which the family identifies.

Importance of Culture for Practice

To understand and to be able to work efficaciously with families from cultures different from one's own, health care professionals must be aware of that culture's unique, distinctive qualities and the variety of lifestyles, values, and structures found within that group. Hence the importance of culture lies in its vital and unique character. Because cultural differences are often at the root of poor communication, interpersonal tensions, avoidance in working effectively with others, and poor assessment of health problems and their remedies, successful nursing care of clients of various ethnic backgrounds is dependent on the nurse's knowledge of and sensitivity to the clients' culture.

In family counseling the importance of culture is paramount. Coddy (1975) points out that in family therapy the health care professional and client must have interlocking cultural patterns. Without knowledge of the differences in cultural norms and patterns, behavior that differs from normative patterns is usually labeled as deviant, crazy, immoral, or illegal (depending on the type of prescribed behavior violated). In the absence of cultural data, it then becomes impossible for the health care worker to recognize the possible cultural meaning of the client's behavior or actions. In addition, Coddy (1975) identifies four other important areas where cultural dissimilarity may permeate and

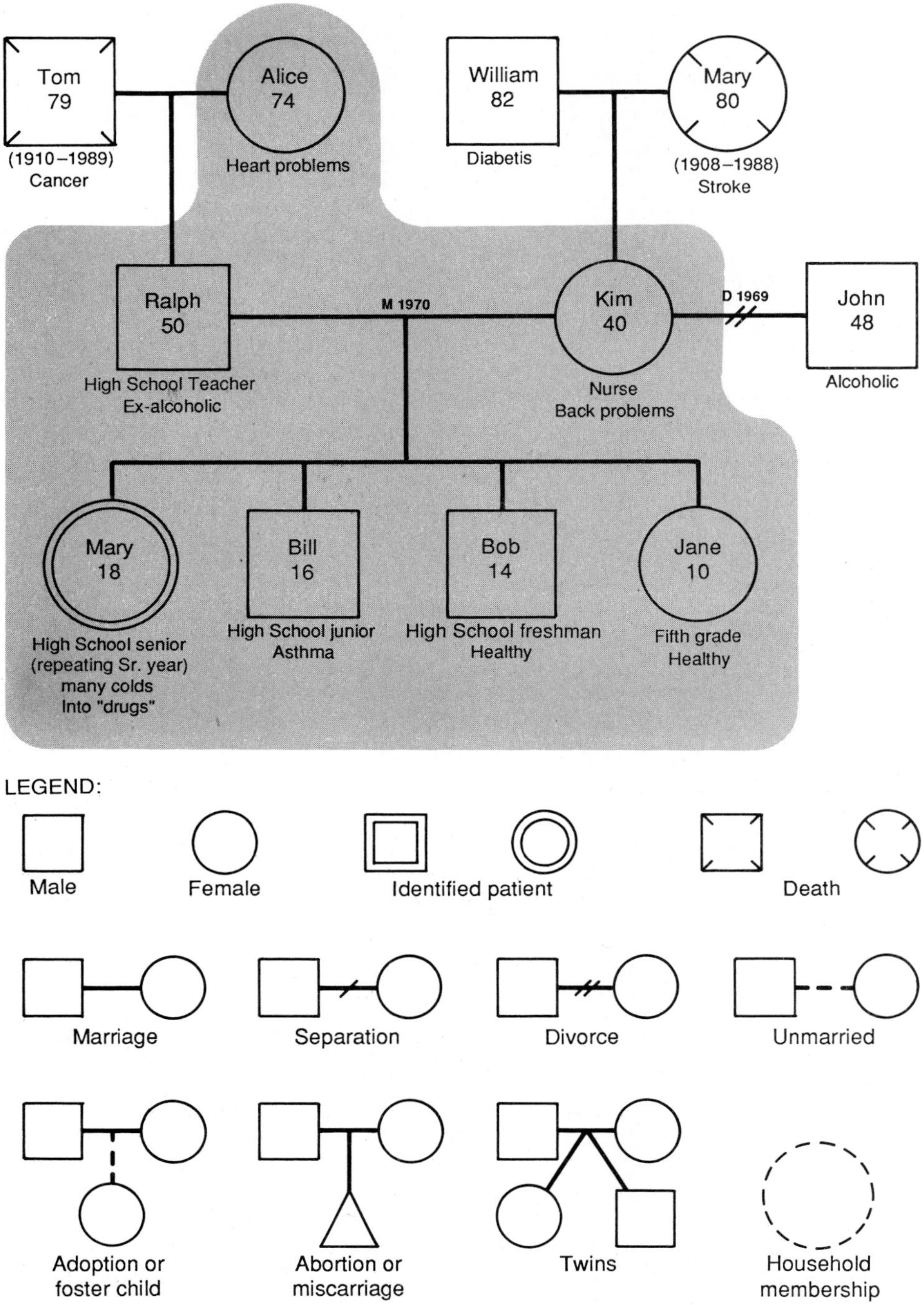

Figure 8–2
Example of family genogram with accompanying legend (symbols used in genograms).

disrupt counseling. These are in the areas of (1) goal expectations, (2) the establishment of rapport, (3) communication styles, and (4) client's acceptance of ideas or recommendations.

The importance of nurse–client cultural congruence is well documented. Several noted authors have pointed to the greater ease and efficacy when the client and the health care professionals have similar ethnic and religious backgrounds (Flaskerud, 1984). When similar frames of references exist in a relationship, the possibilities of greater freedom of expression, deeper identification, and increased empathy present themselves (Coddy, 1975). However, having a health care worker and client of the same ethnic background is, in many cases, an ideal situation. In reality ethnic congruency is not often possible, and perhaps may not even be socially desirable. Otherwise, how are we in a multicultural society to learn to live and relate well to one another?

The critical nature of language barriers also deserves mention. In some regions, where a majority or plurality of one's clients are from a different culture and speak a different language, learning the culture's language will not only result in dramatically improved communication but also in a much greater understanding and appreciation of the culture. Padilla (1976) verifies this assertion in his study of lower-class Mexican-Americans who were being seen in therapy in a counseling center in East Los Angeles. He states that it has generally been assumed by therapists that lower-class persons have difficulty benefiting from psychotherapy because of their nonverbalness, inarticulateness, and lack of ability to think abstractly. Padilla reports, however, that in counseling Chicano clients, this generalization does not hold true when clients were given the opportunity and encouraged to communicate in Spanish, English, or a combination of both in order to enhance the meaningfulness of their communication. He concludes that, "It now seems clear that the Chicano poor are quite capable of verbally expressing themselves in the most intensive 'insight' therapy situation, if they are not forced to communicate in English, a language that may be partly or completely foreign to these individuals" (p. 289).

Cultural–Ethnic Pluralism

Our country is truly a matrix of many ethnic groups or subcultures. Massive waves of immigration have continued to mold and revolutionize the character of the United States throughout the last two centuries. The myth of the American melting pot has been intellectually recognized, though its implications not dissipated. This myth encouraged all diverse ethnic groups immigrating to the United States to succeed in American society by becoming part of the one predominant group. Any differences were typically seen as deviant and inferior. Ethnic variation was perceived as an element of the lower social class and of recent immigrant groups. Moving up the social class ladder to success meant discarding one's ethnic traditions and values and assimilating into the mainstream of society.

The social protests of the 1960s brought about the harsh realization that the society had not, and did not wish to, move toward one homogeneous entity. The civil rights movement and the rise of black consciousness and identity set the model for all other ethnic groups. This model stressed a reaffirmation of cultural differences, a greater demand for equal treatment, and an acceptance of the value of ethnic or cultural diversity in society. This movement was quickly followed by similar demands for ethnic pluralism among white ethnic groups (Jewish, Irish, Italian, and so forth), Asian-Americans, and Mexican-Americans (McAdoo, 1978). Stemming from this push for cultural pluralism, American values have been changing, reflecting a greater tolerance for diversity (see Chap. 13).

Kobrin and Goldscheider (1978), researchers of ethnicity, discuss the salience and meaning of ethnicity for society, family, and the individual:

> Ethnic pluralism is an integral feature of human societies and ethnicity continues to be an organic part of social and cultural changes. The major processes associated with industrialization and urbanization have not resulted in the disappearance of ethnic communities nor the eradication of ethnic differences in major social processes. . . . The conspicuousness of ethnic communities suggests that ethnic institutions and social networks even as they change remain major sources of group identification. (p. 1)

The authors point out that with the recent reemergence of ethnicity, one's cultural heritage and ethnic identity has become an even more tangible and acceptable basis for group cohesion in America. One important reason for placing greater importance and recognition on ethnic or cultural roots is that ethnic identification provides for many persons and families an alternative link to the broader society, partially compensating for the cold, impersonal, and bureaucratic qualities of society today (Kobrin and Goldscheider, 1978). Moreover, ethnicity can be seen as enriching family life and strengthening the bonds of intergenerational continuity.

The reality of the 1990s is that the United States is truly multicultural. A demographic imperative exists for practicing transcultural family nursing. Ethnic minority families continue to migrate in vast numbers. Coupled with a much higher fertility rate among Hispanics, the demographic characteristics of our nation are changing rapidly. The 1990 census projections

TABLE 8–1. PERCENT OF U.S. POPULATION OF ETHNIC MINORITIES ACCORDING TO 1990 CENSUS

Ethnic Group	Percent of U.S. Population
Blacks	12%
Hispanics	9%
Asians and Pacific islanders	3%
Native Americans	.8%

U.S. Bureau of the Census (1991).

(U.S. Bureau of the Census, 1991) illustrate this trend (Table 8–1).

In the largest state in the Union, California, it is projected that by 2030, whites will be an aging minority within the state's population, while ethnic minority people (Latinos, blacks, and Asians/Pacific islanders) will be "the emergent majority" (Hayes-Battista, 1990).

The Cross-cultural Approach

The cross-cultural approach used in anthropology provides a broad comparative picture of human nature and human behavior (Leininger, 1970). This approach to family nursing care is both a practical necessity and a social reality, due to the awareness of the pervasive part culture plays and also to recognition of the growing numbers of people in the United States from different cultural backgrounds. As we become familiar with other cultures and learn to appreciate why certain values and norms are effective through time in those cultures, it is hoped that health care workers will become more sensitive and effective in providing family health care.

Leininger (1970) asserts that it is not only sound for nursing to use a cross-cultural or transcultural approach, it is mandatory: clients have a *right* to have their sociocultural backgrounds understood in thesame way that they expect their physical and psychological needs to be recognized and understood. Whereas health professionals have primarily emphasized psychological principles in their interpretation/intervention of individual health–illness phenomena, the cultural and the social level of analysis and care has been, until only recently, largely ignored (Aamodt, 1978). Even now, as with the use of the family-centered approach, we pay lip service to assessing sociocultural factors.

The following concepts or terms are of fundamental importance for understanding cross-cultural principles and processes.

Culture. Foremost among these concepts is that of *culture*. Culture is usually viewed as a blueprint for man's way of living, thinking, behaving, and feeling. It circumscribes and guides the ways in which societies and ethnic groups solve their problems and derive meaning from their lives. From a systems perspective, culture is defined as systems of socially transmitted behavioral patterns that link human groups to their environmental settings, as well as systems of social change and organization which act to mediate societal adaptation (Leininger, 1976). Culture denotes patterns of learned behavior and values which are transmitted from one generation to the next.

In other words, culture is a mold from which we all are cast. It constrains and regulates our daily behavior, attitudes, and values in many latent and manifest ways. Because people rely on learned behavior or culture for survival, it is the prime source of our adaptability. Hence only through the understanding of culture can one hope to understand our humanity and our personal and social actions and needs.

Ethnicity. *Webster's Dictionary* (1988) defines *ethnic* as an adjective related to people of a particular race or cultural group who are classified according to common traits and customs. In this chapter, ethnicity is used interchangeably with cultural group or subcultural group, even though ethnicity is defined more narrowly (in terms of a group of people) than culture. Subcultures are groups within a society whose members have their own particular set of cultural values, beliefs, and practices, such as an ethnic group. Minority groups have sometimes objected to the term subculture, because some feel this term denotes "less than" or "under" the general culture. Thus this term is used less frequently here, although it is in general usage in the social sciences.

Ethnic Identity. *Ethnic identity* is another related term. This term refers to the way in which individuals classify themselves vis-à-vis other people and the extent to which they associate or fail to associate themselves with people of similar cultural backgrounds.

Variation Within Cultures (Intra-ethnic Variation). Just as there are enormous differences in people between cultures, there is also a great variation in people *within cultures*. Much of the cultural variation we see in families with the same cultural background is a function of the degree to which the family subscribes to the American culture, as well as regional differences in the native culture, social class differences, or simply idiosyncratic variation. Because nursing care is extended to individuals and families, it is of utmost importance to take into account the diversity among individuals within the various ethnic groups (Koshi, 1976).

Unfortunately the tendency is to simplify things by labeling people. Kay (1978) discuss the perennial problem of generalizing about a group of people in anthropologic–ethnographic descriptions:

> Most ethnographies, or accounts of the life style of people who participate in a specific culture, are like still photographs. They describe people staggered in time and space. We call such fixed images stereotypes. Modal personalities are frozen in a changeless place, and subsequently are supposed to represent millions. But if we try to qualify groups by describing certain differences (eg, 72 percent of *barrio* women make their own tortillas as compared with 12 percent who buy Rainbo bread), we end up by describing no one. (p. 89)

We need to be able to generalize about a culture in order to learn about and discuss the culture; but at the same time, remember that cultural characteristics refer to group characteristics only.

Hence the knowledge that the father typically holds primary power in the Mexican-American home, or that the Jewish mother often is "the power behind the throne" in the Jewish culture, serves as a clue about a family's background. However, these culturally derived patterns need to be verified with the particular family the nurse is assessing.

Tripp-Reimer and Lauer (1987) caution family nurses who plan nursing care on the basis of a family's ethnicity. They explain that

> clients may not want traditional beliefs and customs incorporated into their care if alternative approaches are acceptable. Ethnic clients may not wish to remain unassimilated; indeed, it may simply perpetuate another form of stereotype to assume that all members of an ethnic group subscribe to the culture's most conservative position. (p. 96)

Tripp-Reimer and Lauer call this problem the "traditionalist fallacy." We cannot assume we know what the family and its members want simply because we know the family's cultural background.

Stereotyping. Lack of recognition of individual differences or labeling is termed *stereotyping*. Cultural stereotyping involves the nonacceptance or disallowance of individual or group diversity; everyone from a particular culture is viewed as the same and perceived of as fixed in their characteristics.

Acculturation. Exposure of persons from one cultural group to another culture leads to a sociocultural process called *acculturation*. As one of the major causative factors of variation within an ethnic group, "acculturation comprises those gradual changes produced in a culture by the influence of another culture which results in an increased similarity of the two" (Kroeber, 1948, p. 425). In the case of culture groups immigrating to the United States, the influence is usually overwhelmingly one way—that is, the American culture exerts greater influence on the ethnic group to conform to its cultural patterns than vice versa. The resultant *assimilation* may proceed so far as to practically extinguish the ethnic culture (as occurred with the African culture during slavery) or factors may intervene to counterbalance the forces of assimilation and keep the two cultures isolated from one another. For example, language and religious, economic, and geographic barriers have kept Mexican-Americans and Native Americans fairly separate from American society. The strong cultural traditions of Jews and Armenians have to a large extent limited their assimilation. Assimilation denotes the more complete and one-way process of one culture being absorbed into the other.

Kluckholm (1976) hypothesizes that the rate and degree of acculturation of any ethnic group into the dominant culture depends primarily on the degree of congruency between the group's own basic value orientations with those of the dominant (American) culture. Also, certain groups within a particular ethnic subculture are more receptive to social and cultural change. For instance, among urban residents, the more educated, occupationally successful, or higher socioeconomic groups are more likely to experience assimilatory changes. Hence socioeconomic and class factors are crucial elements to consider in learning about a family's ethnicity.

Acculturation, then, implies that members of cultures other than the dominant culture of the society have internalized to a great extent the norms and values of the dominant culture and, moreover, that the wider society has been influenced to varying degrees by its exposure to each of the ethnic or subcultural groups within its boundaries.

Acculturation does not necessarily suggest the loss of ethnic identity—of a detaching of oneself from an ethnic community (Kobrin and Goldscheider, 1978)—nor does it imply the loss of many of the customs related to that culture. Customs that continue, more or less unscathed, are those that are not stigmatizing or illegal, customs such as those involving food, religion, music, and dance. Many times these become the major tangible cultural difference, remnants of cultures quite different. Price (1976) states that sociocultural groups in America become transformed into ethnic subcultures. Although outright destruction never completely occurs, transformation (acculturation) begins immediately on participation in the American economic system—the adjustments necessitated in order to join the work force produce social change. As elements of the old and new culture intertwine, a unique subculture is formed.

Members of ethnic minorities are inevitably part of two cultures. Most ethnic minority families are then bicultural. Biculturalism signifies participation in two cultural systems and often requires two sets of behavior and ways of thinking (Ho, 1987).

Real Versus the Ideal. To understand a family's cultural background we need to understand both its values (what family members say is important or *the ideal*) and its actual behavior (*the real*). Often the variance between the two is striking. It is typically due to the pragmatic adaptation of a family to a particular social and historical context (Friedman, 1990). Sheer practical necessity can often distort one's values in everyday life, so that they become unrecognizable (Graedon, 1985). Numerous examples of the distinction between the real and ideal can be seen in the adaptations ethnic families make to poverty and discrimination.

Cultural Relativism. In working with clients from various cultural backgrounds the aim in the health care professions is to eliminate ethnocentric beliefs and substitute instead a relativistic cultural perspective. *Cultural relativism* refers to the perspective that holds that "cultures are neither inferior nor superior to one another and that there is no single scale for measuring the value of a culture. Therefore, customs, beliefs, and practices must be judged or understood relative to the context in which they appear" (Aamodt, 1978, p. 9). To do this, the health care worker must be flexible enough to assume the cultural perspective of those with whom he or she works (Coddy, 1975).

Ethnocentrism. *Ethnocentrism* implies the lack of cultural relativism. The tendency for health care professionals to be ethnocentric is pervasive when working with families from different sociocultural backgrounds. Due to this unfortunate tendency the importance of studying families from other cultures is even greater—to counter the tendency of believing that the way own families operate is the way in which all (normal) families do and should operate.

Cultural Imposition. A result of ethnocentrism is the problem of *cultural imposition*. Because health workers feel either consciously or unconsciously that their beliefs and practices are superior and proper, they use subtle and/or apparent ways to force their own values, beliefs, and practices on individuals from different cultural orientations (Leininger, 1974).

Cultural imposition may then lead to cultural conflicts—situations in which health care professionals have covertly or overtly tried to impose their health practices on their clients and the clients have reacted negatively. As nurses, we can think of many ways in which clients will "fight back," many times to their own detriment, because of the health system's lack of recognition of their culturally patterned beliefs and practices. The commonly seen reticence of Hispanic families to place one of their members in a hospital because of being forced to separate from the family member is a case in point. If family visiting and participation rights are relaxed to allow for a flexible consideration of client and family attitudes and patterns, both the client and the health care system benefit.

To counter the frequently experienced problems of cultural imposition and cultural conflicts, Leininger (1976) suggests that "the nurse must truly understand a culture before imposing any changes on the people. Sensitivity and foresight are essential to work in diverse cultural contexts" (p. 40). In order to understand a client's culture and provide *culturally sensitive* care, one must first be aware of his or her own value orientation and the health care patterns in one's own culture. The family nurse, to provide culturally sensitive care, must discover—through questions we ask and observations of responses we make—the family member's beliefs about health and illness, particularly of the health problems family members are having. We must assume nothing until adequate validation takes place.

Cultural Shock. Family nurses and students commonly experience feelings of *cultural shock* when visiting with or interacting with families whose culture is (1) at great variance with their own, (2) one about which they are uninformed, or (3) one to which they have had little exposure. *Cultural shock* refers to a condition in which a person, in response to an environment so altered that meaningful objects and experiences have been replaced by those from a different culture, feels confused, immobilized, and "lost" (Aamodt, 1978). Feelings and sensations of discomfort are more pronounced or noticeable when visiting in the home, because the family's differences are much more obvious. Discomfort is also more intense because of the fact that the health care worker is in the client's "territory."

Life-style and value differences are not easy to deal with. Our own values and attitudes will greatly influence our perceptions and nursing assessments and interventions. Therefore, personal feelings, beliefs, and attitudes must be identified, discussed, and accepted before we can effectively help families seeking assistance (Clemen, 1977).

Indigenous Health Care Systems. The last of the more general cultural concepts has to do more specifically with health care practices. Every culture has devised its own *indigenous health care system* as opposed to the Western *scientific or professional health care system.* This indigenous (or folk) health care system uses traditional folk care modalities. Practitioners of an indigenous system are often the first-line, primary care practitioners—the first healers to be consulted by unacculturated ethnic families. As part of the cross-cultural approach proposed earlier, it is recommended that professional systems need to become more culturally attuned to these systems and to learn ways in which to work cooperatively with folk systems, rather than in opposition to them. Health care professionals tend to downplay the significance and value of folk health care and practices. These feelings are both inaccurate and detrimental, however, because much folk medicine is effective (Leininger, 1976).

In fact, in most cases the merits of any treatment depends on whether the sick client recovers or not, and indigenous health care does work in many instances. This is particularly true in illnesses where psychogenic factors are prominent and where effective treatment of the disease depends on a knowledge of the context of the person's cultural belief system. Given this, who knows or appreciates the psychogenic and the cultural context better than the folk practitioner?

Minority Families

Minority families are those families that are classified as belonging to ethnic or cultural groups other than white ethnic groups, such as the Irish, Poles, and Jews. More recently termed "ethnic people of color," this group comprised about 22 percent of our population in 1989. Minority families, then, in contrast to *all* ethnic families (both white and people of color), have certain common attributes and problems. One major thing they share is that while facing all of the same stressors experienced by all other families, they have the added burdens of the effects of discrimination (McAdoo, 1978). Vincent and Ransford (1980) remind us that being an ethnic in America lowers one's status, just as being of lower social class. These sociologists also note that ethnic groups vary in their status, with some groups, such as blacks and Latinos, suffering more status inequality than white ethnics or Asian-Americans.

Cultural Variation or Deviance? Families are not isolated groups that exist independently from the society of which they are a part. Thus if a disproportionately large number of families of a particular minority or ethnic group are poor, unemployed, and "dysfunctional to the whole society," a comprehension of their status can be achieved only through an examination of the role played by the large society. Eshleman (1974) notes that poverty, racism, and/or inferior schools may be due less to an inherent weakness within ethnic groups and families than to:

> 1. Social and cultural systems which place a higher value on moon walks, military strength, and corporate profit than on human needs;
> 2. Religious institutions that stress a chosen ingroup as God's people to the exclusion of "nonbelievers" (ie, anyone who is different);
> 3. Educational systems that admit and serve those who pass "middle-class" exams, speak the "proper" language, and wear the "acceptable" hair and clothing styles, and, in general,
> 4. A society that in many ways places higher values on "things" and goods rather than on the needs and social conditions of people. (p. 203)

If we live in a society in which minority families and their members are devalued and seen as inferior, this message and perception very effectively becomes the perception and beliefs of those people. It is a well-known tenet of social psychology that people develop their identities and perceptions of their worth in interactions with others (Mead, 1934). As the minority family and individual interacts in a white majority world that encourages feelings of inferiority and degrades self-esteem, the minority family and its members begin to believe what the outer world is saying about them. This trap is termed the *self-fulfilling prophecy:* People will conform to other's expectations and perceptions of them by internalizing their beliefs, even negative ones, and thus seem to fulfill the "prophecies" that were made about them (Eshleman, 1974).

Problems within society set up conditions to which minority families and individuals must adapt. Some of these adaptations—such as going on welfare, dropping out of school, joining gangs, or selling drugs—are viewed as "dysfunctional." The tendency becomes one of blaming the victim—the welfare mother, the unskilled, unemployed black male, the black family, the Chicano gangs—instead of looking more broadly at the problem. By seeing the ways in which the entire system is involved (the institutions of society and the individual's interactions within this larger environment), contextual solutions may be identified and the tendency to blame the already stigmatized individual or group will be curtailed.

Controversies About Minority Family Structures. One way in which social scientists have unwittingly stereotyped and stigmatized whole ethnic groups is by attempting to describe a particular cultural group in toto by data actually derived from, and thus only reflective of *poor* segments of that group. In many of these instances, the particular segment of the ethnic group being described is not clearly identified, thereby giving readers an erroneous notion of what the cultural group is like as a whole.

Casavantes (1970) and others have asserted that this overgeneralization has certainly been true within the social science studies of Mexican-Americans in the 1950 to 1970 period. "The net result of this extraordinary scientific oversight is the perpetuation of very damaging stereotypes of Mexican Americans" (p. 22). Willie (1976) and Billingsley (1968) have pointed out the same criticism of studies about the black family and conscientiously differentiate life-styles and values of the black family by the family's social class position. Research has concentrated predominantly on the most oppressed families with findings then generalized to all minority families. In this process biased attitudes are perpetuated and reinforced. As part of this bias, the majority of stable ethnic families, and the processes by which they have become economically mobile, have largely been ignored (McAdoo, 1978).

The importance of social class does not mean, however, that the middle class of a particular American ethnic group is like the white majority middle class. Although ethnic middle-class families are indeed closer to the dominant culture in life-styles, values, beliefs, and so forth, they are still distinctive from the majority culture because of their ethnic identity and sense of peoplehood. Billingsley (1968) explains that families of the same social class but of a different ethnic group show behavioral and value similarities, but not the same sense of historic identification of peoplehood. And conversely, those of the same ethnic group but of different social class manifest a sense of peoplehood, but dissimilar life-styles.

THE PROCESS OF ASSESSING CULTURE

A cultural assessment of a client (individual and/or family) is an essential facet of assessment. Just as a family nurse would not intervene without an assessment of the biopsychosocial aspects of the family and its members, he or she should also not proceed until a cultural assessment has been completed (Leininger, 1976; Tripp-Reimer et al, 1984).

Developing skill in eliciting and recording cultural assessments of the client and the context in which the care is being given (the home, health care setting) is one significant strategy appropriate for nurses working in transcultural settings. As part of the broader assessment process, Aamodt (1978) suggests three additional strategies:

1. Becoming informed about the cultures of the persons with whom one interacts.
2. Identifying alternative coping tactics to use when dealing with clients from a different culture.
3. Continuously reexamining problems and solutions related to sociocultural practices. (p. 15)

Before family nurses work with families of a different culture, it is extremely important that they try to obtain the perceptions, views, values, and practices of people from the particular ethnic group with which they are working. "It is significant to remember that the ability to work with cultural groups is dependent upon the ability to understand the group in terms of their background as they view it and not in terms of our interpretations of their background" (Clemen, 1977, p. 192).

Cultural and Religious Assessment Areas

For many families a thorough cultural assessment is not necessary, and yet assessing the family's ethnic background (as identified by the family) and the degree to which they identify with the dominant American culture or their traditional culture (if different from the dominant culture) is basic identifying information needed in any family assessment. Complicating matters, ethnic backgrounds of parents and spouses may differ, and if this is so, it is important to assess how this difference is handled and how it affects family life.

Information on the family's religious beliefs and practices are intimately related to culture and thus should also be included as part of the cultural assessment (Tripp-Reimer et al., 1984). Religious beliefs often influence a family's conceptions of health and illness and how sick family members are treated. Family roles, rituals, values, and coping patterns are also affected by the family's religious orientation or legacy. The following specific areas are suggested as part of the identifying data about the family:

1. *The family's ethnic background (self-identified).*
2. *The family's degree of acculturation.* The assessment question posed here is, "To what extent has the family retained its ethnicity or cultural heritage?" Or posed in the reverse fashion, "To what extent has the family assimilated American culture?" Table 8–2 presents overall cultural assessment questions that, when answered, give pertinent information on the family's degree of acculturation. Some of the behavioral clues that indicate that the family still retains traditional (ethnic) practices, values, and beliefs follow:

a. Recent migration from another country (first generation).
b. Native culture is very different from American culture.
c. The family's friends and associations are of the same ethnic group (strong ethnic ties).
d. Family lives in an ethnically homogeneous neighborhood.
e. Strong religious affiliation.
f. Social, cultural, recreational, and/or educational activities are within the family's cultural group.
g. Dietary habits and dress are traditional.
h. Traditional family roles are carried out.
i. Home decorations, art, and other visual representations evidence the cultural background.
j. Native language is spoken exclusively or frequently in the home.
k. The territorial complex—the wider community the family frequents—is within the ethnic community primarily.
l. The family uses folk medicine or traditional healers, or perhaps a community health worker in whom the ethnic neighborhood has confidence.
m. Community discrimination (and segregation) against the identified ethnic group of the family exists.
n. Family members are nonwhite (creating obvious racial difference making acculturation more difficult).

Not all members of the family may have the same emotional ties to their ethnic background or religion. The older person and parents who are in the life cycle stages of raising children are usually more traditional than the children and young adults without children. The poor are generally less acculturated than the more affluent classes.

Within immigrant groups the degree of acculturation into the new culture has generally increased with each succeeding generation. An illustration of this phenomenon is the Japanese acculturation pattern. The first-generation Japanese-Americans, the Issei, who came here from Japan between 1890 and 1920, retained almost all of their former traditions. The second-generation Japanese-Americans, the Nisei, occupied an intermediate position on the assimilation continuum, while the third generation, the Sansei, are quite westernized. Interestingly enough, an opposing trend among the Yonsei, the fourth generation, is also being seen. As with other groups, there is a resurgence of interest in

TABLE 8–2. CULTURAL ASSESSMENT GUIDELINES

Assessment Criteria	Questions
Ethnic/racial identity	How does the family identify itself in terms of ethnicity and racial group? Are the parents both from the same cultural background?
Languages spoken	What language(s) is/are spoken in the home? And by whom? What language is preferred when speaking to outsiders?
Place of birth	Where were the parents and children born? If born in the U.S., where were the parents born? If born out the U.S., how many years have parents lived in the U.S.?
Geographic mobility	Where have the parents lived? When did they move to their present residence?
Family's religion	What is the family's religion? Are both parents from the same religious background? How actively involved is the family in religiously based activities and practices?
Ethnic group affiliation	What are the characteristics of the family's friends and associations? Are they all from the family's ethnic group? Are recreational, educational, and other social activities within the ethnic reference group, the wider community, or both? To what extent does the family use services and shop within the family's neighborhood or within the wider community?
Neighborhood affiliation	What are the characteristics of the family's neighborhood? Is it ethnically heterogeneous or homogeneous?
Dietary habits, dress	What are the family's dietary habits and dress?
Household appearance	Are the family's home decorations, art, and religious objects culturally derived
Use of folk systems	To what extent does the family use folk healing practices or practitioners?
Acceptance by community	To what extent is the family affected by discrimination?

Adapted from Friedman (1990).

ethnic "roots," particularly among the Yonsei, with whom the learning of the Japanese language and culture has become increasingly popular. (Peterson, 1981)

In spite of the tendency for persons from immigrant families to become more acculturated over time and in succeeding generations, some values, practices, and beliefs are retained. In the Mexican-American family the importance of the extended family has not waned over time; in fact, research shows that the extended family has grown in structure and functions when studied across generations (Baca-Zinn, 1981).

3. *The family's religious preference and practices.* The family's religious background should be noted, taking into account how individuals within the family differ in their religious beliefs and practices. How actively involved is the family in a particular church, temple, or other religious organization? As we learned from looking at families historically, the function of religion in family life has diminished (D'Antonio and Aldous, 1983). Nevertheless, we have great cultural diversity in our country and are currently seeing a resurgence of fundamental religion among some sectors of society. Hence, the role and importance of religion in families varies tremendously. In addition, it is suggested that an assessment be made of what religious practices the family engages in and what religiously based beliefs appear centrally important to the family.

In addition to the above general assessment areas, cultural assessment questions/areas are integrated throughout the entire family assessment guidelines. By completing the entire family assessment, one should have culled comprehensive data on cultural influences pertaining to the family organization (role, power, values, and communication facets), childrearing practices, affective responses, health care practices and beliefs, and coping strategies.

THE FAMILY'S SOCIAL CLASS

A family's social class is probably the prime molder of family life-style. Family life-style, structural and functional characteristics, and associations with the external environment of home, neighborhood, and community vary tremendously from social class to social class. This variance partially results from differences in preferences and perspectives. More importantly, however, these variations originate in the different conditions of and demands placed on the families of the several social classes. Social class, along with cultural background, exerts the greatest overall influence on family life, influencing family values and priorities, family behavioral patterns, socialization practices, family roles expectations, and world experiences families have.

Social class, social status, socioeconomic status, and occupational level/prestige are often interchangeably used terms (Langman, 1987). Social classes refer to aggregates of individuals who occupy broadly similar positions on the scale of prestige (Williams, 1960). Occupational position, weighted also with education and income, is used as a serviceable index of social class in American society. Generally the work deemed the greatest value to the society receives the greatest rewards, which include not only money but power, prestige, privilege, and autonomy. It has been frequently assumed that the husband's occupational status is the best single index of family ranking. Currently, however, it is being acknowledged that the wife's occupational level and income also have a major impact on the life-style and social class of a family. Family background can also be a factor for determining social class status, especially among the upper classes.

Social class pertains not only to the family's educational level, occupation status, and income, but also to the intricate interplay of these variables. Persons with different basic conditions of life, by virtue of their varied experience and exposure, come to see the world differently, to develop different conceptions of social reality as well as different aspirations, fears, and values.

Every society differentiates and ranks people, styles of life, automobiles, dress, and work in accordance with what it views as most valuable and important. No society, including American society, is classless, although Americans like to believe theirs is an open society with equal opportunity, where people can pull themselves up by their own bootstraps, American society is stratified into classes. Status consciousness is present even among children who begin very early to recognize their "place" and also the "place" of others in their little world.

By identifying a family's social class, family nurses can better anticipate the family's resources and some of its stressors. A family's structure and functions, moreover, are better understood in the light of its social class background.

Social Classes

Six discrete classes have been described by Warner (1953), Langman (1987), and other sociologists: the upper-upper, lower-upper, upper-middle, lower-middle, working class, and lower class. In the American class structure it is the family, not merely the individual, that is ranked. Goode (1964), along with other sociologists, states that the family is the keystone of the stratification system, the social mechanism by which it is maintained.

Presently there is much blurring between the social classes; moreover, within each of the groupings relative to their values and status there is certainly not homogeneity (Kohn, 1969). Other factors are also significant in creating diversity within a social class grouping—religion and ethnicity being two prime examples. The intra-ethnic variation created as a function of the interplay or intersection between the family's cultural and social class backgrounds is called in sociology *ethclass* (Gordon, 1964). Gordon uses this concept to explain the significant role that both the social class membership and ethnicity play in defining the basic conditions of life and simultaneously accounting for differences between ethnic groups situated in the same social class.

Using Warner's schematization of social class in America, the subsequent section of this chapter will briefly describe some characteristics of each of the six social classes, with an emphasis on value differences. Again, these classes are not precise explanations of reality, but are constructs designed to show the patterned relationships and life-style differences.

Upper-class Families. Upper-class families, according to Warner (1953), are divided into two groupings: the established upper-class family (upper-upper) and the "nouveau riche" or newly rich (lower-upper). Families that have possessed wealth for more than two generations are classified in the established group, while families of more recent affluence are placed in the second group.

The established upper-class family and its members were born into wealth and are closely protected and guarded from social exposures involving other social classes. The upper-upper class is very firmly entrenched in its culture, as well as in an extended family and a patriarchal kinship system. Protestant ethic values are subscribed to, to some extent, but these values do not have to be strictly upheld behaviorally, because professional and occupational security and monetary resources are provided by the family.

The New Lower-upper-Class Family. The "nouveau riche" lack the financial security provided by the kinship group in the upper-upper-class family. Its members are able to engage in a life-style resembling that of the established upper class, but they lack the long history of prestige, power, and family lineage.

In contrast with the upper-upper class, the newly affluent families are less likely to inherit their wealth, and more likely to have a greater cultural diversity. Income is earned rather than inherited, and differences in values (eg, spending patterns, which are symptomatic of priorities in values) vary between the two upper-class groups. Whereas upper-upper-class members spend more in the areas of culture and philanthropy, the lower-upper class typically spends more on "conspicuous consumption" of goods and products—automobiles, clothes, expensive recreation, and large houses. Because these families are upwardly mobile, they tend to pursue friendships with socially prominent individuals, rather than maintain close ties with their extended family. Thus, the predominant family structure is nuclear and husband dominated, and its members act independently of kin.

Middle-class Families. The middle class is considered *dominant* numerically and socially, in the sense that they are most able to disseminate their views on what is right, proper, and expected behavior—whether in the family, school, or health agency. This dominance is due primarily to the key positions of the upper middle class in government, education, and mass communications.

The Upper-middle-class Family. This class is comprised of professionals in law, accounting, and medicine; higher-level businesspeople; middle management in corporations; successful entrepreneurs; service professionals, particularly at the university level; mental health workers; and administrators of social service and governmental organizations (Langman, 1987). Being the career-oriented bearers of the "American success syndrome," most in this class are college graduates and comprise the "solid highly respectable" people in the community. Individualism, rationality, personal achievement, and the other secular Protestant ethic values (mastery, future orientation, work, and so forth) are stressed (Adams, 1980; Schultz, 1972).

The number of dual-career, upper-middle-class families has recently increased. In dual-career families, patterns of traditional sex differentiation have blurred and more egalitarianism is seen between spouses.

Upper-middle-class families are often geographically mobile in pursuit of career goals. But in spite of their mobility, extensive visiting, communication, and aid between generations occurs (Lee, 1979).

The Lower-middle-class Family. The lower-middle class is made up of small businessmen, clerical workers, other low-level white-collar workers, bureaucratic functionaries, and salespersons. This class represents a wide variety of national and ethnic backgrounds. Like those in the class above them, the families are relatively stable in spite of problems connected with their economic security and the education of their children. Frequently students report the conflicts that exist between themselves and their parents. The parents work to provide an education for their children, which in turn introduces the children to a set of values that is often in conflict with those of the parents.

The major distinguishing values of the members of this status group are respectability and achievement. Hard work and honesty are also highly valued.

In the lower-middle-class family today, the power structure is usually egalitarian or mildly husband dominated. The wife defers to the husband's authority, yet maintains control over personal and familial household realms. Socially the kinship group is close, and major social activities often take place with relatives from the husband's or wife's family (Schultz, 1972). Families are generally child-oriented (Langman, 1987).

The Working-class Family. Blue-collar or working-class families generally came from rural backgrounds. Families moved to the cities as technology progressed and skilled labor was needed. The blue collar or working class is made up of skilled workers, semiskilled workers in factories, service workers, and a few small tradesmen who usually have steady jobs, even though they often do not pay well. The elite of the working class—electricians, plumbers, and other highly skilled operators—frequently earn more than members of the middle classes and are sometimes viewed as part of the lower-middle-class group. For members of this class who are in trades that depend on the swings of the business cycle, economic stability is lacking.

A considerable proportion of wives are employed outside of the home. Unlike a sizable proportion of female workers from the upper-middle and upper classes, the upper-lower-class wife takes a job more out of economic necessity than from the desire for a career. Family strains are associated with economic uncertainties.

It is within the blue-collar family more than any other class that one still sees many husbands and wives conforming to the traditional husband and wife roles. The husband is often seen as a patriarchial authority. Both of the sexes tend to think that friendship and companionship are more likely to exist between members of the same sex than among marital partners, and see the principal marital ties as involving the sexual union, complementary tasks, and mutual devotion (Adams, 1980; Komarovsky, 1964). Obedience and stricter traditional childrearing patterns are typically seen in this class (Peterson & Rollins, 1987).

When there is need for assistance, relatives are likely to be called on before turning to a public agency. The extended family, the neighborhood peer group, and the informal work group provide much social interaction as well as actual assistance for blue-collar families.

The Lower-class Family. Lower-class families are at the impoverished level of existence, although their degree of impoverishment varies. Wide variations also exist in life-style, as seen in rural versus urban areas, and in different regional and ethnic/social lower-class communities. Generally, however, the common social characteristics of the lower-lower class include the following:

1. A formal education of 8 years or less.
2. The male's occupation is almost always semiskilled or unskilled. His work pattern is often sporadic, with long periods of unemployment. There is also a strong probability that the woman works in an unskilled or service occupation.
3. Because of unemployment or underemployment and low wages, lower-class families make up a large number of those on the public assistance rolls.
4. If they live in the city, their place of residence is typically in the slum areas, often in old, dilapidated homes and buildings converted into small apartments. The ratio of persons per room is often three or four to one, and frequently as many as 20 people share the use of a single toilet (Bell, 1971).

Poverty in America. "The story of the 1980s is that the rich did well and the poor lost ground" (United Press International, 1990). During the period of the Reagan Administration a significant change in the distribution of income and wealth occurred in the United States. (This shift actually began earlier, but accelerated during the 1980s due to the reduction of social programs designed to aid the poor and working and middle classes.) Winnick (1988), a sociologist, calls this a movement toward "two societies, separate and unequal." The gulf in income and resources between rich and poor Americans is wider than at any time since figures were recorded, starting in the 1940s (Kozol, 1990). There is a shrinking of the middle class, with an increasing proportion of the population located in the upper and lower classes.

The effects of certain economic and technological

POVERTY

In 1987 there were 13 million children under 18 years of age living in poverty.

Between 1980 amd 1987, the number of children living in poverty increased by 1.5 million; in contrast, the number of persons 65 years and over living in poverty declined by 3.8 million.

Black or Hispanic children are nearly 3 times more likely to live in poverty than are white children.

*In 1987, a family of four was considered to be living in poverty if its annual income was below $11,611.

Note: Hispanic data not collected prior to 1973.

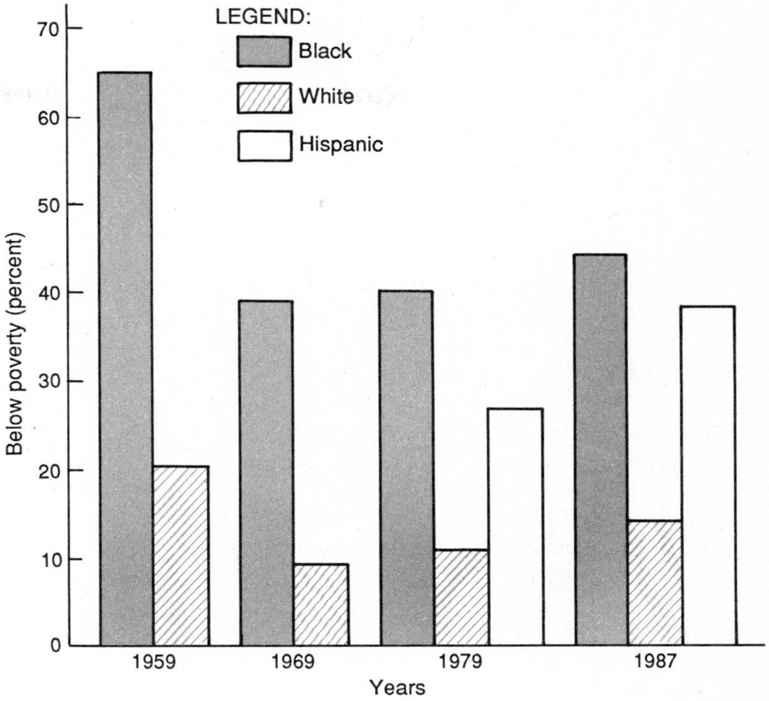

Figure 8–3
Children in poverty. Children under 18 years of age, 1987. (From: U.S. Bureau of the Census, 1989.)

trends, and the last decade of declining domestic and social programs, have had an indelibly harsh impact on poor families. Research findings since the 1930s consistently indicate that economic distress is associated with lower levels of family stability, marital adjustment, family coping, family cohesion, marital communication, and harmonious family relationships (Voydanoff and Donnelly, 1988).

The lower class is disproportionately composed of ethnic minorities and recent immigrants, female-headed households, children, and those with certain personally disorganizing problems: chronic mental illness, alcoholism, and drug abuse. Among families the incidence of poverty is more than three times higher for blacks and Hispanics than for whites (Winnick, 1988). One third of all female-headed households in 1985 were living at or below the poverty level, while among black and Hispanic families over 50 percent were poor. Among children, poverty is widespread. One out of every five children in 1985 was living in poverty, according to Census Bureau statistics. This translates into about 40 percent of all Hispanic and 43 percent of all black children in the United States (Fig. 8–3). The average poor black child today appears to be in the middle of a prolonged poverty period situation for black children than it has been for any year back to the late 1960s (Winnick, 1988).

Both rural and central city areas suffer from high rates of poverty. In 1986, nonmetropolitan (rural) poverty rates were slightly higher than poverty rates in U.S. central cities. The changing economy in farming communities has fueled the growth of poverty in rural America (National Council for Family Relations, 1989).

In summary, current problems of poor families are bleak according to recent national reports and surveys. "Family structures are besieged and weakened by unemployment, poor schools, loss of family support systems, family violence, drug and alcohol abuse and depression" (Family Service America, 1984, p. 77).

It is difficult for most students and teachers to describe the life-style of the lower class without imposing middle-class evaluations. Even the use of the term "lower class" probably imposes a negative connotation and interpretation to people who occupy this class level. As stated by Rodman (1965), "It is little wonder that if we describe the lower-class family in terms of promiscuous sexual relationships, illegitimate children, deserting men, and unmarried mothers, we are going to see the situation as disorganized and chock-full of problems" (p. 223).

In observing social conditions of lower-class life from a middle-class perspective, we should not become so engrossed in looking at the victims that we fail to understand the reasons for the problems. Perhaps it is more realistic to think of these conditions as consequences of, or in some instances solutions to, other issues faced by lower-class people as they experience all the social, economic, political, and legal realities of life (Eshleman, 1974). When working with the poor, family nurses need to accord the same respect and regard for them as for all other clients. Identifying the family's strengths and weaknesses and seeing the family within its own context are important principles for providing care. Oscar Lewis (1961), a noted anthropologist, has termed his class "the culture of poverty." He believed that the lower-class life-style is the direct result of poverty and that this "culture" is not just an American phenomenon, but represents values and patterns that can be found cross-culturally.

In contrast with the working class, the lower class does not have the respect of the larger community. Its members are likely to be stigmatized and characterized as being lazy, shiftless, and dependent. The source of the stigma is usually the inability or lack of fulfillment of our number one cardinal value—productivity.

Poverty in the Family. Directly related to the poverty of the lower-class is the irregularity of employment, and thus income. Because income is irregular, a considerable amount of insecurity exists in regard to food, clothing, shelter, transportation, health care, and other essentials. Children may be forced or encouraged to contribute to the financial needs of the family, and few remain in school beyond the minimum legal age.

Lower-class family life, adapting to scarce resources, is based on assumptions and norms that are different from those of the middle class (Staples, 1976). The poor cannot "afford" such values of the middle class as productivity, achievement, work, and long-range planning. It is interesting to note, however, that parents' aspirations for their children are very "middle class," despite their inability to provide the ways and means for achieving such goals. The modal poor family is large, headed by minority group women who are unemployed or underemployed and dependent on welfare (Langman, 1987). Matrifocality, where the mother is the center of family life, is an adaptation to poverty rather than a desired option.

The American Underclass. A large portion of the poor is now termed "the American underclass" (Russell, 1977; Wilson, 1987). Both stable marriages and legal divorces tend to be luxuries in this class. Toughness is a desirable interpersonal trait. Children are frequently taught to defend themselves physically rather than with mental or psychological tactics.

These are the people who remain more or less permanently at the bottom of the social ladder, completely removed from "the American Dream." The underclass have become increasingly isolated socially from mainstream patterns and norms of behavior (Wilson, 1987). Although its members come from all races and live throughout the United States, the underclass is made up primarily of (1) impoverished urban blacks, who suffer from the heritage of slavery and discrimination as well as the changing economy; (2) Hispanics, primarily Chicanos and Puerto Ricans, who have recently immigrated into cities and rural areas (as migrant workers); and (3) Appalachian migrants who live in dilapidated neighborhoods of some cities. This group now amounts to about 3 to 5 percent of America's population (Russell, 1977).

Their long-term poverty and welfare dependency, plus their bleak environment nurtures values that are often at radical odds with those of the majority—even the majority of the poor. Thus the underclass minority is disproportionately represented among the nation's juvenile delinquents, gang members, drug addicts, physically disabled people, and single parents on welfare. They are "responsible," therefore, for a considerable amount of the adult crime, family disruption, urban decay, and need for social expenditures. The underclass remains a nucleus of psychological and material destitution despite some two decades of civil rights gains in the 1960s and 1970s. Federal reductions in domestic social programs, beginning in 1980, have only magnified the problem.

Even though unemployment decreased in the 1980s somewhat, the underclass is made up of people who lack the necessary education, skills, discipline, and self-esteem to succeed. Long-term unemployment is a common factor here, and large numbers of the underclass are single parents on welfare.

More jobs and a better education are clearly two pressing needs. In our achievement-oriented society, work is more than a source of income. It is also a source of being productive, which brings self-esteem, status, a point of identification with the system, and a satisfying social environment. Stanford University black historian Clay Carson comments: "Permanency of jobs, stability in an economic situation, is important. Even if someone is only a janitor, his job still means stability.

Those who can get established with a job in an urban environment can pass this stability on to their kids" (Russell, 1977).

People from the underclass subculture within our communities, especially our cities, are in the greatest need of our health and social services. In official health agencies, much of the nurse's effort is necessarily concentrated on the very poor. It is only through our understanding and appreciation of some of the major problems and daily realities of the poor that we can even begin to assist these families with the resolution of their health needs.

Economic Status

Economic status, a component of social class, refers to the family's income level and source of income. Geismar and La Sorte (1964) developed criteria and descriptions for assessing the economically adequate, marginal, and inadequate family. Income that is sufficient to meet a family's needs is generally derived from the work of family members or from private sources such as pensions and support payments (nonpublic), while income derived partially from general relief or unemployment is generally marginal, unstable, or barely adequate. The family that is functioning inadequately in this area exhibits these characteristics: (1) income derived entirely from general relief because of failure or inability of adult(s) in the family to work; (2) income derived from welfare by fraudulent means; and (3) amount of income so low or unstable that basic necessities are lacking. Families receiving income from programs such as Aid to the Totally Disabled, Aid to the Blind, Aid to Families of Dependent Children, and Old Age Assistance, although in most cases based on legitimate need, would fall under the marginal or inadequate category, because the level of funding is so low that basic necessities are barely or inadequately provided for.

One of the basic family functions is the provision of adequate economic support and allocation of resources. Hence not only income level should be estimated but also expenditures, focusing on the allocation of resources. Assessing expenditures, again a sensitive subject that should be discussed specifically only when needed, consists of asking about regular financial obligations: rent or mortgage payments, insurance, transportation costs or car payments, phone and utility bills, food expenses, and any special bills the family may have incurred.

Geismar and La Sorte (1964) divided families into four economic levels: adequate, marginal, poor, and very poor. Adequate refers to monies spent on the basis of an understanding that finances are the responsibility of one or both of the parents. The family budgets and realistically manages expenditures. At the marginal level, there is disagreement and conflict over who controls income and expenditures; the family is unable to live within its means; and poor money management resulting in luxuries sometimes taking precedence over basic necessities. Poor money management may or may not endanger the children's welfare, but expenditures and financial needs exceed income. Very poor money management, however, involves impulsive spending and accumulation of excessive debts, and results in the lack of providing for basic family needs.

Social Class Mobility

Another family assessment area related to social class is social class mobility. This refers to vertical mobility upward or downward through the social class strata and is included here because a change in either direction produces considerable stress. Holmes and Rahe (1967), in their social readjustment scale, identify changes of position, status, or prestige, whether positive or negative, as stress producing. Although upward mobility is seen as desirable by most persons, and does often result in new recognition and social prestige, it may also result in rejection and social isolation. The cohesiveness of the extended family most likely decreases. In addition, lower levels of family participation are found in upwardly mobile families. Interpersonal relationships and the degree of personal comfort are also often compromised (Eshleman, 1974).

In America, people expect a move upward as a natural state of affairs. Social mobility seems to be increasing recently but was probably never as widespread as generally believed. Cavan (1969) reports as follows: "A number of studies indicate that about 30 percent of people occupy a different class position than that of their parents, as judged primarily by differences in the occupational rankings of the fathers and sons" (p. 181). The remaining 70 percent of families remain in the same social class, and this stability of social class placement can be seen through a number of generations. Examples of the stability of social class status are found among upper-class families, where their wealth or prestige has continued through several generations. A similar continuity is also observed in the lower classes (Cavan, 1969). In the well-known social class study by Hollingshead (1949), he showed that the lower-lower social class of "Elmstown" had held this position since before the Civil War. Mobility occurs most frequently in the lower-middle, working, and upper-lower classes.

The majority of the vertical mobility in America has been upward, as evidenced by our growing middle class. In some cases, widespread social mobility may result for entire communities or regions as a consequence, for instance, of a prolonged economic depression—producing downward mobility. This process occurred recently in Texas and parts of Colorado with the collapse of the energy/oil industry. At the other end of the continuum, the full employment and prosperity experienced generally in the 1960s and early 1970s may have carried many families upward. Retirement and becoming disabled often result in downward social class mobility. This is because of the marked reduction in income that often accompanies both retirement and becoming permanently disabled.

ASSESSMENT QUESTIONS AND AREAS: SOCIO-ECONOMIC STATUS & SOCIAL MOBILITY

Social Class Status

Based on the family's income level and source of income, and the adult members' occupation and education, identify the family's social class status.

Economic Status

Asking how much the husband or wife earns can be an invasive question, as income is considered a private matter among most families. A question should be asked only if there is an important reason to do so, such as in determining eligibility for assistance or services. Questions relevant to this area include the following:

- Who is (are) the breadwinner(s) of the family?
- Does the family receive any supplementary funds or assistance? If so, from where (eg, retirement fund, Social Security, food stamps)?

From this information, plus information on occupations, one can often estimate weekly or monthly income or ask a question regarding approximate income.

- Does the family consider its income adequate? How does it see itself managing financially?
- What financial resources does the family or could the family have (for example, medical insurance, disability insurance, dental insurance, workman's compensation, food stamps, unemployment insurance, crippled children's services, reduced transportation fares)?

Social Class Mobility

Describe the family's social class mobility—the change(s) that occurred to produce downward or upward mobility, when these changes occurred, and how the family adjusted to the changes.

FAMILY SOCIAL NETWORKS AND SOCIAL SUPPORT: THEORY AND ASSESSMENT

A growing interest by social scientists and health professionals has led to a heightened awareness of the effects of personal and familial social environments and social supports on adaptation and health. Due to the important influence of social support on health outcomes, this concept has emerged as a major variable addressed in health-related research today.

It is widely accepted that people who are in supportive social environments are generally in better condition than their counterparts without this advantage. More specifically, because social supports are thought to attenuate the effects of stress (called a "buffering effect" in research) as well as enhance an individual's or family's mental health directly (called "main or direct effects" in research), social support is a crucial coping strategy for families to have available in times of stress.* Social support also may serve as a preventive strategy to reduce stress and its negative consequences.

Definition of Concepts

In this discussion two closely related key terms are social support and social network. Social network (Hall and Wellman, 1985) refers to a weblike structure comprising one's relationships. Network size, density, accessibility, kinship reliance, frequency of contact, and stability are structural areas of assessment. Within a family's social network are friends and work associates, neighbors, and community networks (church and community groups and agencies); professional networks (including health care providers and other professionals); self-help groups; and extended and immediate kin (Pilisuk and Parks, 1983).

In contrast, social support "focuses on the nature of the interactions taking place within social relationships as these are evaluated by the individual" (Roth, 1989. p. 91). Social support, then, entails an individual or family evaluating whether social interactions/relationships are helpful and to what extent. Cohen and Syme (1985) further clarify the difference between social support and social networks: "While social network may be defined as the structure of the relationship, social support is the function of the relationship" (p. 11).

Most researchers see social support as including both tangible instrumental support (transactions in which direct aid or assistance is given) and emotional/informational support (House and Kahn, 1985;

** Family social support is also discussed in Chap. 17 as an external type of family coping.*

Thoits, 1982). House and Kahn (1985) include these two components of social support in their four types of support: instrumental, informational, appraisal, and emotional.

In the social support/social network literature these terms refer to individuals, not family groups. To focus on the aggregate level of analysis—the family—these terms need to be modified.

Family social support refers to the social supports that are perceived by family members to be available/accessible to the family (the social support may or may not be used, but family members perceive that supportive persons are ready to provide aid and assistance if needed). Family social support can either be internal family social support, such as spousal support or sibling support; or external family social support—the social supports external to the nuclear family (within the family's social network). A family's social network is simply that social network of the nuclear family itself.

Although there are voluminous definitions and descriptions of social support and social network, only a few articles discuss family social support (Friedman, 1985; Kane, 1988). Kane defines family social support as a process of relationship between the family and its social environment. The three interactional dimensions of family social support are reciprocity (the nature and frequency of reciprocal relations); advice/feedback (the quality/quantity of communication); and emotional involvement (the extent of intimacy and trust) in the social relationships.

Family social support is a process that occurs over the life span; the nature and type of social support differs within the various family life cycle stages. For instance, the types and quantity of social support during the stage of marriage (before a young couple have children) is drastically different than the social support types and amount needed when the family is in the last stage of the life cycle. Nevertheless, in all life cycle stages, family social support enables the family to function with versatility and resourcefulness. As such, it promotes family adaptation and health.

Both the nuclear and extended family serve as support systems to its members. Caplan (1976) explains that the family has eight supportive functions including informational support (the family serves as a collector and disseminator of information about the world); appraisal support (the family acts as a feedback guidance system, guides and mediates problem solving, and is a source and validator of member identity); instrumental support (the family is a source of practical and concrete aid); and emotional support (the family serves as a haven for rest and recuperation and contributes to emotional mastery).

In writing about family social networks, Milardo (1988) states that families live in an elaborate system of interactions where they create ties with a broad array of other individuals, families, and larger groups. "Families are profoundly influenced by this web of ties and they are active agents in modifying and adapting these communities of personal relationships to meet ever-changing circumstances" (p. 14).

A deficit and/or impairment in social support within a person's social network is identified by NANDA as the nursing diagnoses of social isolation and impaired social interaction (McFarland and McFarlane, 1989). These diagnoses could well apply to families, as the nature of the problem and the negative outcomes are similar.

Social Support Research

In summarizing an extensive body of social support and health research, Wills (1985) concluded that both buffering effects (social support buffers the negative effects of stress on health) and main effects (social support directly influences health outcomes) have been found. In fact, the main and buffering effects of social support on health and well-being may function simultaneously. More specifically, the presence of adequate social support has been found to be linked with reduced mortality, more favorable recovery from illness, and among the elderly, better physical and emotional health and cognitive functioning (Ryan and Austin, 1989). In addition, the positive impact of social support on adjustment to stressful life events is most often seen in studies where perceived support versus received support is measured.

Family Social Support

Studies of family social support have conceptualized social support as a type of family coping (Friedman, 1985; Stetz et al, 1986). Both internal and external family social supports were found to be utilized.

Extended families provide critical social support to nuclear families today. Most adults live in communities in which they maintain one or more contacts with a living parent or other close relative (U.S. Bureau of the Census, 1989). Recent U.S. Census data (Table 8–3) validate this point (U.S. Bureau of the Census, 1989). Moreover, most family members are satisfied with the frequency and quality of intergenerational relationships (Shanas, 1980).

In the Latino community, extended family ties have remained particularly strong; extended family ties are also stronger in Asian-American and black American families than with white American families. Litwak (1972) referred to the common American form of family as "the modified extended family," emphasizing that it

TABLE 8–3. CONTACTS BETWEEN PEOPLE 65 YEARS OLD AND OVER AND CHILDREN WHO DO NOT LIVE IN SAME HOUSEHOLD

Frequency of seeing or talking with child	
Daily	= 41%
Two or more times/week	= 21%
Weekly	= 20%
Two or more times/month	= 7%
Monthly	= 5%
Less than monthly	= 6%
Traveling time for child to get to parents	
Within 10 minutes	= 26%
10 to 29 minutes	= 29%
More than 30 minutes	= 45%

U.S. Bureau of the Census (1989).

consists of two or more nuclear families, linked to one another by a web of economic interdependence, mutual aid, and social interaction.

Because we have a large proportion of single parents, blended families, and dual-worker families, the various forms of family life today show a wide range in their ability to provide the needed supports during high-demand periods. The management of chronic illness is a case in point. Chronic illness often necessitates greater economic, social, and psychological sacrifices than many extended families are ready and able to make (Pilisuk and Parks, 1983). Family caregiver burden is a major concern here. The role of the extended family varies according to the nature of the need for assistance. Extended kin are reported in research studies to be the preferred source of assistance for disasters, financial assistance, long-term crises, and more extensive problems. Geographic distance of family does not preclude extended family support (Lee, 1979).

Assessing the Family's Social Support and Social Network

Does the family have meaningful ties with friends, relatives, and social groups that provide satisfaction and assistance when needed? If so, who are they and what is the nature of their relationship?

Or does the family have little or no contacts with neighbors, relatives, or social groups, and is it dissatisfied or hostile toward community?

Hogue (1977) suggests that these types of questions be asked to elicit information on the family's support system. She says that it is more acceptable with clients to move from life events already identified and ask:

> "Who helps you with . . . ?" If you had any problems about . . . who would you talk to, get help from?" Asking general, then more specific questions is helpful. For example, "Who helped you through retiring from your job?" (general), "Who or what kind of help have you had with the financial concerns most people have when they retire?" (specific). Another useful question is, "Who has helped you through tough situations in the past?" (p. 77)

To obtain further social support network information, both the genogram and the ecomap are suggested. Figure 8–2 depicts the family genogram. The genogram identifies primary kin within the extended family (these are the parents' siblings and parents).

The ecomap graphically depicts the family's relationships and interactions with its immediate external environment. This tool assists the family and family health provider to visualize the family social network and, to some extent, how family members are perceiving and/or receiving social support. Figure 8–4 is a blank ecomap that family members and the nurse may jointly complete.

To complete the ecomap, place the family in the middle circle, and significant people, organizations, and agencies in the outer circles. The nature of the relationships between the family and its various contacts are indicated by lines. Straight lines show strong relationships, dotted lines tenuous relationships, and slashed lines conflictual/stressful relationships. The wider the straight lines, the stronger the relationship. Arrows may be used to show the direction of energy and resources within a particular relationship (Hartman, 1978; Wright and Leahey, 1984). Figure 8–5 shows an example of an ecomap. By using both the family genogram and family ecomap in assessment, the family nurse is able to get a fuller view of the family and its social network and supports.

FAMILY RECREATIONAL ACTIVITIES: THEORY AND ASSESSMENT

Each family member has his or her own special leisure-time activities, depending on individual interests and needs, age, and available time and resources. In addition to individual leisure-time activities, the family unit itself will also, hopefully, have regular family-centered activities where all members can share and enhance their life together. These activities may be religious, educational, recreational, civic, or cultural in nature.

Recreational activities refers to those activities that are apart from the obligations of work, family, and society and to which individuals turn at will for relaxation, diversion, self-development, or social participation. Family recreation entails the renewing and strengthening of family bonds, having fun together, sharing feelings, reducing tension, and improving fam-

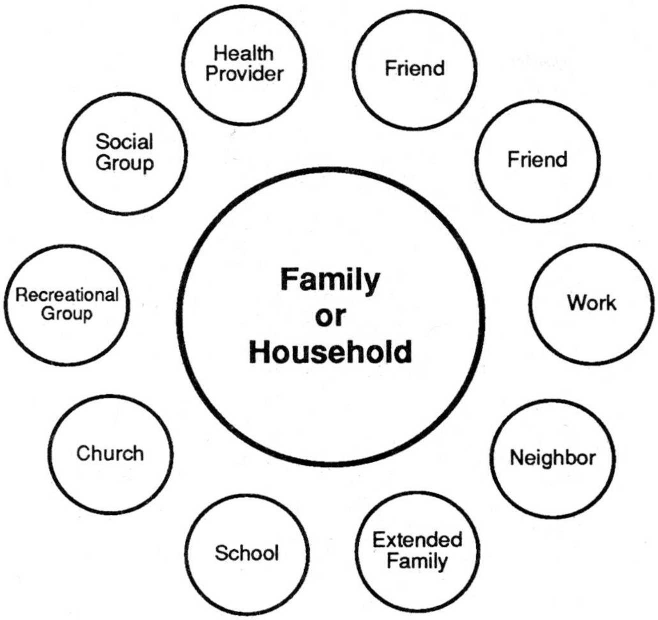

Figure 8–4
Blank family ecomap.

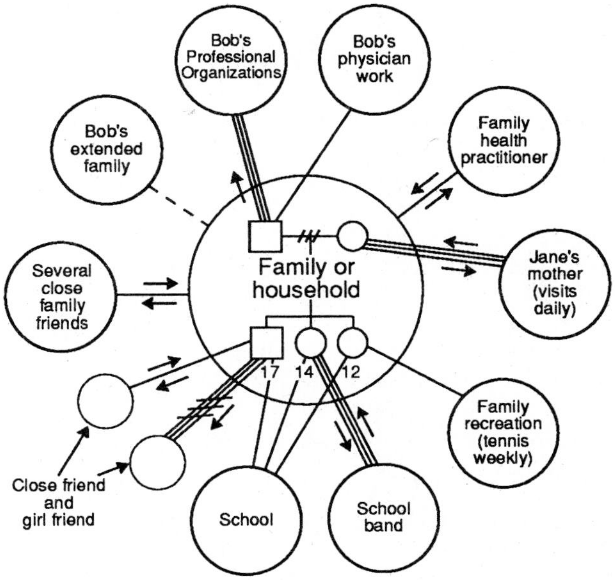

Figure 8–5
Example of family ecomap.

ily members' feelings about their family (Geba, 1985; McCown et al, 1989).

Changing values of society have made quality of life, high-level wellness, and self-fulfillment through work and leisure more prominent today. In the family today recreation has in some ways declined in importance because of competing leisure-time opportunities for individuals. Other factors, however, are responsible for making family recreation a continuing significant family activity: longer paid vacations, shorter working hours, more 3-day weekends, and greater accessibility to recreational facilities, at least for the more affluent social classes. Carlsen (1976) reports that there is considerable evidence that recreation is highly valued among families and that the spouses feel a sense of duty to provide for such activities for the family. Planning and engaging in family recreational activities appear to be a shared role among parents. Researchers report that family members believe that not enough time is spent in family leisure-time activity (Smith, 1985).

Research on family recreation has focused on its positive effect on marital and family satisfaction, family unity, and marital stability (Hill, 1988; Smith, 1985). For instance, Gerson (1960), in studying married college couples, found a positive relationship between a number of leisure-time factors and marital satisfaction. West and Merriam (1969) discovered a positive correlation between outdoor recreation and family solidarity. Hill (1988), applying attachment theory to her study, found that spouses' shared recreational time was predictive of marital stability.

Kelly (1978) concluded that the family is a central social context of leisure. He observed that the home is the most common locale for leisure-time activity and family members are the usual companions for most kinds of weekday, weekend, and vacational leisure. Stinnett (1979), Otto (1973), and McCubbin and McCubbin (1988) validate the important role family leisure-time activity plays in family life by including indicators of family recreational activity in their lists of family strengths—such as spending time together, having common interests, having fun together, and having family traditions, celebrations, and rituals.

Family Recreation Assessment Areas

Suggested assessment areas pertaining to a family's recreational or leisure-time activities include the following:

1. Identifying the recreational/leisure-time activities of the whole family. What types of activities? How often do these activities occur? Who participates in them?
2. Identifying the recreational/leisure-time activities of the family subsystems (spouse subsystem, parent–child subsystems, and sibling subsystems). What types of activities? How often do these activities occur? Who participates in them?
3. Exploring the family members' feelings about the family's leisure-time/recreational activities (satisfaction with time spent and types of activities).

Keeping the family subsystems strong and functioning effectively is crucial to family health. Thus recreational activities involving the subsystems as well as the whole family is viewed as a major family strength.

FAMILY NURSING INTERVENTIONS

This section discusses intervention guidelines associated with the several aspects covered in this chapter—guidelines for working with ethnic minority families, for assisting families with economic difficulties, for promoting adequate social support, and for increasing families' recreational/leisure-time activities.

Sociocultural Family Interventions

Guidelines for providing culturally appropriate family health care to ethnic families are necessarily broad, because more specific intervention strategies are limited to only certain ethnic groups. Four basic strategies suggested in the literature involve (1) selecting the appropriate system to work with, (2) providing more time to work with unacculturated families, (3) dealing with language differences, and (4) taking into account the family's interactional norms.

Selecting the appropriate family system to work with is a crucial consideration. Which system to work with (a family subsystem such as the marital or parent–child subsystem, the nuclear family, or the extended family) can determine the outcome. Understanding and respecting the ethnic minority family's cultural norms and present social context are perhaps the most important skills in selecting a system for counseling (Dilworth-Anderson and McAdoo, 1988; Ho, 1987).

> Considering the intense involvement that ethnic minority families have with their extended family, some family problems can be resolved simply by involving the extended family members, especially the spokesperson, who normally is the grandfather (Asian/Hispanic) or grandmother (black and Indian) (Ho, 1987, p. 258).

A second general intervention guideline deals with the time needed to provide care to ethnic families. If the family is unacculturated, Harwood (1981) stresses the importance of allowing more time for health care interventions. More time is typically required for translation, for discussion and clarification of health information, for explanation of diagnosis and treatment plans, and for socializing the family members to the health care system.

Language use in clinical encounters with members of ethnic families is a third general consideration. In assessing and intervening, the health practitioner should not assume that a foreign-born client and his or her family wish to carry on an interview in their native language. When the language ability of the individual is not apparent, asking what language he or she prefers to use is indicated. Having translators is not without its problems, but usually is preferable to attempting to use a phrase book or a very limited vocabulary to communicate (Harwood, 1981).

Harwood (1981) gives three recommendations that address interactional norms to clinicians working with ethnic minorities. First, he suggests that in ethnic groups that are kin-based or from peasant societies, the elderly are accorded more respect than they are in our society. Moreover, social interaction between sexes is more limited, and standards of modesty more strictly prescribed. As a result, the style of interaction between the family nurse and family member should reflect these interactional norm differences. For example, a younger health care professional should show greater respect and deference to an older family member. Certain potentially embarrassing topics should be discussed only with certain members of the family present. Because the health care professional is usually seen as an authority figure, he or she needs to assume an active, more directive role in the beginning phase of working with an ethnic family (Ho, 1987).

Secondly, due to professional and class status differences, members of ethnic families are often reticent to ask questions or discuss their concerns. Active encouragement to ask questions and bring up concerns is needed to breakdown this barrier.

And a third related approach is to actively listen to what family members have to say. The family nurse should convey an interest in the client and family, personalizing the encounter such as the folk healer might do.

Ho (1987), a family therapist, discusses culturally relevant techniques and skills in the phases of family therapy. Due to cultural barriers to family mental health services, he stresses the cruciality of developing trust with the family in the beginning phase of family counseling. During the early engagement phase, he suggests that the clinician may need to explore with the family ethnic/cultural differences between the clinician and family.

Family nursing interventions that are culturally appropriate during health care treatment include facilitating access to needed health knowledge, consideration of dietary practices and beliefs, family visiting and participation practices, and understanding preferences for home versus inpatient and long-term care.

Harwood (1981) points out that unacculturated ethnic minority families generally have poor access to health knowledge. Especially if they do not speak English, are poorly educated, and have a social network composed of families from their same socioeconomic and ethnic background, they have limited access to accurate, up-to-date health knowledge. As a consequence, these families are much more in need of health education than more advantaged majority families. Health knowledge deficits need to be carefully addressed here.

As part of medical regimes, therapeutic diets must incorporate ethnic differences if they are to be followed. Ethnically acceptable therapeutic diets should reflect both ethnic food preferences and ethnic food beliefs.

Family visiting and participation in a family member's care while he or she is in the hospital also varies from ethnic group to ethnic group. In many cultures, the family plays a major role in patient care. In ethnic groups with strong familistic orientations, such as in Asian and Hispanic families, sickness is a time when relatives display their support and solidarity. Hence, visiting the hospital and fully participating in care are important family activities for the psychological state of not only the patient but also the family (Harwood, 1981).

And a last general guideline to providing culturally appropriate health care addresses the difference in preferences of ethnic minority groups to home care versus hospital care or long-term care. "Many ethnic groups strongly prefer home care over institutionalized care for the incapacitated and terminally ill. . . . Chinese, Haitians, Italians, Mexicans, and Puerto Ricans all manifest this preference, while urban blacks and Navajos do not" (Harwood, 1981, p. 503). Harwood explains that the reasons for this preference among the former groups has to do with their strong extended family ties and the low participation of women caregivers in the work force. The high percentage of urban black and white women in the work force is undoubtedly a major barrier to home care in those groups.

Financial Interventions

Interventions that assist families in ameliorating the financial implications of health and illness problems are often overlooked in family nursing. If family nurses are aware of the financial impact of health problems on families, there is often much they can do to help (Millington and Zieball, 1986), particularly if the nurse is in the primary care or community setting. A family that is at high risk medically is also a family that is at high risk financially, given the need for expensive, specialized diagnostic and treatment procedures, personnel, and long-term care.

Financial stress often permeates the family system and results in family disruption. The medical bills may necessitate that the mother work outside the home, the father take on a second job, and vacation and leisure time activities be eliminated. Strains in the marriage that then "ripple" into the other sets of family relationships are commonplace. Divorce, separation, acting out children, psychosomatic problems, and substance abuse are symptomatic of the long-term disruptive effects financial stress may induce (Millington and Zieball, 1986).

For the most part, nurses have tended to leave financial concerns up to the social worker to handle. Yet in many settings there is no available social worker and the nurse is the appropriate health care professional to intervene. Even if there is a social worker available, only when the nurse assesses for financial problems can he or she then become aware of the problem and make the appropriate referral.

Usually nursing interventions in this area center around providing information to families on health care costs and community resources, as well as making referrals—a case management intervention.

Nurses need to be aware of the costs to families when

TABLE 8–4. FINANCIAL ASSESSMENT AND INTERVENTION STRATEGIES

Assessment Strategies
Establishing trust and rapport with family.
Assessing family's financial costs, resources, and allocation of resources for health care.
Assessing family's coping efforts and resources.

Intervention Strategies
Teaching family ways to reduce health care costs by presenting available alternatives/options.
Teaching family to understand and evaluate insurance coverage.
Referring family to appropriate services within and outside health care agency.
Helping family cope with financial stress.

Adapted from Millington and Zieball (1986).

complex problems arise, as well as the family's financial resources and how the family is and will pay for the needed services, supplies, equipment, and so forth. He or she should be familiar with the types of medical care programs available for the medically needy within the particular target population as well as the community services available free or at reduced costs for all regardless of their ability to pay. Immunizations and screening clinics are examples of these latter types of community resources.

Teaching in the financial area, according to Millington and Zieball (1986) includes teaching families about ways to reduce health care costs, to evaluate their insurance coverage, to determine how their health resources are being allocated and where costs could safely be reduced. Teaching families how to look at their financial situation objectively and problem solve effectively is also suggested. Table 8–4 summarizes assessment and intervention strategies for assisting families at high risk for financial stress.

Social Support and Social Network Interventions

Because of family nurses' commitment to families and family members, the importance of human relationships and support to families is readily apparent. This places family nurses in an ideal position to assess and intervene to enhance clients' social support and social network.

Families need to have available social supports to prevent them from entering into crisis when demands on the family increase. When families do face life events and transitions that challenge their coping skills, social support can be mobilized in several ways: (1) by improving the quality of support received by the family's social network, (2) by reanchoring themselves into a network that is more responsive to their present emotional needs or reorienting themselves to sectors of their network containing more appropriate psychosocial resources (Gottlieb, 1983), and (3) by fostering affiliation among people facing similar stressful circumstances (use of self-help groups).

Family nurses are involved in counseling families to cope effectively by using their social supports to share the burden (Venters, 1981) and provide emotional and informational support (House and Kahn, 1985). Reinforcing positive patterns of help-seeking is an excellent preventive intervention strategy. Helping family members access untapped social support is another helping strategy aimed at promoting adequate family social support.

In the social support literature, two specific strategies are described for mobilizing social support. These are (1) the use of self-help groups and (2) the use of social network family therapy principles and strategies.

Use of Self-help Groups. Nurses are increasingly aware of the value of self-help groups for family members who need support to overcome a stressful handicap or life experience.* Self-help or mutual support groups (terms are used interchangeably) are defined as small groups of peers who come together to share a common problem and through mutual assistance to resolve or ameliorate the problem (Steiger and Lipson, 1985; Trainor, 1983).

Self-help groups have proliferated in the last three decades, and their rapid growth is evidence of their perceived effectiveness. Writers attribute this growth to being a response to a highly technical and mobile society in which ties to naturally occurring support of family, friends, neighbors, fellow church members, and the like are often weakened or absent. Our formal social support system—the health care and human service systems—also are inadequate in terms of providing accessible, effective assistance to the large number of people who are in need of mutual support mechanisms.

Self-help groups are described as being largely self-governing and self-regulating, emphasizing peer solidarity rather than hierarchical authority. They advocate self-reliance and usually require commitment and responsibility to other members. They generally provide material and emotional support to members, offering a face-to-face or phone-to-phone fellowship network, available and accessible without charge. Groups

* *Use of self-help groups is also discussed in Chap. 17 as an external type of family coping.*

are self-supporting and usually occur outside the aegis of formal institutions or agencies (Borman, 1975).

Self-help groups have been established for people and families with almost every conceivable problem. Increasingly, self-help groups are being formed to assist families of those afflicted with a particular illness or disability. Examples of these types of groups are Candlelighters for families with childhood cancer, Al-Anon, for families of alcoholics and Adult Children of Alcoholics. Many groups welcome both the person with the identified problem and family members, such as Make Today Count for clients and family members of persons with life-threatening illness, and Mended Hearts for clients and families of people who have had heart surgery.

Research on the outcomes of self-help group participation has indicated that self-help group participation is useful cognitively, through providing beneficial information, attributing meaning to the problem (Shapiro, 1989), and assisting with problem-solving skills; and emotionally, through providing a network of support for expressing feelings and encouraging grief work. Groups enable its members to pool their experiential knowledge and profit from others' experiences. They provide role models of successful adaptation and reinforcement for successful coping. And lastly, by helping other group members, it is found that those individuals help themselves (Trainor, 1983).

Nursing Interventions. Family nurses are in a key position to encourage family members to mobilize social support by participating in a self-help group. Trainor (1983) summarizes the role of the nurse here by explaining that nurses have a responsibility to:

1. Seek information about groups offering assistance to individuals and families.
2. Collaborate with such groups.
3. Understand how these groups enhance and complement professional services.
4. Refer client and families to appropriate groups.
5. Create new groups or encourage others to do so when there is a lack of a needed self-help group.

In addition family nurses may be engaged in counseling groups of family members who have formed support groups to help themselves with particular problems they are facing.

Social Network Family Therapy. In family therapy, the social network family therapy approach is an innovative strategy aimed at mobilizing family social support. A family in distress is the unit for intervening with this approach. In this approach the family's social network is mobilized—that network of people with whom the family in crises has a social relationship (extended family, friends, neighbors, and other associates). Healing of the distress is believed to come from within this social unit as it is brought together to support the distressed family (Jones, 1980). Family therapy takes place in the home setting with the family and its large social network assembled to create a nurturing and healthy social matrix. More specifically, the family social network is assembled to

> set in motion the forces of healing with the living social fabric of people. . . . We find the energies and talents of people can be focused to provide the essential supports, satisfaction, and controls for one another, and that these potentials are present in the social network of family, neighbors, friends, and associates of the person or family in distress. (Speck and Attneave, 1973, p. 7)

Social network family therapy is a useful strategy for nurses to employ who have more advanced preparation in family systems nursing and who are working with families in crisis. A more limited application of this notion is for family nurses to invite extended family members or close friends to be part of the family unit that is receiving care (Haber, 1987).

Interventions to Promote Family Recreation and Leisure-time Activities

Where nurses, based on a family assessment, find that a family is lacking in cohesiveness or bonding, the fun of being a family, or social supports; or is under stress; promotion of regular, more frequent family recreation and leisure-time activities may be indicated. McCown and associates (1989) identify the nurse's role in promoting active family recreation as consisting of "modeling behaviors, providing an education and a knowledge base, and contracting for client self-care through the nursing process" (p. 227). Hence, family nurses are urged to be good role models of an active, healthy life-style; to act as health educators and counselors for families in need of increasing their recreation and other leisure-time activities; and to use behavior modification and contracting as one mechanism to assist families to acquire additional healthy life-style patterns.

☐ STUDY QUESTIONS

1. Give a brief answer to the question of why it is essential to understand a family's cultural background when providing family health care.

Choose the correct answers to the following questions.

2. One of the assumptions made in dealing with families from different cultures is that we become less judgmental of other people's behavior as we attempt to:
   a. Give up our values and learn to accept people as they are.
   b. Recognize the origins of our own values and understand why we hold them.
   c. Work purposefully to overlook other people's values that are contrary to our own.
   d. Gradually work to change other's values when we consider them detrimental to their well-being.

3. Cultural ignorance and insensitivity lead to the following problems (choose all the correct answers):
   a. Poor communication
   b. Interpersonal tensions
   c. Stigmatization
   d. Inadequate assessments
   e. Professional objectivity

4. Ethnicity is an important resource for individuals and families because (choose all the correct answers):
   a. It guides them in occupational choices.
   b. It compensates for the cold impersonality of modern society.
   c. Its traditions enrich family life and strengthen its continuity.
   d. It facilitates upward mobility.

5. The cross-cultural approach is relevant for family health care because it (select the one best answer):
   a. Provides information about different cultures.
   b. Predicts ethnic minority family behavior.
   c. Provides a broad comparative picture of individual and group behavior.
   d. Assumes a cultural deviant perspective in assessment.

6. Match the proper definition with the corresponding concept.

CONCEPT

1. Cultural conflict
2. Acculturation
3. Assimilation
4. Ethnic identity
5. Ethnocentrism
6. Stereotyping
7. Cultural relativism
8. Cultural pluralism
9. Cultural imposition
10. Culture shock

DEFINITION

a. Blueprint for man's way of living.
b. People of a particular cultural group.
c. Nonacceptance of diversity within cultural group.
d. Gradual changes created as one culture is influenced by another.
e. The way individuals see themselves as to their cultural association.
f. Denotes the more complete one-way process of acculturation.

(continued)

11. Indigenous health care system
12. Self-fulfilling prophecy
13. Culture
14. Ethnic group

g. Culture is viewed nonjudgmentally and understood within its own context.
h. Lack of cultural relativity (seeing one's own culture as superior to others).
i. Local professional health care system.
j. Lay health care system.
k. Primary tactic used in cultural anthropology to analyze cultures.
l. Discomfort and confusion created by experiencing cultural differences.
m. Ethnic diversity.
n. Forcing one's values and practices on another person because of ethnocentricity.
o. A degraded person's tendency to conform to the beliefs and expectations others have about him or her.
p. Negative responses of clients to culturally unacceptable practices of health agencies and health workers.

7. Social class is based generally on three criteria: income, education, and occupational status. Identify which of these is the most important determinant.
   a. Income level
   b. Occupational status
   c. Educational level

8. The primary difference between the "nouveau riche" and the upper-upper class families is:
   a. Wealth.
   b. Spending patterns.
   c. Ethnicity.
   d. Family background.

9. The upper-middle class highly values (choose all the applicable values):
   a. Education.
   b. Productivity.
   c. Materialism.
   d. Community involvement (voluntarism).
   e. Individualism.

10. Lower-middle-class families, in contrast with upper-middle-class families, tend to (choose all correct answers)
   a. Value education highly.
   b. Be more racially and ethnically mixed.
   c. Have closer kinship relations.
   d. Put more emphasis on individualism and productivity values.

11. The blue-collar or working class is often difficult to distinguish from the lower-middle class, especially because there may be little income difference. Nevertheless, the most obvious differences between the two groups are (choose all correct answers):
   a. Wife's employment.
   b. Emphasis on family background.
   c. Spending patterns.
   d. Husband's type of employment—manual versus nonmanual labor.
   e. Education.

12. The lower class consists of the poor. In this social class the following characteristics are prevalent (choose all correct answers):
    a. Most often families live in rural or suburban areas.
    b. Men have unskilled jobs (sporadic and underemployed) or are unemployed.
    c. The family may receive welfare.
    d. A larger percentage of whites are poor in comparison with ethnic minorities.

13. The poor's value system is substantially different from the dominant culture values. Identify three examples of these contrasting values.

14. The definition of social support and social network are closely related, but different. The best description of this differences is (select the one best answer):
    a. Functions versus people.
    b. Micro versus macro perspective.
    c. Family versus individual system analysis.
    d. Quality versus quantity of support.

15. Briefly describe two basic family nursing interventions aimed at promoting family social support.

16. Social support research findings show that social support affects the health status of individuals by (choose the correct answer):
    a. Directly influencing health outcomes (main or direct effects).
    b. Acting as a buffer between stress and health outcomes (conditional effects).
    c. Both directly and conditionally affecting health outcomes.

17. Family nursing interventions appropriate for promoting better family financial health and family recreation include the following (complete the sentence).
    a. Health teaching addressing health-related financial problems of families may be in the area of ____________________
    b. Initiating referrals addressing health-related financial problems of families may be to ____________________
    c. Health teaching aimed at promoting family recreational/leisure-time activities include ____________________
    d. A second strategy to help families to increase their family recreation and other leisure-time activities is ____________________

CHAPTER NINE

Family Environmental Data

Learning Objectives

1. Define and describe the following environmental data and apply content to a written case example.
   a. Physical setting: Home (characteristics, safety hazards, spatial adequacy, provision of privacy).
   b. Physical setting: Neighborhood and community, including geographic mobility patterns.
   c. Associations and transactions of the family with the community and the family's perceptions and feelings regarding the neighborhood and community.
   d. Family's support system.
2. Explain the territorial concepts and apply to case example.
3. Discuss housing and the family's habitat relative to its effects on:
   a. Self-perception.
   b. Stress.
   c. Health.
4. Describe the impact crowding has on health.
5. Summarize research findings relative to the problem of homelessness and its effects on individual and family health.
6. State a family nursing diagnosis within the family environmental area.
7. Propose several nursing interventions aimed at promoting family environmental health.

Families do not exist in isolation, but in constant interaction with the world around them. It is the nature of this family–environment interaction that, in large part, determines the health of the family. In other words, there needs to be a good fit between the family's needs and environmental inputs/resources for the maintenance of family wellness (Holman, 1983; Killien, 1985).

Having an environmental or ecological perspective in family nursing practice is imperative, because families must be viewed within their naturally occurring contexts. Killien (1985) eloquently explains the benefits of incorporating an environmental perspective in nursing assessment and intervention.

> The practice of nursing from an environmental perspective broadens the assessments, diagnoses, interventions, and evaluations made by the nurse to include not only the client but also the environmental systems surrounding the client. As a result, there is increased understanding of client's health behavior, additional intervention strategies become available, and interventions may be more successful than when the focus of practice is exclusively client focused. (p. 259)

This chapter presents some of the basic information about the family's environment and discusses the assessment of the home, neighborhood, and community. Family nursing intervention guidelines for promoting family environmental health are also described at the conclusion of the chapter.

The scope of a family's environment is large. "It consists not only of concrete realities such as food, clothing, shelter, medical care, employment, physical safety, education, and recreation, but also includes social realities in terms of interpersonal relationships" (Holman, 1983, p. 40). For the purposes of this chapter, however, the focus is limited to the previously noted areas, while food, health care, recreation, and social support/social networks are discussed in other chapters (recreation and social support/social networks in Chap. 8 and food and health care in Chap. 16).

THE FAMILY'S ENVIRONMENT

Although the environment is defined in many different ways, the easiest way to think of the family's environment is anything outside of that particular family, including the immediate physical setting in which the family is situated and the family's social environment. Bronfenbrenner (1979) called the specific places where individuals and families engage in specific activities and roles *microsystems* or behavior settings. In systems language, microsystems would be referred to as interacting systems. These are the immediate physical contexts where face-to-face encounters between family members and others occur. At a more global level, the family is situated in environmental *macrosystems*. For instance, the macrosystems of a family could be the educational system, work system, social service system, and so forth. In systems language, a macrosystem would be referred to as a suprasystem. Environmental demands and environmental stress (where the demands exceed the family's resources) can exist both within the family's micro- and macrosystems (Melson, 1983).

HOUSING: FAMILY'S HOME

Provision of a healthy environment in the form of adequate shelter is an aspect of family functioning which is of special concern to the family-centered community nurse. A family's home is extraordinarily significant for its members because it becomes part of their family identity. "Home is that place where things are familiar and unchanging and where people maintain some sense of autonomy and control" (Rauckhorst et al, 1982, p. 159). Homes reflect the influence of a family's life-style, culture, interests, values, and economic status. In a healthy state a family will attempt to create a sheltered, protective, and satisfying environment for its members.

Through home visits nurses are able to observe the physical setting of the home and the particular arrangement of family life space, observations that otherwise would be impossible. Such assessment of the home environment provides a most valuable aid in understanding the family and its life-style. Because the home is its territory, the family behaves more naturally and comfortably, and health care professionals are able to assess more accurately the particular dimensions of family life. The home's sanitary and safety conditions are focal assessment areas (Daniel, 1986).

Before describing actual assessment areas relative to the home environment, this chapter looks at salient literature on housing and its effect on families, the concept of territoriality, the impact of crowding on families and homelessness, and safety in the home.

Housing and its Effects

The placement of houses and apartments in relation to one another and to the larger urban environment clearly influences family and social relationships. In particular, extremely poor housing conditions perceptibly, and adversely, influence behavior and attitudes (Schorr, 1970). The effects of housing and neighborhood can be seen in three major areas. First, there are psychological aspects that affect self-perception and life satisfaction; if these are negative, they can serve as stressors and illness-producing factors. Second are the effects of space—the house's state of repair, its facilities, and its arrangement. Such physical conditions may influence privacy, child-rearing practices, and housekeeping or study habits. Third are the effects of poor housing and its location, such as near a toxic dump, that adversely impacts family members' health.

Psychological Effects: Self-perception. Residents of deteriorating neighborhoods who resist being moved from one location to another make it plain that they do not view their surroundings with contempt. In fact, such neighborhoods may serve functions that are useful to residents, if only that of satisfying their territorial needs or having a place to call one's own. Since house and neighborhood are generally felt to be extensions of one's self, housing is usually a subject of highly charged emotional content, a matter of strong feeling. These feelings about one's habitat are significant factors in determining how individuals and family perceive themselves and are perceived by others. Thus, one evaluates his or her surroundings far from objectively.

If one then calls a house a slum, the tenant is likely to hear that he or she is being called a slum dweller (Schorr, 1970)!

To the middle-class resident, the social elements that are involved in self-identification with his or her housing may be evident. The following questions are common to the process of deciding where to live: Who is accepted there? Are they my kind of people? Is it a step up or down? What will it do for me and my children? Who will I meet?

Hence self-evaluation and motivation influence where a person selects to live, and conversely, living in poor housing influences a person's self-evaluation and motivation. A good deal has been written about the pessimism that is common to the poor, their readiness to seize the present satisfaction and let the future care for itself, and their feeling that one is controlled *by* rather than in control *of* events. Although there is considerable variability in attitudes, not to say aspiration, among even the very poor, studies of families living in deteriorated neighborhoods make the same point: pessimism and passivity present the most difficult barriers to rehabilitating neighborhoods or relocating families. In any case, where vigorous effort has gone into the upgrading of neighborhoods, some families have improved their housing and, as a consequence, feel they have improved their situation and status.

Psychological Effects: Stress. Housing may affect behavior by contributing to or dissipating stress. Some people have more effective adjustive mechanisms than others—patently a factor that influences reactions.

Almost any characteristic of housing that negatively affects individuals may be interpreted as stressful—crowding, dilapidation, vermin infestations, or high noise levels are examples. Two further stressful factors are social isolation and inadequate space. There is some evidence that aged people who live alone are more likely to require psychiatric hospitalization than those living with families. Any environment that tends to isolate an individual from others offers a stress that will lead to distinguishable personality changes. The amount of space per person and the way space is arranged to promote or interfere with privacy have also been related to stress (Schorr, 1970).

Effects on Health. Substantial evidence links poor housing with poor health. It is well understood that certain diseases are correlated with poor housing (see Table 9–1 for examples).

Even though family pets provide tremendous psychosocial benefits, the large number of family pets in homes today also can cause health problems, either directly from animal bites or through animal-transmitted infections (salmonella from dogs, psittacosis from pet birds, fleas from dogs and cats, allergies—eczema and asthma—from the fur of hairy pets).

TABLE 9–1. EXAMPLES OF DISEASES ASSOCIATED WITH POOR HOUSING

1. Acute respiratory infections, related to the multiple use of toilet and water facilities, inadequate heating or ventilation, and inadequate and crowded sleeping arrangements.
2. Minor digestive diseases and enteritis, related to poor facilities for the cold storage of food and to inadequate washing and toilet facilities and sharing of food and drink.
3. Injuries resulting from home accidents related to crowded physical space in home, or inadequate kitchens, poor electrical wiring, and poorly lighted and unstable stairs.
4. Infectious and noninfectious diseases of the skin related to crowding and shared or inadequate facilities for washing.
5. Lead poisoning in children who eat scaling paint from typically poor, old homes.

Territoriality and Families

We recognize that animals, as part of their innate repertoire of behaviors, lay claim to a specific area and defend this area against intruders, while other animals, in turn, tend to respect their claims. A similar type of instinctual characteristic applies to man and family. The human desire to possess and occupy specified areas is very pervasive, even though overt expression of infringement by others is attenuated by socialization. It has been noted that the most sacred prerogative in Western civilization is that of ownership of private property, especially of a home.

The first home visit by a student nurse may therefore seem quite threatening to him or her, partially due to the feeling of intruding into someone else's territory. Families may also feel aggression and/or hostility regarding this intrusion, especially when health care workers have not been specifically invited into the home.

Home territory is an area where the family has relatively much more freedom of behavior and a sense of control and power over both the area and its members. The home is viewed as a "haven in a heartless world," to coin the words of Christopher Lasch (1977) who wrote a book by that name. When a family member leaves home personal space becomes important. Stea (1965) defines personal space as a small circle in physical space, with the individual in its center and a culturally determined radius or "bubble" around the individual. An individual's personal space expands, shrinks, and changes in openness depending on the social situation, the physical context, the culture of the person, and the other persons present (Meisenhelder, 1982).

In public health, one will often observe families that are constricted in their movement due to feelings of fear, discomfort, and/or poverty. They are essentially home-bound and uncomfortable moving from their neighborhood. Other families may be much more at ease moving through a wider geographic complex. The territory that the family feels comfortable in and moves in may in part be a function of income, physical mobility, cultural or personal values, or a result of socialization. In the Los Angeles area, for example, there are many Mexican nationals who are more comfortable in visiting Mexico and receiving health care there than going to a new part of the city and attending an Anglo health clinic.

Within families there are both spatial (physical) and behavioral dimensions of territoriality. The feelings of belonging and cohesiveness among family members make up the behavioral component, while the actual physical space of home, yard, family name and address, and frequently visited community systems—school, work, shopping centers, churches, and community agencies with which the family interacts—are the spatial aspects of territoriality (Anderson and Carter, 1974).

Impact of Crowding in the Home

During the 1970s, well over 200 studies researched some facet of crowding (Epstein, 1981). Schorr (1970), in summarizing the results of "crowding studies," commented that fatigue and too little sleep may be consequences of seriously inadequate, crowded housing. The effect of crowding on intrafamily friction has also been observed in various connections. One of the results of seriously inadequate space in the home appears very often to be that family members spend much of their time outside the home. This tendency may be a particularly serious matter in relation to children and adolescents. It has been observed that poor children from crowded, inadequate homes do not study sufficiently and are not within reach of parental control. "Street life" takes on increasing importance for these children during grammar school years and by the time the adolescent years begin, peer associations "on the street" are commonly very influential.

There appears to be inconclusive findings with respect to the effects of crowding on family members' actual physical health status.

Epstein (1981) found that an important person variable that influences how individuals adjust to crowded conditions was the person's perceived control. If an individual perceived that he or she was able to maintain adequate personal control over his or her environment, this fostered more favorable adaptation to crowding.

Crowding is very strongly associated with socioeconomic status and ethnic background. From Figure 9–1 it can be seen that the percent of racial and ethnic minorities who lived in crowded conditions in 1977 was more than three times that of whites.

Impact of Homelessness

Homelessness as a societal problem has risen sharply in the United States since 1980. Particularly in cities and temperate regions, homelessness has been a major community health concern. The problem is much

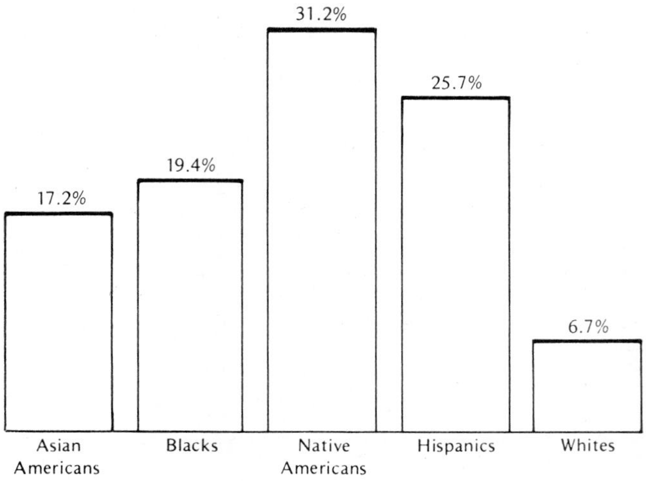

Figure 9–1
Crowded housing conditions by ethnic/racial group (From: United States Department of Health, Education, and Welfare, 1977.)

larger than the absence of a home. A family's entire existence is threatened.

Homelessness is a problem that time will not solve. Numerous cases are not short-term; some studies suggest that the average episode exceeds 3 years (Vernez et al, 1988). Among the most alarming characteristics of this growing population is the rising number of families with children, as well as the increasing proportion of persons who are severely mentally disabled.

Homeless families, in fact, have become the fastest growing segment of the homeless population. The Children's Defense Fund (Kozol, 1990) recently estimated that 500,000 children in the United States are homeless. A case in point about the rising number of homeless families is the New York City experience. In 1987, nearly one half of the occupants of homeless shelters in New York City were children. Their average age was only 6 years old (Kozol, 1990).

While it is accepted that homelessness is a great stress to families and children, little research has been conducted to document the effects of homelessness on families. Several studies have documented, however, the adverse effects of homelessness on the health of children and mothers. Numerous chronic and acute physical and serious mental health problems have been found (Berne et al, 1990; Bowdler and Barrell, 1987). Harsh environmental conditions and health-damaging responses breed demoralization, hopelessness, despair, and all the other problems associated with poverty.

Safety in the Home

One of the most valuable assessment areas relative to the home is the assessment of safety conditions and potential or real hazards, both inside and outside the home. Especially within the home, accidents are a major threat to a family's health status. Each family member is exposed to certain threats from accidents related to his or her developmental stage (Kandzari and Howard, 1981). "Increasing the family's awareness of the chief accident problems, providing factual information, and suggesting ways for the family to improve its level of safety wellness are the goals for the nurse" (Kandzari and Howard, 1981, p. 223).

Home accidents kill about 27,000 and injure more than 4.2 million persons in the United States each year. Of the above deaths, 9800 result after falls; 5700 result from fires; and 2500 are the consequence of poisoning. Furthermore, home accidents kill more children between the ages of 1 and 14 years than all the next six causes of death combined. Nearly all of these deaths and injuries could be prevented by proper protection and safety education (Bete, 1976; McFarlane, 1986).

Assessment Areas: Home

The following questions are suggested for completing an assessment of the home environment; both Kandzari and Howard (1981) and Rauckhorst and associates (1982) provide more detailed coverage of this area.

1. Describe the dwelling type (home, apartment, or rooming house). Does family own or rent their home?
2. Describe the home's condition (both the interior and exterior of house). House interior would include number of rooms and types of rooms (living room, bedrooms, etc), their use, and how they are furnished. What is the condition and adequacy of the furniture? Is there adequate heating, cooling, ventilation, and lighting? Are the floors, stairs, railings, and other structures in good repair? Is the water supply adequate? Is there a telephone in the home or accessibility to a phone? What is the condition of the yard?
3. In kitchen, observe water supply, sanitation, and the adequacy of refrigeration and cooking facilities.
4. In bathrooms, observe sanitation, water supply, toilet facilities, and presence of towels and soap.
5. Assess the sleeping arrangements in the house. Are they adequate for family members, considering their age, relationships, and special needs?
6. Observe for the home's general state of cleanliness and sanitation. Are there any infestations of vermin (interior especially)? Are there pets and any sanitation problems related to their presence?
7. Assess family's subjective feelings about home. Does the family consider its home adequate for its needs?
8. Identify the family's territorial unit.
9. Evaluate the privacy arrangements and how the family feels about the adequacy of its privacy. Privacy functions to protect and maintain an individual's need for personal autonomy; to serve as an emotional release; and to provide an opportunity for self-appraisal and protected communication. Having one's own room, bed, possessions, clothes, toys, and pets are assets. Privacy for an adolescent is especially significant in assisting him or her to achieve the developmental needs of independence. Marital privacy is critical in most families.
10. Evaluate the presence or absence of safety hazards in other areas of the home. Ask about the

storage of medicines and substances containing toxic substances. Are they stored safely away from children and pets and clearly marked? Observe for dangerous objects that might cause safety hazards to children or elderly family members. Are the entry and exits from and into the house barrier free and is there adequate space and lighting to move safely through the house (Daniel, 1986)? Are there any exposed electrical cords or loose rugs on the floor? Are there provisions for emergencies (smoke detector, emergency numbers by the phone)? Is there a swimming pool, and if so, is it adequately fenced in and locked if small children are in the home?

11. Evaluate the adequacy of waste and garbage disposal.
12. Assess the family members' overall satisfaction/dissatisfaction with their housing arrangements.

PHYSICAL SETTING: THE NEIGHBORHOOD AND COMMUNITY

The neighborhood and community in which the family lives exerts a tremendous influence on the family. Using the social systems and structural–functional frameworks for assessing families, the family nurse needs to examine "the family and its universe." Its universe consists of the inner and outer environments of the family. The outer environment includes the territorial concepts previously described. The territorial unit includes the small "home" circle, while territorial cluster and complex pertain to the family's neighborhood and community.

Neighborhood and Community Effects on Families

Most researchers, in describing the effects of neighborhood on families, have looked at the type of social interaction that occurs in different types of neighborhoods. Substantial social and economic homogeneity has existed in most of the communities that have been studied. In homogeneous neighborhoods, because the families' behavior patterns, values, and interests are alike, they naturally tend to form friendships with one another. Homogeneity is found to be more significant in creating a large number of friendships and associations than is proximity (Schorr, 1970).

In working-class neighborhoods, family membership is concentrated in the locality, and the most active ties are with other members of the family. Proximity makes for frequent contacts with relatives and other neighbors, casually in passing and less casually on the sidewalk or in the corner tavern or shop. Neighbors tend to be deeply involved in one another's family lives. There is considerable attachment to the place itself. Relationships are identified with locality.

Working-class neighborhoods have a mood of warmth, security, and identity. It is evident that when these working-class families move, many find it difficult to maintain their neighbor- and extended family-centered patterns of relationships. This necessitates a complex series of adjustments by the family (Schorr, 1970).

Rural Families. It has been noted that rural communities have drastically different effects on individuals and families than do urban areas. Recently there has been extensive interest and concern about the health and other needs of rural families (Bushy, 1990; Weinert and Long, 1987). It seems that the rural environment, in spite of its more personalized social environment and tranquil setting, has some unique, special problems. The rural community is directly affected by the primary economic resources of a region, such as farming, ranching, lumbering, or mining. Inasmuch as farming, lumbering, and mining (three major industries) have experienced recent crises, it stands to reason that the stressors rural communities and families face also have amplified. Rural people are described as being self-reliant and traditional in their values and to have a strong work ethic. Poverty, however, has increased markedly and eroded the ability of families to uphold these values. Accessibility to health care and other needed services has declined due to geographic remoteless as well as economic hardship (Bushy, 1990).

In summarizing social interaction patterns in communities and neighborhoods, it has been consistently found that social class homogeneity, and frequently age, ethnic, racial, and religious similarity, foster social interaction, whereas social class disparity discourages it. People want to live and mix with their neighbors (other families) who share the same, or similar, values and life-styles (Chilman, 1978).

The neighborhood and wider community have definite effects on family health. Noise, traffic, air, and garbage pollution, of course, produce continual, probably low-level stress. Chronic, low-level exposures to toxic substances in the air, water, and food can produce diseases and conditions that have a latency period, an insidious onset, or a diffuse set of symptoms (Wiley, 1989).

Assessment Areas: Neighborhood and Community

1. What are the characteristics of the immediate neighborhood and the larger community?

Type of neighborhood and community (rural, suburban, urban, intercity).
Types of dwellings in neighborhood (residential, industrial, combined residential and light industry, agrarian).
Condition of dwellings and streets (well kept up, deteriorating, dilapidated, being revitalized).
Sanitation of streets and homes (clean, trash and garbage collected, etc.).
Problems with traffic congestion.
Presence and types of industry in neighborhood (air, noise, water pollution problems).

2. What are the demographic characteristics of the neighborhood and community?
   Social class and ethnic characteristics of residents.
   Occupations and interests of families.
   Density of population.
3. What changes have occurred in the neighborhood and community? Is the neighborhood and community in a state of transition or is it stable demographically?
4. What health and other basic services and facilities are available in neighborhood and community?
   Marketing facilities (food, clothing, drug stores, etc).
   Health agencies (clinics, hospitals, emergency facilities).
   Social service agencies (welfare, counseling, employment).
   Family's church or temple.
   Schools. What is the accessibility and condition of the neighborhood school? Are there problems within the school (eg, crowdedness, poor quality of education, gangs, racial/ethnic tensions) that affect children's education?
   Recreational facilities (playgrounds, parks).
   Availability of public transportation. How accessible (in terms of distance, suitability, and hours) are these services and facilities to family?
5. How long has the family lived in the neighborhood and/or community? What has been the family's history of geographic mobility? From where did they move or migrate?
   Many middle-class Americans have few geographic roots and move from city to city and region to region as their jobs and personal preferences dictate. Mobility is highest among young adults, those in middle-income levels, and those in the military or migrant labor jobs. Hence their support systems within the community are probably lacking.
6. What is the incidence of crime in the neighborhood and community? Are there other safety problems?

The rates of certain crimes—robbery, aggravated assault, larceny (pickpocketing), and purse snatching—are much more frequent problems for persons over 65 years of age. More than 60 percent of the elderly live in metropolitan areas, and most of these reside in the central city. For cultural, emotional, and economic reasons, many of the elderly have lived in the same areas for decades. Many cannot afford alternative housing, and they are often dependent on public transportation. Consequently, these urban elderly are close to those most likely to victimize them—the unemployed, the drug addict, and the teenage school dropout.

The psychological impact of fear of crime is very great. A 1974 Louis Harris and Associates national survey of the problems of the elderly found that they rank crime as their most serious problem—above health, money, and loneliness. People with low income and the black elderly were found to experience a higher rate of crime than the nonpoor white oldster (Mallinchak and Wright, 1978).

ATTRIBUTES OF HEALTHY FAMILIES: THEIR ASSOCIATIONS IN THE COMMUNITY

Healthy families are those who are active and reach out in self-initiating ways to relate to various community groups, according to Lewis and associates (1976). They believe that the family that is functioning in a healthy way perceives itself as being related to and part of the larger community. Part of a family's successful coping is its ability to secure compliance from the environment or maintain a good family–environment fit, meaning that within the community the family is able to seek out, receive, and/or accept the appropriate resources to meet its needs for food, services, and information (Hall and Weaver, 1974). Passive acceptance of community services, however delivered, may be an indication of an isolated, estranged family or a dependent family functioning on a much lower level of health.

Assessment Areas: Community Associations

Completing a family ecomap as suggested and described in Chapter 8 is advised to obtain information about family members' associations and transactions with their reference groups and community. These specific questions are also suggested to assess this area.

1. *Who* in the family uses *what* community services or is known to which agencies? For example, the

family with school-age children might be involved with the public school system, a church group, the welfare department, or a scouting organization.

2. How frequently or to what extent do they use these services or facilities?
3. What is the family's territorial cluster and complex?
4. Is the family aware of community services relevant to its needs, such as transportation? Is the family aware of availability of lower transportation fees (monthly card, discount cards for transportation for children and senior citizens) and direct route to health clinics and community resources?
5. How does the family feel about groups/organizations from which it receives assistance? Assess the family's perceptions and feelings regarding association with above community groups and agencies. If the experiences in using community or neighborhood agencies have been positive, these are resources that can be used again and perhaps with even greater success.
6. How does the family view the community? For example, is it a community where the family is worried about having children play outside during the day because of high crime and personal attack rate in the neighborhood? Satisfaction with neighborhood and community have been found to be closely associated with satisfaction with life in general (Chilman, 1978). It is also true that expectations of neighborhoods and communities by people differ, depending on social class status: The higher the social class, the greater the expectations of the community (Rainwater, 1972). These same differences in expectations are noted in all community agencies. The poor demand little, while the affluent have high demands and expectations. The lower expectations are correlated with and result from feelings of powerlessness and learned helplessness.

NURSING DIAGNOSES: FAMILY ENVIRONMENTAL HEALTH AREA

According to Killien (1985) nursing diagnoses related to an environmental perspective focuses on the family–environment fit, "the balance of demands and resources between the client and the environment" (p. 270). The environmental demands can either be actual or potential, making room for preventive, curative, and rehabilitative types of nursing diagnoses. The North American Nursing Diagnosis Association (NANDA) has one family environmental nursing diagnosis listed, that of "impaired home maintenance deficit." This diagnosis is used to describe the array of individual and family environmental problems that result from an individual or family being unable or potentially unable to independently maintain a safe, hygienic, and/or growth-promoting environment (McFarland and McFarland, 1989).

FAMILY NURSING INTERVENTIONS

Many of the strategies for intervention related to environmental health are preventive in nature. Primary prevention should be a primary emphasis here. For instance, working with families to prevent falls in the elderly, poisoning of children in the home, or skin rashes due to vermin infestations, are major accomplishments of the community-based family nurse.

Primary Prevention: Environmental Health Promotion

Teaching family environmental self-care requires that families accurately perceive their vulnerability to accidents, injuries, or illness and "use self-responsibility to prevent environmental stressors and to protect and promote the family's environmental health and safety" (Wiley, 1989, p. 313). By recognizing and anticipating potential and actual environmental threats to their health, there is much families can do to make their home and life-style health promoting.

Promoting Safety in the Home. "Increasing the family's awareness of the chief accident problems, providing factual information, and suggesting ways for the family to improve its level of safety wellness are goals for the nurse" (Kandzari and Howard, 1981, p. 223).

Family teaching in the following safety education areas is recommended when potential or actual problems are assessed:

1. How to prevent falls by arranging furniture to avoid obstacles; installing handrails on all stairs; placing cords for electrical equipment away from walking areas; having adequate lighting for all traffic areas, especially the stairs; keeping scatter rugs away from head and foot of stairs; installing handrails for shower and bathtub; using nonskid mats for bathtub and bathroom floor; and placing lights so that they can be turned on from bed and groping in the dark can be avoided.
2. How to prevent fires by removing rubbish like old newspapers, wastebaskets, trashcans; never emptying ashtrays or tossing matches into wastebaskets unless one is sure they are out; never

smoking in bed; and checking the chimney, fireplace, and furnace to keep free from fire dangers.

3. How to avoid lifting accidents by using good body mechanics in lifting, reaching, and carrying heavy items.
4. How to avoid poisoning accidents. Most poisonings are due to carelessness, so advise parents to keep medicines locked and away from food if small children are in family; give medicine only as prescribed (never give leftovers to other family members); keep medicines in their original containers (label contains vital information); make sure medicine bottles have safety caps; and store and use household cleaners with the utmost care (they can be killers if swallowed by children).
5. Make sure the house is tailored to the safety needs of the age(s) of the children and adults in family. Both the very young and the old have special safety needs. The very young, for instance infants, should never be left unattended on table or in tub and should be kept away from stove. The older person requires excellent lighting, handgrips in bathroom (by toilet, shower, or bath), and stairs that have nonskid surfaces and good, sturdy handrails (Bete, 1976).
6. Point out to families that they should have an emergency plan, so that if an emergency does arise, they will be fully prepared. This includes posting a list of important telephone numbers on a wall by the phone; keeping a first-aid chart accessible and becoming familiar with its instructions; and having on hand in the medicine cabinet the items needed to treat common emergencies.

Secondary Prevention Related to Environmental Problems

Secondary prevention intervention strategies are also indicated. Secondary prevention has to do with early detection and treatment. Teaching families about diagnosis and treatment of common home injuries and exploring with them their proximity to emergency facilities are examples of interventions here.

Tertiary Prevention: Environmental Modification Strategies

Tertiary prevention, as you will recall, involves convalescence, rehabilitation, minimization of the effects of the disability, and maximization of the client's functioning. Tertiary prevention in the form of environmental modification is very important for nurses in home health care who care for the disabled and frail elderly. Assisting families in reducing environmental demands and increasing their environmental resources are goals when recommending environmental modifications. Environmental modification or home improvisation is needed in these situations so that the special needs of the disabled and aged are taken into account. Disabled family members often need modification in their home environment to enable them simply to remain there. Families are often not knowledgeable or may not be present to help (unless the nurse or patient specifically enlists the aid of extended family members). Environmental modification recommendations for the family with a disabled or elderly member(s) include:

1. Modifying the kitchen to make shelves, cupboards, and drawers more accessible and hence functional.
2. Clearing hallways and floors of loose rugs and dangerous objects and rearranging furniture for improving home safety.
3. Modifying the bathroom to improve the safety of the toilet, bath, and shower facilities, such as by adding sidebars and handgrips in shower, bath, and toilet areas.
4. Making entrance/exit modifications, such as adding railings to stairs, building ramps, and widening entrances.

Family nurses who work with the disabled should be familiar with the common types of special adaptive equipment needed to make the home safer and more functional. Moreover, the home health family nurse should understand the ways these special adaptive devices are covered by Medicaid, Medicare, and other third-party reimbursement sources so that this information can be shared with the family.

Interventions to Assist the Homeless

The homeless are in need of a wide variety of services and types of assistance. A comprehensive case management approach (see Chap. 18 for elaboration of this intervention strategy) is suggested due to the complex needs of homeless families. Homeless families need help not only with their multiple primary care needs, but also with subsistence services, alternative housing arrangements, access to entitlements (welfare, Social Security, etc), crisis intervention, ongoing mental health services, transportation, and child care. Assisting families to obtain these services, or initiating referrals and closely following up on the referrals, are suggested interventions. Clinicians working with the homeless stress the importance of showing respect toward these clients, being nonthreatening, assuming a low profile, and minimizing reporting and paperwork requirements (Vernez et al, 1988). Political advocacy is urged by nurses who work with the homeless—to exert pressure on government to expand available housing or housing subsidies to poor families.

☐ STUDY QUESTIONS

1. "Housing affects a person's self-perception." Discuss in what way this occurs.

2. Housing may affect behavior by contributing to or dissipating stress. Several aspects of housing have been identified as frequently stress producing. Name four.

3. Substantial evidence of linkage between extremely poor housing and physical health exists. Identify three health problems associated with poor housing.

Choose the correct answers to the following questions.

4. The most rapidly growing group within the homeless population is:
   a. The mentally disabled.
   b. Substance abusers.
   c. Children.
   d. Women.

5. Which effect(s) of severe crowding have been described?
   a. Increased intrafamilial stress.
   b. Too little sleep.
   c. Fatigue.
   d. Excessive amount of time spent inside home for all children of all age groups.

6. Social interaction in neighborhoods is more a function of (choose the best answer):
   a. Physical proximity rather than homogeneity.
   b. Homogeneity rather than physical proximity.
   c. Satisfaction with community and neighborhood rather than dissatisfaction with habitat.

Are the following statements True *or* False?

7. Where families live close to each other in working-class neighborhoods, the most active social ties are with other members of the family.

8. In working-class neighborhoods there is considerable attachment to the neighborhood itself.

9. Working-class neighborhoods have been described as being warm and as providing security and identity.

10. Territoriality as a concept refers to a person's possession of physical land and the resources on that land.

11. Homelessness is associated with acute rather than long-term mental health problems in children and women.

12. Case management is recommended for dealing with the array of complex health and social welfare problems of the homeless.

13–16. Please read the following case study and answer the study questions following this hypothetical case.

Family Case Study

(Questions are asked here which relate also to Chaps. 6 and 8).

One year ago, the Juarez family moved to Los Angeles from their birthplace, a small agricultural area in northern Mexico. The husband and wife both worked as migrant workers on a large cooperative farm in Mexico and stated life was "hard" (basic necessities—food and shelter—were a struggle to obtain). Mr. J., age 30, and Mrs. J., age 25, now live with their three children, Maria, age 8, José, age 6, and Pedro, age 4, in an older small wooden house in a low-income Mexican-American district in Los Angeles. The district has a paucity of health and social services, although there is a market and shopping center within walking distance.

Their housing is minimally adequate. There are two bedrooms, with parents sleeping in the larger bedroom, two boys sharing the other, and Maria sleeping on a cot in a small room off the kitchen. The living room is small, with two chairs. The family owns a large old-fashioned radio, an older stove, a refrigerator, and washing machine. The rooms are clean, have no carpeting, few lights, and electrical wall heating in living room and hallway that is minimal but functions. The electric wall heater had a protective screen on it at one time, but it has been removed.

Since the family arrived they have pretty much stayed within their immediate vicinity. Mr. J. is employed in a steady job as a dishwasher for a local Mexican restaurant. Mrs. J. has a part-time janitorial job in a small business nearby.

Because both parents speak very little English and are embarrassed because they did not go beyond the third grade, they have not been to school to talk with the teachers, although the children appear to be having learning problems. The parents and children belong to no community groups, but attend mass at the Spanish-speaking Catholic church in their neighborhood. They have no family recreational activities, except that Mrs. J. occasionally takes the children to a neighborhood park.

In spite of isolation from their extended family, which still resides in Mexico, and their language barrier, they like the community, feel they are starting to get ahead, and that the neighborhood is friendly and its people helpful. They are, however, worried about their children's associations (are they associating with "good" children?) and with the high crime rate in the neighborhood.

Only a limited amount of information was gained about the family's history. Mr. and Mrs. J. were neighbors as children and Mrs. J.'s brother and her husband were friends. Both families felt they would be happy together, so they married when Mr. J. was 20 and Mrs. J. was 15. Maria was conceived 6 months later; both parents were very pleased. Each new child was positively accepted as a natural part of the family life. They seem to be quite content in their relationship together, with well-delineated (traditional) roles and functions. Mrs. J. is in the home except for her part-time work; Mr. J. is the breadwinner and "leader" of the family.

Describe the identifying data and appropriate information under these broad headings from the family case study cited.

13. ***Family Identifying Data***

13.1 Composition of family.
13.2 Type of family form.
13.3 Religious and cultural orientation (from Chap. 8).
13.4 Social class status.
13.5 Social class mobility.
13.6 Developmental stage and history of family (from Chap. 6).
13.7 Social support/social network.
13.8. Recreational activities.

14. ***Family Environmental Data***

14.1 Home.
14.2 Neighborhood and community, including geographic mobility.
14.3 Associations and transactions of family with community.
14.4 Family's perceptions and feelings about neighborhood and community.

15. State a family nursing diagnosis related to the family's environment.

16. Propose two family nursing interventions aimed at promoting the family's environmental health.

CHAPTER TEN

Family Communication Patterns and Processes

Learning Objectives

1. Define the following systems and communications terms: information, punctuation, the redundancy principle, and feedback.
2. Identify the content and instruction levels of messages.
3. Compare the effects of negative and positive feedback.
4. Briefly discuss the four basic components of functional communication.
5. Name four primary characteristics of the functional sender.
6. Describe the manner in which listening, feedback, and validation facilitate the receiver's comprehension and response to a message.
7. From hypothetical interactions, identify the use of assumptions, unclear expressions of feelings, judgmental expressions, inability to define needs, and incongruent communication.
8. Given a family case example, use the assessment questions included in this chapter to assess family communication, state a family nursing diagnosis in the area of family communication, and propose two family nursing interventions aimed at promoting more functional communication.

Before beginning to discuss the areas within family structure and how they are assessed, it is helpful to look at the larger picture—the family system structure and functions—and to identify the components subsumed under these dimensions. The structural–functional approach analyzes the family's structural characteristics (the arrangement of the parts that form the whole) and the functions the family performs for society and its subsystems. The structure of the family refers to how the family is organized, the manner in which the units are arranged, and how they relate to each other. The four basic structural dimensions of the family elaborated on in this text are family (1) role structure, (2) power structure, (3) communication patterns/processes, and (4) value system. These elements are intimately interrelated and interdependent. Because the family is a social system, there is continual interaction and feedback between its internal and external environments. A change in one part of the family system is generally followed by a compensatory change

Chapter 10 was first coauthored by DeAnn Young, R.N., M.S., Professor, Department of Nursing, California State University, Los Angeles, and Barbara E. Bailey, R.N., M.S., private practice, Los Angeles, and Marilyn Friedman. It has been revised in the second and third edition by Marilyn Friedman.

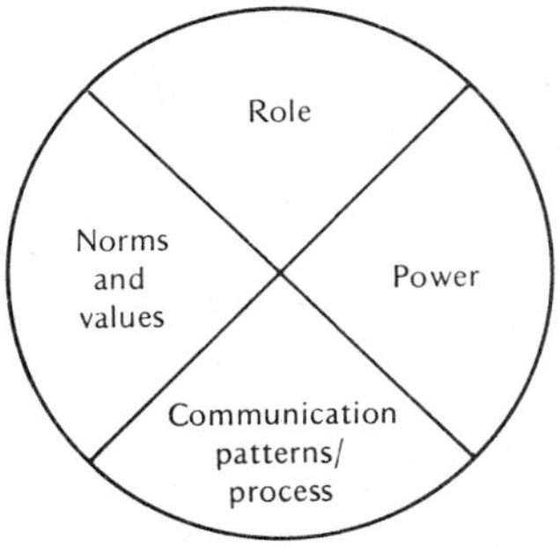

Figure 10–1
The structural dimensions of the family.

in the other internal structural dimensions. Hence, although these dimensions are not separable in real life, they will be individually dealt with in the text for heuristic purposes. The family system may be conceptualized as being structurally organized as shown in Figure 10–1.

In addition to having an organized scheme or structure, the family must have "system" functions—its reason for being. Family structure or organization is ultimately evaluated by how well the family is able to fulfill its general functions (the goals important to its members and society). The family's structure, especially its communication structure, serves to facilitate the achievement of family functions. For example, adequate family communication makes it possible for the family to socialize children, a basic family function.

Family communication can be viewed as both a structural dimension and as a system process. In other words, communications in the family can be considered as patterned content and described as a structural component, or as sequential interactions (as forms) over time and assessed as processes. Eight basic sections are included here: elements of communication, communication principles, channels of communication, functional communication, functional patterns of communication, dysfunctional communication patterns, family nursing diagnoses, and family nursing interventions.

Defining Communication

Communication refers to the process of exchanging feelings, desires, needs, information, and opinions (McCubbin and Dahl, 1985). Galvin and Brommel (1986) in an excellent book titled *Family Communication: Cohesion and Change*, defines family communication as a symbolic, transactional process of creating and sharing meanings in the family. Just as each person has his or her own distinct style of communication, so too does each family have its unique communication style or pattern.

One of the prime tasks the family assumes to assist its members is to provide a nurturing environment in which family members may develop good self-esteem. Clear and functional communication among family members is the crucial vehicle through which the necessary feelings regarding self-worth develop and become internalized. Conversely, unclear communications are believed to be a major contributor of poor family functioning (Holman, 1983; Satir, 1983).

The problem of flawed or problematic communication in families is ubiquitous. Watzlawick and associates (1967), researchers of family communication, estimate that 85 percent of all messages sent in families are misunderstood. With this observation in hand, it is not surprising that in a survey of family therapists 85 percent of couples seeking family therapy reported poor family communication as the primary problem bringing them into therapy (Beck and Jones, 1973, as cited in Goldenberg and Goldenberg, 1985, p. 116).

ELEMENTS OF COMMUNICATION

As a consequence of using a general systems framework, family communication patterns and processes will be defined in this chapter as the processing of information within the family or its subsystems. Family communication patterns and processes are key elements in the fulfillment of family functions. Communication serves as the critical vehicle for binding the subsystems together to form a cohesive whole and maintain the entire system.

In the language of information processing, communication entails a sender of a message, a form/channel of the message, a receiver, and some interaction between the sender and the receiver. The sender is the person who is attempting to transmit a message to another person; the receiver is the target of the sender's message; forms/channels are the routes of the message. They extend from the cognitions (the thoughts) of the sender, through space, to the cognitions of the receiver.

Interaction is a broader term referring to the sending and receiving of messages, including the response of the message causes in the receiver *and* the sender. Interaction encompasses the dynamic, constantly changing process of communication between people (Watzlawick et al, 1967).

Messages initiated by the sender are always somewhat distorted—either by the sender, through the interaction between sender and receiver, or by the receiver. One primary cause of distortion is anxiety of either interactant; the greater the level of anxiety, the greater the possibility of misunderstanding. Another common cause of message distortion is a difference in the frames of reference of the interactants, due to either sociocultural or idiosyncratic dissimilarities. In their daily interactions, family members usually assume that other family members have a similar frame of reference; since this is untrue in many cases, misunderstandings inevitably arise.

COMMUNICATION PRINCIPLES

Watzlawick and co-workers (1967), in their seminal text on family communication (*Pragmatics of Human Communication*), delineate several principles of communication that are basic for understanding family communication processes. First and foremost is the dictum that *it is impossible not to communicate, as all behavior is communication.* In any situation where two or more persons are present, we may not communicate verbally, but we cannot but help to communicate nonverbally. "All nonverbal communication is meaningful" (Wright and Leahey, 1984, p. 18).

A second principle of communication is that communication not only conveys information or content, but is coupled with a command (instruction). Messages therefore contain *two levels of communication: content and instruction.* Content is the literal definition or what actually is being said (verbal message), while instruction or the *metamessage* conveys the intent of the message. The content of a message may be a simple statement, but the metamessage or instruction depends on variables such as emotion, intent, and context, and may be expressed nonverbally by the rate and flow of speech, gestures, body position, and tone of voice. If "I am bored" is whispered in a theater to another member of the family, it may be a comment on the quality of the movie. If the "I am bored" message is sent in an emphatic manner during prolonged family discussion, the meaning differs. In this instance, it probably signifies anger, frustration, and heightened emotionality. Hence emotion, intent, and context have produced very different meanings in a message containing identical content. In the presence of disparity between the two levels of communication, the receiver usually "tunes in" more to the instructional level.

A third principle of communication delineated by Watzlawick and associates is what Bateson (1979), another communications researcher and theorist, calls *punctuations* in the sequences of communication. Communications involve a transactional process, and in the interchange each response contains the preceding communication, in addition to the preceding history of the relationship (Hartman and Laird, 1983). Different members of the family will explain interactional events and sequences differently because they impose their own punctuation into the explaining of a situation. Goldenberg and Goldenberg (1985) give a graphic example of this tendency:

> Each [in this case a mother and daughter] arbitrarily believes that what she says is caused by what the other person says. In a sense, such serial punctuations between family members resemble the dialogue of children quarreling: "You started it first!" and so on. . . . It is meaningless to search for a starting point to a conflict between two people because it is a complex repetitive interaction. (p. 188)

In effect there is no beginning (cause) or end (effect) in communication transactions, because circularity of responses occurs. Family members' interpersonal behaviors (communications) are therefore best understood by taking a circular rather than a linear view of causality (A $\rightleftarrows$ B rather than A $\rightarrow$ B).

To further understand the idea of "punctuations" in communication sequences, the notion of feedback loops needs to be reviewed. Communication serves as an organizing, purposeful, and self-regulating process in families. Self-regulating processes in a system are dependent on two-way communication, termed feedback loops. According to Von Bertalanffy, (1966), feedback loops are "circular, causal chains." As Figure 10–2 indicates, feedback loops in communication trigger necessary change in the family system that keeps the system "on track." A part of the system, (eg, a family member) can alter its communications (output) based on the information he or she receives regarding the effects of his or her previous outputs on other parts/members of the system. Through feedback mecha-

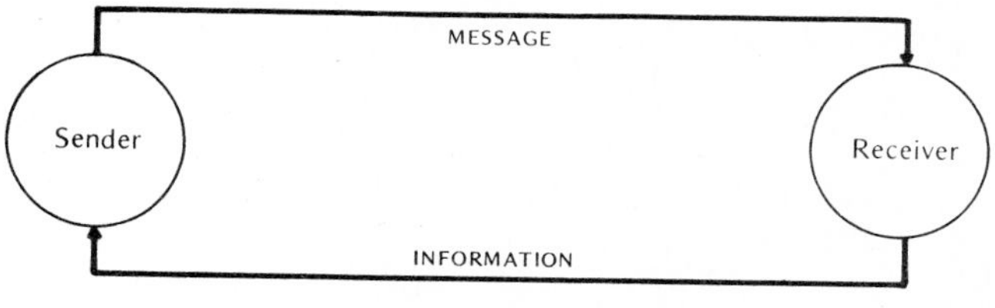

Figure 10–2
Negative feedback loop. (Adapted from Von Bertalanffy, 1968).

nisms, a portion of any system's output is reintroduced into the system as input information about the original output (Goldenberg and Goldenberg, 1985). Feedback loops have been likened to home thermostats. Setting the thermostat at 72° programs a detector device to activate the heating system when the temperature drops below that point. Also a feedback mechanism signals the furnace to cut off the heat once the desired temperature has been obtained.

A continual exchange of communication occurs in families—involving introducing new information, correcting misinformation, problem solving, having and resolving misunderstandings and conflicts, and so forth. The feedback loops entailed in these transactions may be negative or positive.

Negative feedback is the most productive type of feedback because it is corrective; it regulates or modulates communications or information flow so that the system may adjust homeostatically or maintain stability. "Negative" is not a judgmental term, but is simply a reference to the direction in which the information flows (Fig. 10–2). Self-regulating negative feedback is present when a sender initiates an interaction by sending a message and then, because of a new input received, modifies his or her message before a reply is possible or expected. The problem-solving and decision-making process depend on negative feedback. This process begins when a problem arises and is identified. In the family problem-solving situation, the sender or initiator of the interaction usually identifies the problem, family members then explore the problem, various solutions are discussed, and a decision is finally made through one of the processes described fully in the next chapter.

Positive feedback, in contrast, increases instability or deviation from a homeostatic state. In the above case the furnace would continue and the home would get hotter and hotter. Theoretically, if positive feedback continues it has the potential of amplifying deviation to the point that the system self-destructs or no longer functions (Steinglass, 1978, as cited in Goldenberg and Goldenberg, 1985). An argument between parent and child that continues to escalate is an example of a common type of family communication positive feedback situation.

From these examples positive feedback sounds like it always has adverse consequences. This is not so. Positive feedback needs to occur in families for change and growth to take place. There may be immediate instability and tension created in the family system, but in the long run, positive feedback is necessary for change and growth.

A fourth principle of communication described by Watzlawick and co-workers (1967) is that *there are two types of communication: digital and analogic.* Digital communication is essentially verbal communication using words with commonly understood meanings. The second kind of communication, analogic, is where the idea or thing being communicated is transmitted nonverbally in a representational manner (Hartman and Laird, 1983, p. 102). Analogic communication, known commonly as body language, sends messages by means of posture, facial expressions, the rhythm and cadence of the spoken words, "or any other nonverbal manifestation of which the person is capable" (Watzlawick et al, 1967, p. 62). Analogic communication, which conveys the metacommunication, although often ambiguous and imprecise, tends to be a more powerful way to communicate about relationships (Hartman and Laird, 1983).

A fifth communication principle described by the same group of family communication theorists (Jackson, Haley, Bateson, and Watzlawick), is called the *redundancy principle.* It has been consistently observed that a family interacts within a limited range of repetitive behavioral sequences. Hence, if a family observer misses one instance of a behavioral sequence or pattern, according to the redundancy principle, this sequence will soon manifest itself again.

Watzlawick and associates (1967) point out that the repetitive behavioral sequences are circular communication patterns. There are repetitive circular communication patterns that occur in every family. An example of a repetitive communication pattern in a family is the following. In the Jones family, when the youngest child is angry and has a temper tantrum, the mother rushes to his side to console him. The child then responds by demanding his way, and the mother gives in. Wright and Leahey (1984) suggest diagraming circular communication patterns, as the diagrams tend to "concretize and simplify repetitive sequences noted in a relationship" (p. 56). The basic elements of a circular pattern diagram are shown in Figure 10–3, and an example of a diagram is given in Figure 10–4.

The sixth communication principle described by Bateson and associates (1963) is that all communicational interactions are either symmetrical or complementary. In symmetrical communication one interactant's behavior mirrors the behavior of the other interactant (eg, both mates would equally contribute to the decision as to where to go for vacation). In complementary communication, one interactant's behavior supplements the other interactant's behavior (eg, the husband says he has selected a particular place to go for vacation and the wife nods that she has heard him). When one of these two types of communication is used

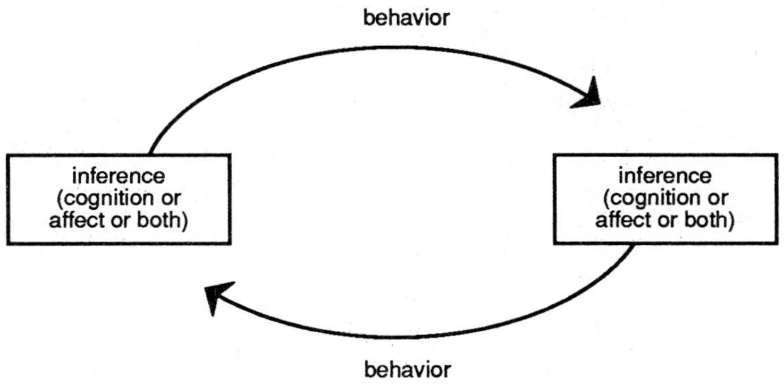

Figure 10–3
Basic elements of a circular pattern diagram. (Wright and Leahey, 1984.)

consistently in family relationships, the communication type is reflective of family values and role and power arrangements.

CHANNELS OF COMMUNICATION

Channels of information flow are the routes that information may take to reach the receiver. In the family, these involve the flow of information between the various sets of relationships. Families have usual channels of information flow, which reveal the family power structure, the closeness of relationships, family roles, and the popularity of individuals within the family. The popularity or centrality of individual members is indicated by a convergence of many channels of information to one person. This person serves as intermediary or "go-between" in families. In contrast, a relative absence of channels to a family member may reveal unpopularity, fear, or rejection. Chapter 11 further explains this process.

FUNCTIONAL COMMUNICATION IN THE FAMILY

Functional communication is viewed as the cornerstone of a successful, healthy family and as such is defined as the clear, direct transmission and reception of both the content and instruction level of any message (Sells, 1973), as well as the congruency between the content and the instruction levels (Satir, 1983). In other words, functional communication in the family setting requires that the intention or meaning of the sender be sent through relatively clear channels and that the receiver of the message have an understanding of its meaning that is similar to that of the sender (Sells, 1973). Effective communication means matching mean-

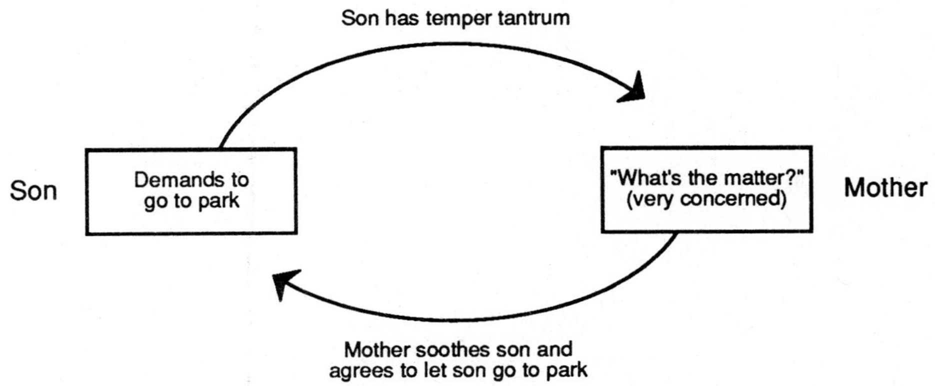

Figure 10–4
Example of circular pattern diagram.

ing, gaining consistency, and attaining congruence between the intended and the received message. Thus effective communication in the family is a process of constant definition and redefinition that will achieve a matching of the content and instructional levels of messages. Both the sender and the receiver must be actively involved and capable of interchanging positions by becoming either sender or receiver during the process.

The communication patterns within the family system have a major impact on the individual members. Individualization, learning about other people, the development and maintenance of self-esteem, and the ability to make choices are all dependent on the information that is passed between members in the family.

Interactional Characteristics of a Functional Family

Functional families have certain characteristics that are revealed in the communications they utilize. A functional family uses communication to create and maintain mutually beneficial relationships. Their interaction reveals a tolerance for error, as well as an understanding of the member's imperfections and individuality. Differentness (Satir, 1967), acknowledgment of the individuality and uniqueness of each member, is encouraged to the degree that is reciprocally beneficial to the family system and each individual. A sufficient amount of overt openness and honesty exists to enable members to recognize the needs and emotions of one another.

The communication patterns in a functional family demonstrate acceptance of differentness, as well as a minimum of judgments and unrealistic criticism of each other. Adjustments in individual behavior necessitated by the stress of external social demands or the needs of the family system or of personal development generate healthy adjustments in the whole family; one person is not expected to do all of the changing necessary for the family to continue in a stable manner, and sufficient cohesiveness and flexibility exist for the family to adapt effectively.

Communication in healthy families is an extremely dynamic two-way process. Messages are not simply sent and received by a sender and a receiver. For instance, as the sender begins a message, the receiver may show a facial expression that will, through "negative" feedback, change the sender's message before he or she is finished speaking. As a result, the sender might change the wording of a message in the middle of the sending action so that the receiver will have a similar frame of reference. This dynamic nature of communication makes functional interaction, however, complex and unpredictable. Communication, even in the healthiest of families, is still many times tenuous and problematic. In functional families it has also been noted that feelings of family members are allowed expression. Satir (1983), a well-known family therapist and writer, believes that the acknowledgment of feelings is vital.

In the following two sections descriptions of the specific verbal behaviors the functional sender and functional receiver uses when communicating are reviewed.

The Functional Sender

Satir (1967) states that the sender who communicates in a functional way can:

1. Firmly state his or her case.
2. At the same time clarify and qualify what he or she says.
3. Ask for feedback, as well.
4. Be receptive to feedback when he or she gets it.

Because each of these four elements is basic to understanding healthy communication, each will be briefly discussed.

Firmly States Case

Congruent Levels. One of the foundations for firmly stating one's case is the use of communication that is congruent on both the content and instruction levels. Satir (1975) calls the person who uses this style of communication a congruent communicator. For example, in the case of a person who is angry, to be congruent not only should the literal message denote anger, but also the tone of voice, body position, and gestures should reflect the same message.

Intensity and Explicitness. When a person communicates, the sender is asking something of the receiver. Such requests include various degrees of intensity and explicitness, both of which involve how firmly the sender states his or her case. Intensity refers to the ability of the sender to effectively communicate internal perceptions of feelings, desires, and needs at the same intensity as he or she is experiencing these perceptions internally. Normally there will be a fluctuation of intensity in the expression of feelings, desires, and needs, instead of a monotone presentation or "reasonableness" of expression. In other words, the functional sender conveys an accurate appraisal of his or her perceptions.

To be explicit, the functional sender informs the receiver of how serious the message is by stating how the receiver should respond to the message. An example illustrating a high degree of explicitness is: "I want to sit in that chair."

Clarifies and Qualifies Statements. A second dimension Satir identifies as an essential characteristic of the functional sender is the use of clarifying and qualifying statements in his or her communication. The use of clarifying and qualifying statements enables the sender to be specific and to check out his or her perception of reality against that of the other person. Specific types of clarifying and qualifying statements include those described below.

"I Want" Statements. A statement that clearly states what the sender wants (Strayhorn, 1977). Example: "Stop contradicting me when I'm disciplining the children."

"I Feel" Statements. The sender directly states his or her internal perceptions of a specific feeling. These feelings may be internally triggered or may be a reaction to another person's behavior (Strayhorn, 1977). Example of internally triggered expression: "I sometimes feel frustrated when my hands ache and I'm unable to do the chores around the house" (a patient with arthritis); externally triggered expression: "When you call me stupid in front of the children, I feel embarrassed and irritated."

"I Intend" Statements. This type of statement implies a concrete independent action will be initiated by the sender. Example: "I'm still experiencing weakness after my surgery and plan to take a nap this afternoon."

"I Like" and "I Don't Like" Statements. These are statements in which the sender states precisely what gives him or her pleasure or displeasure, or what the receiver does or does not do that bothers the sender (Strayhorn, 1977). Examples: "I like it when you clean up your room" and "I don't like it when I have to stay in my room by myself when I'm sick."

Self-disclosure Statements. A self-disclosure statement by an individual refers to an open and honest revelation of an intention, desire, or past action, or a fallibility that is considered private or personal to that individual. Examples: "I'm concerned about my biopsy because my mother died from cancer of the breast" and "I'm scared to show my anger because my husband may leave me."

Direct Questions. This involves asking concrete questions to elicit specific information. Example: "Are your stitches causing you any pain?"

Open-ended Questions. Open-ended questions focus on a general area of interest and encourage the receiver to express his or her own response. Open-ended questions do not structure the receiver's response. Example: "Tell me more about your reluctance to have the surgery."

Elicits Feedback. A third element of a functional sender is the use of asking for feedback, which enables him or her to verify whether the message was received accurately, as well as enable the sender to gain information needed to clarify his or her intent. In the following examples the sender seeks feedback to obtain the receiver's perception or reaction to what the sender has communicated: "I keep asking myself, should we tell the children that I have cancer? What do you think?" "Since you're still on limited activities because of your heart condition, I think your parents should visit at another time. What's your reaction?"

Receptivity of Sender to Feedback. The sender who is receptive to feedback will exhibit a willingness to listen, react nondefensively, and attempt to understand. In order to understand, the sender must not have so narrow a perspective that he or she is unable to comprehend the validity of the receiver's point of view. Thus by asking for more specific criticism or "checking out" statements, the sender demonstrates his or her receptivity and interest in feedback (Strayhorn, 1977). Examples: George's wife has criticized his lack of sexual responsiveness. To gain further information he asks, "What things bother you when we're making love?" Or JoAnn states, "I just bought the children some new clothing for school." Don reacts, "I'm really angry you did that." And JoAnn replies, "Are you angry because of the type of clothing I purchased, or did you want to shop for the children?"

Functional Receiver

People receiving messages generally tune in to the metamessage level of communication, but in the case of the functional receiver there would be an even greater ability to make an accurate assessment of the intent of a message. Therefore, he or she would be better able to correctly weigh the message's meaning and would be able to more precisely assess the sender's attitudes, intentions, and feelings as expressed in the metacommunication. According to Anderson (1974), the functional receiver tries to comprehend the material fully before attempting to evaluate. This means that motivations and metacommunication, as well as content, are analyzed. The new information is checked with that which is already known, and the decision to act is carefully weighed. Each of the communication techniques discussed below facilitate and enable the receiver to comprehend and respond more fully to the sender's message.

Listening. The ability to listen is perhaps the most important quality of a functional receiver. Listening effectively means focusing one's full attention on what is being communicated, thus blocking out all extraneous "noise." The receiver attends to the sender's complete message rather than prejudging the meaning of the communication. Sells (1973) explains:

> To listen is
> to be still
> to expect
> to wait for a response
> to practice restraint. (p. 23)

Many people are passive listeners, responding with blank expressions and a seemingly "couldn't care less" attitude. An active listener responds with gestures that communicate actively listening. Asking questions is a vital part of active listening (Gottman et al, 1977). It is as if the receiver were a student learning a new subject, and as a good student, he or she would ask questions and explore the facts. To actively listen means to be empathetic, to think of the other person's needs and desires, and to not disrupt the sender's flow of communication.

Feedback. The second major characteristic of the functional receiver involves feedback—that is feeding information back to the sender that tells how the message was interpreted by the receiver. The following are examples of giving feedback.

Asking Sender to Clarify and Qualify. These statements encourage the sender to elaborate more fully. Example: "What do you mean when you say I get frustrated too easily with the children?"

Associating. In the process of associating, the receiver makes a relationship between previous personal experiences (Gottman et al, 1977) or past related incidents and the sender's communication at both content and instructional levels. Example: During her last trimester of pregnancy, Susie comments to family nurse, "I have been getting upset quite easily and feel more dependent upon my husband. I never felt this way until I got pregnant."

The nurse responds, "I remember when I was pregnant having the same type of feelings. I would frequently ask my husband to do little things for me which I always did for myself before I was pregnant. In the families I visit the women have often shared these same types of feelings with me."

Paraphrasing and Checking Perceptions. The receiver, by using either a question or a statement summarizes the sender's message (Gottman et al, 1977). The receiver does this by restating the sender's message in his or her own words. The central purpose of paraphrasing is to clarify the sender's message. Examples: "So you're saying . . ." and "What I understand is. . . ."

Validation. Another major technique for facilitating communication is validation. In utilizing validation the receiver conveys the following: "I can see how you think and feel that way" or "It makes sense and is reasonable to feel that way." Validation does not imply that the receiver agrees with the sender's communication, but demonstrates an acceptance of the merit and/or worth of the message (Gottman et al, 1977). Examples:

1. Validation of thoughts. "You're saying that you're spending too much money on food and medication and want help with budgeting?"
2. Validation of feelings. "Sounds like you were hurt when I complained about your mother's behavior." Or, "I sense that you're really frightened that your tumor might be malignant."
3. Validation plus statement of own point of view. "I feel you're really angry with me, although I'm still feeling that your punishment of Tommy was too excessive."

FUNCTIONAL PATTERNS OF COMMUNICATION

As distinguished from the discussion of functional communication, this section covers family interaction more broadly or macroscopically, dealing with patterns of communication rather than specific or discrete interactional exchanges.

Family communication patterns are the characteristic, ongoing, circular interactional patterns of the family, which in addition to influencing and organizing the members of the family, produce the meaning of transactions between family members (Peters, 1974).

Most importantly, it is through interaction that the affective needs of family members are fulfilled. Most family communications take place within the subsystems (the parent–child, spousal–parental, and sibling subsystems), making analysis of subsystem communications in the family the primary locus of interest.

Interaction in families is affected by the roles and tasks of the members as prescribed by the culture. For instance, in some cultures direct sexual assertiveness by women is subject to disapproval; in other cultures, affectional interaction between fathers and children is discouraged. Other types of interactions, such as conflict resolution and decision-making techniques, are also culturally derived. The extent to which family members are verbal is also dependent on the culture as well as the socioeconomic level and developmental stage of the family.

Curran (1983), who extensively studied and described healthy families, writes that the first trait of a healthy family is clear communication and the ability to listen to each other. Good communication is necessary for loving relationships to develop and be maintained. The ability of family members to recognize and respond to non-verbal messages was also identified as an important attribute of healthy families.

Emotional Communication

Emotional communication deals with the expression of the range and variety of emotions or feelings—from the expression of anger, hurt, sadness, and jealousy to happiness, affection, and tenderness (Wright and Leahey, 1984). Lewis and associates (1976), in carefully studying the differences between dysfunctional and functional families, found that healthy families displayed a full spectrum of feelings, while more dysfunctional families were emotionally constricted and rigid in their expression of feelings. For instance, in more dysfunctional families anger may be permitted from parents to children, but not the reverse, or overt expressions of tenderness and affection are not permitted.

Affective communication—the verbal messages of caring and nonverbal, physical gestures of touching, caressing, holding, and looking—is especially important. As Bowlby (1966) demonstrated, physical expressions of affection in early childhood are essential in the development of normal affectional responses. Later in life, verbal affectional communication patterns become more predominant in relaying affectional messages. It should be noted here, however, that cultural background makes a big difference in how much emotional communication takes place.

As part of healthy affective communications, the family members need to be able to enjoy themselves and other family members. When their responses to each other are fresh and spontaneous, rather than controlled, repetitious, and predictable, this enjoyment can be realized.

Open Areas of Communication and Self-disclosure

Functional families, those with functional communication patterns, value openness; a mutual respect for each other's feelings, thoughts, and concerns, spontaneity; authenticity; and self-disclosure. It follows that these families would also be able to discuss most areas of life—both personal and social issues and concerns. These areas are referred to as "open areas of communication." With respect to self-disclosure, Satir (1972) asserts that family members who *level* with each other are people who feel self-confident enough to risk meaningful interaction. People with good self-esteem tend to be levelers who believe in self-disclosure—a revealing of intimate thoughts and feelings.

Satir and other family therapists assume that complete honesty/self-disclosure is ideal. Contrary to this notion, research in marital relationships demonstrates that total honesty and self-disclosure may not work for many couples. Many satisfied couples report that they do not tell one another everything, for fear it would jeopardize the relationship, hurt the partner's feelings, or create more interpersonal or personal stress (McCubbin and Dahl, 1985; Pearlin and Schooler, 1978). Hawkins and co-workers (1980), family communication researchers, observe that very few marital partners have ideal functional communication styles. Apparently most American marriages are suffering primarily from the lack of emotional communication.

It is generally true, however, that the more functional the family, the fewer areas of closed communication exist, and vice versa. Nevertheless, consideration of a family's culture is crucial here, because cultural norms concerning modesty, privacy, and sexual roles play a very large part in influencing areas of open and closed communication.

Power Hierarchy and Family Rules

Family systems are based on power hierarchies or "pecking orders" wherein communication containing "commands or imperatives" generally flows downward. *Functional* interaction in the power hierarchy occurs when power is distributed according to the developmental needs of the family members (Minuchin, 1974), or when power is assigned according to the abilities and resources of family members and is consonant with the family's cultural prescriptions of family power relationships. (See Chapter 11 for a more complete discussion of the family power structure.)

Power communications have characteristics that are readily apparent. The communication, "Joan, I want you to go upstairs and clean your room now or I will not take you to the show this afternoon" is typical of a coercive power communication. It is a command type message, specifying the action the receiver is to carry out and negatively reinforcing alternatives (Miller, 1969).

Family Conflict and Family Conflict Resolution

George Simmel (1858–1918), one of the founding fathers of sociology, was the first scientific observer of the role that conflict played in human interactions. Simmel's central thesis in writing about human interactions was that conflict is one vital form of social interaction. Social conflict is both ubiquitous and essential for group development and maintenance (Coser, 1956). Conflict functions to maintain family communications and interaction in several important ways (Table 10–1).

Verbal conflict is a routine part of normal family interaction. The literature on family conflict indicates that healthy families seem to be able "to strike a delicate balance between enough conflict to realize the positive benefits, but not too much conflict which would disrupt family relationships" (Vuchinich, 1987, p. 591).

TABLE 10–1. SUMMARY OF SIMMEL'S IDEAS ON CONFLICT

1. Conflict is designed to resolve divergent dualisms; it is a way of achieving some kind of unity.
2. Conflict is often necessary to keep an ongoing relationship going. Without ways of venting hostility toward each other, and expressing dissent, family members may feel completely powerless and demoralized, with withdrawal the usual outcome. By releasing pent-up feelings of hostility, conflicts serve to maintain a relationship.
3. Close, intimate family relationships are likely to contain both converging and diverging motivations, both "love and hatred." In relationships where persons are deeply involved, where they are engaged with their total personalities rather than a segment of it (like their work role only), there arise feelings of both love and hate . . . both attraction and repulsion. This great involvement or investment in a relationship also leads interactants to be likely to suppress hostility to avoid risking their relationship.
4. When conflict does occur, the closer the relationship, the more intense the conflict. The more we have in common with another, as whole people, the more easily will our totality be involved. Therefore, if a quarrel arises between people in such an intimate relationship, it is often so passionately expansive.
5. In marriage and family relationships, the absence of conflict is not functional—it is not an appropriate criterion for judging the vitality, strength, or stability of family interactions. In fact, the very absence of conflict may be an indicator of the existence of underlying strain and insecurity. Closeness in family relationships generates frequent occasions for conflict, but if family members do not feel secure in their relationships, they will avoid conflict, fearing its presence might threaten the continuance of their relationship. In this case, the couple's or family members' disagreements, differences, and hostilities go underground, and their communication becomes more covert and indirect.

Source: Adapted from Simmel (1955).

Recent research findings of White (1989) indicate that among white middle class couples there are gender differences in how spouses resolve conflict. Men assume a more coercive (competitive) stance towards their wives, whereas women take an affiliative (cooperative) stance toward their husbands.

Conflict resolution is a vital task of interaction in the family. Spouses need to learn to have constructive conflicts. Although how marital partners resolve conflict varies, functional conflict resolution occurs when the conflict is openly discussed and strategies to solve the conflict are employed, or when parents appropriately utilize their authority to close off conflicts. Parents need to act as role models for their children in terms of expressing conflict/differences and resolving these conflicts.

DYSFUNCTIONAL COMMUNICATION IN THE FAMILY

In this chapter functional and dysfunctional communication have been separated for discussion purposes. In reality, however, this demarcation does not exist, and communication patterns in families are not all totally healthy or unhealthy. Rather, they should be viewed on a continuum from functional to dysfunctional, with all but a small percentage of families falling somewhere between these poles. In contrast to the definition of functional communication, dysfunctional communication is defined as the unclear and/or indirect transmission and reception of either or both the content and instruction (intent) of a message and/or the incongruency between the content and instruction level of the message. The indirect aspect of dysfunctional communication refers to whether the messages go to their appropriate targets (direct) or are deflected and go to other persons in the family (indirect).

Characteristics and Values

One of the primary factors that generates dysfunctional communication patterns is the presence of low esteem of both the family and its members, especially the parents (Anderson, 1972; Satir, 1972, 1983). Three interrelated values that perpetuate low esteem are self-centeredness, need for total agreement, and lack of empathy.

Self-centeredness. Self-centeredness is characterized by focusing on one's own needs to the exclusion of the other person's needs, feelings, or perspectives. In other words, self-centered individuals seek to get something from the other to meet their own needs. When these individuals must give, they do so reluctantly and then in a hostile, defensive, or self-sacrificing manner. Thus bargaining or negotiating effectively is difficult, because self-centered persons believe they cannot afford to lose what little they have to give (Satir, 1983). Some social scientists see this tendency for self-absorption/self-centeredness to be a product of our present society. Lasch, in *Culture of Narcissism* (1979), analyzes this widespread propensity of individuals in American society.

Value of Total Agreement. The family's value of maintaining total agreement and avoiding conflict begins when the marital partners discover that each is different from the other, although what these exact differences are may be difficult to explain. Differentness—as expressed in opinions, habits, preferences, or expectations—may be seen as a threat because it can and does lead to disagreements and the awareness that they are both separate individuals. If marital partners have low self-esteem and feel that it is absolutely necessary to be loved and approved at all times, they try to constantly please their mate. This need to continually please prohibits them from communicating openly when displeased or acknowledging disagreement. The couple perceives that expressions of their own unique thoughts and feelings might lead to conflicts that could then result in a "catastrophe" (Gottman et al, 1977). Distracting and placating tactics are often used to avoid conflict and act as if there is agreement (Satir, 1972).

Thus unwritten rules come into being that forbid open expression of one's own individuality and differentness as a means of staving off this threat. These rules are often rigid and elude conflict or negotiation, so that there is no consideration of alternatives that would enable each mate to interact differently and yet be accepted. As part of the socialization process, the children learn these same values and ways of relating and thus have difficulty in recognizing and interpreting a variety of feelings and experiences. These values and resultant communication patterns constrict the growth of all family members.

Ruesch and associates (1974), in their research of marital relationships, found that in those marriages where conflict was avoided and negative feelings buried, the negative feelings "poisoned" the relationship. They observed that avoidance of conflict may lead to "devitalized marriages"—marriages in which mates feel emotionally detached and indifferent to each other.

Lack of Empathy. Family members who are self-centered and cannot tolerate differentness also cannot recognize the effect of their own thoughts, feelings, and behavior on other family members; neither can they understand other family members' thoughts, feelings, and behavior. They are so consumed with meeting their own needs that they do not have the ability to be empathetic. Underneath a facade of unconcern, these individuals may suffer feelings of powerlessness. Not only do they devalue themselves, they also devalue others. This leads to an atmosphere of tension, fearfulness, and/or blame.

The stage is therefore set for a style of communication that is confusing, vague, indirect, and covert, with defensiveness rather than openness, clarity, and honesty prevailing. Satir (1967; 1983) and other family therapists who advocate the use of family communications theory in practice, assert that the more dysfunctional the communication, the more dysfunctional the family. This is a primary theoretical proposition within this theoretical perspective.

Dysfunctional Sender

Specific verbal behaviors indicating a dysfunctional sender and a dysfunctional receiver are now presented, so that when these behaviors are observed, there is a greater understanding of the dynamics and their consequences.

The dysfunctional sender's communication is often ineffective in one or more of the four basic characteristics of the functional sender: in stating case, in clarifying and qualifying, in eliciting, and/or in being receptive to feedback. The receiver is often left confused and has to guess what the sender is thinking or feeling. The communication of the dysfunctional sender is either actively or passively defensive and often negates the possibility of seeking any clear feedback from the receiver. "Unhealthy" communication in the sender is discussed under five major categories: assumptions, the unclear expression of feelings, judgmental expressions, inability to define needs, and incongruent communication.

Assumptions. When assumptions are made, the sender takes for granted what the receiver is feeling or thinking about an event or person without validating his or her perceptions. The dysfunctional sender is usually not aware of the assumptions he or she is making. He or she rarely clarifies content or intent, thus serving to obscure and distort meaning. When this dysfunction in communication occurs, it elicits anger in the receiver, who is being given the message that his or her own opinions and feelings do not matter much.

The following illustrations represent various forms of the use of assumptions.

Speaking for the Other. The sender acts as a spokesperson for another by telling someone else what the person is thinking or feeling (Gottman et al, 1977). Example: Without checking with spouse, the husband comments to the children, "It is perfectly obvious that your mother never wants to go on walks with us."

What Is Perceived or Evaluated Cannot Be Altered The individual assumes that what he or she has perceived or evaluated cannot be changed. Examples: "Jim has always been messy. I've just had to learn to live with that fact." Or, "Joey's so accident prone, but that's life."

Incomplete Messages. The sender does not finish the sentence or message but assumes that the receiver will complete it. Example: "He said we couldn't agree on . . . you see what I mean?"

Assumes Others Share Same Perceptions, Thoughts, and Feelings. The sender automatically takes for granted that other people share his or her perceptions, thoughts, and feelings (Satir, 1983). Example: "I dislike going to the free clinic; I know you feel the same way."

Generalizations. The content of the message describes behavior or events in general terms instead of citing specific behaviors and observations. The sender assumes that the receiver will fill in the specifics. Example: "You're such a poor father," as opposed to, "I wish you would discipline Sarah when she doesn't put away her toys."

One Instance Exemplifies All Instances. The individual, in failing to learn that thoughts, actions, and sentiments change, falls into the error of overgeneralizing and makes an assumption that one situation is an example of all similar situations to follow. Example: "The nurse at the free clinic was impatient and blunt with me. I'm not going there again to get this same treatment from her and the rest of the staff."

Unclear Expression of Feelings. Another type of dysfunctional communication by the sender is unclear expression of feelings. Due to fear of rejection, the sender's expressions of feelings must go underground or be uttered in such a covert manner that the feelings are not recognizable. In another instance, the sender may express his or her feelings but does so without the same intensity as the feelings were perceived internally, the usual situation being that feelings are understated. Various types of unclear expression of feelings will be presented.

Sarcasm. Sarcasm denotes the use of humorous or witty statements that enable the sender of a message to avoid taking responsibility for his or her hostile feelings. If confronted, the sender can always reply that he or she was just being humorous. Example: "Fathers were made to play with their sons while mothers were made to take all the responsibility for raising them."

Super-reasonableness. Satir (1975) describes being super-reasonable as one of the four modes of dysfunctionally communicating. In this situation the sender's words bear no relationship to how he or she feels. Messages are stated in an unemotional way. This should come as no surprise. In our society men are taught not to reveal their feelings if they are really a "man," and women are cautioned against "sounding aggressive."

Silent Resentment. In the case of unclear expression of feeling, the sender feels irritated with the receiver but does not express the anger overtly and/or may displace the resentment onto another person or thing (Satir, 1983). Example: The children have broken a second window in the period of a week. Joan is infuriated but remains silent. When her husband comes home from work, she coldly stares at him and then leaves the room (displacement of anger onto the husband).

Expression of Hurt As Anger. The sender expresses anger as a defensive maneuver to cover up feelings of hurt, rather than expressing the more basic emotion of hurt. Example: Eileen takes great pride in creating various artistic items for her home. She has just completed a new floral arrangement Land made some new drapes for the living room. When her husband comes home from work she proudly shows him the items, at which he only nods his head and seems preoccupied and disinterested. Eileen angrily states, "I'm sick and tired of trying to share my interests with you." This communication technique is extensively used. If hurt (the underlying emotion) is expressed, rather than the cover-up emotion, anger, the receiver then usually reacts in a more appropriate and positive fashion.

Judgmental Expressions. This category of dysfunctional communication is characterized by a tendency to constantly evaluate messages in terms of the sender's own value system. Judgmental statements always carry moral overtones where it is clear to the receiver that the sender is evaluating the worth of the other person's message as being "right" or "wrong," "good" or "bad," "normal" or "abnormal." It is not only a message that is being evaluated or judged, but also the sender of a message who is being indirectly evaluated or judged. Two types of judgmental expression are put-down statements or questions and "you should" statements.

Put-down Statements/Questions or Blaming. These are statements or questions that carry a negative connotation and value judgment. Judgmental expressions may also involve a covert unmet need or an unexpressed dissatisfaction with the other interactant. Examples: "You are really clumsy." (As opposed to, "I want you to be more careful when carrying a glass of milk.") And, "When are you going to amount to something?" (As opposed to, "I want you to spend more effort doing your homework.") Blaming occurs in families where the blamer wants to let the receiver(s) know who is boss. In families blamers are often called "tyrants" or "dominating husbands or wives" (Satir, 1975).

"You Should" Statements. The words "should" or "ought to" imply that the sender is an authority figure who knows what is "good" or "bad." If the sender is a parent and the receiver the child, this type of communication may be functional and necessary in the socialization process, but must generally be held to be a dysfunctional mode of communication. Example: Family health nurse to mother, "Johnny's too fat! You should feed him less."

Inability to Express Needs. The dysfunctional sender is not only unable to express his or her needs, but due to fear of rejection is incapable of defining the behaviors he or she expects from the receiver to fulfill them. Often the dysfunctional sender unconsciously feels unworthy, with no right to express needs or expect that personal needs will be met. Various examples of the sender's inability to express needs follow.

Silent Need for Nurturance. The silent need for nurturance is defined as an unexpressed need for help, empathy, or some aspect of "being taken care of." This may also include an expectation that others should be able to anticipate the sender's needs and that asking for nurturance or assistance renders the response to such requests inauthentic and unsatisfying (Strayhorn, 1977). Example: After her radiation therapy, Jane sometimes experiences nausea. Jack, not realizing his wife's discomfort, does not offer to prepare dinner. When Jane finally asks for Jack's assistance, she feels angry even though he agrees to prepare dinner.

Covert Requests. These types of requests are made without acknowledging "ownership" (the sender does not overtly admit his or her wishes) (Strayhorn, 1977). Example: "It would do you good to spend more time with the children." (The sender does not directly ask the other to spend time with the children.)

Complaints. In this case the sender appears unable or unwilling to describe the desired behavior needed from the receiver, and the sender expresses these needs in terms of a dissatisfaction. Example: the Smiths, a couple in their seventies, typically complain to their children, "You never visit us." (As opposed to, "Please come over for dinner Wednesday evening.")

Incongruent Communication. In this type of dysfunctional communication, two or more simultaneous and contradictory messages are sent. The receiver is left with the enigma of how to respond.

Verbal–Verbal Incongruency. In this case two or more literal messages sent simultaneously oppose each other. Examples: "Jimmy's such a well-behaved child. Did I tell you last week he had another fight at school?" And, "I don't mind being alone so much when I'm sick; of course, it would be nice if the children would visit me more often."

Verbal–Nonverbal Incongruency. The sender communicates a message verbally, but the accompanying nonverbal metacommunication contradicts the verbal message (Satir, 1983). This is commonly known as giving "mixed messages." Example: "I'm not angry with you!" spoken in a loud, gruff tone of voice with fists clenched.

Dysfunctional Receiver

When the receiver is dysfunctional, a breakdown in communication occurs because the message is not received as intended due to the receiver's failure to listen, the use of disqualification, responding offensively, failing to explore the sender's message, or failing to validate the message.

Failure to Listen. In the case of failure to listen, a message is sent, but the receiver does not attend to or hear the message. There may be many reasons for failure to listen, ranging from willfull inattention to a wish but an inability to listen. This is commonly due to concomitant distraction, such as noise, improper timing, or high anxiety (Sells, 1973). A frequently used way in which individuals do not listen is by ignoring messages.

CLIENT: I keep wondering if I will always be this limited in my activities because of my heart condition.

NURSE: Has the swelling in your ankles decreased?

Failure to listen causes distortion and misinterpretation of the message.

Disqualification. A disqualification is an indirect response that allows the receiver to disagree with a message without really disagreeing.

"Yes-butting." The dysfunctional receiver partially agrees with the intent of the message, yet at the same time finds something wrong with the sender's opinion, feeling, or suggestions (Gottman et al, 1977).

NURSE: When Bobby has temper tantrums, why don't you try going in to see that he's all right, and then leave him alone until he calms down.

BOBBY'S MOTHER: Yes, that's a fine idea, but I'm afraid he would hurt himself.

Evasion. The receiver disqualifies the message by avoiding the crucial issue.

NURSE: Well, how effective was leaving the room when Bobby had a temper tantrum?

HUSBAND: Wouldn't you say it worked, Jean, because the number of tantrums decreased this week?

WIFE: Bobby's constant requests are driving me crazy.

Tangentialization and Distraction. Here the receiver responds to a peripheral aspect of a message and ignores the central intention or content of the message. He or she "distracts" by responding with words and behavior that are irrelevant or unrelated to the message sent or what is going on (Satir, 1975).

HUSBAND (hospitalized for a myocardial infarction 6 weeks prior to the visiting nurse's visit): All of my recreational interests were of a strenuous nature, so all I do now is complain to my wife that I have nothing to do all day.

WIFE: I love strenuous activities myself and have always been interested in tennis.

Offensiveness and Negativity. Offensiveness in communication denotes that the receiver of a message reacts negatively, as if being threatened. The receiver seems to react defensively to the message by assuming an oppositional posture and an attacking position. Statements and requests are consistently made in a negative manner or with a negative expectation (Harris, 1975). The family member receiving the consistently negative communication learns to respond with similar statements or behavior. Habitually conflicted couples behave this way.

Attacking With a Different Issue. Before any progress is made on a threatening issue introduced by the sender, the person receiving the message responds with an extraneous issue that hurts or threatens the sender—that is, the receiver uses a "counterattack."

WIFE: I very rarely see you set any limits on the children.

HUSBAND: After 5 years I keep wondering when you're going to learn to cook a decent meal.

Insulting. The receiver attributes a negative or insulting characteristic to the sender. In other words, the receiver attacks the sender, not the issue (Gottman et al, 1977).

CHILD: Dad, you never play baseball with me anymore.

FATHER: You're so uncoordinated that you can't even catch the ball.

Rebuff. In response to requests to clarify or qualify, the receiver conveys disgust by refusing to elaborate or to comply with the sender's request. Examples: "How many times do I have to repeat myself?" And, "You heard me the first time."

Lack of Exploration. In order to clarify the intent or meaning of a message, the functional responder seeks further explanation. In contrast, the dysfunctional receiver uses responses that negate exploration, such as making assumptions (as discussed previously), giving premature advice, or cutting off communication.

Premature Advice. Premature advice is defined as the offering of a suggestion or solution to a problem before exploring it sufficiently or requesting additional feedback.

PATIENT: This diagnosis of multiple sclerosis has really been a shock.

NURSE: I'd suggest rest periods during the day, and don't overtire yourself by engaging in strenuous activities.

A functional response would have been to explore the emotional impact of the diagnosis on the patient.

Cutoffs in Communication. When the dysfunctional receiver does not want to continue discussing the issue at hand, he or she makes a statement or uses an action that curtails any further discussion of that issue. This technique is often used to avoid dealing with unpleasant or negative feelings (Strayhorn, 1977). Examples: "Let's just forget it" and "It's not that important." In addition, physical actions are another way of cutting off communication. For example, the receiver could leave the room, engage in busywork, or turn away from the sender.

Lack of Validation. As stated previously, the receiver in an interaction often has the difficult task of attempting to correctly interpret both the content and the intent of the message. Validation, as previously defined, refers to the receiver's conveyance of acceptance. Therefore, lack of validation implies that the receiver either responds neutrally (shows neither acceptance nor nonacceptance) or distorts and misinterprets the message. Assuming rather than clarifying the thoughts of the sender is one example of a lack of validation.

NEW MOTHER: My mother has just come to stay with us for 3 weeks to take care of the new baby while I get my strength back.

FAMILY NURSE: How wonderful! I'm sure that your mother will be a tremendous help to you during this time.

This interaction is dysfunctional because the nurse assumes that the client has positive feelings about her mother's assistance without exploring with the mother her evaluation of how helpful the mother has been.

DYSFUNCTIONAL COMMUNICATION PATTERNS

In this type of patterned interaction, two or more family members have established repetitive networks and strategies of dysfunctional communication that attempt to maintain homeostasis and the integration of the family unit. These dysfunctional processes are often subtle, and the intent of the communication is covert or hidden. Thus accurate assessment of this type of unhealthy circular communication patterns becomes more difficult. In this section, three dysfunctional interactional communication processes that are less difficult to assess have been selected.

Self-perpetuating Syndrome

Each individual in the interaction constantly restates his or her own issues without really listening to the other's point of view or acknowledging the other's needs.

WIFE: To discipline the children, I have them spend 15 minutes in their room. I'm not a believer in severe punishment.

HUSBAND: I believe in stern limits. Last week I took Jody's allowance away for a month and refused to let him play outside for a week.

WIFE: Yes, 15 minutes in their room gets the point across.

HUSBAND: If you dish out stern punishment, the children really listen.

In this situation, each partner continued to restate his or her own viewpoint and did not acknowledge that of the other.

Inability to Focus on One Issue

Each of the individuals in the interaction rambles from one issue to another instead of resolving any one problem discussed or obtaining closure.

HUSBAND: I'm tired of your mother visiting without calling first.

WIFE: When are you going to take Jack shopping?

HUSBAND: Soon as you balance the checking account correctly.

Notice how each partner introduces a new problem without any attempts of a discussion of one problem at a time.

Closed Areas of Communication

While more functional families have more open areas of communication, less functional families displaying dysfunctional interactional patterns will demonstrate more closed areas of communication. Families have unwritten rules about subjects that are approved or disapproved for discussion. These unwritten rules are most overtly seen when a family member breaches the family's rules by bringing up unapproved subjects or expressing forbidden feelings.

Unwritten family rules about what communication is open and closed reveal much about other aspects of a family's structure (their values, norms, power, and roles in the family). Communication restrictions may be limited to certain family subsystems: for example, discussion of sexual habits in front of the children, or a parent's alcoholism. Financial issues may be discussed only between spouses but not with the children. Moreover, an area may be closed in terms of expression of feelings but open in terms of expression of thoughts.

Cultural norms of modesty, privacy, and sexual roles probably play a large part in influencing the areas where closed and open communication exist. Thus communication patterns must be evaluated in their cultural context.

A common interactional pattern utilized in families to avoid discussing meaningful issues and/or expressing salient feelings is termed "chitchat." The family, in using "chitchat" consistently, talks about superficial daily occurrences and avoids the meaningful issues of family life.

For example, a mother has been taking her child to a pediatric clinic because of recurrent convulsions. At the clinic the diagnosis of epilepsy was recently confirmed. Since hearing of the diagnosis, the family has never discussed their thoughts or feelings about the diagnosis; their only conversation in this area has dealt with the inconvenient hospital parking arrangements and the long travel time to the clinic.

COMMUNICATION IN FAMILIES WITH HEALTH PROBLEMS

Findings from research that has examined adaptation of families to chronic and life-threatening illness has consistently demonstrated that a central factor in healthy marital and family functioning is the presence of open, honest, and clear communication in dealing with the stressful health and health-related issues (Kahn, 1990; Spinetta and Deasy-Spinetta, 1981). When families do not discuss the important issues they are faced with, emotional distancing in family relationships results, and family stress increases (Friedman, 1985). Increased stress affects not only family relationships but also the health of the family and its members (Hoffer, 1989).

FAMILY COMMUNICATION: APPLYING THE FAMILY NURSING PROCESS

The following assessment questions should be considered when analyzing a family's communication patterns.

☐ *ASSESSMENT QUESTIONS*

1. In observing the family as a whole and/or the family's set of relationships, how extensively is functional and dysfunctional communication used? Give examples of recurring patterns.
   a. How firmly and clearly do members state their needs and feelings?
   b. To what extent do members use clarification and qualification in interaction?
   c. Do members elicit and respond favorably to feedback, or do they generally discourage feedback and exploration of an issue?
   d. How well do members listen and attend when communicating?
   e. Do members seek validation from one another?
   f. To what degree do members use assumptions and judgmental statements in interaction?
   g. Do members interact in an offensive manner to messages?
   h. How frequently is disqualification utilized?
2. How are emotional messages conveyed in the family and within the family subsystems?
   a. How frequently are these emotional messages conveyed?
   b. What types of emotions are transmitted within the family subsystems? Are negative, positive, or both types of emotions transmitted?
3. What is the frequency and quality of communication within the communication network and familial sets of relationships?
   a. Who talks to whom and in what usual manner?
   b. What is the usual pattern of transmitting important messages? Does an intermediary exist?
   c. Are messages appropriate to the developmental age of the members?

4. Are the majority of messages of family members congruent in content and instruction (including observations of nonverbal messages)? If not, who manifests incongruency?
5. What types of dysfunctional processes are evident in the family communication patterns?
6. What important family/personal issues are open and closed to discussion?
7. What internal (familial: values, roles, power, affective socialization patterns and coping; and personal: parents' self-esteem) and external (environmental, socioeconomic, and cultural) influences affect the family's communication patterns?

FAMILY NURSING DIAGNOSES

Although family communication problems are frequent and very significant family nursing diagnoses, the North American Nursing Diagnosis Association (NANDA) has not identified any family-based communication diagnoses. The one nursing diagnosis listed by NANDA is "impaired verbal communication," which is focused on the individual client who is unable to verbally communicate (McFarland and McFarlane, 1989).

A broad family nursing diagnosis may be used, such as dysfunctional family communication or dysfunctional parent–child, sibling, or marital communication (if the problem is primarily located in the subsystem). Other general family nursing diagnoses in this area are impaired family communication or family communication problems. If broad diagnoses are used, then defining characteristics and related factors should accompany the diagnosis, following the NANDA pattern. Some family nurses may identify a more specific family communication problem as the diagnosis, such as minimal affective or emotional marital communication, or incongruent communication patterns of parents.

FAMILY NURSING INTERVENTIONS

Family nursing interventions in the area of communication are focused on all three levels of prevention: primary, secondary, and tertiary prevention. Strategies primarily involve teaching and counseling, and secondarily collaboration, contracting, and referrals to self-help groups, community organizations, and family therapy clinics or offices.

General Family Nursing Interventions

Family counselors often remark that one of the major roles they enact in working with families is to teach them about family dynamics and how to communicate in a more functional way with each other. Much of the teaching that takes place is informal—that which goes on in the spontaneous client–nurse interactions. Role modeling is also a crucial type of teaching. It is through the family members' observation of the family health professional and how he or she communicates during different interactional situations that they learn to imitate healthy communication behaviors. The nurse in role modeling functional communication should listen intently, deliberately, and empathetically, following up with clarifying questions and encouraging further expression of thoughts and feelings. Role modeling becomes a particularly potent teaching method when family members positively identify with the family nurse.

Counseling in the area of family communication involves encouraging and supporting families in their efforts at improving communication between themselves. In counseling the family nurse is a facilitator of group process and a resource person. His or her presence gives families both permission to try out new ways of communicating and the safety of having "a third person" there when they bring out previously closed areas of communication to discuss or break other unwritten communication rules, such as disagreeing or asserting their view.

Specific Family Nursing Interventions

More specific intervention strategies in the area of family communication reflect what we know about functional family communication—promoting functional family communication being the overarching goal here. Wright and Leahey's (1984) classification of the three types of direct family interventions (those focused upon the cognitive, affective, and behavioral levels of family functioning) aid in organizing specific communication strategies that can be applied. Intervention strategies within each of the three domains include both teaching and counseling.

Cognitive-level Focus. Family nursing interventions in this area provide new information or ideas about communication. The information is educational and hopefully encourages family problem solving.

Whether family members change their communication behavior is first largely dependent on how they perceive the problem. Wright and Leahey (1984) affirm the crucial role of perception by stating, "the nurse must help the family to obtain a different view of their problems" (p. 179). Hence, the goal here is to change the family members' perception and beliefs about a specific communication problem.

Helping family members reframe certain messages so that they have a more positive view of a particular situation is very helpful. For instance, helping family members see that when a person in the family gets very angry, that usually means he or she is feeling hurt, pain, and possibly a sense of rejection. Hurt is a much more "acceptable" and positive emotion for family members to respond to than anger and hostility.

Another important "lesson" for family members to learn is that there is no one reality. Multiple realities or perceptions exist about a particular situation or event. Each family member will have his or her own perceptionsor perspective about a particular situation or event. In order to deal with conflicts or situations requiring decision making, family members' perceptions (and feelings) about the situation should be understood and considered.

Affective-level Focus. Interventions in this area are directed toward changing the emotional expression of family members—by either increasing or decreasing the level of emotional communication or modifying the quality of the emotional communication. The specific nursing goals here are to help the family members express and share their feelings with each other so that (1) their emotional needs can be better conveyed and responded to; (2) more congruent, clear family communication occurs; and (3) family problem-solving efforts are facilitated.

Direct interventions aimed at the affective level of family functioning include urging parents to share their feelings, both positive and negative, with their children. And likewise, supporting parents' effort at encouraging their children to share the full range of their feelings with their parents, so that children can be better communicators. (Children learn to express themselves as they see their parents expressing themselves.) In addition, family nurses can point out incongruences in family members' levels of communication and encourage them to be more congruent in their content and metamessages (the metamessage or instruction consists of how content is said, including the feelings with which the words are said).

Behavioral-level Focus. Understanding or having more positive perceptions about a family communication problem is not sufficient for change to occur. There also must be behavioral change (Wright and Leahey, 1984). Rather than search for underlying causes and "whys" to problems, Wright and Leahey suggest that family nurses ask about the "whats" of the problem. For example, when a father decides by himself what movie the family will see, asking what effect that has on the other family members is more helpful than asking why he made that decision himself.

Behavioral changes stimulate changes in perceptions of a family member's "reality" and perceptions stimulate changes in behavior (there is a circular, recursive process involved here). Hence, when the family nurse assists family members to learn new and healthier ways of communicating, he or she is also helping to change family members' perceptions or their construction of reality about a situation.

Some teaching and counseling interventions designed to change family communication (remember, all communication is behavior) or the way family members relate to each other include:

1. Giving the family members instructions on specific behavioral changes. For example, in the case of working with an anxious new mother and her baby who constantly awakens and cries, instruct the mother that when the baby cries to check to make sure his needs are met and then leave the infant in his crib alone and let him cry for 15 minutes before entering the room again.
2. When family members are exhibiting beginning attempts to communicate clearly and congruently, support and compliment them for their efforts—so that the positive behaviors are reinforced and will be attempted again.
3. Monitor behavioral changes that have been suggested at previous meetings. Ask how a particular suggestion worked or if any problems occurred or questions arose when they tried the recommended action.

McCubbin and Dahl (1985), family educators, recommend communication tactics for couples to use to manage conflict productively. A summary of their guidelines follows.

1. Try not to engage in "kitchen-sink fighting" (throwing in all kinds of additional issues into the conflict).
2. Talk in terms of issues, not personalities.

3. Be an active listener" (obtain feedback and ask for clarification).
4. Recognize that your mate's unhappiness is not always your responsibility.
5. Find a way for both sides to win (pp. 187–189).

Self-help groups that are emotionally oriented facilitate open group communications, which in turn assists families in improving their communications. There are numerous community organizations and programs designed to improve marriage and family communication and relationships as well as parenting skills. Communication skills are very much emphasized in these programs and organizations. Referring families and couples to appropriate community groups and family counseling facilities is indicated when the available services are not sufficient to deal with the family's problems and the family wishes to seek further assistance.

☐ STUDY QUESTIONS

1. From the list below select the four primary characteristics that are *not* representative of a functional sender.
   a. Listens
   b. Receptive to feedback
   c. Elicits feedback
   d. Makes assumptions
   e. Firmly states case
   f. Validates
   g. Clarifies and qualifies
   h. Generalizes

2. Name four basic components of functional communication.

3. Match the five major categories of dysfunctional communication in the left column with the specific illustrations given at the right.

CATEGORY	EXAMPLE
a. Assumptions.	1. "I'm not mad at you," spoken in loud, sharp tone.
b. Unclear expression of feelings.	2. "I dislike patients who are constantly complaining."
c. Judgmental expressions.	3. "I don't understand how you can be so dumb."
d. Inability to define needs.	4. "I just love it when you don't come home for dinner, then I have only a few dishes to wash."
e. Incongruent communication.	5. "If you would like to go out for dinner, so would I."

4. Which of the following situations *best* demonstrates that information has been received from a sender?
   a. A parent tells a child to stop playing with his food and the child continues to play.
   b. A parent tells a child to drink his milk and the child looks at the parent.
   c. A parent shows a child how to butter bread and the child states that she knows a better way to butter her bread.

5. Which of the above situations (in question 4) best indicates that interaction has not occurred and the receiver needs more information to make a decision?

6. Punctuation in interactional sequences means (choose the best definition):
   a. When the beginning of the sequence is perceived to have begun.
   b. How the sequence was ended.
   c. Who, in fact, started the interactional sequence.
   d. A poor grasp of expression of ideas by a family member.

7. Feedback is a term used in systems theory to describe the process of information flow (answer *True* or *False*).

8. In the following situations describe both the content and instructional level of the message.
   a. A newlywed couple is watching a movie. The woman caresses the man's arm and hugs it to her while she whispers, "I'm really not interested in this movie."
   b. A child starts to crawl on his parent's lap. The parent pushes the child away and says, "You know I love you, go play with your new toy."
   c. A child is throwing cereal with a spoon. The mother grabs the spoon and cereal bowl and emphatically states, "Stop it! You may not play with your food!"

9. When a transaction between two family members is repeated over and over again, this tendency is referred to as the ____________ principle.

10. A wife, in finding that her husband has not helped with the dishes as he promised to do, expresses her anger at him. He, in turn, yells back that "he will wash the dishes in his own time." She then continues to berate him. What kind of feedback loops does this series of transactions illustrate?

Family Case Study

During the reading of this family case example, jot down your interpretation of the interactions (using the theory presented in chapter), in addition to completing assessment questions at the end of the case description.

A member of the Visiting Nurses' Association is going out to visit Mr. Herman Katz, a Jewish male, age 68, who has suffered a myocardial infarction and has just recently returned home after 4 weeks of hospitalization. The doctor has requested that the visiting nurse review his dietary and exercise regimen and report back her appraisal of his diet and tolerance to the progressive exercise regime.

The nurse's notes on the interagency referral form from the hospital states: Mr. Katz was alert, very conscientious about his care, but was quite reluctant to do any of the activities—and thus was somewhat demanding and dependent on the nurses. He ate poorly and got up to go to the bathroom by himself. During the last week he has had no pain or dyspnea during self-care activities.

The visiting nurse on her first visit learned that Mr. K. had been a business manager for many years and that he had retired 3 years ago. This was his second heart attack according to his wife (the first occurring 6 months postretirement). Past recreational interests had been heavy gardening and remodeling of his home prior to his first heart attack.

Mrs. Sylvia Katz is 65 years old and also Jewish. She has been in fairly good health except for being overweight and having osteoarthritis, which has made walking much more difficult for her. She prepares rich Jewish foods for herself, and her single daughter Marian, age 40, who also lives with her and her husband.

She or her daughter constantly answers for Mr. K. when the nurse asks questions. Mrs. K. is very talkative and complains of being very tired herself.

The Katz family lives in a nicely furnished three-bedroom house. Mr. K. has a college education and is a certified public accountant. They have two grown sons, who live nearby, and an unmarried daughter, Marian, who is temporarily living with them to help her father out.

On the second visit a week later, the nurse observed the following: Mr. K. continued to be unwilling and afraid to do things for himself and had not increased his level of activity. He appeared short of breath and uncomfortable (as though in pain) when talking about his illness and symptoms, but when distracted he appeared to have no dyspnea or pain. Mr. K. has seen none of his social or work friends since he has been home, according to Mrs. K. He has not been getting dressed or taking care of his personal hygiene adequately.

The following interactional vignettes were extracted as the nurse began to discuss Mr. K.'s rehabilitation program:

NURSE (question directed to Mr. K.): What activities did the doctor recommend for you to do this week?

SYLVIA (interceding): I told Herman that he should take it easy because after all this is his second heart attack and the next one will be his last!

MARIAN: Yes, mother's right. He should be taking it easy. Isn't that right? (Looks at mother for agreement.)

NURSE: I understand both of your concerns for your husband's and father's welfare. But, Mr. Katz, I want to know your understanding and feelings about what activities and the amount of exercise your doctor wants you to get.

HERMAN: Well, my understanding is that I shouldn't do anything that upsets or fatigues me. And up to now I haven't felt like doing anything much.

NURSE (again looking at Herman): What specifically did the doctor say you should do?

Herman looks at his daughter and then wife, and Marian immediately jumps up to get his written directions on exercises and diet guidelines. Nurse reads these guidelines and explains the concept and importance of the recommended progressive exercise program. As this is being carefully explained, Mrs. K. looks over to the kitchen as if she is disinterested and then walks out to begin lunch preparation.

As the exercise program continued to be discussed, Herman remarked:

HERMAN: These activities don't use up much of my time and I'm tired of watching TV. I feel restless 'cause I have nothing to do.

NURSE: But, Herman, I understand that you have been refusing to get out of bed or dress yourself every day. We discussed last week that you could go outside and sit on the front porch, socialize, play cards and quiet table games, but you have not been interested in doing any of these things.

MARIAN: Dad, you're just stubborn and unwilling to do anything the doctor says!

MOTHER (looking over at her daughter): Oh, Marian, you're always attacking your father. He's just scared to death to move too much for fear of hurting his heart again.

MARIAN: But you don't help him any by cooking him that rich Jewish food and caring for his every need.

MOTHER: Let's drop it.

From the family case example, answer the following assessment questions involving family communication

11. How extensively does the family use functional and/or dysfunctional communication?

12. How well do members state feelings and needs?

13. Are qualification, clarification, or feedback techniques used?

14. How well do members listen to each other?

15. Are judgmental statements or assumptions used?

16. What values underlie the family's communication?

17. Are affective messages communicated?

18. Describe the family communication network.

19. What variables influence the family interactions?

20. State one family nursing diagnosis in the area of communication.

21. Propose two family nursing interventions directed toward resolving the above family communication problem.

CHAPTER ELEVEN

Family Power Structure

Learning Objectives

1. Describe the importance of understanding the family power structure.
2. Define the following concepts: power, authority, decision making, and family power.
3. Distinguish between the various bases for power and recognize some of the major gender, ethnic, age, educational, and socioeconomic differences in the use of power sources.
4. Identify and explain the role each of the following variables plays in influencing family power: power hierarchy, formation of coalitions, family communication network, social class, family developmental stage, situational contingencies, and family cultural/religious background.
5. Describe the most commonly used typology or classification for family and/or conjugal power.
6. Explain briefly how the overall family power structure and marital satisfaction are associated.
7. Discuss the major contemporary change occurring in the family power structure.
8. Using the family power continuum, identify where "healthy" families typically are situated.
9. Apply the following assessment areas in a written case history:
   a. Who makes which decisions? Who has the "last say?"
   b. What are the decision-making techniques utilized?
   c. On what bases of power are decisions made?
   d. What are the significant variables affecting family power?
10. From your assessment of the above areas in a case situation, classify whether the family is dominated by a family member (and if so, who); is egalitarian (syncratic or autonomic); or is leaderless and chaotic.
11. From the written case history, state a family nursing diagnosis within the power domain. Propose two general family nursing interventions to assist the family in dealing with its family power problem.

Numerous authors in the fields of family sociology and family counseling have written of the importance of the power dimension within the family. Cromwell and Olson (1975), specialists in this aspect of the family system, wrote that "power is one of the most fundamental aspects of all social interaction" (p. 3). Haley (1976), a noted family therapist, believed that power is central to all human relations. He portrayed human relationships as an ongoing struggle for status and control.

All social systems, including the family, have structures that determine who wields power and what the hierarchy or "pecking order" is. Power, as viewed in this text, is one of the four interdependent structural dimensions of the family, and as such is a reflection of family's unwritten family rules and underlying value system. In addition, it is of significance in understanding the interpersonal dynamics within the family and between the family and its external relationships. Power and status dimensions are crucial in the establishment and maintenance of family communication channels and networks. In fact, Blood and Wolfe (1960), who conducted the foundational research in family power, maintain that "the most important aspect of the family structure is the power position of the members." Furthermore, the close interrelationship with family roles is apparent in that a person's roles and positions are basic to his or her capacity to influence others (Rogers, 1974).

Power structures vary greatly from family to family, with differences positively related to the overall health status of the family. Some power arrangements are dysfunctional and thereby contribute to family maladaptation and ill health. Moreover, decision making, as one measure of family power, has been a central concern in family therapy. Satir (1972) notes that "there is probably nothing so vital to maintaining and developing a love relationship (or to killing it) as the decision-making process" (p. 131).

Contemporary changes in the family have created an even greater need for family health professionals to assess the power dimension. As part of the rapid changes in family life, families are not rigidly bound by tradition to relationships as they once were. Decision making and family power are generally more shared in families (Scanzoni and Szinovacz, 1980; Szinovacz, 1987). No change in the American family is mentioned more often than the shift from one-sided male authority to the sharing of family power by the husband and wife. The declining sex role traditionalism in the family results in family decision making becoming increasingly significant, complex, and conflictual (Scanzoni and Szinovacz, 1980).

Knowledge and an appreciation of a family's power structure may be crucial in providing effective health care, especially when families have problems complying with a health regimen or obtaining needed health services. The family member who acts as health leader (being the recognized authority in the area of health or the overall family leader) must be identified, acknowledged, and consulted. For instance, although the mother may be the person with whom the nurse is usually in contact, some channel of communication with the father or grandparent must be found if he or she in fact has the final decision-making power.

Following a presentation of basic definitions and concepts, this chapter discusses the following basic areas in the assessment of family power: (1) the bases for power, (2) power outcomes, (3) the decision-making process, and (4) variables affecting power. A family power typology is then suggested, followed by a description of the attributes of healthy and unhealthy families relative to the family power structure.

FAMILY POWER: DEFINITIONS AND CONCEPTS

Power has numerous meanings, including influence, control, dominance, and decision making. For the purposes of the discussion to follow, *power* is the ability—potential or actual—of an individual(s) to control, influence, or change another person's behavior. Power always involves asymmetrical interpersonal relationships—one interactant exerts greater influence/control in the relationship. Power is also multidimensional in nature, meaning that it includes sociostructural, interactional (process), and outcome components (McDonald, 1980). *Family power,* as a characteristic of the family system, is the ability—potential or actual—of individual members to change the behavior of other family members (Olson and Cromwell, 1975). Major components of family power are influence and decision making. The term *influence* is practically synonymous with power, being defined as the degree to which formal and informal pressure exerted by one member on the other(s) is successful in imposing that person's point of view, despite initial opposition (McDonald, 1977). *Dominance* is also used in the same context. In this chapter power, dominance, and influence will be used interchangeably. *Decision making* refers to the process directed toward gaining the assent and commitment of family members to carry out a course of action or to maintain the status quo. In other words, it is the "means of getting things accomplished" (Scanzoni and Szinovacz, 1980). Through decision-making, power is manifested. *Authority* is another closely associated term referring to the shared beliefs of family members, which are culturally and normatively based and which designate a family member as the rightful person to make decisions and assume the leadership position. In other words, authority is present when the individuals involved feel that it is proper for power to be held by a particular member of the group. Traditional beliefs and values, and their concomitant roles, are largely the basis for such feelings. *Legitimate power* is a synonymous term.

Power and authority do not always go hand in hand. A family member who has the authority to decide or act may not exercise this power for a variety of reasons. Thus there may be an incongruency between the power and authority elements in a family. Comparing the family to a larger social system, one could equate authority with the formal power structure and power with the informal power structure of a bureaucracy. It has long been recognized that within an organization the formal and informal power structures may be quite different from each other. The same situation applies to families. A family member who nominally holds the power may not be the actual power holder. Although family members might tell the health worker that the father is "in charge," he or she might on observation note that the wife–mother is actually the informal power holder (Pasquali et al, 1985).

Power is an abstract, complex, and multidimensional phenomenon and as such is not directly observable. It must then be inferred from observable behaviors and/or from self-reports of family members, conducted through goal-directed interviews. What is observed by outsiders and what is reported by family members in terms of family power, however, are often at odds with each other (Szinovacz, 1987).

Power is a dimension of the family *system* or *subsystem*, in that it is not a characteristic of a family member apart from a social system. Thus family power can be assessed only within the context of the system or subsystems, and more specifically within the context of the circular processes of family interaction. Communication patterns reveal family role and power dimensions. Family power can be seen in family processes ranging from daily routine exchanges to negotiation of complicated conflictual issues involving, for example, decision making, problem solving, conflict resolution, and crisis management. Moreover, family power applies to all of the following situations: the various subsystems within families (eg, the sibling subsystem, marital subsystem, and parent–child subsystems); the family as a total system; and the family system's relationship with the external social systems (Olson et al, 1975). Within the family, according to McDonald (1980), there are five different units that can be analyzed in terms of their power characteristics. These are marital power, parental power, offspring power, sibling power, and kinship power. Most research and theoretical writing about family power, however, has focused on marital power.

MEASURING FAMILY POWER

How does one measure or assess power in a family? This is the key question, and one for which there is no consensus concerning the appropriate methodology and focus.

Relationship of Task Allocation to Family Power

Starting with Blood and Wolfe's large study of 900 families, which was completed in 1955 and reported in 1960, researchers have examined task allocation on the assumption that there existed a positive relationship between whoever was in charge of carrying out a particular task and power in that area. But later investigations of family differences in the allocation of responsibilities for the various decision areas and tasks indicated that such division of responsibility seldom reflected the dominant authority pattern. Reiss (1976) explains:

> We must keep in mind that division of labor does not indicate in any direct way who has power or how a decision was arrived at regarding such division of labor. Rather, such a division of labor indicates that these are the traditional ways that tasks are allocated because of reasons that used to, and in some cases still do, have roots in the differences between the sexes in physical and cultural training. Males are still often trained to be more handy with mechanical tasks and tasks that take muscle power, and females are still trained to know more about cooking and cleaning, and those cultural traditions seem the essential basis of the division of tasks in the family. (p. 254)

Johnson (1975) verified this difference between family power and task and responsibility allocation. She interviewed 104 Japanese-American wives in Honolulu, including specific questions about who was responsible for and made decisions in the major areas of family life. She then asked questions to determine the wives' overall freedom to pursue individual interests, counter to wishes of their husbands.

Interestingly enough, Johnson discovered that only questioning about specific areas often distorted the real source of overall power, because one partner can be delegated responsibility but ultimate power may lie with the other partner. When wives were queried about specific responsibilities and task allocation, they appeared more influential than the husbands. But when asked broadly stated questions pertaining to the wife's evaluation of her overall power as compared to her husbands' power, the data contradicted the responses to the more specific questions. Relative to their husbands' power, most of these wives placed themselves in a subordinate position, largely attributing this fact to their Japanese heritage and its norms regarding male–female roles. Legitimate power or tradition-derived power appeared to be operating here.

Thus while Japanese-American wives played active roles in decision making, they did so by virtue of a delegation of power from their husbands. In this instance, the husband assigned responsibilities while retaining final authority.

Safilios-Rothschild (1976b) makes a very important distinction between the two types of power demonstrated in the above case of the Japanese family. In some families, one spouse has the "orchestration" power, while the other has "implementation power." She explains:

> Spouses who have "orchestration power" have, in fact, the power to make only the important and infrequent decisions that do not infringe upon their time but that determine the family life style and major characteristics and features of their family. They also have the power to relegate unimportant and time-consuming decisions to their spouse who can then derive a "feeling of power" by implementing those decisions within the limitations set by crucial and pervasive decisions made by the powerful spouse. (p. 359)

Hence, in this type of spousal power arrangement the wife is said to have "implementation power." In spite of the fact that implementation power is, in the last analysis, an inferior type of power, having control over implementation still confers power to the implementor. When a family member, the husband, for example, exerts his influence or control and convinces his nonworking wife that she should maintain more discipline of the children, he depends on the wife's commitment to carry out his wishes, as he is typically not in a position to supervise. In this case, the wife, in her central position, has substantial power, because she will decide how and what to implement. In families where the mother is home most of the time and the father is working long hours, the mother is to a large extent in control of family life (Turner, 1970).

Focusing on Decision-making Outcomes

From Blood and Wolfe's (1960) large and influential work came further studies and questions about what constitute the important and valid measures of family power. Family power has primarily been researched by focusing on decision making. But is power identified by determining the outcome of a decision (ie, what was the decision and who decided it), or by the decision-making process itself? Current thinking prevails on the side of process (Scanzoni and Szinovacz, 1980; Szinovacz, 1987). When we look at power as a process rather than the outcome of a decision, our concern shifts to an emphasis on family interaction rather than independent and isolated events (Sprey, 1972). This appears to be an approach more appropriate when working with families.

Studies of family power have been under criticism because of methodological limitations. Researchers have relied heavily on the survey and structured interview schedule, with little direct observation to validate self-reported data. People are notoriously inaccurate in describing their own behavior. A case in point of this tendency is in the area of marital relations. It has been observed that when information has been gathered by interviewing families, a strong tendency has been discovered for couples to report an egalitarian relationship with each other, a characterization that is later not verified by observational study (Cromwell and Olson, 1975). Hence it is suggested that the most accurate way to assess family power is to combine observation of marital, parent–child, sibling, and family interaction with self-reporting by all family members if possible (Szinovacz, 1987).

GENERAL ASSESSMENT AREAS

A comprehensive assessment of family power is provided by Cromwell and Olson (1975), who divide power up into three areas: power bases, power or decision-making outcomes, and power processes. The major variables influencing the above three domains of power are also considered in the following assessment discussion. Using a systems approach, the target system is the family, but in addition, assessment of power within the conjugal (marital), parent–child, and sibling subsystems is suggested.

Power Bases

One salient aspect of family power concerns the bases for power within the family and its subsystems—that is, the source from which a family member's power is derived. Again this information often has to be inferred from observed behavior and by asking relevant questions. The importance of making this determination lies in the fact that the nature of the particular power base significantly affects interpersonal relationships, marital satisfaction, and family stability (Table 11–1).

Raven and associates (1975) and Safilios-Rothschild (1976a) conducted significant studies of family power bases from which they identified the various types of power bases commonly observed in families. A brief description of these types follows.

TABLE 11–1. FAMILY POWER BASES

- Legitimate power/authority
- Helpless or powerless power
- Referent power
- Resource power
- Expert power
- Reward power
- Coercive power
- Informational power
- Affective power
- Tension management power

Legitimate Power or Authority. Legitimate power (sometimes called primary authority) refers to the shared belief and perceptions of family members that one person has the right to control another member's behavior. By virtue of the roles and positions a person occupies, certain rights and culturally derived privileges exist that are associated with these roles and positions. An example would be the "rightness" of parental control or dominance over children. This is a traditionally based authority. Where the husband is traditionally in control of the whole family, a patriarchal pattern exists. When legitimate power is present both the husband and wife accept the husband's dominant role as being "right" and "best," indicating role acceptance. Primary authority has remained the traditional and significant base for power in many families. Turner (1970) underscores this by stating that "the fundamental determinant of family dominance (power) is authority or the belief in the propriety of unequal dominance" (p. 133). For authority to be effective, the whole family must accept and support this ideology.

Helpless or Powerless Power. A variant form of legitimate power that is often overlooked is called "power of the powerless." This type of power is an important form of legitimate power that is based on the generally accepted right of those in need or of the helpless to expect assistance from those in a position to render it. Weeks and Jackson (1982) label the person with this kind of power the victim. They explain that the victim acquires a great deal of quasi-power in families. The victim is able to covertly acquire influence or power from others who often already feel drained of resources. Helpless power may be very effective in families where one member is chronically ill, disabled, or aged. A spouse or a disabled family member may control the family on the basis of his or her frailty or helplessness. This is a commonly seen base for power and, unfortunately may lead to a situation that makes it difficult for other family members' needs to be adequately met. Children's dependency and helplessness arouse feelings of responsibility in parents and make them susceptible to children's control attempts and use of "helpless power."

Referent Power. A third source for power is termed referent power and applies to the type of power persons have over others because of family members' positive identification with them, such as in a child's positive identification with a parent. Children imitate behaviors of family members, usually the parents, who serve as their role models.

Resource and Expert Power. Resource power is the type of power base that comes from having the greater number of valued resources in a relationship. When power is defined as an ability to influence or pressure, resources such as certain attributes, circumstances, or possessions are seen as primary determinants of that ability (Osmond, 1978). The greater resources of one spouse over the other are viewed as the chief alternative source of family power to traditionally based authority (McDonald, 1977). For example, the husband may be dominant because he controls the pursestrings, or the wife may be dominant because she is more practical and goal directed than her husband.

One important resource is the use of interpersonal techniques. It is not uncommon to find one family member who has few of the objective resources that ordinarily facilitate dominance actually controlling much of family life through his or her masterful use of a broad repertoire of interpersonal techniques (Turner, 1970).

The person in a relationship who has the least interest in maintaining the relationship (like the wife having less interest in the relationship than the husband) has a very important resource at his or her disposal.

Waller (1938) explains this case by what he calls "the principle of less interest." This principle explains that exploitation is likely to occur in a relationship where the differences in levels of involvement are great. For instance, the principle of less interest states that within a dyadic relationship, the person who cares least about whether the relationship continues or not has the greatest power over the relationship. He or she usually has less interest and involvement in maintaining the relationship because he or she has many more alternatives or resources. With decreased involvement, the less interested person can use manipulative or coercive techniques at the expense of the other. A commonly seen example may help elucidate this principle. In a marital situation, one member may be quite valued and independent, while the other individual feels dependent and inferior. Decisions are then made by the dominant mate, since he or she has many more options open and there is less interest or involvement in the relationship. In middle-class America this principle still probably operates in favor of the man because of his greater economic resources.

Expert power, a particular type of resource power, exists in a relationship when the person being "influenced" perceives that the other person (the "expert") has some special knowledge, skill, expertise, or experience (Safilios-Rothschild, 1976a).

Reward Power. Reward power stems from the expectation that the influencing, dominant person will do something positive in response to the other person's compliance. Overt bargaining may accompany the use of reward power. Children, according to Szinovacz (1987), possess an important resource in their compliance. Children's "good" behavior is a source of pleasure and pride to parents, and thus constitutes a basis for power (ie, children often use "good" behavior in order to obtain desired benefits).

Coercive or Dominance Power. The effective use of this source of power is based on the perception and belief that the person with power might or will punish through threats, coercion, or violence other individuals if they do not comply. Coercive power is used with coercive decision making (to be discussed later).

Informational Power. This power base stems from the content of the persuasive message. An individual is convinced of the "rightness" of the sender's message due to a careful and successful explanation of the necessity for change (Raven et al, 1975). This type of power is similar to but more limited in scope than expert power.

A variation of this direct information power is "indirect" informational power. This occurs when a more subtle dropping of hints, suggestions, and information influences a person to act without the obvious indication of persuasion (Raven et al, 1975). In the traditional sex-role relationship, women often use indirect informational power to gain influence.

Affective Power. Affective power refers to the power derived through the manipulation of a family member by bestowing or withdrawing affection and warmth, and, in the case of the spouse, sex. Withdrawal of sex has long been discussed in novels as a "woman's hidden weapon." Because they usually lack the socioeconomic weapons of men, this historically has been a source of power for women. A woman's affective resource, including being loved by her spouse, if exercised, can be a powerful resource in a marriage.

Tension Management Power. This type of power base is derived from the control that one spouse achieves by managing the present tensions and conflicts in the family. Using tears, pouting, endless debating, and disagreements to get a family member to "give in" is an example of tension management power.

Power Outcomes

A second area of assessment relative to family power is the area of power outcomes. Here the focus is on who makes the final decisions or ultimately possesses the control. In other words, "who wins" or "has the last say" (Cromwell and Olson, 1975; Szinovacz, 1987). Specific questions can be asked of the family to elicit this information. For instance, one might ask who is responsible for making decisions about and taking responsibility for the areas of major importance in family life. In conjugal relationships power can vary from one domain to the next, with role definitions determining who had power in a given area. For example, the wife might have more power in regard to social and kin relationships and household matters, while the husband has more control over the finances. In other families power may be more equally divided, with a pattern of shared power prevailing.

It must be remembered, however, that specific areas of responsibility and of decision making may not coincide with the more general and dominant power pattern in a family. Recall the distinction between implementation and orchestration power described earlier. That is, Johnson's 1975 findings of power within Japanese-American families demonstrated the significance of differentiating implementation from orchestration power. An assessor can easily be misled by the obvious responsibilities and decisions of one mate rather than realize that these are actually delegated, or relegated, to the weaker partner by the dominant member of the couple. Thus on the surface it may appear that the wife is responsible for grocery shopping, cooking, and child rearing. But these tasks may only be relegated to her by her husband, and should her actions incur his displeasure, her power may be withdrawn. This is the usual case in authoritarian or patriarchal families. The husband's power may derive not only from a traditional value structure but from possessing more resources. Economic resources (money) are particularly important in determining marital power (Blumstein and Schwartz, 1983).

The second type of question dealing with power outcomes is the more global or general question that can be posed to family members. This question entails asking about whose idea or suggestion is finally adopted (who "wins" or "has the last say") when major decisions or choices must be made. In families where decisions are shared and represent the outcome of mutual discussion and exploration, this kind of information is difficult to obtain. But despite the difficulty involved in getting family members to describe the outcome (people remember what decision was made but find it harder to remember who had the last say or made the ultimate decision), assessment of the outcome of an issue, conflict, or argument is helpful in ascertaining the source of power and in whom this resides. Komarovsky (1964) notes that "power is most visible in contested decisions ending in victory of one partner. But it exists irrespective of conflict, because the powerful partner may so influence the wishes and preferences of his mate that a contest of wills does not even arise" (p. 221). Power differentials, then, may function to suppress potential conflictual situations and "silent agreement" is seen (McDonald, 1980; Scanzoni and Szinovacz, 1980).

In regard to decisions and their outcomes, discerning what kinds of problems or issues are involved and how important they are to the family is helpful. Does a decision cut across all the major areas of family life or is it limited to a specific area? Komarovsky (1964) underscores the significance of ascertaining the centrality of the issue by observing that "general decision making in one or two areas of family life may not be a good index of general power. It depends upon the importance of such areas for each partner" (p. 221).

Power or Decision-making Processes

In addition to assessing power bases and power outcomes, the process used in arriving at family decisions is also crucial in the assessment of family power. The decision-making process is a principal index of power (Blood and Wolfe, 1960). In fact, power or dominance patterns are the by-product of the decision-making process. Family decision making refers to "the interactional techniques which family members employ in their attempts to gain control in the negotiation or decision-making process" (McDonald, 1980, p. 843). In assessing this area, the central focus is *how* decisions are made. By understanding the techniques used in family decision making, the assessor will be better able to identify the relative power of each family member and his or her participation in family affairs and decisions.

There are three types of decision-making processes discussed in the literature. Families tend to make use of one particular method of decision making over another, although the secondary use of one or both of the other basic techniques of decision making is also seen. Analysis of the family decision-making process reveals the tremendous interrelationship of these features with the other structural dimensions of the family. For instance, the family that extensively uses democratic methods of decision making (consensus decision making), for example, will generally have an egalitarian role and power structure and a value system in which role sharing and more open communications exist.

Decision Making By Consensus. The first technique of decision making is termed consensus. According to American ideals, this is the healthy way to make decisions. Here a particular course of action is mutually agreed on by all involved. There is equal commitment to the decision, as well as satisfaction, by the family members or mates. Consensus decisions are agreed on through discussion and negotiation. Because a substantial degree of interdependence and egalitarianism among family members is needed as well as an ability to discuss and problem solve, this kind of decision making is more difficult, complex, and unpredictable.

What happens when consensual decision making is utilized by a family after an initial disagreement? A change takes place in the opinions or views of some or all of the family members. This occurs during the decision-making process when those in disagreement eventually perceive that action to be taken corresponds with their personal or shared values (Turner, 1970).

Decision Making By Accommodation. A second type of decision making is termed accommodation. Here the family members' initial feelings about an issue are discordant. One or more of the family members make concessions, either willingly or unwillingly. Some member(s) assent in order to allow a decision to be reached. Hence it may involve voluntary compromising in which concessions are made by all persons concerned or a sacrifice is made by one family member so that others may have their own way. Privately or publicly the conceding member(s) will not be convinced, however, that the decision in question is best (Turner, 1970).

Accommodative decisions are made somewhere on a continuum from coercion to compromising. Differences in the attitudes of participants towards their commitment, as well as differences in the relationship under which the forms of accommodation take place, determine whether the decision making is more coercive or more compromising.

Going from the most functional to the least functional form of accommodating, the several ways in which accommodation occurs, by compromising, bargaining, or coercion are described. *Compromising* refers to the making of concessions by all the family members involved so that the decision reached is not reflective of any of the interactant's original choices, but has some acceptable elements for all concerned. In bargaining one or more members make concessions to another/others and expect reciprocity, so that ultimately the sacrifices of each balance out. The use of *bargaining* in family negotiations demonstrates that a trust exists among the members, along with a belief that others will be fair and honest in keeping up their ends of the bargain. *Coercion* is the least functional technique along the accommodation continuum as it results in an unwilling agreement by one or more family members to which commitment is assured only by the continuance of coercive power. The existence of threat of punishment shows the dominance of one member over others.

To summarize, an accommodation is always an agreement to disagree, to adopt a common decision in the face of irreconcilable differences (Turner, 1970).

De-facto Decision Making. Family members may also arrive at decisions by using a de-facto route. In this case, things are allowed "to just happen" without planning. A decision is forced by events in the absence of active, voluntary, or effective decision making. De-facto decisions may also be made when arguments occur to which there was no resolution or when issues were not brought up and discussed. These decisions, then, are made by inaction rather than by planning.

De-facto decision making is seen in many disorganized, multiproblem families, many of whom believe in fate and feel powerless to control their own destiny. Moreover; de facto decision making may be situationally limited or occur when problems in communication exist, as when significant problems or issues are not discussed. Cultural norms are important to consider here, because obstacles to open communication and active decision making may also have a cultural or ethnic basis. For example, among traditional Latino couples, sexual relations and family planning may be an area of closed communication; pregnancies may therefore become the outcome of de-facto decision making.

Variables Affecting Family Power

In addition to the need to assess the three domains of family power, there are some important variables that act as contingency variables, also influencing the three domains. A listing of these appears in Table 11–2; some will now be further discussed.

TABLE 11–2. VARIABLES AFFECTING FAMILY POWER STRUCTURE

1. Family power hierarchy.
2. Type of family form (single parent, blended family, traditional two-parent nuclear family, etc)
3. Formation of coalitions
4. Family communication network
5. Social class
6. Family developmental stage
7. Cultural and religious background
8. Situational contingencies
9. Person variables (members' gender, ages, self-esteem, and interpersonal skills)
10. Spouses' emotional interdependency and commitment to marriage

Family Power Hierarchy. Each family has a power hierarchy or "pecking order." In the traditional nuclear family and in most nuclear families today, the power structure is clearly hierarchical, meaning that the power structure is tiered and the "pecking occurs downward." In the egalitarian family, however, a clear, generationally based power hierarchy may be absent.

Minuchin (1974) and Haley (1976, 1980) place great importance on the lines of authority or hierarchically arranged power structures in families. Parents constitute the executive subsystem and should not forfeit or diminish that responsibility in any way (Minuchin, 1974).

Minuchin (1974) also mentions variations in the power hierarchy due to differing family forms. In large families, single-parent families, or families where both parents are employed, some allocation of parental power is usually given to an older child(ren). This arrangement may work well, for the younger children are cared for and the parental child can develop responsibility, competence, and autonomy beyond his or her years. The family with a parental child structure may experience problems, however, when the delegation of authority is unclear or if the parents abdicate their authority, leaving the parental child to become the primary source of decision making, control, and guidance. In these situations, the child is given a task that exceeds his or her abilities and that interferes with meeting his or her childhood needs of support and dependency.

Formation of Family Coalitions. One of the ways the power structure of the family is altered is by the formation of coalitions. Coalitions are either temporary, issue-based alliances, or long-term alliances made to offset the dominance of one or more other family members. Subgroups within a family band together to support each other and to increase their power position relative to other members of the family (Stachowick,

1975). Obviously then, coalitions generate more power for the members who join together.

Coalitions in families are most healthy when they exist within the appropriate power levels (Gorman, 1975). It has been pointed out by family therapists (Lidz, 1963; Minuchin, 1974; Satir, 1972) that a sustaining parental coalition is a healthy and a virtually necessary phenomenon to effectively parent children. In contrast, long-term parent–child coalitions are unhealthy, because they disrupt the intact functioning of the parent–child and spouse subsystems. Nevertheless, mother–child coalitions are especially common in patriarchal families, where the father's power is great and together the mother and an older child can to some degree dilute his power. The child in this case can also expect special favors from the mother. Being in a long-term coalition with one parent may, however, keep the child enmeshed with that parent and inhibit or prevent the child from individuating or separating from the family (Stachowick, 1975).

Sibling coalitions are also common. Children join forces to more efficaciously oppose or evade the rules parents establish (Turner, 1970).

The more detrimental forms of coalitions are those that cut across power or generational levels (like mother and daughter) and are long-standing and extensively used (Smoyak, 1975).

One of the difficulties in a single-parent family is the obvious inability to form a parental coalition. Two-parent families tend to have significantly more resources and alternatives available to them than do one-parent families, because partners in the former can support each other and form a coalition. In one-parent families, the strength of primary authority (legitimate power) may be a dominant and necessary factor in controlling the family situation (Jayaratne, 1978).

Family Communication Network. Communication is seldom of equal intensity within each of the pairs of relationships in the family. The husband and wife may communicate frequently, intensely, and over a wide area of topics, while the father and youngest son may have very little communication with each other. Two siblings may have a close, confidential type of relationship. Age and sex characteristics, as well as personality attributes of family members, influence the nature of the family communication network.

When there is unequal communication between family members, intermediaries ("go-betweens") usually exist. The person in the family who serves as an intermediary in communications between others (in many instances the mother), but who is able to interact directly with all family members, holds a central position in the communication network.

Communication networks are mentioned here because of their correlation with the power structure. The greater the centrality of the family member, the greater his or her dominance, due to his or her control over the outcome of the decision-making process. Because the intermediary understands the attitudes and opinions of most of the family members, he or she can use this information to influence family members. The go-between is also able to censor or screen information from the sender to the other family members. This censorship function and ability to alter messages as seen fit gives the intermediary extensive power, at least in some areas. In larger families one may find a secondary intermediary—such as an older son or daughter—who acts as a link between other children and the mother (Turner, 1970).

Social Class Differences in Family Power

Lower-class Families. Besmer (1967) summarizes the frequently seen power characteristics of poor families. The husband is more likely to proclaim authority simply because he is a male, although actually having to concede more authority to the wife due to the paucity of his resources. The father most generally loses influence in the family at the lower levels as a consequence of his social and occupational inadequacy. The authoritarian theme is a strong underlying factor in the interpersonal relationships of the poor. There is a strong belief in the validity of strength as the source of power and on the rightness of existing patterns. An individual's dominance, rather than expertise and the merit of his or her suggestions, is relied on as the common source of decisions.

The lower-class wife has relatively more duties than either the middle- or upper-class wife or the lower-class husband, and thus frequently has more influence in the family decision making than housewives of the other classes. This is especially true in the financial area, where the lower-class wife may feel that earning money is the man's responsibility and spending it wisely is the woman's.

Komarovsky (1964), who studied a group of working-class* families, found that there was extensive variation of dominance patterns within this large group. She reports that the husbands are dominant in 45 percent of the marriages, the wives in 21 percent, and in 27 percent a balance of power exits. Education was found to be the important determinant as to how authoritarian the family power structure was—the higher the education, the more flexible and "middle class" certain ideals and protocols in marriage became. The inci-

* *Working class is defined as the upper lower class of unskilled blue-collar workers and the lower middle class of skilled blue-collar workers.*

dence of dominance by the husband declined with better education of the husband, and in contrast, patriarchal attributes were more prevalent among the less educated.

Middle-class Families. According to Kanter (1978), the most egalitarian or companion-based marriages seem to be found among the lower-middle-class, white-collar workers, perhaps as a result of the greater availability of the husband's time to share chores and act as a companion to his wife. Resource and expert power are more often used as a bases for power in upper-middle-class families (Szinovacz, 1987).

The Family Developmental Stage. The decisions a family makes are also closely associated with the family's life cycle, as is the distribution of power among the family members. Families tend to evolve from where the major concentration of power is in the hands of the adults when the children are young, to a more shared power arrangement as children move into adolescence. More specifically, during the early years of marriage, before children, couples tend to be syncratic—discussing and mutually deciding on major decisions among themselves, except perhaps decisions about the husband's job and housekeeping matters (Blood, 1969). Later in the family's life cycle, when children are being raised and the system is more complex, each spouse usually has clearly defined areas of power and decision making, although major decisions are still jointly made. Corrales (1975) explains that when the dyad changes to a triad with the addition of a baby, some loss in the wife's power is seen. Typically, mates discuss most areas less and less as time goes on, a sign that some estrangement from each other may also be occurring. During adolescence older children assume more power in the family than when they were younger. The shifts in power that take place during the time when adolescents are in the home are never easy, with much of the conflict that arises at this time revolving around the power distribution. In the later years of the family, the marital couple, returning to a dyadic relationship, again share in decision making and power.

Situational Contingencies. Situational changes can also signal changes in the power structure of the family. For example, it has been observed that when a husband is unemployed over a period of time that he usually loses power in the family if resource power has been the basis for his power (Elder, 1974; McCubbin and Dahl, 1985). The chronically ill or alcoholic husband or wife is often shut out of the family decision-making process.

Other situational contingencies also affect family power. Time pressure is one factor that has been studied. Under high time pressure, there is greater likelihood of agreement (the converse is also true). The presence of others while the power exertion takes place also influences the power processes utilized. More "acceptable" power exertion tactics are used in the presence of others. And finally, family stress affects family members' behaviors in power or bargaining situations. Increased stress tends to decrease interactants' tolerance for ambiguity, cognitive flexibility, and problem-solving skills (Szinovacz, 1987).

Cultural Influences. Cultural and religious differences among families also dictate different power arrangements. For instance, male dominance is commonly seen in unacculturated immigrant families from Europe, Asia, and Latin America. Yet some of our stereotypes about male dominance in Hispanic families and female dominance in black families, have come under close scrutiny, and are being seriously questioned (see Chaps. 19 and 20 for elaboration).

Moreover, an older matriarch is sometimes present in these families. In this case, or in cases where grandparents have a strong influence on the family, greater culturally derived power resides in the extended family.

Spouses' Emotional Interdependency and Commitment to Marriage. Recent research (Godwin and Scanzoni, 1989) has demonstrated that partners' emotional dependency (the love and caring for their spouse that each spouse reports) and the degree of commitment to the current marital relationship influences the decision-making processes used in the family. Data were collected via observation and self-reports from 188 married couples. The study found that the more wives love their husbands, the less coercive tactics are used and the more concensus in decision making is likely. And the more committed husbands are to the marriage, the more control the wife has.

OVERALL FAMILY POWER

One of the purposes in analyzing the assessment areas (bases for power, power outcomes and decision-making processes, and the variables affecting power) is to be able to classify a family as to its overall power structure. This involves being able to state whether a family is dominated by one member (usually one spouse), has an egalitarian power structure, or has no effective leadership (is chaotic). Some authors point out that most of the classifications used to describe families are too simplistic and do not adequately reflect the dynamic qualities of family power or its complexity. Although we should retain an awareness that an overall labeling of family power may neither be possible nor entirely accurate, we cannot overlook the value of classification: namely, that it permits a lot to be said in a few words. If a family displays an overall dysfunctional power structure, a statement of this conclusion may serve as a family nursing diagnosis.

Historically, the literature has described generalized, pure types of families—in particular (1) the patriarchal, traditional family and (2), the democratic, egalitarian, or modern family. In the patriarchal, traditional family, the father is the head of the family, with family power vested in his hands; and his wife, his sons, and their wives and children, and his unmarried daughters, are subordinated to his power. In contrast, the democratic modern, egalitarian family is based on the equality of husband and wife, with consensus in making decisions and increasing participation by children as they grow older (Burgess et al, 1963; Scanzoni and Szinovacz,, 1980).

The most frequently used typology today for classifying power in the marital subsystem or family was developed by Herbst (1954). It divides marital power into autocratic, syncratic, and autonomic patterns. *Autocratic* power patterns exist when the family is dominated by a single family member. In these families, decisions on marital activities, and usually family activities also, are made solely by this individual. *Syncratic* power patterns exist when decisions involving the marriage, as well as the family, are made by both members of the marital dyad. In this case there is a greater mutual commitment and involvement in the marriage. An *autonomic* power structure is present when the two partners function independently of one another in both decision making and their activities. Other authors refer to this pattern at the family level as atomistic. Tinkham and Voorhies (1977) observe that today's families are often more atomistic, with decisions being made by an individual on the basis of his or her own needs rather than on the basis of the family's needs.

One of the problems with Herbst's (1954) original typology is that he assumed that the power always rested with one or the other parents (or was shared). This is a constricting approach, because the dominant individual may be a child, grandparent, or other family member if the family is other than a traditional two-parent nuclear family. Most research into family power has, in fact, dealt with conjugal power rather than family power, focusing on only husband–wife interactions to the exclusion of the child's role in the decision-making processes. The relative power of children in families has been found to be substantial, especially in families with older children. For instance, Strodtbeck (1978) found that the power of an adolescent son in a family was almost as great as that of the mother. Thus an adequate assessment must include consideration of the children's power (McDonald, 1977).

In contrast with the analysis and classification of marital power relationships, the categorization of the parent–child subsystem has usually been quite simple: on a continuum from high to low parental control, for example.

In family process literature, which derives largely from family therapy, the categories most widely used are symmetrical (balanced), complementary (submissive–dominant), and metacomplementary (dominant through weakness) forms. Marital role relationships are discussed in Chapter 12.

Lewis and associates (1976) developed a comprehensive model for summarizing a family's power structure that includes the chaotic or leaderless family not identified in the former models. Figure 11–1 modifies the model by Lewis and associates, incorporating the various types of power commonly observed in families. This continuum is suggested for use in assessing overall family power dimensions. Subsystem power (marital, parent–child, and sibling) is also important to consider.

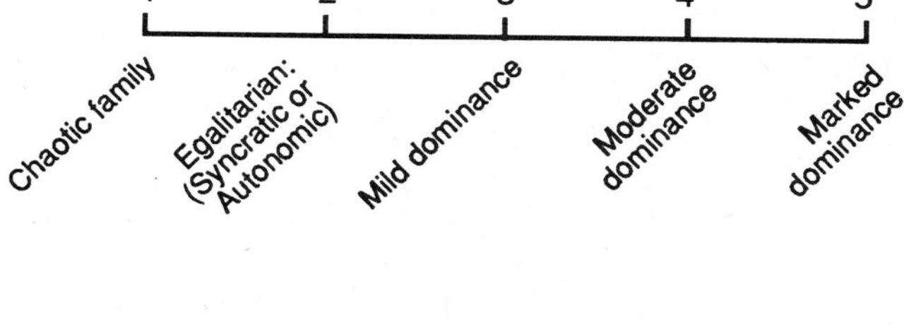

Figure 11–1
The family power continuum. The chaotic family (1) refers to a leaderless family, wherein no member has adequate power to make decisions effectively. In egalitarian syncratic and autonomic families (2), decisions and power are shared. In the syncratic form the decisions are made together; in the autonomic form the decisions are made independently. Dominance or power (3–5) ranges from marked, where there is practically absolute control by an individual and no negotiation, to mild, where there is a tendency for dominance and submissiveness, but most decisions are reached through respectful, mutual negotiation.

Marital Satisfaction and Family Power Type

Research done from 1950 through 1990 consistently demonstrates that family power is significantly related to marital satisfaction. Higher levels of satisfaction are found most frequently among egalitarian couples and couples where the husband was dominant when compared to wife-dominant couples. Wife-dominated couples have generally been found to rate their marriages as less satisfying (McDonald, 1980; Szinovacz, 1987). It is curious that women who were dominant classified themselves as the least maritally satisfied, far below their husbands' satisfaction. The tentative conclusion that may be drawn is that the wife is dominant by default, not choice, being forced to fill the vacuum created by a weak, passive, incompetent husband. Wife dominance also goes against the normative expectations, that is, the cultural prescriptions of either the traditional (husband-dominated) or the modern (egalitarian) marriage. Why are husbands in these marriages not also unhappy? Corrales (1975) speculates that the reason might be because the wife not only makes most of the decisions, but probably also assumes most family roles.*

Women's Roles and Power

When looking at economic, religious, or political power areas, women generally do not have much power. But Kranichfield (1987) points out that in the family domain women in fact have a great deal of overlooked power. Women's power is pervasive when power is defined as the ability to bear, educate, and determine the personality, values, and beliefs of each new human being in society. Women's lives are far more involved in the family than are men's. Women exert more intergenerational influence than do men and hold the position of "kinkeeper" in most families. This situation has not changed, even with the increased participation of women in the work force (Kranichfield, 1987).

CONTEMPORARY TRENDS IN FAMILY POWER

There has been a gradual shift from the traditional, patriarchal family structure toward a democratic, egalitarian family structure. As egalitarianism in the family becomes more prominent, changes in women's base for power are occurring, albeit slowly. Men are often more likely to use expert formal legitimacy or direct informational power as a base for influence in the family, while women use referent power, "helpless" power, and indirect informational power. These bases for power were selected by women because of their greater acceptability to their mates. When women use the modes of expert power and direct informational power, they are sometimes seen as being masculine and aggressive. While the common use of helpless power by women, however, is more acceptable to their spouses; it is not to their self-esteem. As noted, women also use implementation power. Research findings agree that women's work force participation and achievement of higher education has given women more power in the family (Leslie and Korman, 1989).

HEALTHY AND DYSFUNCTIONAL FAMILY POWER ATTRIBUTES

Lewis and associates (1976) conducted in-depth interviews with a group of middle-class families to determine their psychosocial health status and the family structural characteristics with which health status was correlated. From an analysis of these interviews and observations, they grouped families into three categories of health, from the severely dysfunctional to optimally healthy. It was generally found that the most severely dysfunctional families presented chaotic family structures (see Fig. 11–1), and the most competent of families presented flexible structures. These researchers emphasized that "the most direct measure of structure concerned the distribution of power or influence within the family" (Lewis et al, 1976, p. 209).

The power attributes of healthy families were seen to reflect the following:

> In healthy families the parental coalition played a crucial role in the determination of overall family competence. . . . Leadership was provided by the parental coalition as was a model of relating which appeared to be of great learning value to the children. Leadership was shared by the parents. . . . This trend toward an egalitarian marriage was in striking contrast to both the more distant marriages of the adequate families and the marital pattern of dominance and submission that so often was seen in the dysfunctional families. (p. 210)

In the healthy families, the parents acting as a coalition did not exercise their power in an authoritarian or rigid way but, within their style of leadership, left room for options and negotiation. Nevertheless, power and boundaries were clear; there was no confusion as to the position and power of family members. Generally the

** Despite the wife's general feelings of dissatisfaction and the husband's relatively higher level of satisfaction in these marriages, it must be remembered that both of the spouses are intimately involved with establishing and maintaining the power structure within the relationship. Hence the end result is the responsibility of neither spouse exclusively.*

father held the most power, the mother somewhat less, and the child distinctly the least power (Lewis et al, 1976). In contrast, all the severely disturbed families showed that none of the family members had much power. The most inept families, the authors reported, had a powerless father and a strong coalition between mother and child. In families labeled as midrange, a strong, healthy parental–marital coalition did not exist. These families characteristically maintained rigid, authoritarian structures via dominance by one mate.

Family control processes, such as rigid authoritarian structures, affect children in the family. Through modeling, children learn power-relevant behaviors such as coercive, Machiavellian, and violent behaviors (Straus et al, 1980).

Concerning the healthy family's attributes, Minuchin (1974) expresses his belief that the most important aspect of power within a family is the presence of a clear and functioning hierarchy in which the parents function as the executive subsystem and children have different levels of authority. For a family to function effectively, there must also be complementarity of functions, with the husband and wife accepting interdependency and working as a team.

FAMILY POWER STRUCTURE: APPLYING THE FAMILY NURSING PROCESS

☐ *ASSESSMENT QUESTIONS*

In this chapter the various major areas germane to family power are described. Family power is obviously not an easily inferred dimension to assess. In spite of these difficulties, the following summary of the primary facets of power, the areas to observe, and the questions to ask will hopefully make the assessment process more concrete and clear.

Power Outcomes

Who has the "last way" or "who wins"? Who makes what decisions? And how important are these decisions or issues to the family? As some family workers have done, you may wish to ask more specific questions to elicit this information (and validate what you can with your own observations). General questions followed by more specific questions in these areas may be helpful:

a. Financial: Who budgets, pays bills, decides on how money is spent?
b. Social: Who decides on how to spend an evening or which friends or relatives to see?
c. Major decisions: Who decides on changes in jobs or residence?
d. Child rearing: Who disciplines and decides on children's activities? (Johnson, 1975)

It must be remembered, though, when asking these questions, that *overall* power in the family often does not correlate well with specific task responsibilities.

Decision-making Process

What specific techniques are utilized for making decisions in the family and to what extent are these utilized?

a. Consensus
b. Accommodation
    1. Bargaining
    2. Compromising
    3. Coercion
c. De facto

Specific questions eliciting decision-making techniques used would focus on *how* the family makes decisions.

Power Bases

This area deals with the source from which the power of individuals within a family is derived. To enumerate again these various sources:

1. Legitimate power/authority
2. Helpless or powerless power
3. Referent power
4. Resource and expert power
5. Reward power
6. Coercive power
7. Informational power—direct and indirect
8. Affective power
9. Tension management power

Questions asked to elicit information on the source of power might follow either specific questions about who makes certain decisions and how (sometimes how also reveals the source). For example, in speaking to the husband–father: "On what basis was it decided to send the children to summer camp?" Or you may suggest choices, such as, "Was your wife's suggestion agreed on because of her greater knowledge in that area, because of the children's positive feelings and respect for her, or for some other reason?"

Variables Affecting Family Power

Multiple variables were discussed that affect family power. These are:

1. The family power hierarchy.
2. Type of family form.
3. Formation of coalitions.
4. The family communication network.
5. Social class status.
6. Family life cycle stage.
7. Cultural and religious background.
8. Situational contingencies.
9. Person variables (members' ages, gender, self-esteem).
10. Spouses' emotional interdependency and commitment to the marriage.

Recognizing the influence of other assessment areas as listed above will assist the family nurse in more fully appraising and interpreting family power attributes.

Overall Family System and Subsystem Power

From your assessment of all the above broad areas, are you able to deduce whether the overall family power can be characterized as dominated by wife, husband, child, or grandparent; as egalitarian-syncratic or autonomic; as leaderless or chaotic? The family power continuum presented in this chapter can be used for a visual representation of the analysis.

If dominance is found, who is the dominant person? Power arrangements on this continuum in the 2 to 4 range have been found to be healthy and satisfying patterns (if mild dominance is by husband).

To determine the overall power pattern, asking a broad, open-ended question is often illuminating. For example, ask both spouse and children if feasible: "Who usually has the last say about important issues? Who is really in charge and why? Who runs the family? Who wins the important arguments on issues? Who usually wins out if there is a disagreement? Who gets their way when they disagree?"

Another significant follow-up question is, "Are you satisfied with how decisions are made and with who makes the decisions (ie, the present power structure)?"

Subsystem power also needs to be assessed. Observation of marital and parent–child interactions and sibling interactions as well as interview data gathered from family members is used to assess subsystem power characteristics (Olson and Cromwell, 1975).

FAMILY NURSING DIAGNOSIS AND INTERVENTION GUIDELINES

Understanding the power structure in the family is essential in formulating nursing diagnoses and effective nursing interventions. Several prime examples illustrate the importance of including this facet of the family assessment. When health care actions/decisions need to be made by the family, knowing who holds the power for this type of decision and for overall decisions, coupled with knowledge of how decisions are made, will guide the family nurse to speak to the appropriate persons with sensitivity as to how decisions take place.

Where families have a clear, intact power hierarchy that functions well for them, the nurse may want to support or reinforce this healthy structure (this is important in fostering confidence in parents). Where the parental executive subsystem is weak, the nurse may want to plan ways to assist spouses/parents to strengthen this subsystem.

Turning to a third area where nurses can be instrumental, decisional conflicts and other power conflicts need to be identified (McFarland and McFarlane, 1989). If family members are interested in pursuing this problem area, assistance may be provided in helping the family resolve their conflict(s). McFarland and McFarlane (1989) in describing the NANDA diagnosis "decisional conflict," present cogent guidelines for assisting nurses to assist family members to resolve this problem. Chapter 10 also has suggestions for helping families resolve conflictual communication.

☐ STUDY QUESTIONS

1. Power is an important dimension in human relationships and groups because (select all appropriate answers):
   a. It is critical in understanding role relationships.
   b. It greatly influences the establishment and the maintenance of communication channels.
   c. It is the sole determinant upon which an intimate relationship is formed and maintained.

2. Demonstrate your knowledge of several basic power concepts by matching the correct synonyms or definitions with the concepts in the left-hand column.

CONCEPTS	SYNONYM/DEFINITION
__ a. Power	1. Influence.
	2. Legitimate power.
	3. Primary authority.
	4. Dominance.
__ b. Authority	5. May involve individual.
	6. Family group dominance patterns.
	7. One facet is decision making.
__ c. Family power	8. Process whereby things get accomplished.
__ d. Decision-making	9. Assessed within context of family interaction.

3. Identify three limitations cited relative to studies of family power.

4. Match up the appropriate definition with the specific bases for power.

BASES FOR POWER

__ a. Authority
__ b. Referent power
__ c. Reward power
__ d. Coercive power
__ e. Helpless power
__ f. Expert on resource power
__ g. Informational power (direct)
__ h. Informational power (indirect)
__ i. Affective power
__ j. Tension management power

DEFINITION

1. Dominant person's obligation to assist the needy.
2. Dominant person's greater knowledge regarding issue.
3. Legitimate power.
4. Tradition-based power.
5. Based upon positive identification with influencing individual.
6. Belief in ability to inflict punishment.
7. Based on belief in the ability to grant privileges.
8. Way of controlling by managing present stress level in family.
9. Based upon having greater competency in matter.
10. Hinting or "putting suggestions into another's mouth."
11. The giving or withholding of care, warmth, sex.

Are the following statements True or False?

5. In cases where power is maintained by the husband because of his control over money, this type of power is called expert authority.

6. Among traditional patriarchal families, direct informational power is quite common.

7. Primary authority is based on tradition and acceptance of culturally based roles.

8. Identify and describe the three techniques used in making decisions.

9. Describe how each of the following variables affects family power.
a. Family communication network
b. Situational changes
c. Cultural influences
d. Coalition formation
e. Social class
f. Developmental or life cycle changes

Choose the correct answers to the following questions.

10. The most commonly used and well accepted typology of family power is:
a. Democratic–patriarchal.
b. Companionship–authoritarian.
c. Husband-dominated, egalitarian, wife-dominated.
d. Autocratic, syncratic, autonomic.
e. Familistic–atomistic.

11. Which type of overall power structure seems to be the least satisfying to both spouses?
   a. Husband dominated
   b. Wife dominated
   c. Syncratic
   d. Autonomic

12. What is the most outstanding contemporary trend relative to family power?
   a. The upsurge in traditionalism and conservatism.
   b. The atomistic trend in the family.
   c. The rise of the egalitarian, democratic family.
   d. The rise of the matrifocal, matriarchal family.

13. The healthy family, as described by Lewis and associates and Minuchin, is characterized by:
   a. A strong parent–child coalition.
   b. A clear power hierarchy.
   c. Husband having more power than wife.
   d. A strong parental coalition.

14. The following family roles and power relationships are frequently observed in poor families:
   a. Division of marital responsibilities is informal.
   b. Joint planning predominates.
   c. Father is bestowed titular authority.
   d. Father often plays a more passive, minimal role in the home.

15. Komarovsky found that the following factor played a significant role in the type of power structure present in working-class families:
   a. Occupational status.
   b. Residence (city or rural).
   c. Education.
   d. Ethnicity.

Family Case Study 1

From the following example, answer the two questions below.

Mr. G. walked in the door while Mrs. G. was discussing child rearing with the community health nurse. Mr. G. immediately "took over" the conversation, voicing his opinion about every parenting comment made by the nurse or Mrs. G. The children were heard to giggle about a couple of their father's assertions. Toward the end of the visit he shouted to the children to get up and clean the kitchen. The children did not respond, but looked at their mother. She paused and then said, "Children, please go clean the dishes." With this request the children left for the kitchen.

16. In this situation, which one of the following most clearly describes the power and role relationships of the father and mother?
   a. Male dominance.
   b. Children actually manipulate parents, playing one against the other.
   c. Insufficient data to clearly define roles.
   d. Mother acts as final arbiter and dominant one.

17. Data substantiating the above interpretation include:
   a. Father asserting role in an exaggerated manner.
   b. His assertions being responded to by giggles from the children.
   c. Need to show he is "leader."
   d. Children looking toward mother and responding to her request.
   e. No response to father's requests.

Family Case Study 2

Read the family history and then complete an assessment of family power from data presented in vignette by answering questions that follow.

The Simpsons are a middle-class white blended or step-parent family living in a suburban area. John Simpson, age 37, recently (8 months ago) married Sylvia, who had been divorced for 4 years. Sylvia (age 42) has three children, ages 13 (Joe), 10 (Mary), and 8 (Jimmie) from her former marriage. Mr. Simpson had no children from his former marriage. Mr. Simpson is a businessman; he owns and manages a hardware store. Mrs. Simpson is a registered nurse and works at a local hospital. Both have baccalaureate degrees from local colleges and their income level, due to their double income, is "quite comfortable." They live in a lovely, well-kept residential neighborhood. Their home is large and well furnished, containing four bedrooms, a living and family room, and a large, spacious kitchen. They moved to this particular community from the nearby city when they married and formed their new family.

The Simpsons are bringing their 8-year-old child, Jimmie, to the family health center because of bedwetting (enuresis), hyperactivity, and inattention at school. He will be examined by a family practitioner but, because of the nature of his situation, is also being interviewed by a family nurse practitioner who is in the process of completing a family assessment and comprehensive history of Jimmie.

Sylvia, the mother, relates that things in the family have been difficult since John "moved in." "First we had to move and the children lost all their friends. And even though John used to come and take me out for the evening and visit with us—so that the children were able to get to know him—they now resent him terribly and I feel I'm in between the devil and the deep blue sea!"

When asked what seems to be the major area of family conflict and concerns, she mentions disciplining of the children. "John doesn't discipline them, which I wish he did, and when he does set some limits, due to my nagging, the children don't listen to him. Then, I have to come in and settle things myself. I married John because I felt the children needed a father to relate to. Their own natural father lives far away now and seldom keeps in contact with them. The children don't seem to respect John, and the only way he is able to manage them is by promising them something or threatening to punish them."

She says that she never fights or disagrees with her husband in front of the children (believing children should not hear such unpleasant things). But after the children go to bed, she finds herself berating John for not following through with his family obligations—paying bills, repairing house, yard work, and so on. Sylvia sees herself as in charge of the children (primarily), housework, social affairs, cooking, and shopping, and feels that the rest is up to her husband. She does her work, in addition to a full-time job, and expects him to do his.

According to Mrs. Simpson, Joe, the 13-year-old, likes caring for his younger siblings, and Mary and Jimmie turn to him for help and advice if she is not home. She also comments that Joe is the child who really seems to resent John, and speaks to her husband only when necessary, with most messages pertaining to Joe's father going through the mother.

When the nurse asks Sylvia how the family arrived at the major decisions they have made since she and John became involved with each other—such as marriage, moving, and buying the house—Sylvia says that she initiated all three of these conversations. "I'm a practical person. I could see that marriage would be good for all of us, and so suggested it to John!" The nurse then asks, "And what was his answer?" Sylvia replies, "I don't remember exactly. I think he kind of hemmed and hawed around, and then, anyway, agreed, and I started making plans. He didn't want to move from the city or into such a big house, but I convinced him that it would be better economically and that the commuting time was reasonable for him. And I agreed to let him buy a more comfortable car to commute in, in return."

The assessor meets with the whole family twice more to discuss their "identified" problem (Jimmie) and the family dynamics and family problems. At these meetings she notices that twice when she speaks to the parents and the children became noisy or disruptive, the older son, Joe, takes over, scolding them. In their discussion she observes that this is a family in which there is a proliferation of "do's" and "don'ts" about everything—from the time they get up in the morning until the time they go to bed at night. Feelings are not openly expressed, and the two youngest children directly answered the nurse's questions in a short, incomplete manner, looking to the mother for approval. The mother appears quite committed to a particular home schedule. John mentions that it is hard to fit into someone else's schedule and way of doing things. Joe confirms this point with the nurse in his statement, "We all know the rules better than he does, so why do we need him to tell us what to do?" (Mr. Simpson just sits quietly, and neither parent responds to Joe's hostile statement.)

In discussing his own feelings and thoughts about the family, Mr. Simpson perceives that Jimmie may feel confused and insecure because of moving, their marriage, and the new school. He alludes to the difficulty he has faced in parenting his wife's children and to their negative reactions toward him. He also finds disciplining very hard because he never had children before and in growing up was treated very permissively ("anything at all seemed to be okay with my parents"). He comments that "he tries to stay out of child rearing as much as possible."

Mr. Simpson was married twice before and appears to be passive and easygoing with his wife. In contrast, Mrs. Simpson initiates topics, leads discussions, and is quite "definite" and opinionated in her statements.

18. Assess the family power patterns described in the above case.
   a. Who makes what decisions?
   b. What decision-making techniques are utilized?
   c. On what basis is family power derived?
   d. What variables affect family power?
   e. Using the family power continuum (see Fig. 11–1), where would you place this family?
   f. If dominance, indicate dominant family member.

19. State a family nursing diagnosis for this family that focuses on the power dimension.

20. Propose two general family nursing interventions to assist the family with a family nursing problem in the power dimension area.

CHAPTER TWELVE

Family Role Structure

Learning Objectives

1. Define and describe relative to the family:
   Role.
   Position and paired positions.
   Role behavior and role occupant
   Role conflict.
   Role strain/stress.
   Normative dimensions of roles.
   Role sharing.
   Role taking and role making.
   Reciprocal roles and principle of complementarity.
   Role allocation.
   Family homeostasis.
   Role induction and role modification.
2. From the family role studies presented, summarize the findings of these with respect to the basic roles making up the wife–mother and husband–father positions and which roles are shared and not shared according to present trends.
3. Summarize research findings relative to the role of father, mother, and grandparent in the United States.
4. Describe three types of marital relationships.
5. Describe the common role conflict experienced by the working wife–mother and her husband in dual-career families.
6. Define and give examples of informal roles that often exist in families (both healthy and detrimental roles). Describe why both formal and informal roles are assessed in the family, as well as the purpose that informal roles serve.
7. Explain the process and effects of labeling on individuals in the family.
8. Describe the frequently observed role characteristics in lower- and middle-class families, the single-parent family, the step-parent family, and the family during health and illness, including the caregiver role.
9. With the use of a family case example, complete an assessment of the family role structure, state a family nursing diagnosis in the area of family roles, and propose two family nursing interventions directed toward ameliorating or resolving the above role problem.

In all known societies almost everyone lives his or her life enmeshed in a network of family rights and obligations called role relations (Goode, 1964). Family roles are critical, central roles an individual must learn to enact successfully, for adequate role functioning is crucial not only for the individual's successful functioning, but also for the family's successful functioning. It is through the performance of family roles that the functions of the family are fulfilled. In fact, family sociologists often define the family as an interacting, interdependent set of roles that are in a state of dynamic equilibrium (Turner, 1970).

Because of the critical nature which family roles play in the organization of the family, it is imperative for the family nurse to understand role relationships and, from this, be able to promote health role behaviors and identify role problems.

ROLE THEORY AND DEFINITIONS

Because role concepts and terms are fundamental to the discussion that follows, a number of basic terms are first defined. The reader is also directed to the works by Hardy and Hardy (1988) and Biddle and Thomas (1966) for further explanation of these concepts.

Role

According to Nye (1976), there are two basic perspectives on roles—the structuralist orientation, which stresses the normative (cultural) influence associated with particular statuses and their related roles (Linton, 1945), and the interaction orientation of Turner (1970), which emphasizes the emergent quality of roles that generate from social interaction.

In this text, role will be defined in a more structural sense, because normative prescriptions, although certainly variable, are still relatively well defined within the family (Nye, 1976). *Role* is referred to as more or less homogeneous sets of behaviors that are normatively defined and expected of an occupant of a given social position. Roles are based on role expectations or prescriptions defining what individuals in a particular situation should do in order to meet their own or another's expectations of them (Nye, 1976, p. 7).

Position or Status

Position or status is defined as a person's location in a social system. Role is subsumed under the notion of position. While roles are the behaviors associated with one who holds a particular position, position identifies a person's status or place in a social system. Every individual occupies multiple positions—adult, male, husband, farmer, Elks member, and so on (Biddle and Thomas, 1966; Hardy and Hardy, 1988). Associated with each of these positions are a number of roles. In the case of the mother position, some of the associated roles are housekeeper, child caretaker, family health leader, cook, and companion or playmate. Merton (1957) explains:

> A particular social status involves, not a single associated role, but an array of associated roles. This is a basic characteristic of social structure. This fact of structure can be registered by a distinctive term, *role-set*, by which I mean that complement of role relationships which persons have by virtue of occupying a particular social status. (p. 3)

Thus for each position a number of roles exist, each of which is composed of a more or less related homogeneous set of behaviors culturally defined as expected of those in that position or status. They might, however, be shared with other members of a group; in the family, for example, the child-care role is now a shared responsibility of both the mother and father position (Nye, 1976).

Role Occupant

A role occupant is a person who holds a position within the social structure. Role incumbent and occupant are terms used interchangeably.

Role Behavior, Role Performance, or Role Enactment

Role behavior, role performance, and role enactment are all interchangeable terms that denote what a person actually does within a position in response to role expectations. Expectations and/or prescriptions for the sets of behavior appropriate for the basic social positions and their associated roles (family roles, occupational roles, etc) evolve and are developed by society. These expectations are modified in some cases by particular reference groups.

Many of the roles associated with our basic social positions are learned within the family context. Societal role expectations are modified or refined as a result of an individual's exposure to role models and the person's individual personality—that is, his or her capacities, temperament, attitudes, and interests. An individual accepts particular roles based on societal expectation and as modified by his or her identification with role models and individual personality characteristics. The outcome of an individual's role modification is the person's actual role behavior or performance. Figure 12–1 illustrates the process by which role behavior actually develops.

Role Stress/Strain

Role stress occurs when a social structure, such as the family, creates very difficult, conflicting, or impossible

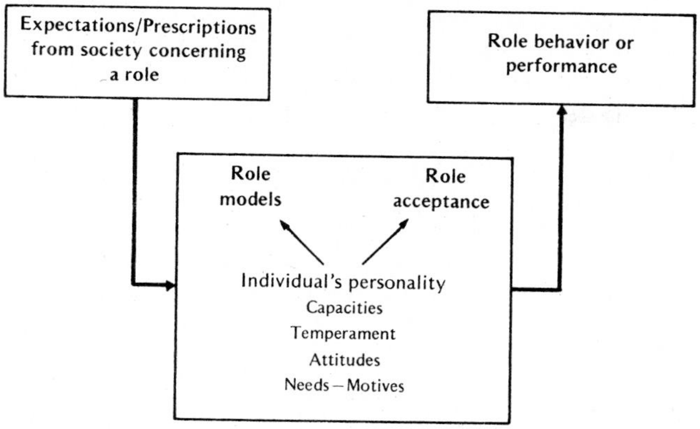

Figure 12–1.
Development of role behavior.

demands for occupants of positions within that social structure (Hardy and Hardy, 1988). It is a characteristic of the social system, rather than of the person in the system. Role stress results in role strain—subjective feelings of frustration and tension. Role strain is also perceived and felt by the associated role partners (Hardy and Hardy, 1988).

Role Conflict

Role conflict occurs when the occupant of a position perceives that he or she is confronted with incompatible expectations (Hardy and Hardy, 1988). The source of the incompatibility may be due to changes in expectations within the actor, others, or the environment.

Several types of role conflict are discussed in the literature. *Interrole conflict* is when the norms or behavioral patterns of one role are incongruent with another role that the same individual simultaneously plays. Interrole conflict occurs when an individual's role complex—that is, the group of roles he or she enacts—involves several roles that are incompatible (Hardy and Hardy, 1988). This type of conflict is due either to the incompatibility of the behaviors associated with the various roles or the excessive amount of energy these roles demand, such as the familiar case of performing the student, housekeeper, cook, marital, and child-care roles all at once.

The second type of role conflict is *intersender role conflict* (LaRocca, 1978), in which two or more people hold conflicting expectations concerning the enactment of a role. An illustration of this second type of role conflict is the presence of conflicting expectations on how one's role as a professional nurse should be performed. For example, the head nurse may expect efficiency of actions; the patient may expect patient-centeredness, based on his or her perceived needs; and the nurse may expect to be able to give individualized care as defined by the standards of her or his profession.

A third type of role conflict is called *person–role conflict*. This type involves a conflict between the person's internalized values and the external values communicated to the actor by others, throwing the actor into a state of role stress. This type of role conflict is similar to the second type, except in this case there is not a disparity in role expectations between people in the outer environment. One can think of the person–role conflict that results in families with young teenagers—when the teenager has one internalized notion of his or her role as a teenager and peers prescribe a very different role.

Normative Dimensions of Roles

As outlined under the description of role, roles are normatively or culturally defined; that is, the culture in which one participates and/or with which one identifies prescribes and proscribes the behavior of the occupants of various positions. However, "not all the family roles are equally normative" (Nye, 1976, p. 15). Jackson (1966) notes that some family roles are more "crystallized"—clearly spelled out as expected behavior—than others. For instance, in the past in the middle-class American family the affective (Nye calls it therapeutic) role of the spouses was not crystallized; that is, it was not *expected* of mates to listen to each other's problems. Today, however, spouses see therapeutic assistance not as optional behavior but as an obligation, because it is a duty to help one's spouse. Thus the therapeutic role for middle-class American spouses has been "crystallized."

One can infer the strength of a role (whether it is a strong norm or not) in a specific position by assessing the sanction(s) applied when the role is not performed. Certainly social ostracism as a sanction against lack of role fulfillment, as in the case where the wife–mother is not carrying out her housekeeper role, is less strong or intense than imprisonment, as might result from failure to carry out the child-care role when it reaches the point of child neglect or desertion. Sanctions provide evidence that the society or parts of the society perceive a particular role to be sufficiently important that conformity to the norm be enforced.

Role Sharing

Role sharing refers to participation of two or more people in the same roles even though they hold different positions. Differentiated, technologically sophisticated societies such as the United States are characterized by their extensive role sharing. Sharply segregated role structures are unusual within families today. An example of normative role sharing in the family is the case of the child-socialization role where both mother and father jointly participate, in addition to school teachers, youth leaders, ministers, and so on. In the older family, the housekeeper and shopping roles are often shared by the retired couple.

Role Taking

Another essential concept within role theory is that of role taking. In order for family members to play roles, they must be able to imagine themselves in the role of a counterpart, or role partner; in this way they are able to assign a role to the other and also better understand how they should behave in their own roles (Turner, 1970). Through socialization family members acquire a repertoire of roles through which they can act and interact with others. "Roles are never learned singly, but always as pairs or sets of interacting roles. Because the individual learns the role of alter [his role partner] while playing his own role, he is able to play the role of the alter when others in the situation are playing his usual role." (Turner, 1970 p. 215). Over a period of time, however, the self-conception incorporates certain roles and denies others, so that the individual no longer plays past roles.

Reciprocal or Complementary Roles

A basic concept in role theory is that of the complementarity of roles. A role is interdependent with and patterned to mesh with that of a role partner. In other words, a role is always paired with a reciprocal role of another person. One can never look at a role in isolation. To use a teacher as an example, one must look at the teacher's role together with the student's role, because both are necessary for either to function. Society specifies behaviors for each person in these reciprocal arrangements so that each will know what is expected of the role partner. Both role partners are constantly influencing each other's role behavior through their many interactions with one another. For instance, if students become more verbal and assertive with teachers, the teacher responds by modifying his or her expectations and behaviors toward the students. Likewise, as society changes and family systems evolve, changes in social and family roles become necessary. Thus if a wife begins working, she may become more instrumental in financial decisions and the husband may become more involved with household tasks and child rearing.

Parsons and associates (1953) coined the concept of "the principle of complementarity," referring to the functional adequacy of roles in social situations that are based on the match between the performances and the expectations of partners in a relationship. The principle of complementarity is of great significance because it is chiefly responsible for that degree of harmony and stability that occurs in interpersonal relations (Spiegel, 1957).

Whenever there is dissimilarity in expectations and performances of family roles—due to cultural, social class, or individual differences—the potential for lack of role complementarity and possible conflict and stress exists.

Role Patterning or Role Allocation

The patterning or allocation of roles provides for definitions of what is to be done in the family, who is to do it, including who is to decide on the allocation of tasks (the leadership role). Role patterning makes provision for carrying out tasks on the basis of age, sex, and personality characteristics; it also provides sanctions for dealing with the neglect or poor performance of agreed-on tasks.

Family role allocation is largely defined by culture and social class, although more latitude and flexibility exist today. Furthermore, family roles are also the result of each member's searching for a viable position for himself or herself (a group of roles that give a person some feelings of satisfaction, competency, and dominance in a "sphere of influence") and of the functional requirements of the family (Turner, 1970).

Family Homeostasis

Roles, both formal and informal, serve a homeostatic purpose in families. Family homeostasis refers to the family's use of regulatory mechanisms to maintain equilibrium in the family. The family achieves this homeostasis through adaptation—by altering family structure including roles or bringing in assistive outside resources, and/or integration (mobilization of inner resources such as cohesiveness). Turner (1970) remarks that once a system of formal and informal roles is established within the family, family processes proceed laboriously unless the members play their expected role. This is because families become dependent on the existence of certain informal roles to be enacted so as to maintain family homeostasis. For example, if the family is used to having the middle daughter act as the mediator in disputes, this enables other family members to be less restrained in their sentiments and assures family members that she will step in to help resolve disagreements. When the mediating daughter is not present, conflicts are handled in a much less effective manner due to her absence.

Role Induction and Role Modification

The techniques families use to "persuade" family members to change their role behavior during times of role conflict, and thus restore family equilibrium, involve the use of either role induction or role modification. In the case of role induction, a family member changes role behavior as a result of coercion, coaxing, or other manipulative techniques. Because role induction is primarily defensive and basic value conflict is only temporarily avoided, the same conflict will reappear. On the other hand, role modification involves a change in both parties to a conflict. Complementarity is achieved through mutual agreement. Role modification, which leads toward insight and mutual agreement usually progresses through several phases: (1) joking; (2) referral to a third party; (3) exploring, a testing phase that may involve the work of the helping person who assists the family to find solutions to conflicts; (4) compromising, the phase in which parties to the conflict perceive the need for a change of goals; and (5) consolidating, or learning how to make the compromises work (Spiegel, 1971).

Criteria for Adequate Family Role Functioning

In respect to role relationships in the family, what does the adequate family look like? If we have an understanding of satisfactory family functioning, we may better be able to understand families that are marginally or inadequately coping. Glasser and Glasser (1970), based on their work with a number of families in which one member of the primary group was undergoing psychotherapy, summarized their findings. From their observations and analysis they identified four general criteria necessary for adequate family functioning. They underscored the importance of role complementarity; compatibility of family roles and norms with societal norms; the presence of roles in families that meet the psychological needs of family members; and the ability of the family to respond to change via role flexibility (Glasser and Glasser, 1970; Messer, 1970). In addition, in a healthy family role allocation is reasonable and does not overburden one or more members. This results in all the necessary family functions being fulfilled.

FORMAL FAMILY ROLES

Family Positions

There are a limited number of positions defined as normative within the most common type of family form, the two-parent nuclear family. These positions are referred to as *formal* and *paired,* and consist of father–husband; wife–mother; son–brother; and daughter–sister. Although a variety of other family positions may be seen today, they can be viewed simply as variations of the two-parent nuclear family structure.

Each of the normative positions of the family group is associated with related roles. Husband–fathers are expected to be wage earners, among the other roles they may possess. Wife–mothers are viewed as homemakers. When a wife–mother is employed outside the home, as often occurs in American society, this role is not viewed as her primary responsibility, whereas the wage-earner role of the husband–father is viewed as his primary role.

In the single parent family the mother often plays the mother–father role with no spousal role. In the step-parent family, the husband will often play husband–father, but because the children are biologically not his own, the father role is a quasi-father role (the role lacks crystallization).

Formal Roles

Associated with each formal family position are related roles, clusters of more or less homogeneous behaviors. The family apportions roles to its family members in a manner similar to the way society apportions its roles: according to how critical the role performance is to the system's functioning. Some roles require special skills and abilities; others are less complex and can be assigned to the less skilled or to those with the least amount of power. Standard formal roles exist in the family, (eg, breadwinner, homemaker, house repairman, chauffeur, child rearer, financial manager, and cook). When there are fewer persons in a family the number of persons to fulfill these roles is limited; thus there will be more demands and opportunities for family members to play several roles at different times. If a member leaves home or becomes unable to fulfill a role, someone else fills this vacuum by taking up his or her role to keep the family functioning (Murray and Zentner, 1975, 1985).

Marital and Parental Roles. Nye and Gecas (1976) have identified eight basic roles making up the husband–father and the wife–mother social positions:

- Provider role.
- Housekeeper role.

- Child-care role.
- Child-socialization role.
- Recreational role.
- Kinship role (maintaining relationships with paternal and maternal families).
- Therapeutic role (meeting the affective needs of spouse).
- Sexual role.

In this scheme the companionship role has been subsumed under the recreational and therapeutic roles.

Many people fail to separate parental roles from marital roles, but in reality the two roles are quite distinct, and marital roles should not be shortchanged due to overinvolvement in the other role.* Marital roles are focused on the husband–wife interactions, while parental roles are focused upon the parent–child interactions and the parental responsibilities. Nevertheless, performance of marital roles will certainly have an impact on parental roles and vice versa.

Marital Roles and Types of Marriages. Minuchin (1974) stresses the importance of the spouse role relationships: the need for mates to maintain a strong marital relationship. Children especially can interfere with the marital relationship, creating a situation where the husband and wife form a coalition with one of their children and diminish the close relationship with each other. Maintaining a satisfying marital relationship is identified as one of the vital family developmental tasks of the family as it progresses through its life cycle. In the previous discussion of family development, the stress that children put on the marital relationship was made quite evident.

What are marriages supposed to be like? In the past, behavioral scientists put together a composite picture of the well-functioning marriage that we now think of as biased, simplistic, and rarely found in reality. Moreover, two fairly well-conducted studies have shown that a variety of relationships present in marriages generally (Cline, 1966), particularly in stable, long-standing marriages (Cuber and Harroff, 1966). In both of these studies the researchers found that no one pattern of satisfactory marital adjustment existed. A wide range of behaviors and marital roles were found among persons who felt content with, or at least remained in their marriages.

One of these classic studies was conducted by Cuber and Harroff (1966). They interviewed about 400 upper-middle-class couples who had been married at least 10 years and had a stable marriage. From this data they devised a typology of marital relationships illustrating the diverse types of stable marriages. These varied from conflict-habituated relationships to devitalized relationships; passive, congenial relationships to vital, total relationships. Cuber and Harroff estimate that roughly 80 percent of the marriages they studied were utilitarian oriented, while only 20 percent were vital or total relationships. Thus it appears that the American ideal of a marriage, where most of one's intimate and social needs are met by a spouse, may be a widespread myth.

Bott (1957) attempted to explain some of the differences found in the extent of involvement and intimacy in marital relationships; she theorized that when marriages were superimposed on a social network of friends, neighbors, and relatives among whom there was frequent and meaningful interaction that met many of the needs of the husband and wife, the impetus for the mates to become deeply involved with each other and share roles was decreased. Thus she speculated that a sharper demarcation of roles would be seen, in addition to a lower value placed on the marital relationship itself. It may well be that the social environment in which the family is embedded influences the nature of the marital relationship. Conversely, the nature of the marital relationship probably affects the extensiveness of the mates' social network.

Types of Marital Relationships. In addition to studies demonstrating the wide diversity of marriages, efforts have also been made to classify the types of dyadic (two-person) relationships. For assistance in assessing the marital and other dyadic relationship in families, one of these typologies will be explained briefly. Described first by Bateson (1958) and later by Watzlawick and co-workers (1967), two types of basic relationships are found in dyadic relationships. These are termed complementary and symmetrical, with parallel relationships being a combination of the two.

Complementary Relationships. Mates in this type of dyad exhibit contrasting behavior. One spouse is the leading, dominant personality and decision maker, whereas the other partner is the subservient follower (a typical "one-up and one-down" position). A strong element of dependency exists between spouses who have a complementary relationship.

The positive element in this type of relationship is that it allows one to give and the other to receive. The inherent danger lies in its tendency to become increasingly rigid, thus stifling the growth of both people.

It is necessary that both partners of a complementary relationship play their "proper" role. If either mate does not continue to perform his or her respec-

** The reader is referred back to Chap. 7, to the section exploring the vital nature of family subsystems and how these need to be kept intact and strong.*

tive functions, the relationship will come to an end, with each feeling disconfirmed by the other.

Symmetrical Relationships. This type of relationship is based on the equality of the partners. The partners demand equality through the character of their mutually exchanged messages and behavior, and each mate has the right to initiate action, to criticize the other's behavior, and to have a voice in family decisions.

The positive aspect of this type of relationship is that it allows for mutual respect, trust, and spontaneity, with the optimal effect being that each partner is free to be him- or herself, knowing that each will be accepted and respected by the other. The danger inherent in this type of relationship is that the competitive aspect of the relationship may become overemphasized. When this happens there is increasing frustration and a decrease in cooperative behaviors (mutual assistance and support). Egocentricity by one or both partners may preclude the mutual accommodation and giving needed to enhance and nurture the intimate, affectional part of a marital relationship.

Parallel Relationships. This third type of marital relationship was later introduced by Lederer and Jackson (1968). In parallel relationships, the spouses alternate comfortably between symmetrical and complementary relationships as they adapt to changing situations. Depending on the situation and the partner's areas of competence, there is an interchange and flexibility in relationship patterns. This switching from one pattern to the other restores the stabilizing properties when either pattern threatens to break down.

Because of the greater flexibility and individual growth-enhancing properties, each partner being able to contribute according to his or her competencies and the situational needs, this type of relationship is seen as the most mature, healthy, and stable form of the three types. Developmentally, if maturation is allowed to occur relationships should evolve in a person's lifetime from being complementary to being symmetrical and then to being parallel. If one visualizes this in terms of the dependency factor, relationships undergo a change from dependency (complementary) to independence (symmetry) to interdependence (parallelism). One qualification needs to be made here, however. The value judgment placed on these types of relationships and their perceived degree of maturity does not take into account the cultural background of the individuals involved—an obvious limitation.

Contemporary Family Role Changes

The roles of family members have become more variable, flexible, and complex. In the past, there was "women's work" and "men's work," and little role sharing existed except under special conditions. The family lived according to relatively rigid, traditionally established rules that were maintained by the social and moral pressures of the entire society. Today, great variation in the roles of both sexes is feasible. The expectations and practices differ tremendously. In one family, both adult members may be expected to work and jointly share in all family affairs and responsibilities; in another family, traditional roles are expected and performed; and in yet another situation, the single-parent family, the adult assumes the roles of both parents.

Because the normative limits of family roles are so broad, a wide range of behaviors are acceptable as appropriate to a particular position. Turner (1962) pointed out that the requirements of the situation and the individuals in it determine specific behaviors found in a role. Thus individuals tentatively construct their roles in response to the cues given by other(s) in the situation (their role partners).

For Aldous (1974), this role taking and social interaction generates much *role making* in marriages and families. She states that "there is a great deal of role-making in families today since changing conditions have rendered suspect or inappropriate age and gender norms" (p. 232). And she points to changing marital roles as a prime example of role making in process.

> When gender norms dictated that men were the breadwinners and women were responsible for the family, a segregated conjugal role organization, in which women saw to the day-to-day operation of the family and men provided the economic resources, made a certain kind of sense. With 65.7 percent of married women presently engaged in gainful employment, including 20.6 percent of women with children under six years of age, people no longer are willing to accept the norms legitimating and prescribing a segregated conjugal role organization. The questioning particularly comes from women who according to gender norms are the most responsible for household affairs even though they are holding full-time jobs. They experience "role overload" with all the attendant problems of mental and physical strain. (p. 232)

Research Addressing Contemporary Family Roles

Research confirms that a spouse's feelings and perceptions about his or her marriage differ from those of the mate. Bernard (1972), a noted feminist sociologist, suggests that there are actually two marriages for each couple: his and hers. The couple's differing reality is evidenced in the wife's more negative appraisal of their marriage. Bernard cites the increased rates of depression and illness among married women (when compared to their husbands) as evidence of these two realities. One probable cause for this increased marital dissatisfaction by wives is that traditionally wives were

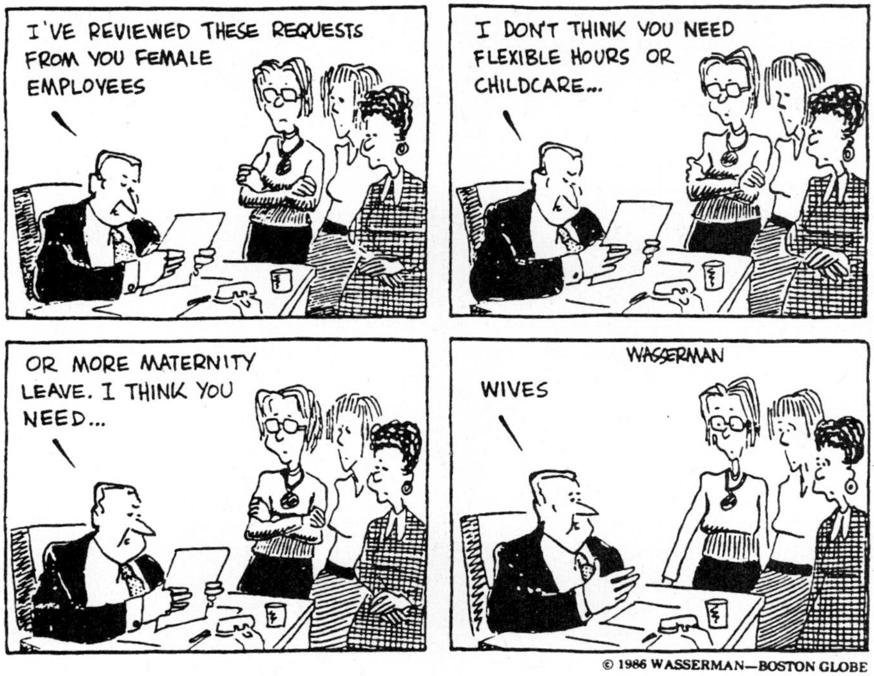
I'VE REVIEWED THESE REQUESTS FROM YOU FEMALE EMPLOYEES
I DON'T THINK YOU NEED FLEXIBLE HOURS OR CHILDCARE...
OR MORE MATERNITY LEAVE. I THINK YOU NEED...
WASSERMAN
WIVES
© 1986 WASSERMAN—BOSTON GLOBE

Figure 12–2.
The traditional view of a wife's role. (From Boston Globe, 1986. Distributed by Los Angeles Times Syndicate. Reprinted with permission.)

taught to meet their husbands' and childrens' needs rather than their own.

Women's Roles in the Family. Research on women's roles in the family has focused primarily on the effects of women's employment on the family and in allocation of roles (Elias, 1987; Spitze, 1988). The extent to which women retain the traditional sex-role obligations (childrearing, housekeeping, and so forth) and simultaneously perform their work role has been analyzed. Role overload, role conflict, and role strain are documented in study after study as women move into the labor force and create careers for themselves. With the widespread advent of dual-career families there are three full-time jobs: the husband's paid work, the wife's paid work, and the family work. "Wives in all social classes do the bulk of family work" (Walker, 1990, p. 16).

When women work they generally expect their husbands to share in the roles of child rearing and housekeeping (Shaw, 1988). (Fig. 12–2). In some studies, men expected role change due to wife's employment, but behavioral change was not forthcoming (Cronkite, 1977). More recent research confirms that the role behavior of husbands with respect to assuming more household activities appears to be changing, albeit slowly (Meissner, 1975; Spitze, 1988). The increased involvement of husbands who have working wives appears to be mainly through increased involvement in child care (Pleck, 1985).

Cronkite (1977) discusses the common dilemmas of the dual-career family and the stresses generated by role changes. She describes how couples see the benefit of the additional income outweighing their objections and reluctance to the wife's working. But at the same time, the husband is anxious about his diminished power in the role of breadwinner, and the wife—though enjoying the challenge of work and adult social interaction—often feels guilty about not spending enough time with her children or fulfilling some of the "traditional" wife/mother functions.

Men's Roles in the Family. During the last 20 years a great deal of literature has appeared about fatherhood. An impetus for much of the research has been the women's movement and the realization that, as women move from the home into the workplace, their roles have changed, and that their role partners' behavior has also changed. Research shows changes are occurring, but at a slower pace than women's movement into the work force. Another factor that has created concern, and thus research efforts, is the rise in divorces, with many children being separated from their fathers. How divorced fathers maintain their fatherhood role with their biological children when separated from them is a major concern. Data show that almost one half of children had not seen their nonresidential parent in the past year (Furstenberg and Nord, 1985). How the father role is enacted when men remarry a woman with children is also being studied.

Kennedy (1989), in his review of the fatherhood literature, reports that three theories of fatherhood are presented. He termed these theories the moral overseer, the distance breadwinner, and the sex role model. The moral overseer role predominated during colonial times. The prime role of fathers during this period was to exert moral leadership in the family. In contrast, the distant breadwinner pictured the primary role of the father as being a provider but uninvolved with child care. The father was supposed to be a good provider, but not have a direct influence on the life of the child. After World War II a new theory of gender identity began to emphasize the crucial role that fathers played in molding children's identity, particularly the son's identity. The "new father" began in the 1980s and is viewed as an extension of the gender identity theory, modified by changes in the woman's role in the family. Kennedy (1989) describes "the new father's" role:

> He is present at the birth; he is involved with his children as infants, not just when they are older; he participates in the actual day-to-day work of child care, and not just play; he is involved with his daughters as much as his sons. (p. 364)

Research on the new father has focused on fatherhood in the family life stages, satisfaction with the new father role, and rural/urban and cultural differences (Bronstein and Cowan, 1988; Kennedy, 1989; Lamb, 1987). Based on several literature reviews (Bronstein and Cowan, 1988; Hanson and Bozett, 1987; Kennedy, 1989; Lamb, 1987, some interesting research findings in this area emerge.

1. Findings from multiple studies agree that attitudes toward family roles are moving in the direction of egalitarianism and that child care and socialization roles are becoming the shared responsibility of both spouses (Araji, 1977; Hansen and Bozett, 1987; Lamb, 1987).
2. Today's fathers are expected to be more actively involved in child rearing with children of all ages than in the past, and to a modest extent this is evidenced in studies. Lamb (1987) points out, however, that paternal involvement may not be beneficial in all family circumstances. Individual circumstances must be considered in order to understand how children are affected by differences in paternal involvement.
3. There is no evidence that maternal employment status affects levels of paternal involvement in child care.
4. In two-parent families where the wife–mother works at home, husband–fathers spend 20 to 25 percent as much time as mothers participating in child care activities.
5. Fathers spend more time on child care when children are younger; they are more involved and interested in child care with their sons than with their daughters.
6. There are variations in the type of interaction fathers versus mothers have with their children. Mothers' interactions are dominated by caretaking activities, while fathers' interactions are more play-oriented.
7. If both parents are equally involved in infant care, there are no differences in parenting skills between mothers and fathers during the newborn period (Araji, 1977; Bronstein and Cowan, 1988).

Health care professionals are increasingly recognizing that pregnancy, delivery, and child care at all ages are family events. As such, the informed father should be an active, involved participant (Hanson and Bozett, 1987).

The Marital Sexual Role. Another apparent change in roles within the spouse positions involves the sexual role. In the past men had the right to regular sexual activity with their wives, but felt under no obligation to be concerned about the wives' feelings of satisfaction. Today the wife's right to sexual enjoyment and equality is growing in importance, changing the nature of the sexual role for both mates (Napier, 1988).

The Kinship or Kinkeeping Role. There is a rather extensive body of literature that shows that women are the kinkeepers in the family. Kinkeeping, or the kinship role, involves maintaining communication, facilitating contact and the exchange of goods and services, and monitoring family relationships (Hagestad, 1988). Women function as kinkeepers for both sides of the family.

With this added family responsibility "the superwoman squeeze"—the overload experienced by middle-aged women who provide assistance to both children and two sets of parents in addition to working—is a real possibility.

Being the "sandwiched" generation and the "sandwiched" sex, middle-aged women are caught between the needs of parents with increasing life expectancies and children who remain dependent for a longer period of time and need extra help during periods of marital and other personal disruption (Spitze, 1988). Just as many middle-aged women think they are getting off the "mommy track," they are finding themselves, due to the aging of their parents, getting back on "the daughter track." Data support this phenomenon. In a U.S. House of Representatives report of 1988 (Beck and Associates, 1990) it is estimated that the average American woman spends 17 years raising children and 18 years helping aged parents.

The Grandparent Role. The role of grandparent and even great grandparent are becoming growing objects of interest. Certainly the growing number of individuals who are grandparents and great grandparents is a potent factor for this increased interest. The empirical research describes grandparenthood as a heterogeneous experience, with wide variation in how the grandparent role is enacted. The historical context, age, ethnicity, social class and gender tend to produce significant differences in terms of what the grandparent role is like.

There is no concensus on whether grandparental involvement has direct positive effects on grandchildren's behavior. In most instances, indirect effects (through helping the child's parents) and symbolic influences play a greater role.

The symbolic expressions of the grandparent role—the functions the role fulfills—are equally diverse and varied. Bengtson (1985) divides these symbolic functions of grandparenthood into (1) simply "being there" (simple presence); (2) acting as the national guard or family watchdog (being there to protect and give care if needed); (3) being an arbitrator (negotiator between parents and children); and (4) being an active participant in the family's social construction of its history (making connections between the families' past, present, and future).

In a study of 510 grandparents, Cherlin and Furstenberg (1985 and 1986) classified them into three styles of grandparenting: "the detached" (26 percent), who were low in both exchange and influence and saw their grandchild(ren) less than once a month; "the passive" (29 percent), who also scored low on both the above criteria but had seen their grandchild(ren) at least once or twice a month; and "the active" (45 percent), who scored high on exchange and influence regardless of their frequency of visiting. Many grandparents developed companionship relationships with their grandchildren—relationships that were easygoing and lighthearted.

Most of the research has been on grandmothers. Relatively little research has focused on grandfathers and virtually none on the growing number of great grandfathers (Hanson and Bozett, 1987). One of the crucial elements that has been found in terms of the grandchild–grandparent relationship is the relationships between the grandparents and their children, because the child's parents determine the frequency of visits and encourage or discourage the development of a positive grandparent–grandchild relationship. Several researchers have observed grandparents are more involved with grandchildren when parents are divorced, especially when the grandparents are younger. Moreover, black children have been observed to profit when grandparents play a more active role in their upbringing (Cherlin and Furstenberg, 1986).

Role Change Problems

The status and associated roles of individuals in a family will change in many ways throughout a person's life cycle and that of his or her two families (family of orientation and family of parenthood). The change in role relationships, expectations, and abilities is referred to as *role transition* (Meleis, 1975). Role transitions occur at clear demarcations of the family life, such as at marriage, divorce, and the death of a parent or spouse, as well as more subtly as an ongoing response to life experience. A role change experienced by one family member necessitates complementary role changes in other family members.*

It should be acknowledged that the advent of role changes in families does not come without a cost to the individuals involved. Families often experience significant stress during role transitions. It is well recognized that when individuals deviate from normative role expectations and/or take on new roles, they may lack the role preparation or previous socialization needed to perform these new roles comfortably and adequately. In addition to lacking the necessary training, a family member may not feel that the new roles meet his or her interests or needs. Role changes such as those brought on by having a new baby, a wife's employment, a husband's unemployment, divorce, or family relocation, may create role confusion, anxiety, and unhappiness in the family and may heighten familial conflict (Aldous, 1974).

The role change necessitated because of having a new baby is a case in point. Ventura (1987), in a qualitative study of middle-class couples, found that 35 percent of first-time mothers and 65 percent of fathers reported feeling stressed because of multiple role demands. Data were collected at the third month postpartum. Mothers described juggling parenting roles with home and work schedules and having very

* *The changes in family roles throughout the family life cycle are explored in Chapter 6.*

little time for themselves. Fathers' portrayed the stresses as being linked to career and work responsibilities.

INFORMAL FAMILY ROLES

As stated previously, there are specific explicit *formal* family roles operating in families, such as husband–father, wife–mother, and child–sibling in the two-parent nuclear family. Within each of these positions are associated roles and clusters of expected, homogeneous behaviors. Family roles can be classified into two categories: formal or overt roles and informal or covert ones. Whereas formal roles are explicit roles that each family role structure contains (father–husband, etc), informal roles are implicit, often not apparent on the surface, and are played to meet the emotional needs of individuals (Satir, 1967) and/or to maintain the family's equilibrium.

Feldman and Scherz (1967) underscore the salience of looking at both types of roles within a family:

> The family operates through roles that shift and alter during the course of the family's life. Roles can be explicit or instrumental; they can be implicit or emotional. . . . The healthy family carries out explicit and implicit roles. . . . according to age, competence and needs during all the different stages of family life. (p. 67)

A family member will play many roles in a family, both covert and overt, with some of these roles being shared. The existence of informal roles is necessary to fulfill the integrative and adaptive requirements of the family group. Kievit (1968) explains that

> Informal roles have different requirements, less likely based on age or sex and more likely based upon the personality attributes of individual members. Thus, one member may be the mediator, seeking possible compromises when the other family members are engaged in conflict. Another may be the family jester, who provides gaiety and mirth on happy occasions, and a much needed sense of humor in times of crisis and distress. Other informal roles may exist and emerge, as the needs of the family unit shift and change. In working with families, awareness of the informal roles may facilitate insight into the specific nature of problems faced and in turn possible solutions. Effective performance of informal roles can facilitate the adequate performance of the formal roles. (p. 7)

The following are some examples of other informal or covert roles described in the literature (Benne and Sheats, 1948; Hartman and Laird, 1983; Kantor and Lehr, 1975; Satir, 1972; Vogel and Bell, 1960). These informal roles may or may not contribute to the stability of the family—some of them are adaptive and others detrimental to the ultimate well-being of the family.

- *Encourager.* The encourager praises, agrees with, and accepts the contribution of others. In effect he or she is able to draw out other people and make them feel that their ideas are important and worth listening to.
- *Harmonizer.* The harmonizer mediates the differences that exist between other members by jesting or smoothing over disagreements.
- *Initiator–contributor.* The initiator–contributor suggests or proposes to the group new ideas or changed ways of regarding group problems or goals. Kantor and Lehr (1975) refer to this type of role as a "mover" role characterized by the initiation of action.
- *Compromiser.* The compromiser is one of the parties to the conflict or disagreement. The compromiser yields his or her position, admits error, or offers to come "halfway."
- *Blocker.* The blocker tends to be negative to all ideas rejecting without and beyond reason. Kantor and Lehr (1975) label this role the opposer.
- *Dominator.* The dominator tries to assert authority or superiority by manipulating the group of certain members, flaunting his or her power and acting as if he or she knows everything and is the paragon of virtue.
- *The Blamer.* This role is similar to the blocker and the dominator. The blamer is a fault-finder, a dictator, a bossy "know it all."
- *Follower.* The follower goes along with the movement of the group, more or less passively accepting the ideas of others, serving as an audience in group discussion and decision.
- *Recognition Seeker.* The recognition seeker attempts in whatever way possible to call attention to self and his or her deeds, accomplishments, and/or problems.
- *Martyr.* The martyr wants nothing for self but sacrifices everything for the sake of other family members.
- *The Great Stone Face.* The person playing this role lectures incessantly and impassively on all the "right" things to do, just like a computer. Satir (1975) calls this informal role the superreasonable.
- *Pal.* The pal is a family playmate who indulges self and excuses family members' behavior or his or her own regardless of the consequences. He or she usually seems irrelevant.
- *The Family Scapegoat.* The family scapegoat is the identified problem member in the family. As a victim or receptacle for the overt and covert family

tensions and hostilities, the scapegoat serves as a safety valve.

- *The Placator.* The placator is ingratiating, always trying to please, never disagreeing, talking out of both sides of his or her mouth—in short, a "yes person."
- *The Family Caretaker.* The family caretaker is the member who is called upon to nurture and care for other members in need.
- *The Family Pioneer.* The family pioneer moves the family into unknown territory, into new experiences.
- *The Irrelevant One or Distractor.* The distractor is irrelevant; by exhibiting attention-getting behavior he or she helps the family avoid or ignore painful or difficult matters.
- *The Family Coordinator.* The family coordinator organizes and plans family activities, thereby fostering cohesiveness and combatting family sadness.
- *The Family Go-between.* The family go-between is the family "switchboard"—he or she (often the mother) transmits and monitors communication throughout the family.
- *The Bystander.* The bystander role is similar to "the follower" except in some cases more passive. The bystander observes but does not involve himself or herself.

Two informal roles that warrant further discussion are the scapegoat and the go-between roles. The first of these is the scapegoat role, a role adopted by a member to preserve the family and maintain homeostasis. The family member who is constantly scapegoated usually serves to divert attention from a disturbance between the spouses. As described by Ackerman (1966), when the marital pair is in conflict, the attention is focused on the scapegoat and the system is preserved.*

The second informal role that is common in families is that of the go-between (Zuk, 1966). The go-between or intermediary role is usually taken by the mother. In this role the person acts as a "switchboard" between family members, relaying communication from one member to another. In so doing, the direct communication between other family members is blocked. As the switchboard through which all communication must go, the go-between assumes a covert position of power, and by passing along only those messages considered suitable, the go-between acts as a censor. She or he thus becomes a central figure in the family, acting as a confidant to its members. And as the center of the family communication network the go-between is typically in charge of settling all disputes and insuring fairness to all sides. However, when disputes or conflicts do not become resolved, the go-between often gets blamed. Consistently having one person act as an intermediary is dysfunctional in that it is an emotional distancing mechanism and promotes estrangement between the other members of the family, because they are discouraged from communicating directly with each other. Satir (1972) discusses the consequences of communicating via a third person.

> If the family habitually transacts business without all the members present, and also has little spare time, then family members get to know each other through a third person. I call it *acquaintance by rumor.* The problem is that most people forget about the rumor part and treat whatever it is as fact. (p. 266)

The presence of a go-between role is revealed in the family's communication patterns. In interviews, it will be observed that the go-between answers for the children or other spouse when not directly questioned. In addition to talking for other family members, he or she usually gets in the way of messages elicited from or received by family members.

Learning Informal Roles

How do family members come to play these various informal roles within the family? Most learning of these roles occurs through (1) role modeling; (2) filling in "vacuums" where they exist in the family (if there is no leader or decision maker playing the instrumental role, a member of the group will naturally emerge to fill this role); and (3) selective reinforcement a child receives to behaviors he or she exhibits in the family when imitating adult members. The child experiments with various roles in play, receives selective reinforcement for certain roles, and eventually finds informal roles that are comfortable.

Through selective reinforcement of certain behaviors by parents and significant others, children are molded to play specific informal, covert roles. This selective parental reinforcement may occur because of early *labeling* of the child; this labeling leads to a self-fulfilling prophecy. Parents label children for a variety of reasons: projection, comparison with siblings, past unresolved personal needs, and so on. A study of large families (Bossard and Boll, 1956) found that there were a number of specialized roles and labels given to the children. Eight informal roles, which result in or from labels, existed: (1) the responsible one, (2) the popular one, (3) the socially ambitious one, (4) the studious one, (5) the family isolate, (6) the irresponsible one, (7) the sickly one, and (8) the spoiled one. These labels are likely to exist in complementary pairs in a family.

* *Chap. 17 discusses this problem in greater detail.*

Thus if a "sickly" child is identified in a family, the family usually labels another as the "healthy one"; if a "dumb one" is present, there is usually a "smart one." Parents are continually comparing their children with each other.

All labeling limits the way an individual may act or develop. True negative labeling—where adverse adjectives are used—occurs when parents and/or significant others label a child according to an attribute or behavior that indicates the child is inferior or unlovable. Because the parents see these labels as bad, the child sees himself or herself in the same light. Initially parents condemn the child; later the child, through identification with parental labels, internalizes the parental label and condemns himself or herself. Negative labeling has been identified as an antecedent to both depression and lowered self-esteem (Mishel, 1974).

As a result of early negative labeling and the internalization of these labels, individuals often develop certain limited ways of perceiving themselves and of reacting to others called "life games" or "scripts"; these restrict and limit a person's adaptability and repertoire of interpersonal skills (Lange, 1970). In other words, a script is formed in early childhood based on messages and labels (both verbal and nonverbal) that a child receives from parents, such as parental perceptions of the child related to his or her worth, lovableness, sexual status, work, responsibility, and dependency. "Life patterns," which include suicide, obesity, and recurrent physical illness—especially when treatable and preventable—are all examples of tragic scripts (Lange, 1970).

VARIABLES AFFECTING ROLE STRUCTURE

As with the family power structure, there are major factors that influence both formal and informal roles. These factors include (1) social class, (2) family forms, (3) cultural background, (4) family life cycle stage, (5) role models, and (6) situational events—in particular health/illness problems.

Social Class Differences

Lower-class Families. The functions of family life in terms of family roles is, of course, greatly influenced by the demands and necessities put upon the family by the larger social structure. Thus, in response to our society's "benign neglect" of poor, lower-class families of all ethnic groups, a variety of family role adaptations have evolved as a means of solving the recurrent problems and issues arising from their disadvantaged class position. Single-parent families are the most numerous type of family form that is poor. Poverty is the most predominant feature of single-parent families. Thirty-five percent of all single-parent families live in poverty (Gelman et al, 1985).

Marital Roles. Marital stability in the lower class is far more precarious than in other social classes, with divorces being two to six times greater among the unskilled labor group than among the professional middle class. The high rate of unemployment among the very poor is a major stressor in the marital relationship and a significant cause of its dissolution.

Several studies have found that lower-class marriages tend to provide less companionship than middle-class marriages. Furthermore, the marital therapeutic role is usually attenuated, or hardly present, in that emotional isolation from each other is expected. Personal and marital happiness are positively correlated with companionship and sociability with the spouse. In studying marriages among the lower class, Bradburn (1970) found that a strong relationship existed between personal happiness and marital satisfaction and that the marital relationship was much less satisfying to mates among the lower social class.

The lower-class family is a relatively loose-knit structure, although the roles of the marital partners and their division of responsibilities are formal. In many poor families there is a sharp demarcation of family roles based on whether the jobs are located inside or outside the home. These firm lines of authority serve to reinforce the emotional distance of the mates. The husband generally plays a minimal role in the low-income family, often conceiving of his role as being simply the provision of money to meet material needs. The lower-class wife's role, in turn, is expanded, and she often performs the majority of functions in the home, in addition to child rearing (Besmer, 1967).

Parental Roles. Because typically the affective and social needs of women are not met by their husbands, they develop greater emotional attachment to children as compensation for the emotional distance and lack of communication with their husbands. A peer relationship often develops between the mother and her children of either sex. A son may be expected to contribute economically at an early age and become the man of the family (Besmer, 1967).

In the poor family, the parenting role is of central importance to the mother, with mother being more traditional in her outlook toward child rearing (eg, a greater emphasis on respectability, obedience, cleanliness, and discipline of young children) when compared with the middle-class parent, who centers more on developing self-reliance and independence in children and takes more cognizance of developmental and psychological principles in the parent–child relationship. In other words, the focus of parenting in the poor family is on fulfillment of maintenance functions—providing food for the children, making sure they eat, have adequate rest, bathe, get to school on time—and on the maintenance of order and discipline in the home (Besmer, 1967).

Sibling Roles. When the children are older, the sibling roles acquire significance as a socializing agent far beyond that seen in the middle class. When there is a breakdown in communication between parents and children, the sibling subsystem tends to encourage expression of opposition to parental control (Besmer, 1967). Peer groups are also very important, especially for boys who seek masculine models, given the central role of the mother and the more passive role of the father in child rearing.

Working- and Middle-class Families. Komarovsky (1964) found in her qualitative study of unskilled and skilled blue-collar workers and their families that the more educated the husband, the greater the degree of emotional closeness and companionship in marriage. This was confirmed by later studies. In middle-class marriages companionship is a strong reason for the initiation and continuance of a marriage, an aspect that is stressed by a large number of families as being the chief end of marriage. In Blood and Wolfe's (1960) large study of the marital relationships of working-class and middle-class families from both urban and agrarian settings, about one-half of the wives from both environments identified "companionship in doing things together with the husband" as the most valuable aspect of marriage. Additionally, middle-class couples report more sexual satisfaction in their marriages than do partners of the lower class.

Working-class families generally tend to have more traditionally based family roles than middle-class families—the husband being more authoritarian in his role as head of the household. There is less joint planning and less of an egalitarian role relationship than in the middle-class family, but again there is wide variation, with the educational level of the spouses a prime factor (see Chap. 11).

Child rearing is now generally a shared role of middle-class parents, and their role behavior toward their children differs qualitatively from the lower-class family. It has been pointed out that one major reason for this may be the unconscious molding of a child to survive in the world as experienced by the parents. For instance, if a family is poor, parents expect that their boys will probably have to work in a menial position where obedience, respect for authority, and conformity are stressed. Hence, training that promotes creativity, questioning, and independence would be counterproductive to what the child needs when he matures and has to relate and survive in society. In contrast, middle-class parents are more concerned with psychological growth, individual differences, independence, and self-reliance in their children. These traits encouraged by middle-class parents are functional to success in the middle-class occupational life (Kohn, 1969).

Family Forms

The majority of the families we serve are not the typical "idealized" two-parent traditional nuclear families. The 1990 National Census (U.S. Bureau of the Census, 1991) confirmed the decline of the two parent family household. In March, 1990, 26 percent of all U.S. households consisted of married-couple families with children under 18 years of age. Another 30% of married couples had either adult children or no children living with them. About 12 percent of family households were maintained by women alone. Twenty-nine percent of households were non-family units, one third of these consisted of persons living alone. The type of family form, as explained in more detail in Chapter 1, greatly influences the family's role structure. Because single-parent and step-parent families are probably the two most common variant family forms, these two types of family forms will be described in terms of their unique role arrangements and role stresses.

Roles in the Single-parent Family. The number of single-parent families has swelled rapidly in the last decade. Fifty percent of all black families, 20 percent of all Hispanic families, and 15 percent of all white families in 1985 were single-parent families (U.S. Bureau of the Census, 1985). The three primary streams swelling this number are divorces, births out of wedlock, and desertions of spouses. Most single-parent families are headed by mothers, although fathers are increasingly heading single-parent families. About 20 percent of single-parent families are headed by a man (U.S. Bureau of the Census, Feb. 1991). Fathers as single parents are much better situated economically than mothers. One reason for this is the father's higher educational attainment (Nortan and Glick, 1986).

Two prominent role features of these families are (1) role overload and role conflicts and (2) role changes of the single parent. The parent must fulfill both mother and father roles, in addition to lacking the support of a marital relationship. Single parents tend to be either overloaded with roles or in conflict over their various role commitments, because they have double tasks to assume. With a spouse to depend on, there is some role flexibility (if the child-care and housekeeping roles are shared). And even though the single parent is freed from the responsibilities of marital roles, other adult relationships often enter in and create demands on the single parent's precious time. About 80 to 90 percent of the mothers who are single parents will eventually remarry, necessitating another role change—relinquishing the father's role and forming new marital and parental roles (Le Masters, 1974; Macklin, 1988). Because most single parents also work, high job/family role strain and reduced levels of wellness were found in a study conducted by Burden (1986).

Significant research has been generated by behavioral scientists who have studied the single-parent family with a view to determining whether the single-parent family is detrimental to children. Mueller and Cooper (1986) and Nock (1988), in summarizing research findings in this area, point out that there is abundant evidence that the *mere absence* of a father in a family has a detrimental effect on a child's educational and occupational attainments. Factors such as how competently the mother handles her child-care roles, however, are often cited as being very crucial here.

Roles in the Step-parent Family. With the tremendous increase in the number of divorces (the divorce rate for first marriages in 1984 was between 40 and 50 percent) and remarriages (75 percent of the divorced remarry, one-half within 3 years) we have a tremendous increase in step-parent families (Family Service of America, 1984). In 75 percent of these cases, this type of family form denotes the entry of a new husband and surrogate father (step-father), rather than stepmother, into a previously established female-headed single-parent family.

Step-parent families are at higher risk of serious problems than families of "first marrieds" or "second marrieds" with no children: 60 percent of all second marriages end in divorce (Kantrowitz and Wingert, 1989). One of the primary reasons for this is the greater complexity involved with integrating the stepfather into an already established family, coupled with the mixed allegiance the wife–mother experiences—to her new husband on the one hand and to her children on the other.

There has been growing research interest on the step-parent family and the adjustments and the roles of its members. In a groundbreaking study, Fast and Cain (1966) identified role confusion as a major familial problem. The step-father and mother were both uncertain about whether the step-father should assume the role of parent or nonparent. These authors noted the following problem areas: (1) denial that any interpersonal problems were present; (2) hypersensitivity of step-parent to suggestions or criticism; and (3) the newly formed couples' scapegoating of the children, perceiving them to be the source of all their conflicts and marital problems.*

Perhaps the underlying issues creating role confusion for the step-father and the resultant family disequilibrium are the issues of child rearing and disciplining of children. As discussed in Chapter 15, the diversity in child-rearing practices and values is great. Each parent draws on his or her own family background when defining child-rearing beliefs, practices, and discipline. And it is difficult to compromise in these values and beliefs, because many of them are not objectively based. When parents enter into a relationship in which the step-father heads the household but is not really the parent, synthesis of these values and rules is problematic. Furthermore, the children, through exposure to their natural parents' child-rearing practices, have developed their own behaviors and expectations of what is acceptable or unacceptable behavior, for both themselves and their parents. In the step-parent family the step-father has no biological rights over the children, and whatever parental rights he may have must be granted him by his wife. This places the step-father into a rather untenable position. When conflict arises over the disciplining of a child, the mother feels a natural right to decide the issue. If the step-father goes ahead and disciplines the child, the mother will often either directly become angry, or more often, indirectly strike back by undermining him. This latter course is particularly devastating to the entire family and often exacerbates the conflict, with the mother being torn between the loyalty to her children and to her husband.

Children in step-parent families also have major difficulties in adjusting to their new households. Generally step children have more developmental, emotional, and behavioral problems than children in intact families (Kantrowitz and Wingert, 1989).

Cultural Variation

Culturally derived norms and values strongly influence how roles are carried out within a given family system. Knowledge of the core values, customs, and traditions are important for interpreting whether family roles in a family are appropriate (Holman, 1983).

In some cultures, formal family roles are performed by extended family members who hold other family

* *It is clear that if conflict exists between step-father and child (due to lack of clarity as to whether he should be a parent or not), the entire family is negatively affected, including the marital relationship.*

positions. A common example of this situation is when an uncle acts as a father surrogate in a single-parent family. Members of the extended family (such as a grandfather, uncle, or older brother) may, in some cultures, act as surrogate fathers even though the father is present, without causing any conflict or strained relationships. The maternal grandmother may also perform formal family roles, especially in black single-parent families.

Because so many married couples are culturally heterogeneous, a major problem in these types of marriages is often one of role incongruency. Because of the couple's dissimilar cultural backgrounds, the expectations the spouses have of their roles and their spouse's roles differ. Each marital partner may criticize the other for failure to carry out the marital or parental role as expected, while at the same time feeling guilty for not meeting the other's expectations (Hartman and Laird, 1983).

Family Developmental Stage

It is quite clear that the way in which family roles are enacted substantially differs from one life cycle stage of the family to another. The parental roles are a blatant example of this change. Being a parent to an infant requires 24-hour care of a totally dependent baby, while parenting an adolescent requires letting go of the adolescent while still providing guidance and support, as the adolescent differentiates from the family.

Role Models

When a family member is exhibiting or experiencing role problems (role transitions or role conflicts), assessing the role models of the troubled family member is helpful. This analysis is aimed at finding out about the early life of the family, when the individual was learning both his or her role and the counterpart's role (such as learning the role of a daughter, as well as a mother), and how those early experiences have affected his or her present role behaviors and difficulties. Our role behavior as parent or marital partner often imitates the roles we observed our parents playing. For example, it is not uncommon to find people tending to treat their children as their parents treated them in the past. With this observation in mind, family therapists have recently placed great importance on looking at the intergenerational aspects of clients' marital and parental roles.

Situational Events

Major situational life events confronting families unavoidably affect their role functioning. These situations are usually stressful events such as natural disasters, unemployment, or the wife–mother returning to work. The one situational factor to be described here is that of the impact of health–illness problems on family roles.

FAMILY ROLES DURING HEALTH AND ILLNESS

Although Chapter 16 elaborates on the entire area of the family's involvement in health care and health practices, one aspect of this broad area is what happens to family roles when family members are sick or disabled, and what factors influence the family role structure during illness. When a family member acquires a chronic, disabling illness and is taken care of at home, another role becomes primary—that of the caregiver. Summarization of this issue as well as the two above questions are addressed in this section.

Role of Mother in Health and Illness

It has become increasingly clear that in most families an important role subsumed under the mother–wife position is that of health leader and caregiver. Whatever criteria have been used in studies to measure health decision making and roles–including such measures as illnesses incurred and treated, medical and health services used, and primary source of family assistance—the pervasive and central role of the mother as prime health decision maker, educator, counselor, and caregiver within the family matrix has remained a constant finding (Litman, 1974). In this role, the mother defines symptoms and decides the "proper" disposition of resources. She also exerts substantial control over whether the children will receive preventive and curative services (Aday and Eichhorn, 1972; Diosy, 1956; Rayner, 1970), and acts as the main source of comfort and assistance in times of illness (Litman, 1974).

One of the ways one can surmise the importance of the mother's health leader role is by observing what happens to her and the family when she is ill and unable to carry on her roles. First of all, the mother–wife has been observed to assume the sick role only when it is absolutely mandatory, and then only reluctantly. Because her role performance is considered essential to family functioning, her illness tends to be quite disruptive and disorganizing (Mechanic, 1964). Usually, severe illness or prolonged incapacitation of the mother–wife is seen as a more serious blow to the family's functioning than is the incapacitation of the husband–father (although if his illness is prolonged, adverse economic reverberations are felt) (Litman, 1974).

The Caregiver Role

Numerous clinical observations and extensive research publications have recently made family nurses more aware of the serious issues facing caregivers because of the number of frail elderly and chronically ill receiving care in the home today. Studies have consistently documented the stresses and burdens that families, particularly caregivers, face when providing care to frail elderly and chronically ill members. Providing continuous home care may produce serious negative consequences to caregivers (Treas and Bengtson, 1987).

Hoenig and Hamilton's (1966) longitudinal study encapsulates the caregiver burden problem. They found that 66 percent of the families in their sample reported adverse effects on the household due to the patient's chronic illness. Providing physical nursing care was most burdensome, while the patient's excessive demands for companionship were second on the list.

It is well recognized that women assume a much greater burden of caregiving for aging parents than men do. Finley (1989) studied the reasons for this gender difference in caregiving and concluded that the caregiver role, like the household role, is institutionalized in society as being women's work. Society expects women to carry out this role in the family and the lack of contributions of males to family caregiving is not seriously challenged. Wives are the most common caregiver, and then daughters. Caregiving women tend to experience more health strains than caregiving men (Miller, 1990).

In some families, where two or more siblings are present, shared filial responsibility is seen. In Matthews and Rosner's (1988) study, they found that siblings formed a network in which each sibling took the actions of the other(s) into account. Some adult children provided regular assistance, some acted as a backup, some were circumscribed in their help (highly predictable but bounded), some were sporadic with their help, and some dissociated (could not be counted on). Styles of participation by adult children, then, varied tremendously, with number of siblings and gender composition of sibling group making the major difference in how extensive sibling participation in caregiving was.

Elderly people prefer to live in their own home; when an elderly person requires help the expectation is that the spouse will provide it. However, spouse caregivers, who are usually elderly themselves, are at high risk for developing health problems or exacerbating existing conditions because of the strain of caregiving and because of their own advanced age (Blieszner and Alley, 1990).

Role Changes During Illness and Hospitalization

In a period of crisis, such as that caused by the serious illness of a family member, the family structure is modified, the extent of modification depending on (1) to what degree the sick member is able to carry out his or her usual family roles and (2) the centrality of the family roles or tasks that are vacated. The roles taken on by the mother are, as discussed previously, a good example of the centrality of a member's roles. When illness results in the vacancy of critical roles the family often enters a state of disequilibrium in which role and power relationships are altered until new homeostasis is achieved (Fife, 1985; Hill, 1958).

The role changes which occur due to the loss or incapacitation of a family member may be of two basic types. First, the remaining family members have enough inner and outer resources that they are able to take on the basic and necessary role obligations and tasks that the sick family member is unable to assume—this is the functional way the situation is managed. Or second, they lack the needed inner and outer resources, and as a consequence, certain basic and necessary roles in the family are not performed or are performed unsatisfactorily. In other words, the adequately functioning family can either flexibly modify family roles to meet the demands of the situation or may call in resources and assistance from the outside to fill the vacuum. In dysfunctional families, however, this does not happen.

Because of the role changes necessitated due to the loss or incapacitation of a family member, role conflicts and role strain are often present, especially during the stage of family disequilibrium immediately following the loss or incapacitation, when family structure is in the transitional period. Either interrole or intrarole conflict may exist, as the family members are "forced" to accept new roles and have had little opportunity to learn these roles or to rearrange all their other role responsibilities. Role strain/stress is often the outcome. The family members burdened with the acquisition of new roles may feel worried, anxious, and guilty because of feelings that they are not doing a competent job in their new roles or that with these added responsibilities, their role complex is excessively demanding and unmanageable.

Once a family has achieved a new equilibrium in response to a sick member's inability to perform his or her roles adequately, a similar reintegration must take place when that member resumes his or her place in the family unit. Understandably, having once gone through the process of adapting, the other members may well be reluctant to again "reshuffle" family roles and tasks, despite the recovery or reentry of the "lost" member. One sees this reluctance even in the most well-functioning families, because the process of reintegrating a family member entails the difficulties and problems that are part of any disorganization before a new (in this case, renewed) balance is achieved.

FAMILY ROLE STRUCTURE: APPLYING THE FAMILY NURSING PROCESS

□ ASSESSMENT QUESTIONS

An assessment of family roles primarily focuses on the characteristics of the formal and informal role structure, coupled with a consideration of how sociocultural and situational factors affect family role structure. There are four broad areas for the assessment of the family role structure:

1. The formal role structure.
2. The informal role structure and types of relationships.
3. Role models.
4. Variables affecting role structure.

Formal Role Structure

Each family member's position and roles are described by addressing the following questions:

1. What formal positions and roles do each of the family members fulfill? Describe how each family member carries out his or her formal roles.
2. Are these roles acceptable and consistent with the family members' and family's expectations? In other words, are there any conflicts present?
3. How competently do members perform their respective roles?
4. Is there flexibility in roles when needed?

Informal Role Structure

Questions pertinent to this area include:

1. What informal or covert roles exist in family, who plays them, and how frequently or consistently are they enacted? Are members of the family covertly playing roles different from those that their position in the family demands that they play?
2. What purposes do the identified covert or informal roles serve?
3. If the informal roles are dysfunctional in the family, who enacted these roles in previous generations?
4. What is the impact on the person(s) who play this (these) dysfunctional informal family roles?

Role Models

1. Who were (or are) the models that influenced family members in their early life, who gave feelings and values about, for example, growth, new experiences, roles, and communication techniques?
2. Who specifically acted as role model for the mates in their roles as parents, and as marital partners, and what were they like? From this information a family member can be helped to see how past models influence his or her expectations and behavior (Satir, 1983).
3. What is the impact on the person(s) who play this (these) roles? (Hartman and Laird, 1983).

In analyzing the informal role structure, an important area to describe relates to the types of role relationships within the subsystems of the family. Role relationships can be observed and assessed within each of the family subsystems, thus adding further information on both the adequacy of those sets of relationships and also the informal roles played within the subsystems. In assessing marital, parent–child, and sibling relationships, it is suggested that reference be made to the types of dyadic relationships discussed previously (complementary, symmetrical, and parallel), which will assist in describing the nature of the subsystem role relationship.

In identifying the formal and informal roles that family members play, Satir (1972) questions patients about their roles by asking: "You wear three hats . . . individual, marital partner, and parent. I can see the parent, but where are the other two?" "Before marriage you were Miss So and So. What happened to her?" (pp. 174–175). Satir also explicitly teaches family members about their roles by listing the three basic roles—individual, marital partner, and parent—on a blackboard and explores their responses to interactions in these different roles and what other response options are available.

Variables Affecting Role Structure

- **Social class influences.** How does social class background influence the formal and informal role structure in the family?
- **Cultural influences.** How is the family's role structure influenced by the family's cultural and religious background?
- **Developmental or life cycle influences.** Are the present role behaviors of family members developmentally appropriate?
- **Situational events, including health and illness changes.**
  1. How have health problems affected family roles? What reallocation of roles and tasks have occurred?
  2. How have the family members who have had to assume new roles adjusted? Is there evidence of role stress and/or role conflicts as a result of these role shifts?
  3. How has the family member with the health problem reacted to her or his change or loss of a role(s)?

FAMILY NURSING DIAGNOSES

Families are continually bombarded with demands for change—either because of normal developmental transitions or because of the various situational stressors families experience. Health stressors are one prime example of demands families face. Stressors/demands require family role changes. If family members do not have the requisite knowledge, skills, or emotional readiness for adjusting to the needed role changes, then role stress, role strain, role conflict, role overload, role loss, role insufficiency, and so on, may result. One important role of the family nurse in this regard is to assist families to identify role transitions so that information about the new role may be provided to prevent role problems.

Role problems are frequently observed by family nurses. They may not, however, be identified as role problems, because there are so many interrelationships and overlaps between problems. Any of the above role problems may be stated as a family nursing diagnosis, remembering that role problems involve at least two people: the role occupant and his or her role partner(s). Because these role problems are still very general, defining characteristics and related factors should also be stated.

In reviewing the list of nursing diagnoses approved by the North American Nursing Diagnosis Association (NANDA), the diagnoses given in Table 12–1 relate to role problems (McFarland and McFarlane, 1989). It should be noted here that only one of these diagnoses mention "role" in the diagnostic title, but actual and potential role problems could be one of the related factors within the nursing diagnoses. Included under altered role performance are four more specific role problems: role transition, role distance, role conflict, and role failure. Defining characteristics of each of these types of role problems are seen on Table 12–2.

TABLE 12–1. NANDA NURSING DIAGNOSES RELATED TO ROLE TRANSITIONS/ROLE PROBLEMS

NANDA Nursing Diagnoses	Role Problems
Anticipatory grieving	Related to role loss
Dysfunctional grieving	Related to role strain
Social isolation	Related to role change
Alteration in family processes	Related to role conflicts
Potential alteration in parenting	Related to role overload
Alteration in parenting	Related to role change
Potential for violence	Related to role conflict
Altered role performance	Related to role loss and strain
Impaired home maintenance management	Related to role failure or role distance
Body image disturbance	Related to role loss
Family coping diagnoses	Related to role insufficiency or role ambiguity

*These are only samples of role problems which could be associated with the accompanying nursing diagnoses.

In *Handbook of Nursing Diagnoses,* Carpenito (1987) also lists nursing diagnoses associated with medical diagnostic categories. For instance, for spinal cord problems many associated nursing diagnoses are listed, but in particular three dealing with role problems are identified. They are alteration in family processes, potential social isolation, and potential alteration in parenting (altered role performance should also be listed). The NANDA diagnoses are helpful guides. Because they are predominantly oriented toward the individual client, however, they are not sufficiently inclusive.

FAMILY NURSING INTERVENTIONS

Assessment and diagnosis guides health professionals in their planning and implementation strategies. Role transitions and role problems can create substantial disequilibrium and stress throughout the entire family system, even though on the surface only one or two family members seem to be affected. This is due to the high degree of interdependency between the subsystems and "the ripple effect." Hence, teaching and counseling strategies, as well as coordination/case management and referral strategies, are often used to ameliorate role transitions and role problems.

Johnson (1986) summarizes the general nursing interventions appropriate for role transitions and role problems. She refers to these interventions as "role theory strategies." Johnson's role theory strategies include:

- Helping the family members identify the significant cues of the other family members (eg, teaching parents how to distinguish between hunger crying and crying for attention in newborns).
- Clarifying expectations about the needed roles (family members identify their expectations for new roles).
- Strengthening the family members' abilities to enact a new role. Teaching strategies are used here.
- Rewarding the new role-taking behaviors.
- Helping the family member to modify the new role by helping him or her see how the role fits into his or her role complex.
- Reinforcing the feedback of the "relevant others."

Role Supplementation Strategies for Role Transitions

Role supplementation consists of a set of interventions suggested by Meleis (1975) and Meleis and Swendsen (1978) for facilitating role change and preventing role failure or role insufficiency. Role supplementation strategies can be either preventive, used to clarify role insufficiency, or therapeutic, used with individuals who are experiencing role insufficiency (Morehead, 1985).

TABLE 12–2. TYPES OF ALTERED ROLE PERFORMANCE (NANDA DIAGNOSIS AND DEFINING CHARACTERISTICS

Role Transition
- Change in capacity to perform role.
- Change in other's perception or expectations of role.
- Change in usual pattern of responsibility.
- Feelings of anger and depression.
- Inability to achieve desired role.
- Refusal to participate in role.

Role Distance[a]
- Uncertainty about role requirements.
- Lack of knowledge of role.
- Different role perceptions.

Role Conflict
- Frustration in role or conflict of roles; intra- or interrole conflict.
- Ambivalence about role.
- Incongruent or incompatible role expectations.
- Confusion.
- Inadequate problem-solving skills.

Role Failure
- Loss of role skills.
- Difficulty learning new roles.
- Withdrawal.
- Inability to achieve desired role.
- Refusal to participate in role.

[a]Role distance is present when a person's role behavior differs from socially prescribed expectations.
From: McFarland and McFarlane (1989).

Role transitions involve adding new roles and dropping others. Role transitions are created because of developmental changes and situational changes including health-related stressors. The result of unsuccessful role transition is role insufficiency, role failure, and role distance. Role transitions involve role loss; hence some reactions to loss or grieving should be expected.

Role supplementation consists of components, strategies, and process. The two components are (1) role clarification, understanding the specific information and cues needed to enact the role; and (2) role taking, being able to imagine yourself in a particular role and assuming the perspective of the other person. Roles are paired and learned in pairs. Hence, if an individual learns the expectations of a parenting role, theoretically he or she should also know the role of the role partner, in this case the child.

The strategies used to accomplish role clarification and role taking are role modeling, role rehearsal, and reference group interactions. Role modeling is a very useful teaching strategy. Through modeling, the desired behavior is performed by the health professional for the family member to imitate; the imitation eventually becomes part of the family member's own behavioral repertoire (Goldenberg and Goldenberg, 1985). For example, a family nurse may serve as a role model for a caregiver by showing how to help the stroke patient ambulate and to praise every little improvement that is made.

Role rehearsal is a second role supplementation strategy suggested by Meleis (1975). Here the role behavior and reactions of significant others are mentally enacted. This strategy is very helpful when a new role can be anticipated. This mental practice prepares the individual for a future role change. The nurse can effectively use role reversal with parents, marital partners, and in parent–child and sibling relationships. Helping family members to rehearse their interactions is good anticipatory guidance. For instance, there may a helpful strategy to use when helping a step-father deal with his step-children who are displaying anger and resistance toward his parenting efforts.

The third role supplementation strategy is reference group interaction. Reference groups are groups with which an individual or family identifies. Self-help groups can become powerful reference groups for individuals and families. Self-help groups assist their members to adapt to their new roles by sharing feelings and perceptions in the group and offering practical solutions to vexing issues related to the new role. Nurses often initiate referrals of family members to a self-help group and, in some cases, lead a self-help group or act as a consultant to the group.

The process used in role supplementation is communication. Through communication new information needed to enact the new role or role options can be shared. Feelings can be ventilated—such as feelings of anger, depression and frustration over difficulties in learning the new role. Exploration of family members' perception of what has changed and how the role change has affected them is a vital area to discuss. And lastly, through communication clients should be encouraged to seek out new information and explore role options themselves.

Interventions for Role Strain

Several ways have been suggested to deal with role strain. Family nurses can explore the following options with family members who are experiencing role strain:

1. Redefining the role in terms of what behaviors are considered adequate role performance.
2. Examining an individuals's role complex (the various roles the role occupant plays) and setting priorities within a role and among roles.
3. Role bargaining or role negotiation with role partners so that role occupants achieve a set of positions that collectively are relatively equitable and rewarding. Role negotiation involves influencing the members of one's role set so that they agree to changes in the role and the allocation of resources.
4. Reduced interaction with role partners. If role partners have a high interdependency on each other this tactic usually leads to unsuccessful role bargaining and role distancing. Partial withdrawal from interaction may not relieve role stress (Hardy and Hardy, 1988).

Interventions for Role Fatigue of Caregivers

Respite care and participation in self-care groups are recommended for those primary caregivers who are strained in their caregiver role (Dell Orto, 1988). Studies of caregiving role strain and reports from family support groups indicate that regularly scheduled periods of respite are essential to counter role fatigue and stress (Pallett, 1990). Respite care refers to temporary care of disabled individuals for the purpose of providing relief to the primary caregiver (Dell Orto, 1988). Friends and family sometimes serve as surrogate caregivers. Nurses can assist families in locating community resources for respite care, such as adult day care, temporary nursing home placement, and/or intermittent home care. Unfortunately there is a scarcity of funding for respite services. Pioneering efforts have been made by groups and organizations to implement respite care programs for the developmentally disabled, the physically disabled, and the mentally ill. Some family caregiving situations are very intense, and if left without intervention such as respite or home care, increased family stress and accelerated deterioration in family functioning may result.

Participation in a formal self-help support group for caregivers has proved to be important in boosting morale. Family caregiver groups have been found to be very helpful in a number of research studies (Pallett, 1990). Feelings and frustrations, as well as practical solutions, are shared in groups.

Interventions for Role Distance or Role Inadequacy

Role distance or role inadequacy refers to a role occupant not fulfilling the role behaviors that are a part of that role. The role expectations are set by society and they are in conflict with the role's occupant's behavior.

Teaching strategies should be used here. Family members need to understand role requirements; they very much need information, because knowledge deficits are usually present. Focusing on clarifying perceptions and fostering awareness of prevailing expectations is recommended. In addition, showing respect for role behaviors that are culturally derived and comparing the role occupant's customs with current practices here is suggested.

Many fathers in our society have a role distancing problem—that is, they are not undertaking the father role that the culture today expects of them. Hanson and Bozett (1987) and Kunst-Wilson and Cronenwett (1981) recommend several tactics for nurses to use to promote greater active participation by fathers in family health care. These suggestions include:

1. Encourage fathers to attend clinics with their children and to attend prenatal clinics and family planning clinics with their wives.
2. Encourage fathers to join men's support groups and resource centers if they feel they need support to undertake new father roles.
3. Encourage fathers' participation in birthing and parenting classes.
4. Encourage spouses to negotiate infant and child care roles. Role sharing and role negotiation can help reduce role stress. Role negotiation involves an agreement among involved persons regarding the behaviors that are expected in an associated role.
5. Support fathers' active involvement in labor, delivery, and newborn care in the hospital.

Interventions for Role Conflict

Interventions for role conflict cover both intrarole and interrole conflicts. Guidelines for this problem include the following.

1. Before beginning to intervene, plan strategies to reduce or resolve role conflict. To do this, determine sources of stress and type of role conflict.
2. Encourage expression of frustration with role conflict.
3. Encourage family members to discuss their feelings about the roles in question.
4. Encourage family members to discuss their feelings and perceptions together and problem solve on their own behalf.
5. Assist family to set priorities.
6. Incompatibilities of roles may require family members to meet together. The nurse, acting as a facilitator, encourages the family members to explore role incompatibilities and to come up with a different allocation of roles or perhaps different role expectations.

Interventions for Role Failure

Role failure implies that the client has tried to carry out the role, but has failed. Role failure addresses the lack of knowledge and skills for a particular role. Strategies are aimed at resolving role failure problems and assist family members to achieve satisfactory role competence. Here teaching is a primary strategy. Teaching about role requirements is paramount. Counseling involves encouraging family members to voice their concerns and questions about their new role(s). Because clients' are often disappointed and frustrated about the new role, recognizing and praising each successful behavior is important. Strengths and resources the client possesses should also be recognized and supported. Behavior modification and contracting may be used here. Setting up a behavioral therapy plan involves tasks analysis (defining the tasks within the role), breaking the tasks into small chunks of information or skills, and then consistently reinforcing each small chunk of behavior or information as it is learned.

In conclusion, family nurses are able to intervene effectively to assist families with role transitions and role problems. Another benefit in assessing family roles is that the knowledge of the formal and informal role structure improves our understanding of family strengths and resources. This supplies us with important data for planning interventions to resolve health problems.

☐ STUDY QUESTIONS

1. Match the correct definition or description with the appropriate term.

TERMS

a. Role
b. Role taking
c. Position
d. Role making
e. Role enactment
f. Socialization
g. Role conflict
h. Reciprocal role
i. Role strain
j. Role patterning
k. Family homeostasis
l. Role sharing

DEFINITIONS

1. Status
2. Described as being empathetic.
3. Incompatibility of the role(s) (intrarole or interrole).
4. A set of behaviors of an occupant of a particular social position.
5. The process of learning family and adult roles in preparation for societal responsibilities.
6. Balancing in family structure to maintain stability.
7. Joint participation in fulfilling same role.
8. Complementary role.
9. The worry or guilt felt as a result of difficulty with role enactment or presence of role conflict.
10. The actual behavior exhibited in a role.
11. Allocation of roles and their associated tasks.
12. The generation of new behaviors for a certain position, based on ongoing feedback within a relationship.

Are the following statements True *or* False?

2. The most functional way of maintaining equilibrium in a family in the face of change is by use of role induction.

3. The principle of complementarity states that there must be a match in expectations and performance of roles by role partners in order for stability and harmony to be present in the relationship.

4. Paired relationships in the family refer to father–son and mother–daughter relationships.

5. For each of the roles making up the wife–mother and husband–father positions listed in the following table, indicate whether in the American family these roles are normatively shared or the primary responsibility of one or the other partner. If the trend is toward sharing or being more or less a single partner's role, indicate this with an arrow pointing up (increasing emphasis) or down (decreasing emphasis). A check (✓) indicates that role remains the same.

Role	Shared Role	Role of Wife–Mother	Role of Husband–Father
Provider			
Housekeeper			
Child care			
Recreational			
Kinship			
Therapeutic			
Sexual			
Companion			
Health leader			

6. From the two studies presented on the observed types of marriages (by Cline, and Cuber and Harroff), which conclusion would be the most accurate and practically significant?
   a. Well-functioning or long-standing marriages are distinguished from poorly functioning marriages.
   b. It was discovered that diverse patterns of marital relationships existed.
   c. A wide range of behaviors and roles existed in the marriages studied.
   d. Because there is no one type of marriage which fits the needs of most couples, acceptance and understanding of this diversity among couples is indicated.

7. When a wife is employed in a two-parent nuclear family with children, what are common role changes and conflicts experienced by the husband and the wife?

8. Identify three commonly seen differences in role structure between the lower- and middle-class families.

9. List five examples of informal roles seen in the family, indicating which of them could be functional.

10. The maintenance of informal roles is vital to the family because (select the best answer):
    a. It relieves the role overload of some members.
    b. Without covert roles the family could not exist.
    c. Each formal role has an associated informal role.
    d. Through the assumption of informal roles, family homeostasis is maintained and individual socioemotional needs are met.

11. Why are both formal and informal roles important to assess?

12. Give reasons why labeling is restrictive to an individual's growth and development.

13. Identify two role characteristics of single-parent families that act as stressors to the family and its members.

14. What are two prominent role problems within the step-parent family?

Are the following statements True *or* False?

15. When a family member is ill, the functional way of handling the situation is to leave the roles unfulfilled until he or she returns.

16. Role flexibility suggests that family members have the motivation and capacity to shift and reenact new roles when needed.

17. Middle-class parents are generally more concerned with promoting self-reliance and independence in their child-rearing practices, while lower-class parents stress respect and obedience.

Family Case Study*

After reading the following case study, answer questions 18 through 23.

Mr. and Mrs. G. are a young couple, married for 3 years, with a 2-year-old son. The 23-year-old husband is a garbage collector, earning $18,000 a year. He completed 2 years of high school; his 22-year-old wife is a high school graduate. (But the family nurse commented: "It is hard to believe in view of her poor vocabulary and illiterate handwriting that she had completed high school." The husband said: "She was sort of a dumbbell at school, but people liked her and she got through.")

Mr. G. is a slim tall man, slow moving and soft spoken. When asked what he liked about himself, he replied, "People tell me I'm easygoing but not a chump." The assessor observed his deceptively lazy attitude as the manner of a man who thinks that most people, particularly women, become too excited about things and foolishly so. He reports that he quit school at 14 because he did not like it. Since then he has held a number of unskilled jobs. Concerning his present occupation as garbage collector, he stated: "People laugh at you for being in this line of work. I don't know what's so funny about it. It's got to be done. There is no future in it, though, and the pay is terrible. I'm going to make a break for it as soon as I can. Everybody's looking out for me now, and something is bound to turn up pretty soon."

Both Mr. G. and his wife express satisfaction with their sexual relations and with the marriage in general. Mr. G. is in charge of the outside of house and repairs to their home, and Mrs. G. is in charge of the interior of the home and child.

A good deal of the communication between them is nonverbal. This type of communication pattern began during their courtship. When asked whether her husband had said he loved her when he proposed, Mrs. G. answered, "He just got softer and softer on me and I could tell that he did and we got to necking more and more and he wanted to go all the way and I didn't want to unless we were going to get married." The nurse asked whether he had ever said out and out that he could go for her or wanted her or anything like that. Mrs. G. said, "No, we don't go in for that kind of stuff." When she told him she was pregnant, "He looked a little funny when I told him, but he didn't say much. You know that's what's going to happen. After a while, when I began to show a lot, he asked me sometimes how I felt."

Mrs. G. was asked to describe their quarrels. She said they quarrel little, but when they do, it is about such things as his failure to help move the furniture or her failure to do something he demands. "We just get over it." He might "crab around and then he would know that he had been mean to me and makes it up." There is no conversation about such quarrels, but Mr. G. helps to dry the dishes or asks her if she likes a television program or wants something else. Mrs. G. felt that talking does no good, since it might worsen things.

When asked whether they like to talk about what makes people tick or to discuss the rights and wrongs of things, each said in separate interviews, "No, we don't hash things over." Mr. G. added, "It's either right or wrong—what is there to discuss?"

This "conversation of gestures" between Mrs. G. and her husband contrasts sharply with the communication characterizing her relationships with female relatives and friends. On many counts Mr. G. reveals her emotional life to the

* *Adapted by permission of Random House, Inc., from Blue-Collar Marriage, by Mirra Komarovsky with the collaboration of Jane H. Phillips. Copyright 1962, 1964, 1967 by Random House, Inc.*

latter. And this extends to spheres of experience beyond the "feminine world" of babies, housework, or gossip.

Mrs. G. sees her sister and her mother daily. "Oh yes," she said about her sister, "we tell each other everything, anything we have on our minds. We don't hold nothing back. We discuss the children, the house, cooking, and 'female things.'" But when asked whether she can talk to her husband, she answered, "Sure, I can talk to him about anything that has to be said." Her view is that "men and women do different things; he don't want to be bothered with my job of cleaning and children and I don't want to be bothered with his. He makes the big decisions and I don't have to bother with it. Sometimes we got to do the same things, something around the house and we have to tell each other."

When asked what helped her when she was in the "dumps," Mrs. G. replied, "Talking to my sister or my mother helps sometimes." When asked directly whether conversations with her husband ever have a similar effect, she replied, "No."

Mr. G. enjoys an active social life with his male friends and relatives, Mr. G. revealed to his father and his brother he fears that Mrs. G. was making a "sissy" out of their son, and he regularly consults with them about his occupational plans. He does not discuss the latter topics with his wife because "there is no need of exciting her for nothing. Wait until it's sure. Women get all excited and talk too much."

Mr. G. thinks the world of the fellows in his own clique whom he sees after supper several times a week and on Saturday afternoons. Mrs. G. does not always know where he meets his "friends" when he leaves in the evenings. Mr. and Mrs. G. testified independently that having a beer with the fellows is the best cure for his depressions.

Select the one *best answer referring to the family case study.*

18. This marriage was characterized as "happy" by both marital partners. This was because:
   a. Both come for same social class.
   b. Both shared same marital role expectations.
   c. Both were denying how really alienated they were from each other and how unsatisfactory their marriage was.
   d. Their sex life was adequate.

19. This marriage illustrates:
   a. The mates' lack of understanding of one another.
   b. An insufficient amount of communication in meaningful areas of family life.
   c. That marital companionship is not essential to make a satisfactory marriage.
   d. That both mates did not communicate openly with anyone.

20. This type of marriage is frequently seen in:
   a. Lower-class families.
   b. White, skilled working-class families.
   c. Disorganized families.
   d. Middle-class white families.

21. Through the couple's communication we can gather that:
   a. Both mates carry out traditional male–female roles.
   b. Mrs. G. would rather move out and be with her sister and friends.

c. Mr. G.'s occupational role is of central concern to him.
d. Mr. G. desires to raise his son to be "a man."

22. Which type of relationship does this marriage most closely fit?
a. Symmetrical
b. Parallel
c. Complementary

23. Complete a brief description of the couple's formal roles from what can be inferred from the narrative.

24. In the above case study, are there any potential or actual role problems manifested?

25. If the wife was going to vocational school and began to question her husband's traditional sex roles in the family, what kind of role problems might result? (Name at least one).

26. Suggest two strategies to ameliorate or resolve the role problem identified in question 25.

CHAPTER THIRTEEN

Family Values

Learning Objectives

1. Define the terms values, norms, and family rules, and give their significance relative to family assessment.
2. Describe the common outcome of a disparity in value systems between health worker and client.
3. Identify and briefly explain four important changes that have taken place in society and in family values in recent years.
4. Discuss the major value orientations of American society in terms of their significance today and their interrelationships with each other.
5. Identify four of the variables that influence the family's value system and that create value conflicts.
6. Given a case situation and using the value assessment process, identify the salient values operating within the hypothetical family and state a family nursing diagnosis in the area of values.
7. Describe the meaning and purposes of the value clarification process.

Family health assessment is not complete without an analysis of a family's central values, because the value system is one of the four highly interdependent structural dimensions of a family. Understanding what is important to a particular family is vital in terms of assessment, diagnosis, and health care intervention, for we know that what a family believes and values affects both the family's and its members' behavior. Moreover, when family values and beliefs are identified, we may better understand the family dynamics and behavior.

It needs to be recognized that as health care professionals we have the tendency to diagnose or label a family as pathological when they deviate from the dominant cultural values and norms. Most research on families is based on the majority culture (described below), and we must be particularly cautious about extrapolating these findings to all social classes and cultural groups, whose life conditions and traditions differ greatly from those of the dominant culture.

An accurate assessment of a family's value system should help us tailor our nursing interventions to a particular family or groups of similar families. We need to work within the family's value system and relate our services to goals that are important to the family being assisted. For instance, it is well accepted that "ideas and methods which least affect the patient's habits, beliefs, and values meet less resistance than those that attempt to alter existing behavior patterns and values (Dougherty, 1975, p. 441).

In assessing a family's value system it is also imperative for us, as health care providers, to recognize our own priorities and values and to examine carefully how our values and attitudes subtly—and sometimes not so subtly—affect our family-centered care. One ultimate goal in assessing family values is to demonstrate to families an appreciation of the inherent worth of different value systems (Clemen, 1977).

BASIC DEFINITIONS

One of the most developed definitions of *value* is by Rokeach (1973): "A value is an enduring belief that a specific mode of conduct or end-state of existence [such as freedom] is . . . preferable to the opposite or converse mode of conduct or end-state of existence" (p. 5). Values are central features of an individual's belief system due to their enduring quality; they are not short-lived attitudes. Values serve as guides to action (Rokeach, 1973).

Family values are defined as a system of ideas, attitudes, and beliefs about the worth of an entity or concept that consciously and unconsciously bind together the members of a family in a common culture (Parad and Caplan, 1965). The family's culture is a prime source of a family's value system and norms. In turn, the family group is a prime source of the belief systems, value systems, and norms that determine individuals' understanding of the nature and meaning of the world, their place in it, and how to reach their goals and aspirations.

Values serve as general guides to behavior and within families guide the development of family norms or rules. For instance, if a person values health and feels it is a desirable state, he or she is much more likely to engage in preventive health care and salubrious health habits. In addition, there will be a moral injunction (a norm or family rule) against "bad" health habits.

Values are not static. The potency, or primacy, of a family's values change over time, as the family and its members are exposed to different subcultures, as societal values undergo continual change, as the family developmentally evolves over time, and as particular situations demand a shift of priorities by the family.

Furthermore, families and individuals rarely behave according to consistent value patterns. Certain values we hold compete with other values we simultaneously hold, like the competition between valuing individualism and freedom versus valuing familism (meeting of the family's needs before personal needs).

Also certain values are amenable to conscious identification, whereas others are less susceptible to conscious expression. Simply put, some values are consciously held while others are not.

There is a hierarchical nature to values. Some values are more central, molding or influencing most aspects of our lives, while other values are more peripheral and have less influence, involving only certain aspects of our life-style and daily functioning. In other words, certain values have a greater priority or potency than other values, particularly when looking at a family at a given point in time.

A family's configuration of values ascribes meaning to certain critical events and at the same time suggests ways to respond to these situations. This configuration of values provides definitions of the time dimension; contains concepts concerning the responsibility and worth of the individual members of the family; ranks certain commonly held life goals; imposes a framework within which the pursuit of risks connected with the pleasure impulse takes place; defines what messages, thoughts, and feelings should and should not be shared and with whom; and lastly, involves a system of sanctions.

Values are learned from the family of origin, which is the basic transmitter of societal or cultural values from one generation to the next. The family of origin assimilates societal and cultural values and modifies them somewhat to match with its own values. Societal values change, with some values becoming more important than others; these value changes and swings greatly affect the family, profoundly affecting its own family values, norms, and ultimately its behavior.

Family values are not only a reflection of the society in which the individual or family resides, but also of the subculture(s) with which the family identifies. Most persons belong to a number of subcultures based on social class, ethnic background, occupational groups, peer groups, religious affiliation, and so forth. Subcultures exist within the larger, dominant culture, and so aspects of that value system also pervade the subculture. Thus members of a particular subculture respond to both subcultural and dominant value systems, although at different moments the values of one or the other may be more relevant to the individual or family. Obviously the greater the degree of congruence between a family's subcultural values and the community's values, the easier the individual's and family's adjustment, and the greater degree of success the family will meet in relating to the community.

Families will often have values that are not realizable. Sheer practical necessity can often distort a family's values in everyday life so that they become unrecognizable (Graedon, 1985). In assisting families, both their values and actual behaviors need to be understood—for what families say is important may be at striking variance with their actual behavior. In anthropology this is referred to as the real (family's actual behavior) versus the ideal (the family values espoused). The variance between the ideal and real is typically due to the family making a pragmatic adaptation to a particular social and historical context. Poor ethnic minority families often have had to compromise their values or ideals due to the harsh realities of their world.

Norms are patterns of behavior considered to be right in a given society and, as such are based on the family's value system. They are also modal behaviors. In other words, norms prescribe the appropriate role behavior for each of the positions in the family and society and specify how reciprocal relations are to be maintained, as well as how role behavior may change with the changing ages of occupants of these positions.

Family rules are an even more specific reflection of the family values than family norms. They refer to the specific regulations the family maintains as to what is acceptable and what is not. The family rules, guided by more abstract values, provide the stability, commonality, and guidance family members need. Holman (1979) suggests that family rules form the family culture, the shared meanings that define the individual character of each family as different from all other families.

An example of how family roles express the value system by which the family operates is the case of the Latino family. The high value of familism among Latino families translates to the norm and family rule that members of the extended family are all part of the "familia," and are to be treated as such. Values are also determinants of family rules about communication—perhaps what is discussed and not discussed and with whom. Recall the high value that respect for elders, especially fathers, has in some families, with a resultant family rule being to not openly challenge the father's decisions or actions.

Family rules are reflective of the family's level of functioning. Whall (1986b) corroborates this association by stating that in general "it is fair to say that dysfunctional families have dysfunctional rules since one begets the other" (p. 100).

DISPARITY IN VALUES SYSTEMS

Between Client and Health Care Professional

One of the primary stressors in relationships between health care workers and clients (family) is the social distancing created because of social class and/or cultural value differences. When the professional and client do not possess the same basic beliefs and values, the results are often divergent goals, unclear communication, and interactional problems. As professionals working within the health care system, we generally uphold the values of the white, Anglo-Saxon Protestant (WASP) dominant culture. Brink (1976) described the American nurses' value system thusly:

> The American nurse, educated in the United States, falls within the "Old Yankee" classification of value systems. American nurses are future-oriented, belong to a doing-oriented profession, are individualistic in decision-making, but lineally-oriented in the health institution, believe that disease is controllable, and view the human being as neither good nor evil, but ill (pp. 63–64).

This picture of health providers' having one common value orientation does not negate the reality that many nurses and nursing students come from diverse cultural and social class backgrounds and possess their own configuration of more particular values and goals, although also conforming to the central values of the health care system of which they are a part. Clients, on the other hand, come from all walks of life and more often than not hold different values than the health care worker. Because the class and cultural backgrounds of many clients differ from those of the health care professional, the possibility of value conflicts is present (Lauver, 1980).

The Danger of Stereotyping

As family nurses, we need to have basic information on social class and cultural differences, but must at the same time realize that studies and descriptions address *group* tendencies, not individuals. Therefore, our assessments must be individualized, recognizing the unique attitudes and qualities of the client involved. Yet to have any practical significance, one must be able to generalize and synthesize from relevant studies.

Murillo (1976), in writing about the Mexican-American family, speaks to the problem of generalizing and perhaps "stereotyping." In pondering on how to describe a traditional Mexican-American family, he writes:

> In an effort to solve this problem (there being no uniform pattern of family life), I have tried to temper my description of the "traditional" Mexican-American by describing it also in the context of a comparative cultural value system. . . . I will go further, however, and make explicit that the values discussed must be viewed from a probabilistic approach. That is, every value I attribute to a Mexican-American person or family should be understood basically in terms of there being a greater change or probability that the Mexican-American, as compared with the Anglo, will think and behave in accordance with that value. . . . In the final analysis, one must come to know and accept the uniqueness of the individual or specific family. Many Mexican-Americans are not only bilingual,

> but bicultural, and it is very worthwhile to ascertain the special blending of cultures one may encounter in a person or family in order to acquire a realistic understanding. (p. 17)

VALUE CHANGES IN AMERICAN SOCIETY

Since the 1960s the United States, as well as the world at large, has witnessed a profound revolution in ideas, values, and norms. Most of the literature suggests that the Civil Rights Movement marked the beginning of the cultural revolution. Because of other turbulent events in society and the family, a widening social stratification and rise in poverty and growth in consumerism and materialism (Samuelson, 1986), has continued to shape and change American cultural values. "All these events and more have shaken our society and its social institutions" (d'Antonio, 1983, p. 81). Although the family has been widely perceived as threatened by these multiple events and concomitant value shifts, turning the tide back to "the good old traditional days" appears futile, in spite of the fervent efforts of fundamentalist groups and other reactionaries.

Profound physical and social changes have also taken place. For example, in the last 200 years, the United States quadrupled in physical size and its population grew 52 times greater. We have gone from an overwhelmingly rural society to become a highly urbanized nation. Whereas only 1 percent of Americans were high school graduates in 1800, 76 percent of Americans now graduate from high school. And more recently, the country changed from an overwhelmingly white, Anglo-Saxon Protestant country to one with increasingly significant Catholic, Jewish, Asian, black, and Hispanic populations.

In recent years a number of authors (Aldous, 1987; Koten, 1987; Glick, 1989; Schwartz, 1987; & Yankelovich and Gurin, 1989) have suggested that the vitality of the traditional values (the Protestant ethic, essentially) has declined. Despite the continual clash between the new and traditional values and the resultant modification in values and priorities, a substantial amount of continuity in the American value system has, however, prevailed.

A discussion of American society's core/major value orientation, coupled with the recent value shifts, provides the foundations for understanding our primary family values today. The core values that appear to have continued salience are productivity/achievement; individualism; materialism/consumption; the work ethic; education; equality; progress and mastery of the environment; a future orientation; efficiency, orderliness, and practicality; rationality; quality of life and health; a "doing orientation;" and a tolerance for diversity. Some of these values are of lesser importance today and some are of greater importance. A discussion of this shift in priorities follows.

The more recent surveys of Americans and their values and life-styles indicate that Americans, particularly middle-class Americans, are a very heterogeneous group today. There is no one overarching core value orientation today like there was in the 1960s and 1970s. Koten (1987) of the *Wall Street Journal* agrees that there is no longer one set of values to which the middle class subscribes. "There are fewer things that everybody wants and fewer things that everyone feels compelled to do" (p. 25).

Shifting values have fueled institutional changes throughout society. Both Family Service America (1984) and Scanzoni (1987) describe surveys in which Americans, according to the values they reported, were divided into three groups. At one end of the continuum were the "traditionalists," those who espoused traditional values, such as preserving the good old days, duty, obligation, and hard work. At the other end of the continuum were the "new wave," the "progressives," those espousing emerging values of self-fulfillment, freedom, and individualism over authority. The middle-of-the-continuum group was composed of the vast majority of Americans. They valued some of the old and some of the new values and goals. Scanzoni (1987) reports that in one national survey 20 percent were traditionalists and another 20 percent new wavers or progressives, while 60 percent were middle-of-the-roaders. Most sociologists explain that our values are in a state of flux or transition. The increasing proportion of families that are either single-parent, blended, or cohabitating families, coupled with the widespread practice of divorce, lends evidence to the shifting from traditional, conventional values to individualistic, utilitarian values (Glick, 1989).

MAJOR VALUE ORIENTATIONS

In spite of the declining state of the Protestant ethic and the existence of other strongly conflicting values, a cluster of core values still molds and shapes, to a varying degree, American society, and thus also shapes family life and the behavior of health care professionals. Figure 13–1 depicts the most important personal values described by Americans in a large national survey conducted by Yankelovitch, Skelley and White.

Productivity/Individual Achievement

Individual achievement and productivity have been consistently identified as key traditional values in this society (D'Antonio, 1983; McKinley, 1964; Williams,

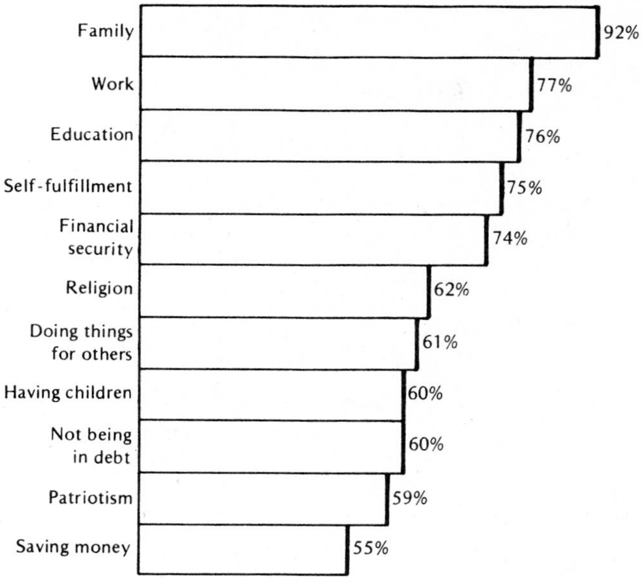

Figure 13–1.
Most important personal values. (From: Yankelovitch et al, 1975.)

1960). Success and achievement, the reputed outcomes of being productive, are corollary social values. In the middle class extensive stress is placed on personal achievement, especially occupational achievement. Each person, particularly the adult male, must prove himself or herself basically worthy of approval by acting in a productive manner toward some higher goal—for the male, in his occupation.

Because so much apprehension surrounds choice of occupational goals, there is an anxious postponement in selecting one's career. Many Americans also have not learned how to relax and enjoy life, as seen by their anxious preoccupation with activity and productiveness and the enormous numbers of people suffering from stress-related illnesses. Another behavioral consequence of our achievement value is its effects on individuals who do not have the required position and role adequacy for productiveness. For those people, the emphasis on achievement often leads to a lack of goals and norms and to alienation.

In order for a value to continue to mold a person's goals and behavior, a powerful system of social sanctions and rewards must be present. According to McKinley (1964), there are four major rewards available to the "successful," which are referred to as the "American Dream": material possessions, interpersonal approval and status, control over others, and control over self (autonomy).

Various types of interpersonal sanctions are employed against those individuals who are "unproductive," including the unemployed, those on welfare, or those who choose values markedly different from society's values. These responses range from gossip, laughter, and ridicule to social ostracism, isolation, or rejection. Members of society will vary their reactions depending on the society's evaluations of where the responsibility for unproductiveness lies and how important the deviation is. As a result of society's disapproval, many times the individual adopts those same attitudes toward himself or herself (ie, low self-esteem, lack of self-worth), a phenomenon referred to as "the self-fulfilling prophecy."

Individualism

In the numerous writings about value changes in American society and the family, there is agreement about the rising importance of individualism today (Glick, 1989; Schwartz, 1987). Individual freedom of choice is one of our central social values in Western societies according to Lesthaeghe (1983). The trend toward more individualism and away from familism has weakened but not killed the ideal of permanence in marriage.

Part of individualism and individual freedom of choice is the shift from a child-centered to a self-centered culture. This transformation indicates that people are becoming less firmly rooted in the traditional institutions of family, community, and church and more committed to individual goal attainment—unfettered by traditional obligations (Rossi, 1986).

Other authors, based on demographic trends, also emphasize that people in Western societies are becoming "averse to long-term commitments and increasingly focused on individual autonomy and detachment" (Rossi, 1986, p. 123). Lasch called our society the *Culture of Narcissism* (1979).

Individualism is a reversal of the traditional Catholic doctrine of the ethic of reciprocity in which "you are your brother's keeper," or of familism (where family needs take precedence over family members' needs). Individualism suggests that every person has to make it on his or her own merits. Whereas in the traditional Catholic culture, the extended family is expected to assist a needy cousin or adult brother, the WASP family typically would meet such a situation with questions, only responding under "justifiable" circumstances.

Individualism also involves the associated values of self-reliance and self-responsibility. The prevalent belief remains that "strong" persons can control their own lives and that lack of such control is evidence of their own weakness. Self-fulfillment is another value closely associated with individualism.

Materialism/The Consumption Ethic

The possession of money and goods is not only an essential reward for being productive, but is also a central value of society in and of itself. This value is referred to as materialism. Materialism declined somewhat in the 1960s, but is again on the rise." Samuelson (1986) writes about "the discovery of money" and society's increasing preoccupation with wealth as a measure of achievement. Money and wealth are both the foundation for power and prestige and the primary symbol of success and achievement. Money has been consecrated as a value over and above its use in procuring goods and services or for its enhancement of power. Society, through its major institutions, reinforces this cultural emphasis except perhaps among the lower class. These institutions join to provide the disciplining and training required for an individual to retain this elusive goal and be properly motivated by the promise of gratification.

Along with materialism has come a relaxation of prohibitions against expressiveness and hedonism. In a society in which the consumption of goods has become a fundamental issue, people are required to cease being ascetic and self-denying and to abandon guilt about spending and expressing their pleasure impulses.

The moral values of thriftiness and saving were parts of the Protestant ethic. As with other traditional values, their importance arose partly from the short supply of material goods and money that existed in the past. In fact, often the ability to save and conserve was critical to survival.

In more recent times Americans seem to have entirely disregarded these values (except perhaps by members of the older generation) as evidenced by our wasteful habits of acquiring vast goods and constantly replacing material items. Toffler (1970) calls this "planned obsolescence." We have acted as if there were a limitless supply of goods and resources. This consumption ethic has now largely replaced the thrift ethic, and the "put-away" society has become the "throw-away" society (Inkeles, 1977).

We may now be seeing a modest swing back to "conservation" goals, however. There is a noticeable attitudinal change, among some Americans that our habits of waste and enormous consumption of the world's resources must be altered. More concern is voiced about ecology, dwindling resources, and environmental impact (Harris, 1984). In spite of these encouraging signs, however, Americans continue to consume goods and resources at increasingly high levels.

Work Ethic

The rule of "He who does not work should not eat" expressed the deadly struggle of the early settlement and frontier days and explains the primacy of this ethic as due to the objective conditions of want that existed historically. As part of Puritanism and the Protestant ethic, however, work literally became an end in itself not the means to an end. Americans were obsessive about work, and even today we meet individuals who are "workaholics." Although the work ethic has lost much of its potency today, it is still part of our dominant culture and upheld by our societal institutions. The success of modern industrial states remains dependent on work-oriented individuals.

According to Inkeles (1977) and Glick (1989), in the 1960s and 1970s the ethic of hard work was fast eroding. Increasing numbers of Americans during that period considered the most important attributes of a job to be high pay and short hours, not the intrinsic importance or a promise of advancement. Yet Yankelovitch and Gurin (1989), surveyors of American values, noted a change in this trend in the 1980s. They observed many Americans returning to the workplace as a site for self-expression of competence, creativity, and satisfaction. The 1960s preoccupation with leisure and the inner self drew attention away from work. A resurgence in entrepreneurship accompanies the resurgence of the work ethic. The scarcity of work and jobs has certainly augmented the return of the work ethic. Several noted authors have written that when jobs were easily found and available, as in the 1960s, they were less valued. As jobs become scarcer, work will correspondingly become more valued. Even if work is not the central overriding value today that it was in the past, it would be premature to prepare for a demise of the Protestant ethic of work and the desire to "get ahead."

Education

Education is seen by the middle class as the means by which to achieve productivity, and the value placed on education is therefore closely aligned with the work ethic, materialism, individualism, and progress. Although education is much more emphasized among the middle and upper classes, its value has also become more prominent within the working class (Inkeles, 1977).

Equality

The value of equality has become more important in American society, although it is only a partially realized value.

The dominant culture values equality in personal relationships much more than many other cultures. Antiauthoritarianism is also still a very important characteristic of present-day American society. Flacks (1971) found that children were dissatisfied about the use of arbitrary or coercive power, feelings that are derived from the family values favoring a power structure based on egalitarianism, as well as expectations resulting from parental fostering of participation, independence, and autonomy.

On the other hand, a strong hierarchical and authoritarian emphasis exists in large-scale organizations. Individual achievement and status are more valued than equality. And running through the whole of our society is the thread of nonequalitarian beliefs and practices concerning interpersonal relations with people of different ethnic groupings and women, recurring manifestations of prejudice and bigotry.

Smelzer and Halpern (1978) clearly point out the clash between individualism/individual achievement and equality. If the priority in the society is on individual achievement this produces greater inequality and a call for equality. Prioritizing equality generates a counterreaction also. The fact that these values are inherently "at odds with each other" is not so surprising—what is, however, is the oscillations that have occurred in recent times concerning the saliency of these two competing values or cultural themes (Smelzer and Halpern, 1978). During the 1960s and early 1970s, equality, as seen in the liberal ideas and programs of the "Great Society," the Peace Corps, and affirmative action and civil rights programs, was prioritized. Beginning in the late 1970s, the pendulum swung back again—with a dismantlement of programs that fostered the value of equality, and a return to the more conservative values of achievement and individualism.

In spite of the resurgence of conservativism, individualism, and achievement values, equality still is recognized as a central cultural value. The importance of equality is closely linked with an increasing tolerance of diversity and the growing tendency to pursue individualistic personal goals, where freedom, independence, and autonomy, as well as greater expression of feelings, are paramount.

The rise of egalitarianism is a major change in family life. According to Toynbee (1955), the noted historian, the most vital revolution of our time is the emancipation of women, because ultimately women's emancipation will affect everyone's life. "Above all, it is going to demand an immense and disturbing psychological adjustment on the part of men, because it implies a revolutionary change in the traditional relations between the sexes" (pp. 52–53). In addition to the women's movement and the affirmative action programs, there has been considerable progress in protecting the rights of the mentally ill and of children. These legislative trends demonstrate the continued potency of equality as a value.

Progress and Mastery Over One's Environment

Kluckholm (1976) refers to this value orientation as involving the "man–nature relationship issue"—whether man is viewed as subjugated to nature, as part of nature, or as lord over nature. Traditional Spanish-American culture in the American Southwest illustrates the first relationship. To the average rancher in the Southwest, there is little or nothing that can be done if a storm damages range lands or disease destroys flocks. He or she simply accepts these events as inevitable. This fatalistic attitude may also be found in dealing with illness and death in a statement such as, "if it is the Lord's will that I die, I shall die" (p. 69). The second relationship, in which man and nature are viewed as aspects of a harmonious whole, is found in many of the North American Indian tribes and traditional Chinese cultures. The dominant American culture, however, views this relationship in the third way—that of man against, or over, nature. Natural forces are seen as things to be overcome, mastered, and utilized by people. We build bridges, blast through mountains, create lakes and massive dams, and exploit all of nature's resources—all to serve mankind (Kluckholm, 1976).

It is this general attitude of being able to problem solve and overcome seemingly impossible obstacles that is referred to as progressiveness. Change is seen as progress or going forward, even though it sometimes seems that the pendulum swings backward. Inkeles (1977) reported that innovativeness and openness to new experiences is widespread, coupled with an optimism or the confidence that striving and change are positive.

Future Time Orientation

Obviously all societies must deal with three time dimensions—past, present, and future. All cultures have some conception of the past, all have a present, and all give attention to the future time dimension. They vary, however, in the emphasis they place on each dimension. For example, Kluckholm (1976) and Murillo (1976) report that in contrast to Americans, unacculturated Mexican-Americans are more present oriented. Historically, China and Japan, on the other hand, were societies that put their main emphasis on the past. Ancestor worship and strong family traditions were both expressions of this time orientation. Many modern European countries, such as England, have also tended to stress the past much more than America.

Americans place their emphasis on the future—which we anticipate optimistically will be "bigger and better." Past ways are considered "old fashioned," and we are seldom content with the present. With the trend toward self-expression and self-satisfaction there is also a greater emphasis on the present and on meeting of short-term goals (Lasch, 1979; Yankelovitch et al, 1975). The value put on the future correlates closely with the value on change and progress. A Frenchman, Servan-Schreiber, wrote, "We Europeans continue to suffer progress while Americans pursue it, welcome it and adapt to it" (Inkeles, 1977).

Efficiency, Orderliness, and Practicality

In frontier society, being practical—learning to improvise and make the best out of one's resources—was tied up with survival. Individuals and families concentrated on obtainable goals in the immediate situation—"If it works, it must be good." Today, this same kind of pragmatism views technical advances with great appreciation, especially those resulting in savings of time and manpower—after all, "time is money." Science is highly valued as an endeavor through which efficiency, practicality, and progress can be achieved. The way we treat food and the manner in which we consume it are expressions of values we hold. Seventy percent of households today have microwave ovens. The purchase of fast foods proliferate. What we value is speed and efficiency.

Rationality

In order to be efficient, orderly, progressive, productive, and practical, one must be rational and able to react by problem solving and by logically thinking through one's situation and goals. Foresight, deliberate planning, allocation of resources in the most efficient way, and long-term gratification is necessary. Rationality became a prime value during the Enlightenment in the late 1700s and early 1800s. Science was a natural outgrowth of this rational philosophy, because it depends on the same logical cognitive approach to the world and its problems. Applied science is highly esteemed in the dominant culture as a tool for controlling nature and the environment.

This value has led to the "rational scientific man" becoming the exemplar of our society. Women, in contrast, have historically been stereotyped with the opposite of these desirable attributes; women have been deemed irrational, illogical, and emotional, albeit this stereotyping is losing its potency as women move into cognitively challenging fields and succeed admirably.

Quality of Life and Maintaining Health

People today are becoming increasingly interested in making qualitative changes in their lives. These include such life-style improvements as curtailing smoking, making dietary changes, and partaking in self-help stress reduction and other mental health programs*; people are also making environmental alterations such as moving from city and suburbia to small towns and rural environments, and participating in creative and leisure endeavors. All these signify a basic modification of values to a more introspective orientation where personal and familial happiness and personal independence in decision making have greater priority. While it is difficult to measure how highly health is valued and how widespread this shift is, available evidence suggests that maintaining health is becoming a major value within the American hierarchy of values (Harris, 1984; Yankelovitch and Gurin, 1989). The importance of this value is probably influenced not only by social class, but also by age and ethnicity.

The "Doing" Orientation

Kluckholm (1976) refers to the normative interpersonal behavior valued in American society, or its national character, as being exemplified in the "doing

** Since 1975 U.S. mortality figures have shown significant decreases in cardiovascular deaths. This has been largely attributed to a decrease in smoking among those at risk for heart disease (U.S. Department of Health & Human Services, 1988).*

orientation." Its most distinctive feature is its demand for action in terms of accomplishment and in accord with external (societal) standards. Again, the person who "gets things done" is seen as productive. The person who finds ways to do something, and is the rational problem solver is much esteemed.

Tolerance of Diversity

Although it may be stretching it to be including this value in the central values of Americans, it has been included because of the notable change toward greater tolerance in recent years. Perhaps due to the civil rights and antiwar movements of the 1960s and/or because of the increasing number of minorities in the United States, a greater tolerance of diversity has been noted (Koten, 1987). This diversity includes greater acceptance of ethnic peoples and women. Increasing tolerance of diverse life-styles and family forms has also occurred* (Boulding, 1976; Koten, 1987).

Weaver (1976) states that the major and most significant result of the women's movement and growing ethnic consciousness has been the growth of popular questioning of cultural assumptions held by Americans for generations. "Rather than having values of a subcultural group dissipated and absorbed by the dominant culture, these two groups have undermined the values and assumptions of the dominant culture" (p. 123).

Foremost among the numerous assumptions made in America has been the myth of the "melting pot." The pot never really melted out the differences, but the myth has tended to downgrade these differences and elevate and validate the standardized middle-class white values and norms. This cultural imperialism (as opposed to cultural pluralism) is a result of racism, technological advances, urbanization, and a progressiveness that holds everything scientific and new is good and roots and traditions obsolete (Weaver, 1976).

FAMILY VALUES

The family's value system is thought to be heavily influenced by the society's core values, as well as by the values of the family's subcultural and other reference groups. Because families have their own special functions within the larger societal context, they also subscribe to certain values—which guide family life.

David Reiss (1981) has written about families creating their own family paradigm—an enduring structure of shared beliefs, convictions, and assumptions about the social world. These shared beliefs are largely based on the family's past experiences. Families develop their own paradigm as an extension of how they deal with hardships and crisis. Family belief systems can have a more internal locus of control (mastery over nature) or external locus of control (situations are governed by external factors beyond the family's control).

A family's value and belief system shapes its patterns of behavior toward problems families face. Family values and beliefs shape the views families have of stressors and how they should respond to stressors. In other words, family beliefs and values determine how a family will cope with health and other stressors. A family with a mastery orientation may believe it can control and solve almost every problem it faces. In this case the family would use more active, assertive coping strategies, like seeking out new information or community resources to resolve or control the problem. Conversely, a family less oriented toward mastery and control and more oriented toward passive acceptance may believe in accepting whatever happens. They may cope by resigning themselves to God's will. These families are often called "fatalistic" (Boss, 1988). Fatalism needs to be distinguished from acceptance according to Boss (1988). Fatalism is the belief that everything is predetermined by a higher power and the family is powerless to change what is preordained to happen. Families that are fatalistic are those that because of their cultural and environmental conditioning, feel a sense of powerlessness to change the course of events.

In situations that are hopeless, with loss inevitable and control impossible, the mastery-oriented and fatalistically oriented families typically behave quite differently. The mastery-oriented family will be less likely to give up hope, even with terminal illness, but will experience much more stress than the fatalistically oriented family, which will passively accept the situation.

MAJOR VARIABLES AFFECTING FAMILY'S VALUE SYSTEM

There are several important variables or factors that greatly influence whether a family assimilates the "major value orientation" of American society, or whether differences in priorities and values or divergent norms continue to operate. A most important variable is social class, which is discussed in Chapter 8. Other important variables include a family's cultural heritage, including religious background; degree of acculturation to the dominant culture; development stage; and familial and personal idiosyncrasies.

Cultural background makes a major difference in how important each of the core American values are to

**There appears to be some backlash or reaction to this growing tolerance of differing life-styles, as seen in the areas of women's rights, especially abortion.*

the family. For instance, Irish-American families place a high value on independence. Irish culture is replete with many sayings that illustrate the importance of this value. "You've made your bed, now lie in it" tells a married family member not to bring his or her problems home to the parent. In contrast, the Italian-American family could hardly imagine this being uttered (Foley, 1986, p. 191).

Whether a family resides (or has resided for a long period of time) in a rural, urban, or suburban community also plays a significant role in shaping a family's values. In terms of country versus city residence, rural dwellers tend to be more traditional and conservative than their urban or suburban counterparts. Suburban communities are primarily residential and middle class, and usually espouse middle-class cultural values. In contrast, urban, inner-city populations are diverse, generally containing families from the whole social class spectrum, as well as families from various ethnic and racial groups; thus urban families usually show a greater diversity of values, although generally tending to hold more liberal social and political views.

Another variable influencing the values and norms of a family is the life cycle of the family and age of its members. Certain values were predominant when persons were in their early adulthood years in the 1950's. These individuals are now most likely in the phase of retirement/aging or the contracting family phase, and they retain many of their traditional work-oriented Protestant ethic values (values that have more potency in their lives than for younger adults). Slater (1970) illustrates the drastic differences in values when he compares the value of the "youth generation" with the old values of the dominant (adult) culture.

VALUE CONFLICTS

Diverse Social Values

Because there are so many factors which serve to alter an individual's or a family's values and norms, conflicts inevitably exist. Issues or unresolved conflicts are present because the traditional and emerging sets of norms exist simultaneously, both within and outside of the family. Within communities certain groups and individuals resist the emerging norms and cling vehemently to the more traditional patterns, whereas other individuals and groups find the traditional patterns unacceptable and adhere to the new set of norms and values. The result of this social change is that areas of major conflict arise. Although our society values its pluralism, where both traditional and emerging value systems and patterns can exist side by side, this social diversity played out in the family results in conflict and confusion. A very common family value issue is that concerning the meaning of marriage. Whereas traditionally marriage was viewed as sacred and binding, today among those espousing emerging social values, marriage is increasingly viewed as a contract to be voided when either or both parties have legitimate grievances (Eshleman, 1974; Scanzoni, 1987).

Clash of Values Between Dominant Culture and Subculture

Another common source of value conflict is a clash between the values of the dominant culture and a family's cultural reference group. Larrabee (1973), a Cheyenne Indian, describes this clash of values and one of its effects:

> In trying to teach our young about themselves, we must tell them about the Indian values of compassion, respect for elders, sharing, and wisdom. We want our children to have these values and to know about them. When our children go to school and are told by the teacher that they must learn to be saving instead of sharing, the child becomes confused. This terrible conflict of values contributes to the high suicide rate among our youth.

When we consider the family as the mediating agent between the culture (or the wider society) and the individual, it follows that a basic incompatibility in values between the family's reference group and wider society generates certain value conflicts, which increase stress within the family as a system and also negatively affect family members.

The findings of Cleveland and Longaker (1972) confirm the disruptive effects value conflicts have on the family. They examined the impact of cultural factors on the mental health of family members by analyzing the transmission and mediation of values in a family setting. Based on extensive data collected from interviews, home visits, testing, and therapeutic sessions, they concluded that the emotional problems in family members studied were a function of two processes: (1) a value conflict between the society the family resided in and the family and (2) a culturally recurrent mode of self-disparagement linked to the failure of individuals to adjust to incompatible value orientations.

Clash of Values Between Generations

A third source of value conflict within families lies in generational differences in values, as mentioned previously. A family may be composed of several generations of individuals, each bringing to the family group his or her generationally based values. When the grandparents hold traditional values, the parents a combination of traditional and emerging (progressive) values, and the children emerging values, value conflicts are inevitable, especially if the family household is an extended family or a family with adolescents.

FAMILY VALUES: APPLYING THE FAMILY NURSING PROCESS

☐ ASSESSMENT QUESTIONS

An understanding of the prevailing value system of American society and how societal values affect the family, as well as an understanding of some of the variables influencing family values, provide the foundation for assessing family values. Assessing specific values to which a family adheres and the generational, cultural, and developmental value differences among family members will lead to detection of intrafamilial value conflicts.

Assessment of a family's values is also very helpful in motivating a family to take preventive or restorative health action or to make health decisions. Elkins (1984) reminds us that the basis for motivation is derived from a family's value system—what is important and unimportant to it and how important different values are. Although health for its own sake may not be a high value in a family's list of priorities, helping the family see that other very important values will be adversely affected if health actions are not taken (such as a parent not being able to work) may be a way of motivating a family. Elkins (1984) explains this motivational strategy:

> A client's value system can serve as a guide in choosing positive reinforcers for client progress toward goals. The client must believe that the behavior change will result in something of greater value to him—a good return on his investment. The nurse can help the client see the results. Any behavior change requires an investment of self, time, and possibly money, all of which are high on the value scales of most people. In reinforcing newly acquired behavior, the community health nurse, by understanding the client's values, can direct the intrinsic and extrinsic rewards so that the client perceives them as being more valuable than the old behavior patterns. (p. 279)

Values cannot be seen directly, but must be inferred from observations and assessment of family roles, power structure, and communication patterns, because these dimensions are strongly influenced by the underlying values held by family members. When family values and beliefs are identified, this information will help the family nurse to better understand the reasons for family communication, power, and roles.

It is suggested that one way of simplifying the assessment of family values is for nursing students to make use of a "contrast and compare" method. This involves comparing and contrasting a specific family's values with those of the dominant culture. This enables the assessor to identify various areas that need assessment and to appraise how much conformity or disparity in values exists between the dominant culture and the family under consideration. If an assessor is familiar with the values and norms of a specific ethnic group, then this same comparison process could be applied, using the family's cultural reference group as a basis for comparison (see Areas to Assess on Table 13–1).

TABLE 13–1. PROCESS TO IDENTIFY FAMILY VALUES, PRIORITIES, AND VALUE CONGRUENCE WITH REFERENCE GROUP AND/OR WIDER COMMUNITY

1.	Identify family's and individual family members' values and beliefs.
2.	Estimate how important a particular value is to the family and/or individuals within the family.
3.	Estimate the extent of compliance and rewards a family is receiving from its reference group and society in general. (Lack of compliance and rewards will be present if there is moderate or marked value disparity, as well as stigmatization of the family by the community.)

To illustrate this process more concretely, it is suggested that a list of central values be utilized as a guide for this assessment. Using a list of central values of the dominant culture on one side of the assessment form and the family's values on the other side, the assessor can then discuss a family's particular values in each of these areas. This listing should help in identifying the specific values to which the family adheres.

AMERICAN SOCIETAL VALUES	THE FAMILY'S VALUES
1. Productivity/achievement	
2. Work ethic	
3. Materialism	
4. Individualism	
5. Education	
6. Consumption ethic	
7. Progress and mastery over environment	
8. Future time orientation	
9. Efficiency, orderliness, and practicality	
10. Rationality	
11. Democracy, equality, and freedom	
12. "Doing orientation"	
13. Patriarchal authority	
14. Family's interests	
15. Family as a haven	
16. Health	

Following this listing, the following questions should be addressed:

- Is there congruence between the family's values and the family's reference group and/or the wider community?
- Is there congruence between the family's values and the family subsystem values?
- How important are the identified values to the family? (Rank order the family values.)
- Are the values consciously or unconsciously held?
- Are there any value conflicts evident within the family?
- How do the family's social class, cultural background, and developmental stage influence the family's values?
- How do the family's values affect the health status of the family?

FAMILY NURSING DIAGNOSES

Family nursing diagnoses in the area of values are not seen so commonly. This is because family value problems are generally considered to be underlying causes (related factors) of other problem areas that are more behaviorally oriented.

The one family nursing diagnoses that has been identified is "value conflicts." If a value conflict diagnosis is made, then the system in which the problem resides (between "whom") must be specified—such as, "value conflict between grandparents and grandson"—and defining characteristics and related factors included. Value conflicts are often seen as a contributory factor to family problems in the other structural dimensions (communication, power, and roles) or in the functional areas (affective, socialization, and health care) and coping.

FAMILY NURSING INTERVENTIONS

Knowledge about family values is important data for the nurse to have in order to establish realistic goals and intervention strategies with the family (Elkins, 1984). In addition, understanding the relation of the family's values to the values of community agencies will help the nurse suggest more value-appropriate community resources when making a referral.

In the nursing literature only one intervention strategy is discussed in the area of values—that is, value clarification. The family nursing interventions described under role conflict (see Chap. 12), however, with slight modification should also be appropriate for value conflict problems.

Value Clarification

Value clarification is a technique or process used to increase a family's awareness of value priorities as well as the degree of congruency between family member values, attitudes, and behavior. Because values are a basis for decision making and coping, helping families reaffirm their existing values, clarify their values, or reprioritize their values will help them become more autonomous and responsible for their own health (Wilberding, 1985).

In addition to moralizing (telling a person, usually a child, what is right and wrong) and role modeling, the value clarification process assists both children and adults to critically think about their values and undertake the process of valuing (Raths et al, 1978). Value clarification, Kirschenbaum (1977) explains, is an approach that uses questions and activities designed to teach the valuing process. These exercises help people to apply the valuing processes to value-rich areas of their lives. Once values become clearer, it is easier to see dissonance between values and behavior; if an individual values health, the dissonance should be reduced by changing his or her health-related behaviors.

A perplexing issue occurs when value clarification is used and the client's values differ greatly from the nurse's values. Is the nurse able to accept differing values without resorting to moralizing? This is an ethical question that must be addressed before undertaking value clarification. According to Wilberding (1985), the ultimate issue is whether the family nurse can accept the client as being an autonomous self-care agent.

There are numerous value clarification tools mentioned in the literature. Pender (1987, pp. 162–181) has developed, as well as adapted from others, tools and exercises to help individuals and families clarify their values. Pender believes that the nurse interested in health promotion should assist clients with value clarification and value changes. She explains that

- Value clarification is increasing personal or group awareness of value priorities and the degree of consistency among values, attitudes, and behavior.
- Value change is the reprioritization of values, abandonment of existing values, or acquisition of new values and subsequent attitudes and behavior change.

Assisting family members with value changes is an intervention discussed in rehabilitation nursing. Disabled persons and their families need to reprioritize their values when certain values are no longer possible to operationalize. This process is a crucial one for a disabled client and family to accomplish in adapting to the disability in a functional manner.

Pender (1987) adds one caveat about the use of value clarification. She states that value clarification should be used cautiously with individuals who have emotional problems or with families who are markedly dysfunctional.

☐ STUDY QUESTIONS

Choose the correct answers to the following questions.

1. It is true that:
   a. Values are defined as a system of ideas and beliefs that bind families together.
   b. Values serve as general guides to behavior.
   c. The family is the basic transmitter of values.
   d. Values are relatively fixed and change very little over time.
   e. All values have the same or similar weight as far as their influence and centrality in a person's life are concerned.

2. The best definition of norms is:
   a. Patterns of personal behaviors.
   b. Modal behaviors.
   c. Role behaviors or expectations.
   d. Clustering of attitudes and beliefs.

3. Family rules are related to family values in which of the following ways?
   a. Family rules generate family values.
   b. Family rules are specific manifestations of family values.
   c. Family rules and family values are distinct concepts and have no overlapping meaning.

4. List and briefly explain four major, recent value changes that have occurred in society and within families.

5. In American society, the most dominant or unifying standard or set of values is (select the best answer):
   a. Puritan ethic.
   b. Catholic ethic.
   c. Protestant ethic.
   d. Middle-class culture.
   e. Secularized Protestant ethic.

6. Value clarification is a process that helps people to (choose the one correct answer):
   a. Identify their values.
   b. Change their values.
   c. See the difference between their values and family rules.
   d. Question the rights and wrongs about their values.

7. In today's family there is greater emphasis on family interests and goals, rather than individual interests and activities (answer *True* or *False*).

8. Several values cluster together, comprising the central configuration of values in the dominant culture. List six values.

9. There are four variables that influence the family's value system. List these. Which is most important generally?

Choose the correct answers to the following questions.

10. Which of the following are sources of value conflicts?
    a. Past versus present mores
    b. Social class differences
    c. Acculturation differences
    d. Idiosyncratic (personal) differences

11. One of the concepts germane to social class is that when a family and its reference group do not subscribe to the central core values of a society:
    a. The adjustment to wider society is relatively easy.
    b. The family is able to gain compliance from society.
    c. The more difficult the family adjustment to community life becomes.
    d. The family experiences social stigma.

Family Case Study—the Gardiners*

After reading the family case study, answer the questions that follow.

* *Family case study adapted from Sobol and, Robischon (1975). This compilation of family case studies is designed to cover the range of families and common health problems family-centered nurses face. These case studies are excellent teaching tools.*

The Gardiner family members are Harry, age 37; May, 28; Len, 11; Joanie, 7; and Ann, 3. The family, black Americans, came to the attention of the public health nurse working in a pediatric outpatient clinic when appointments arranged for Len at the diabetes and urology clinics were repeatedly not kept. Although appointments to the diabetes clinic were kept occasionally, no urology visit was made, and the chart showed that the mother at one time had reported continual bedwetting.

Len was originally diagnosed as having juvenile diabetes when he was hospitalized at age 6. After the child was diagnosed and stabilized, the family was counseled as to treatment regimen. Subsequent to this time, four hospitalizations had occurred because of diabetic crises.

During the nurse's first visit, Mrs. G. appeared very anxious, explaining that she always anticipates "bad news" about Len. In response to inquiries about Len's missed clinic appointments, Mrs. G. seemed indifferent, stating that they have been too busy and that arranging child care for Ann was a problem. On a later visit other factors, more covert, which contribute to the family's reluctance to keep Len's appointments were noted. The mother's statements clarify these factors: "When they told me what was wrong with Len I worried day and night and wouldn't let anyone play with him or take him any place. I was constantly with him. Then I decided I couldn't worry like that anymore. I know he really isn't sick. No one could play as hard as he does and still be sick!" Mrs. G. seemed unwilling to discuss Len's fainting episodes except to say they were Len's way of getting attention. She also refused to discuss his four diabetic crisis hospitalizations.

Data concerning the health status of other family members were also noted. Mrs. G. was of average weight and neatly dressed. She was quite gregarious as long as she could control the conversation. Her knowledge about nutrition and other aspects of family welfare important to her—shelter, cleanliness, adequate child care arrangements, regular school attendance—were satisfactory. Mrs. G. claims good health, although she has not received any preventive care from a physician, with the exception of prenatal care in the past, and even this was obtained late in the pregnancy.

Mr. G. had been in the Army many years ago and since this time has been under the care of a Veterans Administration Hospital. Here he regularly receives tranquilizers and occasional counseling. His wife reported that his physical health is average, stating: "He doesn't get sick or go to the doctor, but he sure is tired all of the time."

Joanie, the 7-year-old, was reported to be in good health, attended school regularly, and was doing all right there. Her mother termed her "a good girl." Ann, the preschooler, was active, friendly, and healthy appearing. Mrs. G. complained of her "overactivity." She explained that Ann was constantly into things and interfered with her efforts to keep the house clean and picked up. Ann's health supervision is irregular and her immunizations incomplete. After well-baby care was completed at 1 year, health care has been sought only for acute illnesses.

The family's economic situation has been unstable. Mr. G. works irregularly in a factory, while Mrs. G. works off and on at a car-washing business. To supplement their insufficient earnings, they receive welfare.

Mrs. G.'s primary expressed concerns had to do with her husband's lack of responsibility for helping with the household and child-care tasks, as well as his overall neglectfulness and his irregular employment. She openly berated her husband in front of him, the nurse, and their children, complaining that he did not bring home enough money for the family to live on and lacks interest in the home, the children, and money matters. Mr. G. sat silently as his wife verbally assaulted him.

There was an impression of little communication or companionship among family members, except in those areas related to the daily activities of living and taking care of the apartment. The children's play was kept at a minimum due to the noise they created. Most communication was in the form of commands, emanating from the mother to the husband and children. Mrs. G. states she is constantly working to keep the home clean, meals ready, and children cared for. The home was viewed as a place to be kept clean and organized, so that everything was put away; the children were expected to be "seen but not heard"; they were to be home exactly on time; attend school regularly; keep themselves and their surroundings clean; and obey and respect their mother. There were no toys or reading materials visible. The only discernible source of recreation for the entire family was the television set, which was on constantly. Family recreational pursuits were practically unheard of. Life was virtually task oriented, and no enjoyable and fun activities were included.

The family lives in a low-income housing project, for which they are charged a minimum rent. Kitchen equipment, food, and clothing storage facilities are adequate as are their furnishings. Although the outside appearance of the housing project is dirty and visually in a state of disrepair, the inside of their apartment is orderly and well maintained.

Mr. and Mrs. G. dropped out of high school in the ninth and tenth grades, respectively, in order to start working to help out their parents. No further education or skill training has been received since that time. Relatives do not reside near them, nor are they affiliated with any religious or other community groups.

The community in which the family lives is part of a large inner-city area that is deteriorating rapidly. Transportation and social, health, and welfare facilities are easily accessible. Shopping for food and other necessities is limited to small neighborhood shops in the area, since they do not own a car. The schools and churches are nearby. The mother feels the neighborhood is crime-ridden (which the nurse confirmed), and hence she has kept the children indoors most of the time.

12. From the limited information contained in the family case study, what are the salient values operating in this family? (Use the assessment process that was suggested in this chapter.)

13. How important are these identified values to the family?

14. Are these values consciously or unconsciously held?

15. Are there any value conflicts evident within the family itself?

CHAPTER FOURTEEN

The Affective Function

Learning Objectives

1. State three reasons why the affective function is a vital family function.
2. Explain briefly the three components of need–response patterns.
3. Discuss how mutual support and emotional warmth originate and continue in a family as an inherent part of the "spiral phenomenon."
4. Describe the aims of a family in achieving a mutual respect balance.
5. Define concepts of bonding or attachment, response bonds, identification, and crescive bonds, and their significance to the family's fulfillment of the affective function.
6. Discuss the prime task of parents in assisting their children to form a stable, sound identity in the area of separateness and connectedness.
7. Compare and contrast the marital therapeutic role with the affective function of the family.
8. Name two underlying values and/or priorities present in energized families related to the affective function area.
9. Identify several NANDA nursing diagnoses that could be appropriate when a family's affective function is being inadequately fulfilled.
10. Using the family case situation, complete an assessment of the affective function. Propose a family nursing diagnosis in the area of the affective function. Suggest two family nursing interventions to ameliorate and/or resolve the above affective problem.
11. Describe several interventions that are helpful to families when a family member is dying.

It is generally recognized that the family exists so as to fulfill certain basic functions that are necessary for the survival of the species (societal needs), namely, procreation and child rearing. Additionally, it acts as the necessary mediator between the society and the individual and forms the matrix in which personal needs are met.

The family is more specialized today, and activities that traditionally took place within the home and/or involved the whole family now take place elsewhere and engage only segments or individual family members. For example, the economic activity in which the whole family was traditionally engaged is now the purview of the father and increasingly the mother, and takes place outside of the family home. In addition, social organizations and institutions such as the school and social services agencies now share in many of the traditional functions of the family. A number of extremely vital functions, however, remain. Of these socialization (see Chap. 15) and affective functions are perhaps the most important. Another significant family function also remaining is the health care function, covered in Chapter 16.

IMPORTANCE OF THE AFFECTIVE FUNCTION

The affective function deals with the internal functions of the family—the psychosocial protection and support of its members. The family accomplishes the task of supporting the healthy development and growth of its members by meeting the socioemotional needs of its members, starting with the early years of an individual's life and continuing throughout his or her lifetime. Adams (1971), a family sociologist, describes the family function in this way: "The family has become a specialist in gratifying people's psychological needs—the needs for understanding, affection and happiness" (p. 92). Fulfillment of the affective function is the central basis for both the formation and continuation of the family unit (Satir, 1972).

The individual's self-image and his or her sense of belonging is derived through primary group (family) interactions. Moreover, the family serves as a primary source of love, approval, reward, and support.

In attempting to fulfill the role of meeting its members' socioemotional needs, the family assumes a heavy responsibility, especially in view of the fact that families move frequently and often do not have the social support systems they need. Moreover, today's families are generally smaller in the number of members, and thus there are fewer members to share the tasks of meeting each other's needs for companionship, love, and support.

Loveland-Cherry (1989) points out that affection among family members produces a nurturing emotional climate that positively influences growth and development and a sense of personal competence. Family nurturance is related to health promotion behaviors and healthy outcomes.

In view then of the increased emphasis on the importance of family relationships, it is not surprising to find a parallel rise in divorce rates. Permissive divorce laws making divorce more accessible to all sectors of society, and a concomitant lessening of social stigma, along with other factors such as gains made by the women's movement, have also facilitated this national trend. Because divorce is an available option in many families today, most families that remain together do so because of the satisfaction that being a family brings rather than out of necessity or because of coercive social pressures.

The importance of assessing a family's affective function is self-evident. Because the affective function is so vital for both survival and the functioning of the family as a whole and its individual members, assessment and intervention in this area are crucial. Both health counseling and education are critical strategies to employ in helping families shore up their relationships and better meet each other's needs. Consideration of the affective function is particularly vital in working with young families with newborns and infants, where parent–infant relationships are so significant in terms of their long-term impact on the individuals' and family's future.

COMPONENTS OF THE AFFECTIVE FUNCTION

The affective function involves the family's perception of respect for and care of the psychosocial needs of its members. Through fulfillment of this function, the family serves the major psychosocial purposes of building within its members the qualities of humanness, stabilization of personality and behavior, relatability (ability to relate intimately), and self-esteem (Table 14–1).

Maintaining Mutual Nurturance

First and foremost fulfilling the affective function involves creating and maintaining within the family a system for mutual nurturance. Recall that in Chapter 13 on family values, one important family value was valuing the family as a haven for warmth, support, love, and acceptance. A prerequisite to achieving mutual nurturance is the basic commitment of a couple to each other and a nurturing, emotionally satisfying marital relationship. This becomes the emotional foundation on which the parents build their supportive structure. The nurturing attitudes and behavior flowing from parents and siblings to younger children will result in a return flow from children to parents as well.

TABLE 14–1. SOCIOEMOTIONAL ATTRIBUTES OF HEALTHY FAMILIES

- A social milieu for the generation and maintenance of affectional bonds within family relationships, where one is first loved and given to, and in turn learns to love and give in return.
- An opportunity to develop a personal and social identity tied to family identity.
- An opportunity for individuals to be themselves. The family provides a home base or haven where its members are permitted to be themselves—to express their true feelings and thoughts (eg, hostility with less fear of consequences) and to experience security and love without fear of rejection.

Brown (1978) views this flow as a spiral phenomenon. As each member receives affection and care from others in the family, his or her capacity to give to other members increases, with the result being mutual support and emotional warmth.

The key concepts here are *mutuality* and *reciprocity.* Parents give emotionally to children; this, in turn, is received and fed back to parents and siblings. (The opposite also occurs: rejecting and angry parents breed angry and rejecting responses in their children.) By maintaining the kind of environment in which its members' needs are adequately responded to, the family provides the opportunity for individuals to form and maintain meaningful relationships not only with family members, but with other individuals also.

Development of Close Relationships. Through the family's fulfilling of the affective function, individuals develop the ability to relate intimately or closely with others. Intimacy is vital in human relationships, because it fulfills the psychological need for emotional closeness with another human being and allows individuals in the relationship to know the full range of each other's uniqueness (Andrews, 1974).

A person usually first experiences an intimate relationship with his or her parents, beginning with early mother–infant bonding. The relationship continues to grow and develop during the years that follow in the family of origin. When achieved, this sense of closeness and trusting gives the person the confidence to reach outside the family confines and establish close and emotionally satisfying relationships with others. As young adults then start their own family, this sense of intimacy and closeness is passed on to the next generation. Conversely, if early bonding and a sense of trust and intimacy does not occur in the family of origin, the individual will not have the confidence and ability to relate intimately with others. Unfortunately this inability is usually passed on to the next generation also, unless some intervening factor such as personal experiences and growth at a later stage in life occurs (Paul and Paul, 1975).

We are reminded by Satir (1972) that it is impossible for a family to meet the emotional needs of its members without the presence of functional, clear family communication patterns. Hence communication becomes the vehicle through which the psychological needs of family members are recognized and responded to.*

**This statement provides a cogent basis for health care or welfare professionals working with families to direct their efforts toward helping families shore up and improve their interactional patterns.*

Mutual Respect Balance

The literature of parent–child guidance presents a well-respected approach to parenting termed the mutual respect balance (Colley, 1978). When operationalized it helps family members to fulfill the affective function. The primary thrust of this approach is that families should maintain, an atmosphere in which positive self-regard and the rights of *both* parents and child are highly valued. Thus it is acknowledged that each person in the family has his or her own rights as individuals, as well as developmental needs specific to his or her age group. A mutual respect balance can be achieved when each family member respects the rights, needs, and responsibilities of other members (Colley, 1978).

Maintaining a balance between the rights of individuals in the family means creating an atmosphere in which neither parents nor children are expected to cater to the whims of the other. Parents need to provide sufficient structure and consistent guidelines so that limits are set and understood. Yet enough flexibility must also be built into the family system to allow for the freedom and room to grow and individuate (Turner, 1970). Mutual nurturance is also made possible when a mutual respect balance exists.

Bonding and Identification

The sustaining force behind the perception and satisfaction of the needs of individuals in the family is *bonding* or *attachment* (used interchangeably). Attachment, according to Wright and Leahey (1984) refers to, "a relatively enduring unique emotional tie between two specific persons" (p. 40). Bonding is first initiated in the marital relations. This is when a couple discovers common interests, goals, and values and finds that the relationship validates each of them, carries with it certain tangible benefits (prestige, among friends, community privileges, etc), makes possible the meeting of certain goals that could not be accomplished alone (having children and a home), and provides a mutual enjoyment and comfortableness due to their sustained contact with each other (Perry, 1983; Turner, 1970). Bowlby (1977) called the development of this emotional tie "falling in love."

This same kind of bonding or attachment develops later between parents and children and between siblings as they continually and positively relate to each other through the process called identification.

Mother–newborn and infant attachment is crucial, because early parent–infant interactions affect the nature and quality of later attachment relationships, and these relationships influence the child's psychosocial and cognitive development (Ainsworth, 1966). Identification is the critical element in bonding, as well as the heart of family relationships. Turner (1970) explains that in its most uncomplicated definition, identification refers to "an attitude in which a person experiences what happens to another person as if it had happened to himself" (p. 66). In other words, when a family member identifies with another member, he or she experiences the joys and sorrows of the other as if these experiences were his or her own.

In order for bonding or attachment to occur in family relationships, positive identification must first be present. As the most pervasive aspect of attachment, it may be based on sympathy or libidinal mechanisms or be solely derived from the internalization of the attitudes of the other whom he or she cares for and depends on. Once established, the long-term consequence of identification and bonding is a change in the individual's self-image toward the characteristics of the other person with whom he or she has identified. Through identification, children attempt to imitate the behavior of their parents (the parents with whom they identify become their role models). As the child's identity is thus enhanced by the learning of behaviors, attitudes, and values of parents, a bond is formed. Through identification and bonding, parents obtain referent power over their children.

The identification or identity bond depends on positive, giving responses from people in the relationships. Even an infant gives or rewards mother in its earliest beginnings of their relationship by feeding, snuggling up, letting the mother comfort him or her, and so forth. Thus, for bonding to be effective there must be support and enhancement of a person's identity through his/her association with another. "Whenever a child shows admiration towards his parent or spontaneously gives affection, the gratification that the parent feels activates a response bond" (Turner, 1970, p. 72).

One facet of the response bond is the general sensitivity, caring for, and responsiveness of the other member(s) in the relationship. When one's communication is accepted, and appreciation and feelings supported this leads to a closeness and a desire to continue sharing together. Bonding may also exist because of special needs that one person meets for the other person. For instance, a dominant, controlling person may bond with a submissive type—with both having their special needs satisfied in the relationship.

Duration of close relationships is also a factor to be considered. Even though the bonding between newlyweds is intense, and the relationship between mother and a newborn child profound, loss of the newly married mate or newborn will generally not be felt as severely as if the relationship had persisted for several years prior to the loss. As family members closely involved with each other continue their relationship, old bonds become intensified and new, stronger bonds emerge; and these stronger bonds unite these individuals together in a unique, sustaining relationship. These attachments are not substitutable—that is, no other person(s) can replace a particular member. Because these enduring bonds are not initially present, and grow through a close, sustained involvement, Turner (1970) terms these bonds *crescive bonds*.

Although crescive bonding sounds like a natural phenomenon, it is not inevitable, and in some situations crescive bonds do not develop. Turner (1970) discusses two factors that inhibit their growth. First, bonds that are situationally based (based on the existence of certain specific needs or circumstances), such as those bonds that meet certain developmental needs that an individual will possibly outgrow, or task-oriented bonds, are far more vulnerable to weakening and eventual breakage. Second, bonding relationships based on contractual agreements, rather than sacred linkages, are also more vulnerable to dissolution, because contracts involve mutual obligations. In this case if one partner fails to live up to his or her part of the contract, the contract can become invalid. Marriages are seen by many in this light. In sacred linkages, the basis for staying together is felt to be God, family, tradition, and/or one's duty. The bond of parent–child is still seen as sacred and immutable. (A case in point: States do not legally permit a parent the right to disown their minor children.)

Assessing the nature of the attachment and quality of the affectional ties between each set of relationships in the family has been suggested by several family therapists and nurses (Minuchin, 1974; Wright and Leahey, 1984). The focus here is on the various affective relationships rather than on the individual members. Later in this chapter, in the assessment questions, the use of an attachment diagram (Fig. 14–1) is recommended.

Separateness and Connectedness

One of the central, overriding psychological issues involving family life is the way in which families meet their members' psychological needs, and how this affects the individual's identity and self-esteem. During the early years of socialization, families mold and program a child's behavior, thus forming his or her sense of identity. Minuchin (1974) explains further: "Human experiences of identity have two elements—a sense of belonging and a sense of being separate. The laboratory in which these ingredients are mixed and dispensed with is the family, the matrix of identity" (p. 47).

Children's sense of belonging comes from being a part of, or connected to, a family—playing the roles of

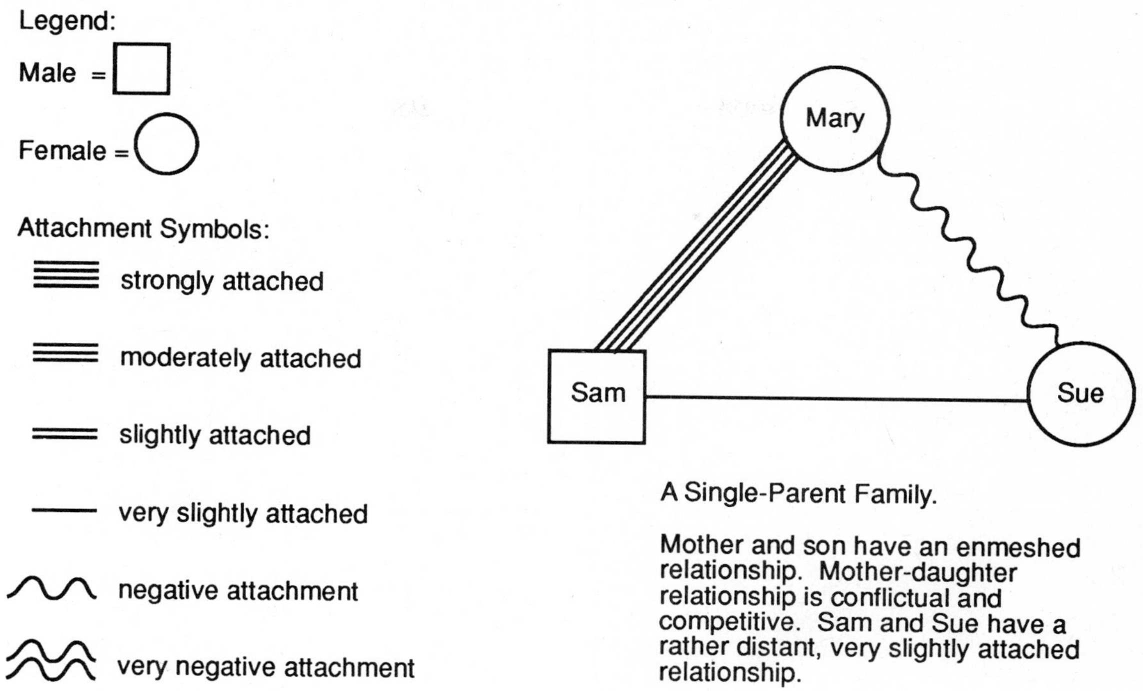
Legend:
Male =
Female =
Attachment Symbols:
strongly attached
moderately attached
slightly attached
very slightly attached
negative attachment
very negative attachment
Mary
Sam
Sue
A Single-Parent Family.
Mother and son have an enmeshed relationship. Mother-daughter relationship is conflictual and competitive. Sam and Sue have a rather distant, very slightly attached relationship.

Figure 14–1.
An example of an attachment diagram. Shows a single-parent family. Mother and son have an enmeshed relationship. Mother–daughter relationship is conflictual and competitive. John and Sue have rather distant, very slightly attached relationship. (Adapted from Wright and Leahey, 1984.)

child and sibling. The development of a sense of separateness and individuation occurs as children participate in roles within the family and in different family events and situations, as well as through involvement in activities outside of the family. As children grow the parents progressively give them more autonomy to develop and to meet their own unique needs and interests (Minuchin, 1974).

Thus in order to perceive and meet the psychological needs of family members, the family must achieve a satisfactory pattern of *separateness* and *connectedness*. Family members are both connected to and separate from one another. Each family handles the issues of separateness and connectedness in a unique fashion, some families placing much more emphasis on one facet than on the other.

Both conditions are basic and constitutive of family life. The young infant begins the separation process at about 6 months. Through the formative years, he or she forms an identity; but individuation and growth continue throughout his or her lifetime. Nonetheless, connectedness is equally basic, taking a variety of forms:

> Connectedness can range from physical proximity and rudimentary child care, to an intensity of mutual involvement which all but excludes all other interests. . . . In one family intense emotional exchange is sought; the members need to relax defenses and public facade, and they respond freely. In other families such confrontation is threatening, though the wish to feel themselves together in binding ties may be great. A family of this kind may be able to approach its desire only through much formalized action or ritualized action, such as giving gifts (Handel, 1972, p. 13).

The family needs to provide opportunities for the mastery of this duality. On the one hand, it must help its members want to be together and to develop and maintain cohesiveness or connectedness. On the other hand, it must gradually provide appropriate amounts of freedom and avenues of expression for members to individuate and become separate individuals.

How much of family life is regulated by power considerations is important here. Parental authority—its scope and the manner of its exercise—is one of the forces shaping the patterns encouraging individuality (separateness) and cohesion (connectedness). Parents differ in how extensively they impose their image on their children. When parents expect children to do all the adapting, there is little room for negotiating, and the chances of promoting individuality are hampered.

Also, families vary in how fast they push their children toward separateness and how intensively they encourage connectedness—that is, how soon they expect their children to grow up and to separate from parents. Some parents encourage babyish, dependent behaviors in their children, while others pressure their children to act more adult at an early age. The pace set for their children's growing up is often based on the parents' aims for themselves and their children. For example, if both parents are working and see dependency as a burden and frustrating to their goals, they will push their children at a faster pace to become self-sufficient and independent. As in other dimensions of family life, parental ideas about child growth and development and the acceptability of various behaviors are also influenced by the family's culture and social class background (Handel, 1972).

In assessing separateness and connectedness within in a family, Hartman and Laird (1983) look at the characteristics of the family in terms of enmeshment–disengagement (a continuum). Minuchin (1974) generated the notions of enmeshment and disengagement in families. An enmeshed family is one in which individual and subsystem boundaries (like spousal subsystem boundaries) are continually violated by members outside those boundaries. In enmeshed families, family members interpret or speak for each other and are supersensitive to family members' signals for help. Enmeshed families are families that don't allow room for separate opinions or autonomous behavior. Members tend to be too close (overinvolved) and too restrictive of individual freedom and personal identity. Conversely, in disengaged families, there are closed, rigid boundaries between subsystems and individuals, and very little sensitivity to members' calls for assistance. In these types of families relationships are too distant and there is little recognition or meeting of family members' personal needs. Moreover, there is an absence of involvement with each other. Neither extremes on the continuum are healthy.

Minuchin and associates (1978), in their studies of troubled families, find that certain types of families are generally enmeshed, including psychosomatic families and families with school phobic and schizophrenic children.

Need–Response Patterns

The affective component of family relationships needs to be evaluated in terms of the extent to which family members seem to care for and about each other (Hartman and Laird, 1983). Parad and Caplan (1965) address this concern in their discussion of the assessment of the *need–response patterns* in families. This concept is essentially synonymous with that of the family affective function. Mutual nurturance, respect, bonding, and separateness–connectedness aspects emerge as vital prerequisites or necessary corequisites to satisfactory need–response patterns in families (Table 14–2).

TABLE 14–2. THE SOCIOEMOTIONAL NEEDS OF FAMILY MEMBERS

1. Love for one's own sake.
2. A balance between support and independence with respect to tasks.
3. A balance between freedom and control.
4. The availability of suitable role models.

Adapted from Parad and Caplan (1965).

Three separate and interlocking phases are inherent in a family's affective response to these needs. First, family members must perceive the needs of the other individuals, within the constraints of the family's culture. Next, these needs must be viewed with respect and seen to be worthy of attention (as discussed under mutual respect balance). And lastly, these recognized and respected needs must be satisfied to the extent possible in light of family resources. It is especially propitious if family members each have confidants within the family with whom they can unburden themselves.

This triad of perception, respect, and satisfaction of family members' needs is very much influenced by American sociocultural perspectives—viewing individuals as separate persons who are deserving of recognition and respect as well as a fair share in the family's resources. This tendency to view family members as unique, evolving individuals corresponds with the high value this society places on individualism.

In working with families it was observed that the family's sensitivity to, and thus perception of the individual members's actions and needs, varies greatly. Most families usually fall somewhere between being extremely sensitive (sign of enmeshment), and thus highly responsive to an individual member's input, and being extremely insensitive and unresponsive to individual members' inputs (sign of disengagement).

The extent to which basic psychological or socioemotional needs are met also varies depending on the family's social support system. Some families have a greater, more involved social network, such as an extended family, from which to draw support. In these families the meeting of family members' psychosocial needs can be accomplished by individuals who are both inside and outside of the nuclear family. In contrast, families that are truly isolated from social support systems—closed families—have limited outside resources and hence depend primarily, or solely, on family members to meet all their psychological needs. Naturally, this latter state imposes a great burden on family relationships, because probably no one person, such as a mate, can meet all of the other person's needs.

A recent study by Barber and Thomas (1986) found that emotional ties varied depending on the gender of the child and parent. The researchers surveyed 527 largely Mormon college students about their relationships with their parents. Fathers were found to be more physically affectionate to daughters, while mothers showed the same amount of physical affection to children of both sexes. Mothers typically had more companionship with daughters, and fathers with sons. Physical affection was found to be positively associated with self-esteem in both sexes.

The Therapeutic Role

In Chapter 12 the therapeutic role of spouses was discussed as one of the emergent roles increasingly expected of mates entering into marital and family life from all social classes, but particularly in the middle class. This role is quite similar to the mates' role in meeting the affective needs of their mates. While the affective function describes the broad mental health function of the family—as a group designed to meet the psychological needs of its members—the therapeutic role describes an important socioemotional role within the marital subsystem. This role has been explained by Nye (1976): "The behavior . . . is therapeutic in assisting the spouse to cope with and, hopefully, dispose of a problem with which he is confronted" (p. 111). When this role is extended to include the rest of the family, children and adults alike, some very important elements of family behavior come to light. Nye (1976) continues: "Listening and giving the family member an opportunity to verbalize, acting as a 'sounding board' for the ideas or reactions of the other, supplying additional information, concepts, or insights, and taking concrete actions in sharing the solution of the problem are all involved" (p. 115). Some of these behaviors, of course, would not be appropriate (therapeutic) in relating to a young child or infant, but with older children, much of the same therapeutic, assistive relating can occur.

Primarily, the therapeutic role spouses play is problem oriented. It involves listening to the problem, sympathizing, giving reassurance and affection, and offering help in solving the problem. In Nye's (1976) study of spousal roles, he reported that over 60 percent of both husbands and wives indicated that mates have the duty to enact this role, the remainder indicating the desirability of this role in marriage. Moreover, Nye found that 63 percent of wives usually engage in this role. More women than men enacted this role well, and also valued it more highly.

THE AFFECTIVE FUNCTION IN ENERGIZED FAMILIES

It is important to know how healthy, functional, or, as Pratt (1976) calls them, "energized" families achieve their affective function, because this will give us an optimal standard to use for comparative purposes.

> A feature of energized family structure . . . is the tendency to provide autonomy and to be responsive to the particular interests and needs of individual family members. . . . This includes the tendency not only to accept, but to prize individuality and uniqueness, and to tolerate disagreement and deviance. Respect and acceptance are given unconditionally, without continuous comparison of the person to others or to prescribed standards. . . . The family members are encouraged in their various endeavors, especially in seeking new areas of growth and in developing their creativity, imagination, and independent thinking. (pp. 84–85)

The one limitation of this description is that it was based on a study of largely middle-class white families. Obviously, the social class and cultural variability must be considered in evaluating what is healthy and less healthy behaviors or patterns in a family.

THE FAMILY UNDER STRESS: THE AFFECTIVE FUNCTION

Maintaining a nurturing familial environment is often a formidable task, as many stressors tend to disrupt family homeostasis and make family members less sensitive and loving toward each other. One of these stressors is the health/illness stressor. Brown (1978) explains that when family stressors occur, "the system for mutual nurturance is subject to disruption; once such disruption occurs, there is a strong tendency for interpersonal tension to reverberate throughout the family system and for the disruption to escalate" (p. 25).

When the psychological needs of family members are not being adequately perceived and addressed, the usual consequence is the overt appearance of symptoms in the form of distress signals from one or more family members. These symptoms of family dysfunction in the family "symptom bearer" include various emotional responses such as anger, anxiety, and depression; delinquent or acting-out behaviors; and somatic complaints and illness. This dysfunction, in turn, further inhibits clear, functional communication within family relationships, resulting in a downward-spiraling process until some positive step is taken to curtail further disorganization and reverse the tailspin.

Parad and Caplan (1965) do not believe that the temporary periods of low response to members' needs are necessarily harmful to their mental health. However, persistent, long-standing need frustration is deleterious, and even a temporary inattentiveness to a family member's needs may be harmful if the loss occurs when that individual is particularly vulnerable, such as during a critical phase of his or her development.

It is often observed that in families with childhood chronic illness, the sick child receives most of the parent's attention and care, and the other children do not have their needs met. A red flag is thrown up when healthy siblings become angry, resentful, or demanding.

Doherty and Campbell (1988), family health professionals, note that family problems and dysfunctions generally become worse or more apparent during the terminal phase of an illness or during bereavement. When the family is grieving, conflicts in the family often become overt and the affective needs of family members are usually not acknowledged.

The death of a family member is probably the most catastrophic event for a family member or family (Crosby and Jose, 1983). The seriousness of this event is demonstrated in the higher mortality rates of spouses up to 2 years after the death of a mate. Bereaved persons are at higher risk for multiple diseases. These are primarily the chronic diseases of middle and late age. The excess risk of mortality due to bereavement is higher among widowed men than women (Kosten et al, 1985). A recent study found that middle-aged people who lost spouses, siblings, and siblings-in-law generally adjusted more poorly than younger or older individuals and were more prone to health problems in the bereavement period (Perkins and Harris, 1990).

Along with death comes the aspect of loss. People who are closest to the person who has died are immediately affected by the loss. Eventually, as in an earthquake, the whole system of relationships is shaken (Gelcer, 1986). Family members' psychological needs for support are much greater during the period when the family member is dying and after the death. If the member's death is unexpected, stress and grief will be more extreme. When death is prolonged over a period of months or even years, stress is continuous and circumstances ambiguous. Family members are often left emotionally depleted in terms of helping themselves or supporting others in the family. Other stressors occur after a death in the family (numerous arrangements that must be made, settling the estate, medical bills, and family role transitions); it is easy to see that the adult member(s) have difficulty supporting the child members of the family. This is often a time when the family's social support system (both formal and informal) can play an important role in supporting grieving families. Functional families also pull together during this period and try to share their grief and support each other.

The affective needs of family members during the time of a major loss is to be able to grieve for the loss. Constructive grief work depends on the ability of the social support network (family and the family's social network) to be permissive of feelings, positively accepting and supportive. Family members' energies should be directed at the actual loss as experienced collectively and individually. When feelings are shared there needs to be an open stage for discussing, recalling, memory associating, and reliving of past events. Moreover, certain beliefs may need to be confronted, especially when guilt is expressed based on irrational assumptions of a person's responsibility for events that were beyond the control of that person.

Children also need to be able to grieve. Sharing feelings and thoughts with children and communicating with them at their cognitive and emotional levels of maturity are most important. The parents' handling of death with children and adolescents is most significant in terms of helping them with their psychological needs (Crosby and Jose, 1983). Those families who are open to expressing their emotions are more successful in adjusting to the loss of a family member (McClowry et al, 1989).

Several recent articles have been written about the similarity between divorce and death in a family in terms of adjustment to the loss. Increased risk of illness and distress among both the recently divorced and widowed has been found. The impact of certain factors upon adjustment to widowhood and divorce (economic, social support, cause of divorce/death, timing of event, and attachment) makes a difference as to how difficult both divorce and widowhood are (Kitson et al, 1989).

FAMILY AFFECTIVE FUNCTION: APPLYING THE FAMILY NURSING PROCESS

□ ASSESSMENT QUESTIONS

The following questions have been included to assist the assessor in appraising the family affective function.

Family Need–Response Patterns

1. Do family members perceive the needs of the other individuals in the family? Are the parents and spouses able to describe their children's and mate's needs and concerns? How sensitive are family members in picking up cues regarding other's feelings and needs? Do family members each have someone they can turn to within the family, to unburden themselves—that is, a confidant?
2. Are each member's needs, interests, and differentness respected by the other family members? Does a mutual respect balance exist? Do they show mutual respect toward each other? How sensitive is the family to each individual's actions and concerns?
3. Are the recognized needs of family members being met by the family, and if so, to what extent?

For questions 1 through 3 it is suggested that a list of the family members be included with their needs identified (as perceived by family members) and the extent to which these needs are being met.

Mutual Nurturance, Closeness, and Identification

4. To what extent do family members provide mutual nurturance to each other? How supportive of each other are they?
5. Is a sense of closeness and intimacy present among the sets of relationships within the family? How well do family members get along with each other? Do they show affection toward each other?
6. Does mutual identification and bonding or attachment appear to be present? Empathetic statements, concerns about others' feelings, experiences, and hardships are all indications of this being present.

To answer questions 5 and 6, use of an attachment diagram is recommended. Attachment diagrams depict both the strength and quality of the affective relationship or emotional ties between members of the family. The focus is on the relationship and the reciprocal nature of the affectional tie.

The evidence gathered to depict the bonds between family members is largely subjective. Both observational and interview data can be used. Observations about relationships include expression of feelings toward a family member as well as signs of affection or distancing (kissing, hugging, eye contact, smiling, comforting, cuddling, sitting close or far away). Verbal (interview) data include responses to questions about how close member A is to member B. For example: How do A and B get along? What's their relationship like? Which of the siblings is closer to parent A? Also historical information often gives clues as to how close a relationship is. An example is the case where the mother constantly has cared for the chronically ill child in hospital and home, while the father and older child rarely became involved in caregiving.

Figure 14–1 illustrates an attachment bond and the symbols used in these diagrams. The present relationships are diagrammed rather then past relationships. Bonds that are very close or very negative (conflictual) are typically maladaptive, although situational crisis sometimes forces very close relationships on a short-term basis and these very close relationships serve a necessary supportive purpose.

Separateness and Connectedness

7. How does the family deal with the issues of separateness and connectedness? How does the family help its members want to be together and maintain cohesiveness (connectedness)? Are opportunities for developing separateness stressed adequately, and are they appropriate for the age and needs of each of the family members?

FAMILY NURSING DIAGNOSES

In families where the psychological or affective needs of family members are not being met, a myriad of family problems may be manifested. A number of North American Nursing Diagnosis Association (NANDA) diagnoses may be appropriate when there is altered family affective functioning (Table 14–3). In these cases, inability to meet the psychological needs of all family members would be a defining characteristic.

FAMILY NURSING INTERVENTIONS

Family nursing diagnoses for this area were addressed by using NANDA's classification of germane nursing diagnoses (Table 14–3). For interventions related to the NANDA diagnoses mentioned previously, the reader is referred to Carpentino (1987) and McFarland and McFarlane (1989). General suggestions for assisting families to better meet the psychosocial needs of their members are briefly explained in the present section.

Interventions Aimed At Need–Response Patterns

The assessment of this area (asking members to tell the nurse about each family member, what his or her psychological needs are, and if family members are responding to these needs) is an education for families in and of itself. Some teaching should preceed this exercise, such as explaining to the family that each person has his or her own individual needs; that many of these needs are based on the person's developmental stage; and that family members need to recognize these and respond to them as well as possible—without interfering with other members' needs. In large families or families that are not psychologically oriented, this may be new information. In fact, there is a misperception by some parents that children should be treated exactly the same, so that no favoritism is involved. With this belief parents often don't see their children's uniqueness. Teaching the family members about individual and family growth and developmental characteristics may be very helpful for sensitizing parents to their children's needs.

Another strategy for helping family members, especially the parents, become more sensitive to individual family members' needs is by asking, "What is Johnnie like?" When parents respond, and the nurse asks further questions about the child's differentness, comments can then be made that interpret a child's behavior so that parents better understand their child. By commenting on a child's behavior, this helps reframe their children's actions in a more positive, informed way. (Example: A mother labels her son's incessant talking as indicating that he is a spoiled brat. The family nurse relabels the behavior, helping the family see the son as anxious and wanting parents' attention).

Maintaining Mutual Nurturance

To help families maintain or initiate mutual nurturance, communication patterns in the family need to be analyzed. Parents need to feel that they are the ones who must stop circular patterns of angry, rejecting, or dysfunctional messages. For instance, they can do this by not responding to messages that start the dysfunctional pattern going or they can learn not to initiate these interactions themselves and instead communicate so that mutual respect is shown. It is not easy to

TABLE 14–3. NANDA DIAGNOSES FOR ALTERED FAMILY AFFECTIVE FUNCTIONING

Diagnosis	Example
1. Altered family processes. Definition: This is the state in which a family that normally functions effectively experiences a dysfunction.	The family is under stress and all the family members' energies are being diverted to handle the stressor, thereby neglecting or overlooking family members' psychosocial needs.
2. Altered parenting. Definition: Occurs when the ability of the nurturing figure(s) to create an environment that promotes the optimal growth and development of another human being is compromised.	A family with marked dominance by the mother (mother is very controlling) and marked passivity by father does not allow oldest adolescent son to individuate or separate from the family, thereby not meeting his psychosocial needs.
3. Potential altered parenting. Definition: Same as above, except that "potential" is added to compromise.	The same as the above family example, except the oldest son is in fifth grade and has not entered puberty. Because of the mother's controlling, overbearing mothering, the potential for a problem occurring when the son reaches adolescence is very great.
4. Dysfunctional grieving. Definition: A maladaptive process that occurs when grief is intensified to the degree that the person is overwhelmed, becomes stuck in one phase of grieving, and demonstrates excessive or prolonged emotional responses to the significant loss.	Dysfunctional grieving is being extended to include the grieving family—which is grieving dysfunctionally. The usual family dysfunction is the *denial* of the death in the family. (Ineffective denial could also be stated.) A family rule is established that it's not alright to talk about the loss, to express feelings about the loss, or to recall memories of the loved one or events where the loved one was there. The memories, feelings, and thoughts are not shared, leading to other problems: psychosomatic illness, depression, pseudomutuality, emotional cutoff, and distancing of member from family.
5. Ineffective family coping, compromised. Definition: Is insufficient, ineffective, or compromised family support, comfort, assistance, or encouragement that may alter the family member's or family's competence in adaptive tasks related to the presenting health challenge (may be short or long term).	Mother has been hospitalized for 1 week due to having surgery. She is the primary nurturer in the family—to both the husband and children. The husband–father has attempted to give the children attention and love, but they (age 2 and 3) are upset and resentful that their mother abandoned them.
6. Ineffective family coping, disabling. Definition: Is the behavior of one or more family members that incapacitates the family (or individual members) to therapeutically adapt to the existing health challenge.	Within this family the wife and husband (both are remarried) have two children—a son, age 10 from the husband's previous marriage, and a daughter, age 5, from the mother's previous marriage. The son has been labeled the troublemaker in the family, and is outwardly called this. The daughter is labeled the "sweet one," and comparisons of the children's personality differences are made when the parents' get angry at the son.
7. Potential for violence. Altered role performance. Social isolation. Self-esteem, low. Altered growth and development.	These problems could also be present given the situation where family members' psychosocial needs are not being adequately met.

Source: Adapted from McFarland and McFarlane (1989).

break repetitive communication patterns. However, if parents understand the dynamics of problematic interactional patterns and are aware of what is happening, they can make definitive steps to change dysfunctional communications. (See Chap. 10 for more elaborate discussion.) Nurses can act as communication role models to families, to help them see that a more healthy mutual respect balance can be achieved in family interactions.

Assisting Families With Closeness–Separateness Issues

Closeness–separateness problems may be due to parents' knowledge deficit, but this is rarely so. These types of problems often have to do with the way the parents themselves were raised and unresolved intergenerational problems. In health settings, overcloseness or enmeshment is a much more common problem than disengagement. This is because there is a tendency in some families for the adult member(s) to become oversolicitous and protective of a family member who has a serious or disabling illness. In some cases, the whole family may be highly resonant (or hypersensitive) to the "identified patient's" needs.

If over-closeness is a long-standing problem in a family and is of the intensity that family members' growth and development is being significantly impeded, then usually family therapy is needed, and a referral should be initiated if the family also believes this is necessary. Minuchin (1974), a noted family therapist, would work to restructure the enmeshed family, while Bowen (1978), another noted family therapist, would work on helping family member(s) become more differentiated.

Assisting Families With Grieving

Several authors have presented guidelines to facilitate grief resolution following a loss or death in the family (Crosby and Jose, 1983; McClowry et al, 1989; Kahn, 1990). In order to help family members who are in anticipatory grief (family member is dying) we need to understand tasks of family members during this difficult time. Rando (1986) describes the tasks of family members:

1. Family members should keep the dying person involved in family decisions as long as possible, so that he or she feels some sense of control and that his or her opinions still matter.
2. The well family members need to remain separate—to individuate from the dying family member. They must come to grips with reality that the loved one will die, and to start contemplating the future without the loved one.
3. Family members need to begin dealing with the reallocation or shifting of roles in the family to establish a new family homeostasis. This shifting of roles is very difficult and family system functioning is often precarious.
4. Family members need to learn to manage the feelings aroused by the terminal illness and death. Sadness, guilt, anger, memories, and reactions to past losses are common emotions that need to be shared and managed.
5. Family members need to face reality in terms of discussion of what needs to be done when death occurs (medical requirements, funeral arrangements, finances, etc).
6. Family members need to "say goodbye." This should be done by each family member—verbally or nonverbally. This critical area requires support and role modeling from caregivers. Family members need to know when death is imminent.

Turning to the role of the family nurse during this period, a central thrust of her or his care should be to help family members achieve patient–family member comfort. Rando (1986) suggests that to achieve this end family nurses can assist by helping to "maintain the relationship between the dying person and family by encouraging open communication to the extent the family style allows" (p. 75). Another intervention family focused nurses make is assisting the family to assume new roles (having family conferences is one way to assist family members to adjust and take on additional duties and make practical plans). A third exceptionally important intervention is to facilitate the expression of emotions, and support the family members in their grief. Family members need to know that their feelings are normal and part of the grief process that has to occur. And lastly, assisting the family to understand and absorb pertinent medical communication about the course of illness and treatment is a central role of the family nurse. Holding family conferences to explain illness and treatment concerns is very helpful and encourages family cohesiveness.

☐ STUDY QUESTIONS

1. Give three reasons why the affective function is so important.

2. In order for families to adequately function in the need–response pattern area, the family members would need to demonstrate (name the three components in sequence):

3. The spiral phenomenon relative to the generation and continuance of emotional support and warmth among family members can be explained as (select the best answer):
   a. Hate begets hate; love begets love.
   b. I'm okay, you're okay principle.
   c. Self-fulfilling prophesy.
   d. Marital role modeling, plus mutual nurturance.

4. The results and goals of achieving a balance in familial mutual respect are (select appropriate answers):
   a. Members of the family do not encroach on the rights of the other individuals in the family.
   b. No family members are expected to cater to the whims of other family members.
   c. Parents treat children as people, not "inferiors" (objects to be manipulated and dominated).
   d. Children do not develop "brat" syndrome, where they seek and receive gratification for their needs, but consider the needs, rights, and responsibilities of parents.

5. Match the four terms and/or concepts in right-hand column with definitions and descriptions in left-hand column.

DEFINITIONS/DESCRIPTIONS	TERMS/CONCEPTS
a. Responsiveness of other member(s) to a family's positive feelings toward them.	1. Bonding or attachment
b. Empathy or role making.	2. Identification
c. Sustaining force behind perception and satisfaction of family members' needs.	3. Crescive bonds
d. Develops in familial relationships where there is continuity and positive interaction.	4. A response bond
e. Grows in intensity with time.	
f. Identification precedes it.	
g. Parents obtain referent power when this is present.	
h. Receiver's reaction to sender's affection and warmth.	

6. Answer briefly: What is the parental task relative to dealing with connectedness and separateness?

7. The spousal therapeutic role differs from the family affective function in that (select all appropriate answers):
   a. They do not differ; both are synonymous terms.
   b. The spousal therapeutic role deals in a subsystem rather than entire family system.
   c. The therapeutic role is largely problem focused, whereas the affective function covers therapeutic aspects and other supportive and nurturing elements.
   d. The family affective function deals only with being sensitive to family members' feelings, while the therapeutic role suggests more skilled assistance.

8. Pratt describes energized families and how they can achieve their affective function. From her description, list two salient values or priorities that energized families display relative to this area.

Family Case Study

A family case study is presented with the study questions in Chapter 17. From this family study, answer the following questions concerning the assessment of the family's affective functioning.

9. To what extent do family members perceive and meet the needs of other family members?

10. Does a mutual respect balance exist, where each member shows respect for the other's feelings and needs?

11. To what extent do family members provide mutual nurturance to each other? How supportive of each other are they?

12. Is a sense of closeness and intimacy present among the sets of relationships within the family? How compatible and affectionate are family members toward each other?

13. Does mutual identification and bonding appear to be present?

14. How does the family deal with the issues of separateness and connectedness?

15. Propose one family nursing diagnosis in the area of family affective function.

16. Recommend two family nursing interventions to resolve or ameliorate the above problem.

CHAPTER FIFTEEN

The Socialization Function

Learning Objectives

1. Define and identify the tasks of socialization.
2. Explain how the family's involvement in socialization changes during the life cycle of the child-rearing family.
3. Discuss the role culture plays in socialization patterns, particularly child-rearing practices.
4. Describe the findings of McClelland and associates relative to their study of child-rearing patterns.
5. Explain the role social class plays in socialization and give some broad differences found between working-class and middle-class parents.
6. Explicate the relationship between a society's value system and that society's child-rearing and socialization patterns.
7. Identify several important issues and/or changes in modern society that have directly affected socialization patterns.
8. Correlate the stage of child development with the stage of parent development and parent tasks according to Friedman's model.
9. Explain one's own biases regarding child-rearing practices and socialization patterns.
10. Using a hypothetical family situation:
    a. Assess the family's socialization function.
    b. Identify one family nursing diagnosis in the area of family socialization.
    c. Propose two family nursing interventions aimed at ameliorating or resolving the problem.

It is generally accepted that the family is more specialized in its function today than it has ever been. Although the family performs many functions that have changed over time, one vital responsibility has remained a primary focus of the family: socialization or the rearing of children. The nurse is frequently in a position to influence, support, and assist the socialization process in families. In an attempt to provide the knowledge needed for assessment and interventions, this chapter defines and identifies tasks of socialization, discusses the influence of culture on parenting patterns, reviews some contemporary trends in child-rearing practices, and examines socialization theory. The chapter concludes with nursing practice guidelines (assessment areas, family nursing diagnoses, and intervention).

Chapter 15 was first written by Maxene Johnston, R.N., M.A., Executive Director, Weingart Center, Los Angeles. It was revised in the second and third editions by Marilyn Friedman.

SOCIALIZATION: A FAMILY AFFAIR

Definition of Socialization

Socialization begins at birth and ends only at death. It is a lifelong process by which individuals continually modify their behavior in response to the socially patterned circumstances they experience. It includes internalizing the appropriate sets of norms and values for the teenager of 14, the bride of 20, the parent of 24, the grandparent of 50, and the retired person of 65.

Socialization embraces all those processes in a specific community or group whereby humans, by virtue of their profound plasticity, through significant experiences encountered in their lifetime, acquire socially patterned characteristics (Honigman, 1967). Translated into role terminology, the concept of socialization refers to "the process of development or change that a person undergoes as a result of social interaction and the learning of social roles" (Gegas, 1979, p. 365). The roles can be as diverse as a child learning manners, a convict "learning the ropes" in prison, or a student learning to become a nurse.

Most often, socialization proceeds informally and inexplicitly, so that changes made in response to altering cultural and environmental conditions go quite unnoticed. Through socialization, people learn to live with others in groups and come to play appropriate sex- and age-linked roles. This occurs within the larger context or process of development.

Child-rearing practices are subsumed under the rubric of socialization and are the primary focus of attention of this chapter. The terms "socialization," "child rearing," "parental behavior," and "parent–child interaction" are used interchangeably in both this chapter and in the child socialization literature in general (Gegas, 1979).

The term socialization most often refers to the myriad of learning experiences provided within the family. These experiences are aimed at teaching children how to function and assume adult roles in society, such as those mentioned above. Reiss (1965) points out that although other functions such as reproduction are deemed necessary to, and performed in, all societies, the nurturant socialization of children is found universally only within the nuclear family structure.

Because this function is now shared with other institutions and is influenced by many extrinsic factors, the family has a reduced role in socialization. The family has never had complete and total control over the socialization of children, despite the fact that parents still try, and do, transmit their cultural knowledge to the next generation. Contemporary changes in the level of shared responsibility are such that today, outside influences may even negate the primary value system of the family.

What has not changed is the fact that the family continues to have the primary responsibility of transforming an infant, in a score of years, into a social being capable of full participation in society. The child has to be taught language, the roles he or she is expected to assume at various stages of life, sociocultural norms and expectations of what is right and wrong, and relevant cognitive structures. Additionally, the child must learn appropriate sexual roles and a sense of creativity and initiative.

One aspect of the socialization process of particular relevance for the nurse involves the child's acquisition of health concepts, attitudes, and behaviors. Typically, the mother is the family's primary health educator and leader. She has the responsibility for deciding who is sick, whether or not to initiate treatment, and what kind it should be. She is also responsible for teaching her children basic health habits and attitudes and, as they grow older, how to care for themselves.

Another important and integral task of socialization is the inculcation of controls and values—giving the growing child (and adult) a sense of what is right and wrong and the internal controls needed for self-discipline. The development of morality has been described by Kohlberg (1970) as a developmental process similar to the stages of emotional and cognitive development of Erikson (1959) and Piaget (1971), respectively. By identifying with parental figures and being consistently reinforced both negatively and positively for their behavior, children develop a personal value system and a set of morals that is greatly influenced by the family (Committee on Public Education, 1973).

Socialization involves learning, which entails the use of social control mechanisms such as discipline. The use of discipline as a means of socializing children includes both positive and negative sanctions. Positive discipline encourages a person to exploit his or her resources for growth and serves as a positive reinforcer of behavior. Different societies and social classes have their own values regulating what sanctions to employ. For example, middle-class mothers in a New England town in the United States preferred incentives like praise to those of rewarding children materially with candy or prizes for being good (Honigman, 1967). Many American mothers present themselves as models to their children to illustrate what they want them to be and not to be.

Negative sanctions, on the other hand, imply punishment and involve a great variety of methods. One of the most consistent claims in the literature is that there is a greater reliance on the use of physical punishment as a means of child disciplining in lower-class families than in middle-class families (Gegas, 1979). Middle-class parents tend to use reasoning and "psychological techniques" (eg, shame and guilt) more frequently. Although we know that punishment often succeeds in eliminating children's undesirable behavior, in itself it lacks direction and does not teach alternative behavior.

One way to measure family success in socialization has been to evaluate the outcomes of the child-rearing process—that is, to evaluate how successful or well adjusted the children are or have turned out to be. Not only are there comparative standards by which we measure a child's progress and hence the family's, but there are also age-related standards; that is, we expect certain socialization skills will be learned at particular ages. Today this measure is no doubt biased and inaccurate, because parents share the socialization function with the school system, peers, other reference groups, and the wider community.

Often, even in the most dedicated and healthy families, children have trouble adjusting and learning socially approved behaviors. Woodward and co-workers (1978) state that parents today often feel powerless in the face of institutional interferences: "The growth of social services, health care, and public education has robbed them of their traditional roles as job trainers, teachers, nurses, and nurturers. And their control over their children's lives is threatened by the pervasive, and increasingly authoritative, influence of television, schools and peer groups" (p. 64). Lasch, in *Haven in a Heartless World* (1979), reiterates this same theme. He believes that outside institutions have robbed the family of one of its central functions, child rearing and thus, have immeasurably weakened its foundations. He describes the parents' quandary over child rearing and their faltering confidence in their own judgment and ability to parent.

> The family struggles to conform to an ideal of the family imposed from without. The experts agree that parents should neither tyrannize over their children nor burden them with "over-solicitous" attentions. They agree, moreover, that every action is the product of a long causal chain and that moral judgments have no place in child rearing. This proposition, central to the mental health ethic, absolves the child from moral responsibility. . . . It is not surprising that many parents seek to escape the exercise of this responsibility by avoiding confrontations with the child and by retreating from the work of discipline and character formation. (pp. 172–173)

Many parents, frightened by the prospects of perhaps damaging their children due to their own parental mistakes, have turned to "recipe books," "how to" parenting tools, and child counseling, searching for the right technique that will make them perfect parents. It is not surprising that by turning to outside counselors, parents may lose even more of their parental authority and confidence in their ability to parent.

From another perspective, it has also been suggested that institutional "overseeing" of the training needs of children has resulted from parents' disenchantment with traditional family roles, as well as their waning commitment to child rearing. Part of this decline in enthusiasm for raising children stems from the difficulties parents feel in trying to fulfill their primary roles due to increased economic and daily living pressures and increased personal needs for their own development, self-expression (Harris, 1984), and socialization.

Most families have two working parents. A substantial number of fathers hold two jobs to make ends meet. Of the more than 15 million women in the labor force, a large number of them are heads of households (U.S. Bureau of the Census, 1988b). In today's busy world even affluent and privileged parents feel overburdened and pressured by the simultaneous demands of work, achievement, information overload, parenting, and being a wife. Feminism has made women conscious of many more options in women's lives and so has contributed to the "overloaded" feeling of modern women—given that they are still expected to carry out all their old roles, in addition to any new ones (Woodward, 1990). Experts tell parents to spend "quality time" and "meaningful" time with their children, but even this is difficult to squeeze in between a multiplicity of other priorities.

Despite societal change in women's and men's roles in the family (fathers have increased the time they spend in child care activities), the mother usually has the primary responsibility for socializing the child through the preschool years. Siblings and the father often play supportive roles during this time. The responsibility is later shared among schools, parents, peer groups, and to a lesser degree, recreational, social, and religious institutions. In the United States today, socialization may also be shared with day-care nurseries, nursery schools, and organized after-school programs. These remove parents from and dilute their involvement in their child's socialization experiences at earlier and earlier stages of child and family development.

Changes in traditional socialization patterns, responsibilities, and time-honored methods are now occurring at a greater rate than ever before. The dilemma of who will teach children important sociocultural traditions, how and where these are to be learned, and at what age and stage, are the questions we have struggled with in the past and will continue to debate into the future.

SOCIETY'S ATTITUDES TOWARD CHILDREN

No matter which society we observe, the attitudes and approaches to the care and rearing of children are congruent with the social, moral, religious, and economic values of that society at a particular period of time. Over time, the place of children in our society has changed. Extraordinary gains have been made in the understanding and care of children. But along with such advances, new social and economic pressures and realities have introduced other attitudes and concerns.

Goodman's (1978) observations of these current events suggest that we are witnessing warnings that something is changing in the most basic relationship in any society: the relationship between its adults and its children, between its present and its future. Goodman (1978) has commented on the reemergence of a hostile relationship between adults and children, and expresses a concern for the untoward effects of this generational conflict:

> Now, increasingly, parenthood is regarded as a personal, individual decision—a "lifestyle," whatever that may be—made apart from community interests. Kids are listed not as economic assets, but as financial liabilities. Each year, someone tallies up the cost of raising them as if they were sides of beef. And each year, someone else tallies up their cost to the local town or city and wonders if they are worth it. In many places, the voters are saying "no."

Child development experts mirror Goodman's concern about societal attitudes toward children. Elkind, a child development expert, states, "There are times in history when children fare better than others. But there's no question about it. Children are not well cared for in our society today" (Libman, 1988). Child advocacy organizations cite statistics that show the declining lot of children (increased poverty, infant mortality, delinquency, teen pregnancy, and so forth).

The professional advice given to parents may be a reflection of the child's changing status in a particular time in society. When one examines the shifts in the advice given to parents over the past 60 years, the fluctuating philosophies and anxieties of a highly industrialized society appear evident:

- 1910—Spank them
- 1920—Deprive them
- 1930—Ignore them
- 1940—Reason with them
- 1950—Love them
- 1960—Spank them lovingly
- 1970—The hell with them!

The sarcasm expressed in the 1970s, which probably also reflects the 1980s, may indeed be an expression of the despair and depression parents feel about their ability to successfully parent. Perhaps the old folk proverb sums up many parents' thoughts today: "Once I had six theories and no children. Now I have six children and no theories."

An examination of the various historic and contemporary attitudes and approaches to children illuminates the obvious; children have always generated an "air of ambivalence" that permeates society and influences its values and beliefs in the care and rearing of its young. Certainly the ambivalence that exists regarding children extends throughout society. The increased use of drugs and alcohol among school-age children and adolescents, along with their myriad of other health and social problems, only increases this feeling of ambivalence. Still, in the middle of conflicting values and beliefs about children and their place in society, an attempt is also being made to adapt to such ambivalence, change, and conflict by emphasizing the importance of the family in child rearing and "revaluing" the parent–child dyad relationships.

INFLUENCE OF CULTURE ON CHILD REARING

Cultural factors in socialization are exceedingly difficult to disentangle from environmental, social, and psychological considerations. In fact, the relative influence of each is often a matter of conjecture and speculation. Over the years, however, specific cultural responses have been studied and have added to our understanding of the variety of socialization patterns among various ethnic and culturally divergent groups.

Cultural Conditioning

The context in which child-rearing and socialization patterns occur was identified by Kardiner (1945) and follows some basic postulates:

1. [The] techniques which the members of any society employ in the care and rearing of children are culturally patterned and will tend to be similar, although never identical, for various families within the society.
2. [The] culturally patterned techniques for the care and rearing of children differ from one society to another. (p. vi)

Studies confirm that parents from different ethnic backgrounds often use child-rearing techniques that are derived from their unique set of cultural values and role expectations. Because the process of child rearing is cross-culturally so intricate, social scientists have specialized in studying different age groups and different cultures, with some researchers conducting longitudinal studies. Work in this area has revealed that despite individual variation, children demonstrate patterned behavior that is linked to the culturally patterned behavior of their caretakers.

Cross-Cultural Comparisons

Caudill's comparative research (1975) on middle-class families in Japan and the United States is one example of studies done in this area. Caudill found that mothers in the two cultures engage in subtly different styles of caretaking that have, however, strikingly different effects. Generally, the American mother seems to encourage her baby to be active and respond vocally, whereas the Japanese mother acts in ways that she believes soothes and quiets her child. By the age of 3 to 4 months, the infants of both cultures seem to have already learned responses appropriate to these different patterns. The striking discovery, however, is the fact that the responses of the infants are in line with certain broad expectations for behavior in the two cultures: in America the expectation that individuals should be physically and verbally assertive, and in Japan that individuals should be physically and verbally restrained.

In middle-class America, the mothers perceive their babies as separate and autonomous beings who are expected to learn to do and think for themselves. The baby is seen as a distinct personality with his or her own needs and desires, which the mother must learn to recognize and care for. She does this by helping her infant learn to express these needs through her emphasis on vocal communication; the baby can thus "tell" her what he or she wants so that the mother can respond appropriately. In contrast, the Japanese mother views her baby much more as an extension of herself; psychologically the boundaries between mother and infant are blurred. As a result of this emphasis on close attachment, the mother is likely to feel that she knows what is best for the baby. There is then no perceived need for the infant to tell the mother what he or she wants. Because of this orientation, the Japanese mother does not place much importance on vocal communication and instead stresses physical contact.

Although there are few such cross-cultural observational studies on infants reported in the literature, it should be noted that Reblesky (1967) obtained similar results in her study of Dutch and American infants. The Dutch mothers were like the Japanese mothers in that they engaged in less talking to and stimulation of their infants.

These two studies should be evaluated carefully before making sweeping generalizations. For example, cross-class studies of infants in the United States have often found that middle-class mothers talk more to their infants than mothers in lower socioeconomic groups. Therefore, the results of the cross-cultural studies may not apply to the child-rearing techniques of mothers in different socioeconomic groups within various cultures.

One interesting cultural difference in childhood training has to do with modesty. In the United States in comparison with many other parts of the world, we place an emphasis on modesty. Immediately at birth Benedict (1938) observed that:

> we waste no time in clothing the baby . . . in contrast to many societies where the child runs naked until it is ceremoniously given its skirt or its pubic sheath at adolescence. The child's training fits it precisely for adult convention. (p. 161)

We are rarely aware of how deep and with what precision feelings of modesty are embedded in our culture until we see and feel the response of medical staff and patients dealing with this issue. For example, modesty may be one of the key factors in resistance to cervical examination in cancer detection programs (Alpenfels, 1969).

All cultures must deal in one way or another with the child's natural cycle of growth from infancy to adulthood. From a comparative point of view, Benedict (1976) has described the extreme contrast Western culture has given to expectations of children versus adults. Children are considered to be sexless, whereas adult vitality is measured in terms of sexual activity; children must be protected from the ugly facts of life, while adults are expected to meet them without disruption; children must be obedient, adults must command. In our society the transition and the conditioning of children to assume adult roles takes place primarily during late school-age and adolescent years.

Thus in Western cultures, a real difficulty in employing our cultural norms in training children stems from the fact that an individual conditioned to one set of behaviors in childhood must adopt an opposite set as an adult. In other cultures, family practices allow the child to engage in some of the same forms of behavior that he or she will rely on as an adult. Benedict (1976), for example, sees this as one major discontinuity in Western child-rearing practices. A child who is at one point a son must later be a father, or a daughter later a mother. In many cultures, behavior is not polarized into this general expectation of submission for the child and dominance for the adult. The child is conditioned to assume a responsible status role by a variety of child-rearing techniques that depend chiefly on arousing the child's desire to share responsibility in adult life. To achieve this, praise and approval may be stressed, whereas the need for obedience would be given little attention.

In cultures where children are not required to be submissive, punishment disappears. Many American Indian tribes are especially explicit in rejecting the idea that a child's submissive or obedient behavior is valuable. For example, if a child is seen as docile, he or she is thought to eventually become a docile adult, an undesirable characteristic. An example of this belief was observed many years ago when a Crow Indian father was heard boasting about his son's obstinate behavior even though it was the father himself who was the target. The father, in commenting on this, remarked that there was no need to be concerned, as his son's behavior was proof that "he will be a man."

Many modern parents have never been taught as children how to care for infants and other small children. In contrast, Whiting (1974) notes that in traditional societies where women have important roles in the subsistence economy, children are required to act as nurses to their younger siblings. In all the agricultural societies she studied, mothers designate a child, usually between 7 and 8 years of age, to be their assistant.

Ideas and beliefs about the capabilities of children are also part of a parent's culture. For example, mothers in these same subsistence cultures need to be freed to return to work in the fields, and therefore believe that 7- or 8-year-old children can be trained to be capable caretakers for younger children. The opposite has been observed in mothers who have leisure time. They have been reported to underestimate the capabilities of their children. Whiting reports that Indian mothers in Khalapur, Uttar Pradesh, or Bubeneshaw in Orissa have been observed bathing and feeding their children beyond the age when societies with working mothers have long since taught their children to care for their own hygiene activities (Whiting, 1974). She points out that at one extreme is an Okinawa child of 4, who was observed washing her own hair and clothes; at the other extreme is the Indian mother who was seen hand-feeding a child of 8 and bathing a son of 9.

These examples indicate the need for a cross-cultural approach to our understanding of families and their child-rearing patterns. Ho (1987), a family therapist, believes that a cross-cultural perspective is crucial in working with families. He states that the parental functions of traditional Hispanics and Asians in the United States follow the cultural prescriptions for the husband–wife relationship. "The father disciplines and controls, while the mother provides nurturance and support" (p. 239). One unique strength characteristic of all ethnic minorities is the involvement of the extended family in the rearing and guidance of children (Ho, 1987).

Within cultural groups it also needs to be noted that considerable intra-ethnic variation exists. For example, Martinez (1988) reported on a descriptive study she did of Mexican-American families. She found that mothers' child-rearing patterns varied considerably, with most mothers using authoritarian or authoritative child-rearing techniques.

The role of the father from culture to culture also varies widely. The many roles fathers play in the family are socially and culturally defined (Lamb, 1987).

INFLUENCE OF SOCIAL CLASS ON CHILD REARING

Although it is now well accepted that a child's socialization is influenced by the social class position of his or her family, most of us have only a superficial acquaintance with the distinctions that exist between the classes in child-rearing practices. We often develop ethnocentric or stereotyped notions about the differences that exist between the poor and the middle class. It is not uncommon to find that in dealing with families in a health care setting, variations from a white middle-class standard are often seen as deviant, interpreted as pathology, or treated as deprived. Acceptable child-rearing practices and parent behavior by lower-class standards are seldom taken into account, because most practitioners continue to evaluate others in terms of their own middle-class standards. Nurses are often bothered, uncomfortable, or shocked by behavior they perceive as careless, overdependent, aggressive, pretentious, or uninhibited. Class differences in definitions of what is considered to be good or bad child rearing, normal or abnormal, acceptable or deplorable, present possible barriers to the therapeutic relationship between the nurse and the family.

Research dealing with social class differences in socialization style continues to show that parents from middle- and lower-class social structures, by virtue of experiencing different conditions of life, go about rearing their children with different conceptions of social reality, different aspirations, and different conceptions of what is desirable. Gegas (1979) completed an extensive review of the investigations that have identified ways in which middle-class families differ from lower-class families with respect to child rearing

Stemming from evaluations of recent child-rearing studies that examined the social class differences in parenting, Gegas (1979) and Peterson and Rollins (1987) identified findings where there has been consensus in a number of studies and where the relationship between social class and child-rearing behaviors are strong enough to be convincing. Their major empirical generalizations follow.

1. One of the most consistent results in the literature is that lower-class families rely heavily on physical punishment as a means of disciplining and controlling the child. Interestingly, earlier studies showed a greater difference between the two classes than later studies.
2. Findings dealing with social class differences with respect to the nature of the parent–child relationship reveal that in middle-class families a more democratic or equalitarian relationship is likely, while in lower-class families, a more authoritarian or autocratic relationship is likely.
3. The third set of findings focus on the affective dimension of the parent–child relationship—the degree of support, affection, and involvement the parent shows. Social class is found to be positively related to parental affection and involvement, indicating that the higher the social class, the more likely that parental affection and involvement will be greater.
4. There is a strong positive relationship between the parents' emphasis on independence and achievement for their children and social class. (Bronfenbrenner 1969).
5. Language (linguistic ability) is more highly developed in the middle-class child. Lower-class parents rely more on the use of commands and imperatives, whereas middle-class parents tend to explain the reasons for a rule or request.

Kohn (1969, 1977) points out that child-rearing practices are related to parents' values and to their idea of what behaviors they need to instill in their children to learn to successfully function as adults in the world as they see it. While the middle-class parent values and perceives that independence, achievement, and verbal ability are attributes that their children need to succeed, working- and lower-class parents value and perceive that respect and obedience to authority are behaviors needed to "make it" as adults in society.

Social class, of course, is only one variable that influences child-rearing patterns (albeit sociocultural variables appear to explain the most variance in child-rearing practices). We should also consider that parental behavior and socialization techniques are influenced by the amount of stress and strain parents experience, parents' more idiosyncratic ways of coping and parenting, and the resources available to assist, counsel, and support them. A great deal of parents' child-rearing behavior also results from their own socialization experiences as children, and so may or may not reflect merely their social class status.

SOCIALIZATION IN A CHANGING WORLD

No sooner did we begin adjusting to the importance of mother–child relationships than the definition of that relationship, and of the nuclear family in general, as the crucial socializing agents became open to the challenges of contemporary change. The variety and degree of social change that is occurring in the world has laid these concepts open for criticism and investigation.

There is a real need to assess the changes that have occurred in the environment. Single-parent families, father as primary caretaker, working mothers, families migrating to new cultures, and a host of other social changes have given rise to many concerns and calls for a dynamic and flexible approach to our traditional notions of socialization.

We do not yet know the long-term effects of these new social relationships and arrangements. Nor can we say with certainty what the impact will be of increased equity in parenting roles, reassignment of traditional male–female parenting practices, fragmentation of the family into single-parent–child units with the possibility of several nuclear configurations, or realignment of traditional cultural values with those of new host cultures. These changes suggest issues that we will inevitably face in caring for today's children and the emerging families of the future.

Changing Socialization Patterns

Methods of child rearing have changed drastically over the decades (Table 15–1). In the 1920s, influenced by Watson, a behaviorist, firm, controlled child-rearing practices were in vogue. In the 1960s and 1970s there was a return to a permissive, more relaxed way of child rearing. In the 1990s it is difficult to decide what the present fad in child rearing is. But what child care experts are saying is that parents are worried and confused. Middle-class parents tend to be well versed in child psychology and many have the tendency to push their child to overachieve (Roack, 1988), to become "superbabies" who have supermoms and superdads.

Discontinuity with prior practices is evident in many aspects of child rearing. But perhaps the one change that has the most profound impact on socialization patterns is that of sex-role behavior and expectations. Masculine and feminine adult roles are changing in families, especially among the middle class, and as

TABLE 15–1. CHANGING VIEWS ON CHILD REARING

From one generation to the next, parents and pediatricians have altered the way they feed, teach and discipline their children. Some examples across the decades:

1900s–1910s	1920s–1930s	1940s–1950s	1960s–1970s	1980s
		Breast-feeding		
Nursing popular although many well-to-do women preferred wetnurses.	Commercial formulas marketed and became all the rage as a convenient and sophisticated means of nourishing infants.		A return to nursing promoted by women's groups and pediatricians as healthier and more natural.	Nursing overwhelmingly preferred by middle-class white women, less popular with blacks and Latinos.
		Thumb-sucking		
Attitudes not uniform, although often discouraged.	Forbidden by most parents and doctors.	Allowed along with pacifiers.	Encouraged, along with pacifiers.	Offered, along with pacifiers but neither discouraged nor encouraged.
		Potty Training		
Enemas and bowel irrigation popular methods of "cleaning" babies.	Begun as early as 2 months of age.	Delayed until 6 to 18 months.		Child determines time to begin, usually between ages 2 and 3.
		Discipline		
Children expected to act like small adults.	Strict and early discipline advocated.	Common sense and nuturance urged.	Permissive era of child rearing.	Moderate discipline at appropriate ages.
		Learning		
Moral training began early.	Nursery schools proliferated as early education became popular.		Early reading advocated along with early training for disadvantaged children.	"Super babies" urged to be treated normally; day care increasingly becomes a national issue.

Roack (1988). Copyright, 1988, Los Angeles Times. Reprinted by permission.

they change, so do the socialization experiences of children. Because motherhood has come to occupy a less significant aspect of many women's adult life and because there are so many married women working, socialization practices are changing. There are fewer sex-based differences in socialization patterns (Hoffman, 1977; Scanzoni and Szinovacz, 1980).

Most parents today are being encouraged to socialize their children in a more androgynous fashion, that is, not as identified with a specific gender. Previous values supporting traditional masculine and feminine roles are still alive in working-class families, however, creating a diversity of child-rearing patterns in American society.

There is a question as to whether the push for a "unisex' upbringing may not also cause some problems in later life (Johnston and Sarty, 1977). Whatever the ultimate adaptive value, our children may be getting inappropriate preparation for an adult world that may still remain sexist.

Another change that seems to be widespread because of the preponderance of married women working today is the phenomenon called the "hurried child." Child development experts believe that today's child is being pushed to act like an adult long before he or she is developmentally ready to do so. Children are being pressured to read before kindergarten and are left unsupervised after school. Some hurried children develop into "harried teens," expected not only to achieve in school but to shop, cook, and care for the family as well (Libman, 1988).

A seemingly conflicting trend with the hurried child

WORKING MOTHERS

*In 1985 nearly half of the mothers of preschool children (under 6 years of age) were in the labor force, an increase of 75% since 1970.

*Although mothers of older children are more likely to be in the work force, between 1970 and 1985 the greatest increase in workforce participation has been by mothers of children under 6 years of age.

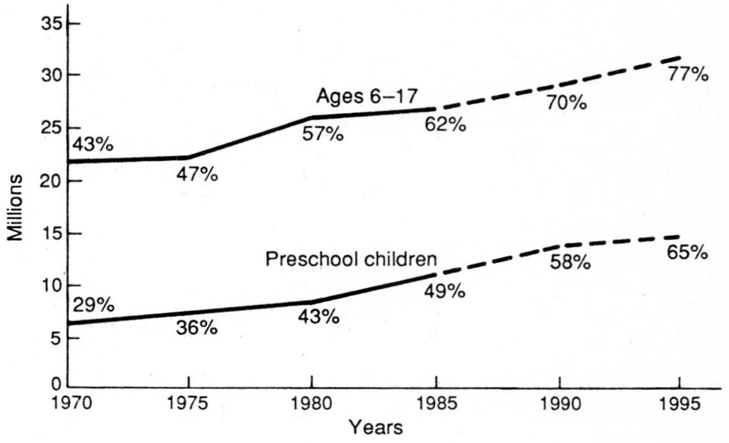

Figure 15–1.
Children with mothers in the work force. (Hofferth and Phillips, 1987.)

is the trend of extended adolescence. Increasing numbers of young adults are taking longer to get their degree, longer to establish a career, longer to leave home and become independent, and longer to get married. Many more young adults are living at home after they graduate from school or are cohabitating so as to avoid commitment. With the unprecedented rise in cohabitation 50 percent of all men and women in their 30s lived together before marriage (Woodward, 1990). Premarital sex and part-time employment (they are not related) at minimum wage during high school have also risen sharply. Only about 11 percent of adolescents in school save rather than spend their earnings from part-time employment. These changes reflect a change in values—values adults put in place: consumerism, narcissism, and instant gratification (Woodward, 1990). These values are learned through role modeling and other socialization experiences in and outside of the home.

The Child Day Care Issue

The proportion of women working who have children continues to rise (Fig. 15–1). Rapid growth in women's participation in the work force means a concomitant growth in child care for preschool through school-age children (after-school programs for those in school). Figure 15–2 shows the growth in day care programs.

Many of today's mothers, confronted not only with the complexities of how to raise their children but also faced with the economic and social realities of living in a highly industrialized and mobile country, are forced to decide who can assist them in terms of day care. Just at the time when mother–child attachments are seen as critical, most mothers are having to deal with the need for day care.

Mothers and some social scientists share the concern that day care is ultimately not as good for the child as the mother's care. For instance, Levine (1988) argues that there is compelling evidence that "day care" children suffer more from diseases and emotional problems (separation anxiety) than children who remain at home with mother, and are poorly socialized when they are sent to day care too soon or for too long. Kagan (1978) disagrees, pointing out that in the studies he reviewed there were no differences in child outcomes between those children staying home with mother and those regularly participating in child care.

Hofferth and Phillips (1987) reported their own evaluation of the research on employment of the mother. They found that employment of the mother has no consistent positive or negative impact on the child. The neutrality of these research findings has clearly had a major impact on reassuring working mothers that it is all right to work.

Legislation Affecting Child Care and Children

The issues surrounding legislation and children are perhaps the least remembered but the most influential in terms of their impact on child rearing. There have been dramatic changes in this century in the laws concerning child care and protection, as well as numerous changes in the concepts of children's rights, parental rights, duties, and responsibilities.

The legal system presents a sometimes contradictory picture of our expectations of parenting. Based on earlier patriarchal patterns of family organization, the

CHILD CARE

*In 1985 over one fifth of children under six years of age whose mothers worked outside of the home wrer in day care centers.
*The largest shift in child care arrangements in the last 20 years has been away from relative and sister care toward child care at day care centers.

*Women who work full time tend to use day care centers while women who work part time are more likely to use family care homes.

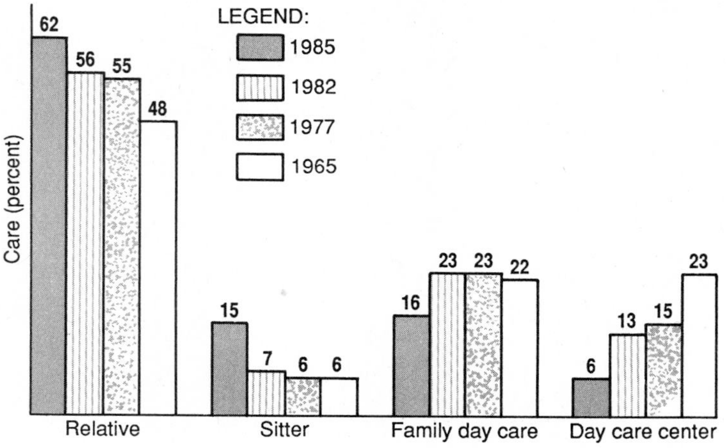

Figure 15–2.
Child care arrangements of preschool children, 1965–1985. (Hofferth and Phillips, 1987.)

father in the past was regarded as the "natural guardian" of the child and was free to punish his child within reasonable boundaries. Loss of parents' rights over the care and discipline of their children could occur only in extreme cases when a "fit person" order was made by the court.

Our laws have evolved considerably from these earlier notions, so much so that the Children's Act of 1975 evidenced a present disenchantment with the natural family as inevitably providing the best care for the child. This change was brought about following the death of a child after being returned to her natural mother. This situation served to strengthen the rights of foster parents, as well as directing the appointment in appropriate circumstances of a person to act as guardian of the child or young person in order to safeguard his or her interests.

Legally, children's rights are now widely recognized by the American courts. For instance, in many states children are entitled to the protection of a lawyer if they are accused of committing a delinquent act and have to appear in court. Greater civil rights for children make clear to parents that children are no longer considered their property and that outside authorities and agencies have the legal right to question parental actions.

Making Parenting a Science

The degree of stress and passion parents have about doing a good job raising their children has not changed over the years; but the focus of parents' anxiety has. At a time when 50 percent of all marriages fail, maintaining family life is a high-risk business. Stressed families are searching for guidelines for rearing their children (Brazelton, 1989).

Our fascination with the notion of parenting, proclaimed in a flood of handbooks, implies a new formula for a scientific recipe to raising children (Johnston and Sarty, 1977). It often appears in this literature that it takes a professional to know the right way to do things.

Today's parents tend to be overwhelmed with parenting issues, as well as with conflicting advice from many sources. Pediatricians and other child care specialists have become the grandmothers of the 1980s. The tendency for parents to rely on the judgment of others may have been carried to the extreme. "One image that repeatedly struck me," says Beckman, a child development researcher, "was a picture of a mother who hearing her child cry, rushes for the book rather than the baby" (Roack, 1988, p. A24). Another example of this trend is from an article in the *Los Angeles Times* by Dr. Joyce Brothers (1990), a psychologist, on "Testing Parenting Philosophies." Dr. Brothers asks her readers eight questions about "What does being a good parent mean?" Scientific answers are then supplied to correct any faulty information the reader might have; from this it is clear that scientific knowledge is the foundation for Brothers' common-sense answers.

SOCIALIZATION IN SINGLE-PARENT AND STEP-PARENT FAMILIES

Most of the research and literature on child-rearing patterns applies to the two-parent nuclear family (with the wife working at home or outside of the home). The

*In 1988, 15.3 million children in the U.S.–24.3% of all children under 18 years of age–lived with one parent only, an increase of 12.4% since 1970.

*In1988, the vast majority of single parent families (88%) consisted of children living with their mothers.

*In 1987, almost half (46%) of the children living only with their mothers were poor.

*Black children are nearly 3 times as likely as white children to live in a single parent household.

*Other living arrangements include foster home placement. The number of children in foster homes increased 29% nationally in three years, largely due to increase in child abuse and neglect.

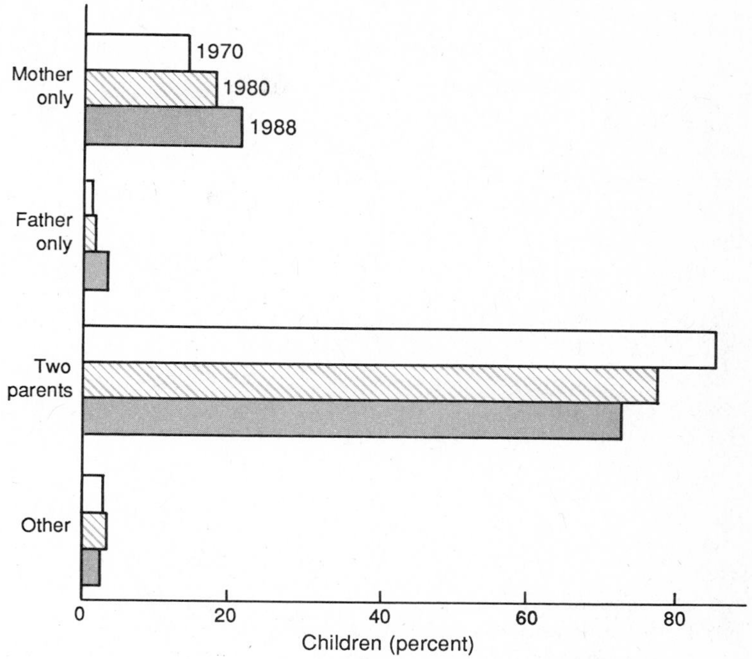

Figure 15–3.
Living arrangements of American children under 18 years of age. (From: U.S. Bureau of the Census, 1988b.)

single-parent family and the step-parent family are two other major types of family forms that should also be addressed in terms of child-rearing patterns and outcomes, because family structure is an important factor affecting socialization.

Single-parent Families

In 1988, 15.3 million American children (24.3 percent of all children under 18 years of age) lived with one parent only, an increase of 12.4 percent since 1970 (Fig. 15–3). the growth of single-parent families is due primarily to a high rate of divorce and out-of-wedlock births.

Child rearing among single parents is difficult, especially if there are no other adult caregivers available to assist the parent. Single parents struggle against the dual demands of providing financial and emotional support for their children. Poverty and employment of the single parent (usually the mother) add to the difficulty in child rearing.

There has been extensive research conducted on the effects of the single parent family on the children—their educational attainment, work, and income. Abundant evidence now exists that demonstrates that children from single-parent families have less success in school, lower earnings, and lower occupational prestige than children reared in intact two-parent families. This has been found even when such factors as income level of the single parent, educational attainment of the single parent and many other background factors are controlled (Mueller and Cooper, 1986; Nock, 1988). Children from mother-only families are also more likely to become single parents themselves (McLanahan and Booth, 1989). Moreover, the difficulties mother-only families have are reflected in the finding that single mothers report less satisfaction in their parenting role (Fine et al, 1986).

Step-parent Families

In the step-parent family two of the underlying issues creating role confusion for the step-father and resultant family disequilibrium are the issues of child rearing and disciplining of children. Each parent draws on his or her own family background when defining child-rearing beliefs, practices, and discipline. Child-rearing practices are quite diverse from family to family, and once set are difficult to change, because they are not objectively based. When parents enter into a relationship in which the step-father heads the household, but is not really the parent, synthesis of these child-rearing rules is problematic. Furthermore, the children, through exposure to their natural parents' child-rearing practices, have developed their own behaviors and expectations of what is acceptable or unacceptable for both themselves and their parents.

In the step-parent family the step-father has no biological rights over the children, and whatever parental rights he may have must be granted to him by his wife. This places the step-father into a rather untenable position. When conflict arises over the disciplining of a child, the mother feels a natural right to decide the issue. If the stepfather goes ahead and disciplines the child, the mother may either directly become angry, or more often, indirectly strike back by undermining him. This latter course is particularly devastating to the entire family and often exacerbates the conflict, with the mother being torn between the loyalty to her children and to her husband (Furstenberg and Nord, 1985; Visher and Visher, 1979).

In a study of 232 remarried families, Hobert (1987) found that depending on whose children they are, children had different statuses in the family. For instance, first-class children were those born to the remarried couple, second-class children were those from the wife's previous marriage, and third-class children were those from the husband's previous marriage. Parents reported that the most positive relationships were with their shared children. Parent–child relationships varied considerably in the remarried families; these relationship problems were also perceived as affecting the spousal relationship.

THEORIES RELATED TO SOCIALIZATION

Developmental Theories

Erikson's Stage of Generativity. The most important socialization task for parents is in establishing and guiding the next generation. Erikson's (1963) concept of generativity demonstrates an understanding of the importance of socializing for continuity. In his discussion of generativity versus stagnation, he describes the mature person's need for and dependence on the younger generation. Erikson asserts that when this stage is not fulfilled, regression to an obsessive need for pseudo-intimacy takes place, often with a pervading sense of stagnation and personal impoverishment. Bronfenbrenner (1974) embellishes on the importance of this developmental stage in his comment that we must bring adults back into the lives of children and children back into the lives of adults.

Achieving the motivation for continuity between the generations has become something of a dilemma, because it is difficult to foster the concept of continuity in a time of discontinuity and change. Past traditions, values, and social norms to many parents seem emptied of their utility for the day-to-day functioning of their families. The lack of traditions in families may have subtle, yet important disruptive effects on the ability of parents to socialize children for continuity.

Stages of Parent Development. In light of the array of available information on child rearing, the nurse frequently is one of the health care professionals assisting parents to sort out and understand their children's needs and their own responsibilities. In this regard, Friedman (1957) suggested five definitive stages through which parents progress and the appropriate child-rearing task for the period. Each stage reflects the major problems in the child's development with which the parent is grappling. These stages have been observed in a wide variety of sociocultural settings and ethnic groups, as well as in single-parent families, and the basic concept appears to be universal. The five stages of parent development are outlined in Table 15–2.

TABLE 15–2. STAGES OF PARENT DEVELOPMENT

Stage of Child Development	Stage of Parent Development	Parental Task
I . Infant	Learning the cues.	To interpret infant needs.
II . Toddler	Learning to accept growth and development.	To accept some control while maintaining necessary limits.
III . Preschooler	Learning to separate.	To allow independent development while modeling necessary standards.
IV. School-ager	Learning to accept rejection without deserting.	To be there when needed without intruding unnecessarily.
V . Teenager	Learning to build a new life—having been thoroughly discredited by one's teenager.	To adjust to changing family roles and relationships during and after the teenager's struggle to establish an identity.

Adapted from Friedman (1957).

Theoretical Developments in Socialization Theories

Probably the biggest theoretical breakthrough in the area of child socialization has been the recognition that parent–child relationships are dynamic and interactive (Rollins and Thomas, 1979). Most research and theoretical discussion up until recently presented a static unidirectional model of parent causation; that is, parents had certain child-rearing techniques, and with these they molded the behavior and attitudes of the child. This one-sided static perspective ignored the prior history of interaction between parent and child, as well as the specific immediate antecedent responses of the child to the parents. This social mold theory blamed the mother for children's later problems. Chess (1983), a well-known child development researcher, explains:

> Although the mother's role in child development is significant, development proceeds through a series of interactions with many others, including the father, siblings, teachers and peers. Other factors that influence child development include individual neuro-chemical, genetic and temperamental characteristics of the child. The point, then, that no one factor is overriding makes linear unidimensional models of child development obsolete. (p. 6)

Today, using a systems circular causation model, where feedback loops exist, children are viewed as active organisms who contribute significantly to the nature and course of the evolving parent–child relationship. Children are viewed as shaping parents' behavior and parents are viewed as shaping children's behavior. For successful parenting to occur, there needs to be a "goodness of fit" between the child and his or her environment (the expectations and demands of caregivers are consonant with the child's skills and potentials) (Chess, 1983).

CHILD-REARING RESEARCH

It has been years now since Sears and co-workers (1957) completed one of the most thorough studies of child rearing ever done in the United States. They were particularly interested in how a mother handled a range of developmental problems. Did she cope with these problems by physical punishment, by withdrawing her love, or by depriving her child of privileges? Perhaps more importantly, they began to probe the crucial question in socialization: Did the way the mother treated the child really make a difference in adulthood? What was the impact of whether or not the mother punished, rejected, or smothered her child with love?

Despite all the attention given to these questions over the past years, and the multitude of subsequent child socialization studies, many of these questions remain unanswered today, although some empirical generalizations can be made.

There has been an extensive amount of research in the area of parent–child socialization. Earlier research studies based their investigations on social mold conceptualizations, while later research has emphasized bidirectional systemic models (the preceding theories section explains the difference between the two theoretical positions) (Peters and Rollins, 1987).

Rollins and Thomas (1979), in an in-depth review and analysis of child-rearing research, state that there is sufficient empirical evidence to support the following propositions:

1. Especially for boys, the greater the supportive behavior of parents toward children, the greater such culturally valued child behaviors as self-esteem, academic achievement, creativity, and conformity (p. 322).
2. In most instances, a positive relationship is found between parental support and cognitive development in children (p. 329).
3. The greater the parental coercion, the less the creativity in the child (p. 329).
4. The greater the parental support, the greater the moral behavior of children (p. 331).
5. The greater the parental support, the greater the self-esteem in children (p. 333).

In summary, parental support was consistently found to have a positive association with all aspects of social competence in children, with the exception of creativity. Here a curvilinear relationship was revealed. Creativity increases in conditions of low to moderate parental support and decreases in moderate to high parental supportive conditions.

Several psychologists (McClelland et al, 1978) have argued that parents have very little control over the formation of their child's personality and character and contend that most adult behavior is not determined by specific techniques of child rearing in the first 5 years. They suggest instead that the way parents *feel* about their children matters.

In their study of child rearing, McClelland and colleagues (1978) found that when parents, particularly mothers, "really" love their children, the children were likely to achieve the highest levels of social and moral maturity. The other dimension that was significant for later social adaptation was how strictly the parents controlled their children's expressive behavior. A child was less apt to become socially and morally mature when his parents tolerated no noise, mess, or rough-housing in the home, and when the parents reacted unkindly to the child's aggressiveness toward them, to his or her sex play, or to expressions of dependency needs. Moreover, when parents were concerned with using their power to maintain an adult-centered home, the child was not as likely to become a mature adult. All in all, it appears that mothers' affection relates to more adult outcomes, while physical punishment is not significantly related to any of the outcomes examined. Thus a mother's affectionate demonstrativeness or warmth toward her child was found to be a crucial determinant of adult social and moral maturity.

It is acknowledged that there is no longer an "approved" way of "parenting." Nor is there one "best method" of discipline. (Because how to discipline appears to be one of the most perplexing aspects of parenting, nurses are often asked for their opinions on what to do.)

Ideally, the parents' goal in disciplining is not punishment for wrongful actions, but to assist children to control their own behavior, develop self-discipline, accept responsibility for their own behavior, and consider the needs and feelings of others (McCubbin and Dahl, 1985). In most cases discipline works best when it is tailored to the individual child and the specific situation. Both Spock (1974) and Jolly (1975) advocate the use of moderate methods of discipline—stating that extremes of too much or too little discipline are less effective.

Baumrind (1978) classifies parental styles of discipline into permissive, authoritative, and authoritarian. The permissive parental style is characterized by being accepting and nonpunitive in dealing with the child's behaviors. In contrast, the authoritarian style of discipline stresses obedience to rules and parents' authority. Finally, the authoritative style of discipline stresses a rational, issue-oriented "give and take" way of dealing with the child. Of the three styles, Baumrind (1978) advocates the third, asserting that it can produce reasonable conformity without loss of autonomy or self-assertiveness.

One last focus of research has addressed the influence of family size on child-rearing patterns and child outcomes. There is strong research evidence to suggest that small and large families constitute qualitatively different developmental experiences. Children from small families tend to receive more attention than children from large families. Research has linked these differences to intellectual development and school performance (Feiring and Lewis, 1984).

CHILD REARING IN HIGH-RISK FAMILIES

There are a number of situations described in the literature that are likely to produce excessive stress on parents and families. Families under stress are high-risk families. Based on systems theory, we know that a ripple effect occurs when stress is experienced by a member or subsystem. Due to the ripple effect, the whole family system is eventually affected. Parent–child interactions and relationships are always affected to some extent, and when parent–child relationships are affected, so are parenting behaviors (child rearing).

Stressors that create high-risk families may originate in the mother (like the teenage mother), the child (like a child with a life-threatening illness), or the family environment (like a local disaster). Examples of high-risk situations follow. When there is a dysfunctional marital relationship, this negatively affects the parent–child relationship. Moreover, it is clear from many studies that when mothers are severely disturbed, their parenting abilities are correspondingly diminished (Shapiro, 1983). When parents have seriously ill children, the care of that child becomes so involved that there may be time for little else. The child and mother then may become enmeshed in their relationship and the other children neglected. Child rearing in both the healthy and ill siblings is thereby impeded. Parents often treat their ill or disabled children differently—as special or vulnerable. This creates particular problems when parents attempt to return to normal parenting practices.

FAMILY SOCIALIZATION FUNCTION: APPLYING THE FAMILY NURSING PROCESS

☐ *Assessment Questions*

Before discussing the assessment of family socialization patterns, it is important that you, as a family nurse, be very clear about your own biases, attitudes, and expectations that might interfere with assessing family child rearing accurately.

How do you see the way you were raised and the way the families you work with are raising their children? How reasonable are your expectations of parents? For example, is it reasonable to expect a mother of five children never to prop a bottle? In determining the appropriateness of a particular family's child-rearing methods, it is helpful to ask yourself how functional or adaptive the approach is for the particular family being assessed. Another example would be to ask yourself if a family's form of child rearing or discipline is culturally derived or influenced.

Question your expectations of compliance with the advice and instructions given. Are your instructions and advice practical or ideal? How should you adapt your routines and nursing methods to achieve a successful outcome with a particular family?

An important issue for nurses to consider in working with parents and children is the possibility of role confusion. Taylor (1970) reminds us that most adults are protective toward children and that all adults feel some responsibility for children, particularly the very young or the ill. It is therefore difficult for most adults not to interfere when a mother or family seem to be mishandling or abusing a "defenseless" child. This natural response has tremendous survival value for the species but does pose a problem for the family nurse. In one instance, such feelings make it possible to work with families and children who are personally unattractive to the nurse, while on the other hand such feelings make it difficult to remain detached enough to function in the professional capacity of the nursing role.

Because families have diverse sociocultural backgrounds, some families will have child-rearing styles that the nurse has been conditioned, socialized, and taught to recognize as "good" and some as "bad." Most health care specialists who deal with the pediatric client tend to assume that the parents are somehow at fault when a child acts in a "socially unacceptable way" or is sick. This covert attitude is a poor one, making it difficult for the nurse to sustain an objective and effective role. Although the nurse often does things for his or her clients that a mother does for a child, it is tremendously important for the nurse to remember the public and social capacity of the nursing role, and avoid replacing the mother or displacing one's own childhood frustrations on the mother by blaming her for the child's condition. The nurse's ability to support the mother without becoming a surrogate for her is critical for the child, as well as for the self-esteem and potential growth of the parent.

In your assessment of families, the following questions will provide useful data from which to identify potential or actual problems and plan care accordingly.

1. What are the family's child-rearing practices in the following areas?
    a. Behavior control, including discipline, reward, and punishment.
    b. Autonomy and dependency.
    c. Giving and receiving of love.
    d. Training for age-appropriate behavior (social, physical, emotional, language, and intellectual development).

2. How adaptive are the family's child-rearing practices for their particular family form and situation?
3. Who assumes responsibility for the child-care role or socialization function? Is it shared? If so, how is this managed?
4. How are children regarded in the family?
5. What cultural beliefs influence the family's child-rearing patterns?
6. How do social class factors influence child-rearing patterns?
7. Is this a family that is at high risk for child-rearing problems? If so, what factors place the family at risk?

8. Is the home environment adequate for children's needs to play (appropriate to children's developmental stage)? Is there age-appropriate play equipment/toys?

Subsumed under the first assessment question is the area of *behavior control.* Because this is the area of child-rearing that seems to pose the most problems for parents, some elaboration of this area follows. Epstein and associates (1982), family researchers and clinicians, have developed the McMaster Model of Family Functioning. This model evolved from studies of both normal and clinical populations, and thus defines family health and family dysfunction. The model postulates that family functioning is based on six dimensions, one of which is behavior control. Behavior control is defined "as the pattern a family adapts for handling behavior in three areas: physically dangerous situations, situations that involve the meeting and expressing of psychobiological needs and drives and situations involving interpersonal socializing behavior" (p. 128). The central focus here is on the standards or rules the family sets to deal with the above three areas and the flexibility they allow around the standards they set. In the families Epstein and co-workers observed, they found four styles of behavior control based on variations in the standards and the latitude with which standards are upheld.

1. Rigid behavior control, with narrow standards and minimal room for negotiation or situational modification.
2. Flexible behavior control, with reasonable standards and an opportunity for negotiation and change depending on the situation.
3. Laissez-faire behavioral control, where no standards are held to and total latitude of behavior is allowed.
4. Chaotic behavior control, where unpredictable and arbitrary shifting of standards and styles occurs, to the point that family members do not know what standards or rules exist.

Epstein and associates believe that the flexible behavior control style is the most effective (this style is more likely to be found in normally functioning families) and the chaotic behavior control least effective (this style is more likely to be found in dysfunctional families). It should be noted that there were variations within normally functioning families. A family may be clear about family rules of behavior in general, but indecisive, unclear, or conflictual about specific, minor areas. This description of the range of behavior control styles observed in families and which styles are associated with healthy and dysfunctional families gives family health professionals some criteria by which to compare the families they are assessing.

FAMILY NURSING DIAGNOSES

Family problems within the area of a family socialization are very common for family nurses in schools, pediatrics, community health, family primary care, and mental health, making family nursing diagnoses within this area most germane. Recalling that the family socialization function covers child rearing, parent–child relationships, and parental behavior, the area is quite broad.

As with the other family dimensions, North American Nursing Diagnosis Association (NANDA) diagnoses were reviewed to identify which diagnoses appear to incorporate actual and potential family socialization problems. Below is a list of the NANDA diagnoses, as described by McFarland and McFarlane (1989), which are appropriate either as the diagnosis or as the outcome or consequence of a problem in this area; in the latter case it could be listed as a defining characteristic.

NURSING DIAGNOSES

Altered family processes
Health-seeking behaviors (health-promotion diagnosis)
Knowledge deficit
Parental role conflict
Altered parenting
Potential altered parenting

POSSIBLE OUTCOMES OF SOCIALIZATION PROBLEM (POSSIBLE DEFINING CHARACTERISTIC)

Altered growth and development
Altered health maintenance
Self-care deficit
Knowledge deficit
Low self-esteem
Social isolation
Impaired social interactions
Potential for violence
Noncompliance
Personal identity disturbance

Two NANDA nursing diagnoses that appear to be directly related to a family socialization problem are Altered Family Processes and Altered Parenting (actual and potential). Altered Family Processes is a more general family nursing diagnosis, but can be used when specific defining characteristics are included. Defining characteristics that McFarland and McFarlane (1989) list are:

- Parents do not demonstrate respect for each other's child-rearing practices.
- Rigidity in function and roles.
- Family does not demonstrate respect for individuality and autonomy of its members.
- Inappropriate or inconsistent family roles (p. 730).

The other nursing diagnosis, which is more specific to child-rearing problems, is Altered Parenting (actual or potential). The defining characteristics of this diagnosis directly apply to the areas subsumed under family socialization. Table 15–3 is included in this text because this diagnosis is so appropriate here. As previously mentioned, defining characteristics and related factors should accompany the diagnosis.

Identifying parents at risk for child-rearing problems—indicating Potential Altered Parenting—is critical. To name some high-risk groups, they include parents in crisis or under stress; teen parents; single parents with limited financial or personal resources or inadequate social support; parents with serious physical or psychological problems; and parents who have premature infants or infants or children with serious or chronic health problems.

FAMILY NURSING INTERVENTIONS

Supporting Parents

The primary thrust of the nurse's approach in working with families is to reinforce or support parents' natural parenting abilities. This, I believe, is the central intervention strategy for nurses working with parents in child-rearing areas. It is essentially a health-promotion focus. We must assume that all parents want to be good parents. By building up their confidence to deal with their children—who they know best—this approach will prove foundational to all the more specific ways of assisting parents.

Notwithstanding the importance of the above general approach to helping parents, specific parent education strategies are advocated. Advice, counseling, and teaching about parenting is considered to be the responsibility of pediatricians, nurses, teachers, child development specialists, and other professionals. It is not unusual to find "socialization failure" or "inadequate or altered parenting" used as fairly common diagnoses today. Often an attempt is made to involve parents in some type of parenting program in order to assist them in dealing with their children.

Making Interventions Socioculturally Appropriate

In all nursing care, assessments and interventions based on appropriate sociocultural data are important, whether counseling a mother, teaching a child, supervising a medical therapy, or coordinating community resources to resolve identified problems. In each case the nurse should focus on the relevance to the family and not on his or her own values or child-rearing techniques. For example, some families can accept and respond to instructions for improving the diet of their children if the parents are given an explanation that ties in with their own values (eg, if the children are fed better, they will behave better and the family will be less stressed). In other families, however, having well-nourished children is valued in and of itself, and so a direct teaching approach is used.

Specific Family Nursing Intervention Strategies

Role supplementation strategies are suggested for parents struggling with becoming parents or with rearing a child in the various developmental stages or during

TABLE 15–3. ALTERED PARENTING (NANDA) NURSING DIAGNOSIS

Defining Characteristics

- Lack of parental attachment behaviors.
- Inattention to infant/child needs.
- Inappropriate caretaking behaviors (eg, feeding, sleep and rest, elimination patterns, clothing, shelter, safety).
- Physical or psychological abuse.
- Abandonment.
- Inappropriate visual, tactile, or auditory stimulation of the child.
- Frequent verbalizations of dissatisfaction or disappointment with the child.
- Frequent identification of negative characteristics of the child.
- Frequent attachment of negative meanings to characteristics or behavior of the child.
- Verbalization of resentment toward child.
- Verbalization of frustration with parenting role or role inadequacy.
- Inappropriate or inconsistent discipline.
- Growth and developmental lag in the child.
- Frequent accidents or illnesses of the child.
- Signs of depression, apathy, disturbed or bizarre behavior in the child.
- Rejection of caregiver or overcompliance by the child.

Related Factors

- Families in which either parent is absent or unable to function because of physical or emotional illness
- Families in which either parent is unable or unwilling to assume parenting responsibilities.
- Families in which the child is unwanted, displays undesired characteristics, or is physically or emotionally ill.
- Families developmentally lacking parental skills.
- Families lacking external resources, such as contact with or support from own parents or others in the extended family, contact or support from community resources.
- Families in which the parents acknowledge a history of ineffective or abusive relationships with own parents.
- Families in which parents demonstrate a lack of knowledge, cognitive functioning, or role identity as a parent.
- Families in which one or both parents hold unrealistic expectations for self, spouse, or child.
- Families in which the role relationships appear chaotic or inappropriate among the members.
- Families experiencing crises (eg, financial, emotional, developmental).

Source: McFarland and McFarlane (1989).

an health/illness crisis. Role supplementation involves teaching, supporting, and role modeling (see Chap. 12 for further information on role supplementation). Parents want information about normal developmental behavior of children. Parents should be referred to some of the books about children and parenting concerns if this is a way they use to gain information.

Behavior modification principles are also used in helping parents with child behavior control problems. (Chapter 16, nursing interventions section, discusses some of the principles of behavior modification). Because behavior modification is based on the premise that all behavior is learned, this intervention is likewise based on behavioral learning principles. After gaining a baseline of a child's problematic behavior, so that the frequency of behavior and antecedents to the problem behavior are known, a structured program of reinforcements is implemented. Positive, negative, and neutral reinforcements may be used; although most behaviorists primarily recommend the use of positive reinforcement. This approach can be quite helpful if there are specific child behaviors parents want to eliminate or modify, and the parent can understand the program and have the resources to follow through with the planned, structured approach. Written contracts are developed that detail the planned intervention, so as to guide the parents and health professional (Johnson, 1986; Jones, 1980).

Family nurses also *initiate referrals* to parenting programs, recreational and preschool educational programs, and other community programs or services.

Working closely with the schools, health and other social agencies, family nurses coordinate a variety of resources and a wealth of necessary information to assist families in coping with the complexities of raising children in a changing world of challenging expectations.

Parenting Programs

Often an attempt is made to involve both parents in some type of parenting program in order to assist them in dealing with their children more successfully. Smoyak (1977) has identified three different parenting programs that provide advice and support to parents on child rearing. One program aims at helping parents accept their role with less anxiety and guilt. This is known as the parent-effectiveness approach. Another program focuses more directly on improving specific parenting skills. The third program supports a family counseling approach, assuming that after disturbing relationships in the total family system are rectified, parents can more successfully parent. This latter group is called a parent support group. Support occurs in the building of a support network, in the reduction of isolation, and in the encouragement of sharing among peers.

By discussing parents' expectations of their role, the family nurse may identify sources of frustration, confusion, and gaps in their information. By initiating parent education programs, conducting parent groups and client education sessions, and providing support and encouragement, parental role transition and improved confidence can be facilitated.

Counseling Single-parent and Remarried Families

Child-rearing or parenting problems are generally more problematic in these two alternative family forms. The stressors on parents are greater than in the two-parent nuclear families, and thus the counseling and educational needs are greater. For guidelines for counseling various family forms, including single-parent and remarried families as well as gay and lesbian couple families, dual-career families, and cohabiting heterosexual couple families, Goldenberg and Goldenberg, two family therapists, have written a recent, excellent book entitled *Counseling Today's Families* (1990).

Early Intervention Programs

For families at risk with children with special needs, early intervention has become one of the cornerstones of treatment. Intervention that is interdisciplinary and comprehensive is incorporated in these programs. Regional developmental centers are examples of such services. Family nurses often serve as coordinators of interdisciplinary services and assessors of the home and family environment, as well as health educators and counselors to families about their children's health care needs. Counseling here is directed at providing family support; it can involve helping families obtain food stamps and other community resources, becoming a case manager, or counseling parents about child rearing of children with special needs and disabilities (Healy et al, 1985).

□ *STUDY QUESTIONS*

1. Which of the following is the best definition of socialization?
   a. The act of learning to relate to people.
   b. The training provided to function in a social environment.
   c. The social and psychologic development of a child.
   d. Child-rearing practices.

2. The central task involved in socialization of children revolves around teaching them how to function and assume adult roles in a society. Subsumed under this main task are several more specific tasks. Name three of these.

3. American families have retained primary and almost exclusive responsibility for socializing their children during what life cycles of the family (select all appropriate answers):
   a. Stage of marriage.
   b. Childbearing (stage of expansion).
   c. Families with preschool children.
   d. Families with school-age children.
   e. Families with teenage children.

4. Culture plays a dominant role in socialization. Explain briefly.

5. McClelland and associates conducted a study of child-rearing patterns and their outcomes among American families. They found that (select the best answer):
   a. Strict limit setting and clear boundaries produced well-behaved, obedient children.
   b. No one approach to child rearing was superior over another approach.
   c. Parental love and acceptance was the crucial determinant in the child's acquisition of social and moral maturity.
   d. Parents have very little control over the formation of their child's personality and character.

6. Social class is another vital variable influencing a family's socialization patterns. Social class makes a difference because (select the best answer):
   a. By virtue of experiencing different life conditions, families from various social classes have varying conceptions of social reality and what is desirable, feasible, and most important.
   b. Social class determines how parents deal with the world and their children.
   c. Being in one social class or another gives a family a limited view of the world and consequently limits their child-rearing techniques to those with which they are familiar.

7. Research concerning social class differences in child-rearing patterns found that (answer *True* or *False*):
   a. The white-collar family stresses respect and obedience more than the blue-collar family does.
   b. Conformity and individualism are both emphasized more by middle-class families.
   c. Middle-class families rely more on reasoning and talking things over with children, while the lower-class families tend to use punishment more as a way of disciplining children.

8. The attitudes and approaches to the care and rearing of children in a society (select all appropriate answers):
   a. Will be congruent with the society's dominant value system.
   b. May or may not be related to the society's dominant value system.
   c. Will be positively associated with the society's dominant value system.
   d. Will be related to the traditions but perhaps not the current values because of cultural lag.

9. Identify several important changes and/or issues affecting child rearing in our society.

10. Match the appropriate stage of parent development and parental tasks in the right column with the child's stage of development in the left column.

a. Infant	1. To allow independence.
b. Toddler	2. To accept rejection without deserting the child.
c. Preschooler	3. Learning to build a new life for parents.
d. School-ager	4. Learning the meaning of the cues.
e. Teenager	5. Learning to accept child's growth and development.
	6. Learning to master anger and frustration.

11. Self-examination of child-rearing biases: What particular beliefs and attitudes do you hold that might limit your effectiveness in working with parents and children in the area of parenting or child rearing?

Family Case Study

From the following family vignette assess the family's socialization function using the questions provided at the conclusion of the vignette as assessment guidelines.

Mr. and Mrs. Chin, ages 50 and 45, respectively, moved 10 years ago to San Francisco from Hong Kong. The Chins operate a small cleaners, and the family income has always been low despite the long, hard hours of work of both parents.

They have four children: Harold, 23, who is at the California School of Technology studying engineering; Lee, 22, who is a registered nurse; John, 17, who is in high school and an excellent student; and Joe, 10, who is attending fifth grade. All the children (including the older ones) are always busy working. John and Joe work extremely hard on their studies, and with school work and home chores there is little time left over for playing or getting into "mischief." The parents have greatly encouraged their children to pursue higher education and academic achievement. Through their accomplishments, the Chins feel the children have brought honor to them.

During the home visit all the children were observed to be respectful of their parents' authority. In the presence of their parents, the two youngest were quiet and did not interject comments or express themselves until directly asked a question, at which time they answered quickly while looking to their mother for approval.

Mrs. Chin states that her husband is strict in child rearing and that if the two younger boys still living at home disobey, he administers immediate corporal punishment. Mrs. Chin relates that a misbehaving child in the Chinese community is considered "not trained," meaning that the parents are to blame; thus a child's wrongdoing brings shame and dishonor to the whole family.

When Mrs. Chin was asked how she raised her children, she related that she cuddled and fondled them a lot while they were little. But as soon as they became preschoolers she gradually withdrew her expressions of love and physical hugs and kisses. From school age on, she and her husband have pushed her children to become independent and responsible. Both parents said that they had emotionally removed themselves somewhat from their children lest their children might lose respect for them.

The parent–child relationships appear to be more restrained and formal than in most American families. However, though muted, one was still able to feel the obvious respect and caring they feel for each other.

12. Describe how the family dealt with the following areas of child rearing: discipline, reward, punishment, moral training, autonomy, initiative, creativity, dependency, giving and receiving of love, and training for age-appropriate behavior (social, physical, emotional, language, and intellectual development).

13. How adaptive are the family's child-rearing practices for their particular situation (social class, culture, environment, etc)?

14. Who assumes responsibility for the child-care role or socialization function? Is it shared and if so, how?

15. How are children regarded in the family?

16. What cultural beliefs are operating in their child-rearing practices?

17. Based on the brief hypothetical family situation that follows:

- Identify a family nursing diagnosis in the area of family socialization.
- Propose two family nursing strategies to ameliorate the problem.

Mrs. Cabrillo is in the pediatrician's office for an infant check-up. She is seen by the pediatric nurse practitioner who, after she has checked the baby, asks Mrs.

Cabrillo how she is managing at home with the two children. Mrs. Cabrillo brings up the problem she is having with Mary, who refuses to go to kindergarten.

Family background: Mr. and Mrs. Cabrillo, ages 35 and 25 respectively, have a daughter, Mary, age 5½ years old and a newborn son, John, age 3 months. The daughter Mary started kindergarten 3 months before the baby was born and went to school pretty regularly at that time. Since John has come home, however, she "is a changed little girl." She hits the baby, shouts "no" to her mother when she tries to discipline her or give her commands, refuses to dress herself to go to school, and throws temper tantrums at the breakfast table when her mother says she has to go to school. Mary is so upset and defiant that the mother can't make her go to school, and so she has been staying home with mother.

Mr. Cabrillo (John Sr.) is very impatient about the situation, because, according to his wife, he doesn't understand. "Mary is different with him. She obeys her father, who is very firm with Mary." Mr. Cabrillo works long hours during the weekdays and doesn't get very involved with the children when he is home.

The parents are both from an Italian family—the mother immigrated just before Mary was born and speaks broken English. She has never worked outside the home. John Sr. was raised in the United States and his family lives nearby. Mrs. Cabrillo is fairly socially isolated because she doesn't drive and speaks limited English. Her only friends are her husband's family, who "always take John Senior's side in discussions."

CHAPTER SIXTEEN

The Health Care Function

Marilyn M. Friedman
Irene S. Morgan

Learning Objectives

1. Recall the various ways in which the family carries out its health care function.
2. Identify three salient factors that influence a family's conceptualization or definition of health and illness, and whether they seek health care.
3. Discuss Baumann's study relative to the three criteria or orientations used to define health and illness, and the group differences found.
4. Explain Koos's central findings in terms of the influence of socioeconomic status on illness recognition and health-seeking behaviors.
5. Diagram the health belief model, explaining the several important components of the model and their relationships to each other.
6. Discuss the significance of each of the cognitive–perceptual primary motivation mechanisms found in Pender's Health Promotion Model.
7. Compare and contrast the Health Belief Model with the Health Promotion Model.
8. Summarize Pratt's findings and conclusions concerning how adequately the American family performs its health care function.
9. Enumerate the basic aspects that need to be assessed when completing an appraisal of a family's (a) dietary practices, (b) sleeping and rest practices, (c) exercise and recreation practices, (d) drug practices, and (e) self-care practices.
10. Identify potential environmental practices that could negatively affect family members' health.
11. Describe the basic specific preventive measures recommended for adults and children.
12. Explain what effect race, income, and education have on health care service utilization.
13. Discuss four health education areas of which families need to be cognizant in order for them to provide adequate dental self-care.
14. Describe what should be included and recorded in a family health history.

For the family health professional, the health care function is a vital consideration in family assessment. To place this function in perspective, it is one of the family functions and entails the provision of physical necessities: food, clothing, shelter, and health care. Shelter (housing and family's neighborhood and community) was discussed previously in Chapter 9 as part of environmental data.

From the perspective of society, the family is the basic system in which health behavior and care are organized, performed, and secured. Families provide preventive health care and the major share of sick care for their members. Furthermore, families have the prime responsibility for initiating and coordinating services rendered by health care professionals (Pratt, 1977; 1982).

There has been a pervasive assumption that as the family has become more specialized in its functions, its health care function has been lost—being transferred to the doctor's office and hospital (Adams, 1971). And yet the tremendous role families play in the provision of health care to family members is clearly evident to health care professionals.* With the acknowledgement that major improvements and maintenance in health occur primarily through environmental and personal life-style modifications and commitments, the family's central role in assuming responsibility for its members' health is strengthened (Pratt, 1982). Therefore, it is the belief of these authors, supported by Pratt (1976) and Forrest (1981), that the provision of health care is indeed a vital and basic family function. If family-centered nurses agree, how health care is delivered to families should be altered considerably; that is, education and counseling for *family self-care* will be a primary goal of family nursing practice.

FAMILY BEHAVIOR RELATED TO HEALTH AND ILLNESS

Health practices and the use of health care services vary tremendously from family to family. Family differences in both conceptualizations of what constitutes health and illness and the degree of motivation needed to seek health care services and improve health constitute the main reasons for the observed diversity of health care practices.

Conceptualizations of Health and Illness

Conceptualizations of health and illness vary widely from culture to culture, region to region, and family to family, as well as among the several social classes and as a result of the degree of technological development that has occurred in a family's community.

People from the same cultural background and/or from a similar socioeconomic status often share comparable attitudes, myths, and values concerning their health. This has been particularly documented in poor communities (McLachlan, 1958). Some health problems endemic to whole communities or groups may be taken as a matter of course rather than defined as illness. Social customs and norms often determine whether particular behaviors are considered sick or healthy (Jahoda, 1958).

It follows that a family, neighborhood, community, or society must label a condition or certain behaviors as an illness or disability before that illness or health condition can be considered a health problem to that group. The frequency of a condition often influences whether the condition is labeled an illness or not. For instance, if practically everyone in a community is suffering from malnutrition, the associated fatigue will probably be considered normal. A case in point: in America today we accept colds and dental caries, which occur so frequently, as annoyances that are a part of normal living, and most sufferers of colds or toothaches do not consider themselves ill.

Kane and associates (1976) point out that the interpretation given to "health" by the poor is a natural consequence of the living conditions in which they find themselves. Irelan further explains:

> Their entire orientation is colored by the fact that they live with other poor people; they take on the perspectives of those around them and reinforce each other's beliefs and values. The way they cope with health problems is "traceable either to the material situation of poverty itself, to the social structure of poverty, or to the aspects of the life outlook of poverty—the ideals, values, and beliefs to which the poor man adheres. (Irelan, 1972, pp. 56–56)

Hence people have different ways of defining whether they are sick or well. Some people feel they are sick only when they can no longer work or carry on their usual daily activities and roles; others are very attuned to their physiological functioning and recognize even minor symptoms or signs as an indication of disease and illness; a third orientation to illness is that people are sick when they are not feeling well.

Baumann (1961) demonstrated these differences in an early study she conducted of middle-aged and older chronically ill clinic patients from working-class and lower socioeconomic backgrounds and freshmen medical students in their first 3 years of medical school, who were generally from middle- and upper-middle-class backgrounds and in their early 20s. She compared the

** The reader is referred back to Chap. 1, which discusses in depth the role of the family in relation to the entire spectrum of health and illness concerns.*

two groups according to their definitions of health and illness. Baumann found the three prevailing basic orientations to wellness and illness alluded to above existed in the two groups: (1) a subjective feeling of well-being or ill health (the feeling-state orientation), (2) an absence or presence of general or specific symptoms (symptom orientation), and (3) a state of being able or unable to perform usual activities (a performance orientation). Consistent with American society's productivity value orientation, both groups (representing both age and socioeconomic differences) mentioned an activity orientation in their conceptualization of health and illness. The clinic patients tended to identify subjective feelings as being a significant factor in their definition (supporting Koos's findings (1954) that the less educated were less articulate in their thoughts about illness), while the freshman medical students identified the presence or absence of symptoms as the second criterion in their definition of health and illness.

Koos (1954), in a classic study, demonstrated that socioeconomic position greatly influences an individual's interpretation of symptoms—that is, whether symptoms are perceived as symptoms of illness or not, and when present, whether they constitute indications that medical care should be sought. He found that as one descends the social class ladder, less symptom recognition and perceived need for medical services exists among the study population. Thus the middle-class worker was found to be much more knowledgeable about disease symptoms, while the working-class and lower-class person showed less recognition of symptoms as being signs of ill health and therefore did not view these symptoms as indicating a need for medical attention. Generally, the poor must reach a stage of being incapacitated before they define themselves as ill. Blatant symptoms of health problems such as loss of appetite, persistent coughing, shortness of breath, and the swelling of hands and feet were recognized by less than one fourth of the lower-class participants in Koos' study.

Social class differences are also quite pronounced relative to a family's overall priorities. In the lower class, health is often found lower on the list of necessities unless a crisis is present. Jobs, food, and shelter are pressing priorities for the poor.

How a family or family members define health and illness has important ramifications for nursing practice. The family's definition of health needs to be clarified so that we as nurses know what goals are important to the family, as well as what possible areas of health education are present.

Knowledge of Health

The family, as part of its task of protecting the health of its members, sets up and carries out health maintenance activities based on what the parents or adult members believe to be healthy and possible. Most middle- and working-class families seek out information regarding health education, with a combination of physicians, dentists, and mass media sources being most commonly cited (Yankelovitch et al., 1979). A considerable amount of health information is also shared among the family's social network of friends and relatives. Feldman (1976) found that the only health area a majority of parents did not cover with their children involved reproduction and sexuality.

As illustrated by the previously mentioned studies of Baumann (1961) and Koos (1954), the more educated a family is, the better the family's knowledge of health usually is. This expectation would have to be validated with a particular client. Also, certain family members, generally the mother, are better informed. Women have consistently been found to have acquired more health education information due to their health role responsibilities in the family.

Yankelovitch and co-workers (1979) in their third General Mills national survey of families, where a representative sample of 2181 members of households were interviewed, found that even though a majority of Americans expressed a growing interest and concern about health, they did not feel well informed. Yankelovitch and associates confirmed respondents' low level of health knowledge, and citing the demonstrated correlation between an individual's own assessment of his or her level of knowledge about health subjects and actual behavior, called for more effective health education programs.

Importance of Personal and Family Health Beliefs

What factors lead to the readiness and intention of an individual to seek health care services or improve his or her life-style (ie, change personal health behaviors)? Are the variables different for explaining preventive health actions (personal health practices and use of health services) versus explaining the seeking and receiving of curative health services or complying with the medical regimens?

The most comprehensive scheme for looking at these questions is the Health Belief Model (Berkanovic, 1976), which has been subjected to testing in a wide variety of preventive and curative health areas. Although modified since its inception, it is believed to be a useful tool for systematically analyzing personal health behavior, predicting such diverse activities as preventive health actions, medical care utilization, delay in seeking help, and compliance with medical regimes (Becker, 1974).

The Health Belief Model utilizes Lewin's theories stressing that it is the world of the perceiver that deter-

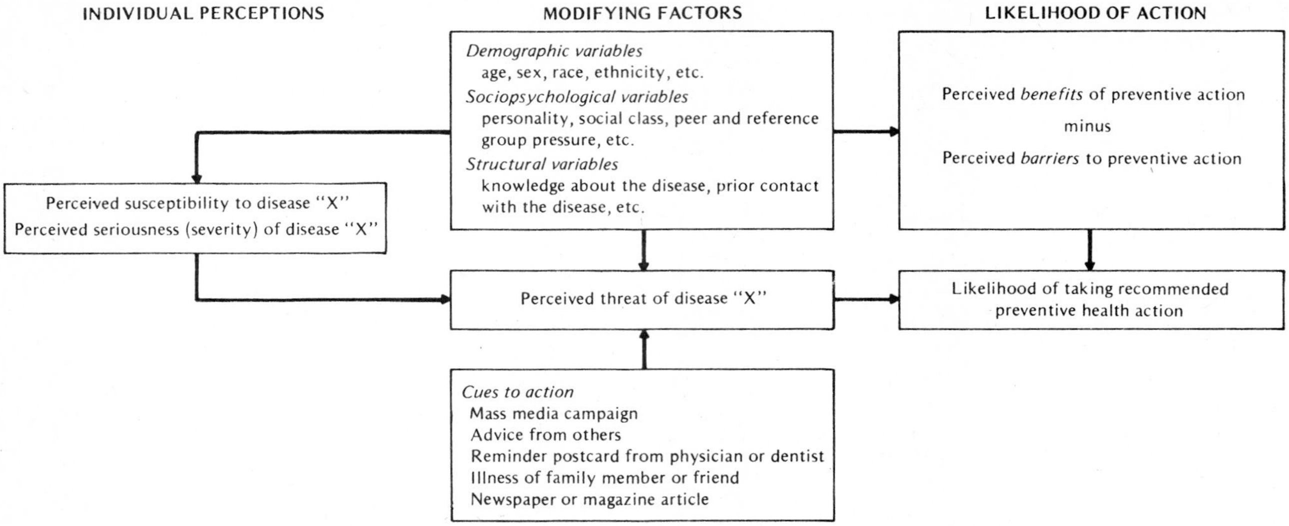

Figure 16–1
Diagram of the (original) Health Belief Model. (From: Rosenstock, 1974, p.7.)

mines what he or she will do, not the physical environment, except as this environment is viewed by the individual. Lewin identifies some aspects of life as having negative valence (negatively valued), some having positive valence (positively valued), and some neutral valence. Individuals seek to avoid the negatively valued aspects, whereas they try to incorporate the positive aspects into their lives.

The original model (Fig. 16–1) deals with explaining preventive health actions—that is, strategies for avoiding the negatively valued regions of illness and disease. In order for an individual to take preventive action to avoid disease he or she would need to believe that (1) he or she was personally susceptible or vulnerable to the disease; (2) the illness was at least moderately severe, so that the consequences of acquiring the disease would significantly disrupt the person's life; (3) taking a particular action would be beneficial in that it would reduce susceptibility to or the severity of the disease; and (4) the benefits outweighed the barriers, such as costs, pain, time, inconvenience, and embarrassment.

The susceptibility and seriousness of the disease are perceived factors, not dependent on fact but on the person's personal beliefs. Both of these individual perceptions become the "readiness" factors leading to the perceived threat of a disease. In this model there are modifying factors (demographic, sociopsychological, and structural) that are posited to modify perceived susceptibility, severity, perceived benefits versus costs, and cues to action. Cues to action refer to the immediate stimuli needed to trigger recognition in the person's mind of the susceptibility and seriousness of a disease (the threat), and the need for taking action to reduce the threat (Rosenstock, 1974).

In newer, modified health belief models, the readiness factors have been extended to include both the perceived feelings of the susceptibility and seriousness of the health problem (the threat) and positive motivation to maintain, regain, or attain wellness. This motivation include concern about and the salience of health matters in general, willingness to seek and receive medical direction, plans to comply, and existence of positive health practices (Becker, 1974 and Pender, 1987).

Pender (1987), extending the Health Belief Model, has proposed a Health Promotion Model that is complementary to the other models of health protection. Health promotion focuses on movement toward a positively valenced state of enhanced health and well-being. The negatively valenced states of illness and disease appear to have minimal motivational significance for health-promoting behavior. Pender suggests that a desire for growth, expression of human potential, and quality of life provides the motivation for health-promotive actions.

Pender's Health Promotion Model (Fig. 16–2), derived also from social learning theory, emphasizes the importance of cognitive–perceptual factors as the primary motivators. Seven cognitive–perceptual factors

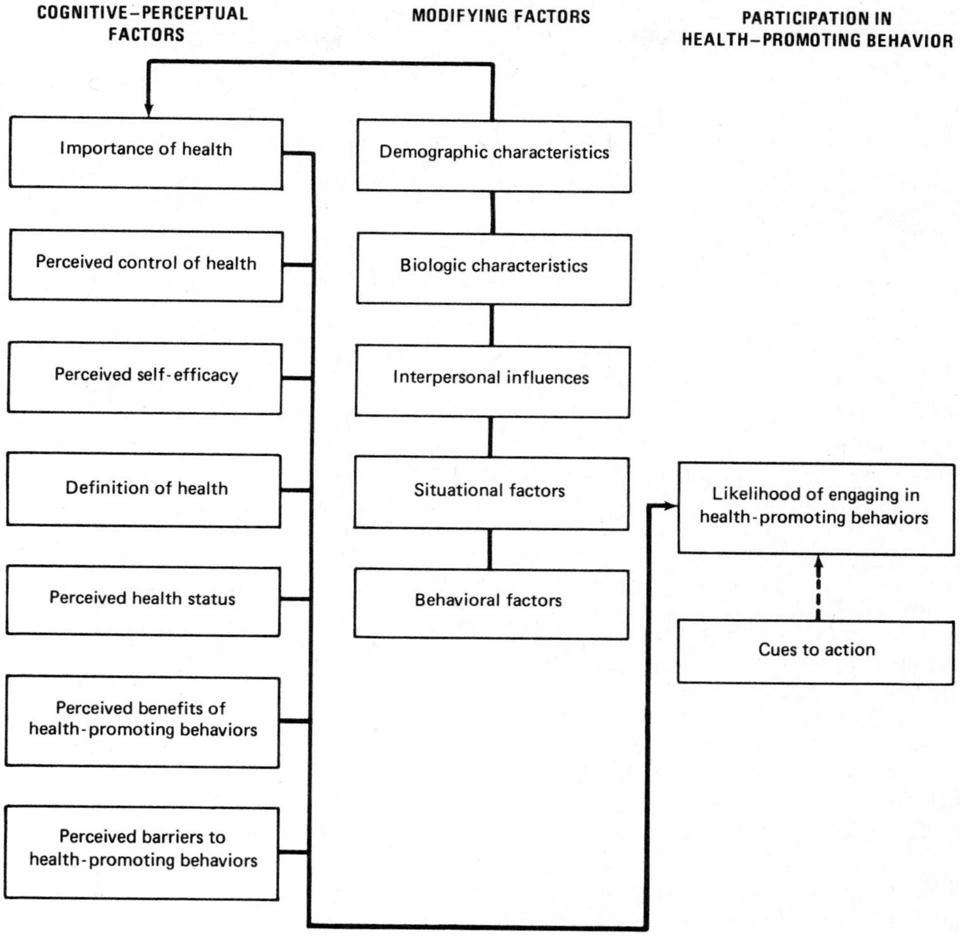

Figure 16–2
Health Promotion Model. (From: Pender, 1987, p. 58.)

affecting predisposition to engage in health–promoting behaviors have been identified within the model. They are the importance of health; how health is defined; and the following perceptions: locus-of control of health; self-efficacy that health-promoting required behaviors may be successfully carried out; health status; benefits of health-promoting behaviors; and barriers to health-promoting actions.

Cognitive–perceptual factors that are hypothesized to be positively correlated with actions that increase personal health status include placing a high value on health; defining health as high-level wellness; having an internal locus-of-control of health and a strong sense of self-efficacy, generally "feeling good"; believing in the long-term rather than short-term benefits of health-enhancing behaviors; and overcoming barriers of availability, convenience, or difficulty of health-promoting activities (Pender, 1987).

The modifying factors of demographic and biological characteristics, interpersonal influences, and situational/behavioral factors are proposed as indirectly influencing patterns of health behavior, as described in the Health Promotion Model. These modifying factors exert influence through the cognitive–perceptual mechanisms that directly affect behavior. Additionally, the likelihood of taking health-promotion action is thought to be activated by cues derived from positive feelings within, or stemming from external influences as a result of personal contacts or exposure to the mass media. The cue intensity required to stimulate action depends on preparedness to engage in health-promoting activities.

In summary, the most important aspect to remember about these models is that they are rational decision-making models in which the occurrence of personal health behavior is thought to be influenced by factors identified in Becker's Health Belief Model and Pender's Health Promotion Model.

In regard to implications for family health care, these models were introduced to emphasize the significance of the family's belief system. If a family perceives a threat and if avenues are then presented to the family for reducing the threat, such as accessible and effective screening, health services, life-style improvements, education, and so on, the family will be more likely to act positively on its behalf. A health practitioner should not use the fear tactic, so as to build up anxiety and thus readiness, without offering an effective and accessible remedial action to handle and reduce the threat.

HEALTH CARE FUNCTION

The health care function is not only a vital and basic family function but one that assumes a central focus in healthy, well-functioning families. Pratt (1976, 1982) underscores the significance of effective functioning in this area by stating, "The more numerous and vital the functions the family performs successfully for its members, the stronger the family system" (1976, p. 122). This section focuses on the question of how well families fulfill their health care function.

Pratt (1976) assessed how well the contemporary American family is functioning as a personal health care system among 510 members of families of New Jersey. She examined the families' adequacy of health practices and home care for ill members, use of professional health care services, level of health knowledge, and attitudes about good health. Pratt found the family to be lacking. For instance, there was a serious breakdown between what should take place to maintain family members' health and what usually occurred. Significant indiscretions were present in the family's pattern of nutrition, exercising, rest, smoking, dental hygiene, communication, and self-care practices. Medication problems were commonplace. Care of dependent, sick, or disabled family members was often not possible or was inadequately carried out. And a significant number of families either failed to utilize health care services or used the service improperly, as in the misuse of emergency rooms for primary health care. Preventive health care was spotty, and although the level of health information was improving, it was still not sufficiently high to serve as a sound foundation in most families. Pratt (1976) concluded that "the composite picture is one of fundamental failure in caring for health" (pp. 45–46).

She suggests that the reasons for the ineffectiveness of families to provide health care for their members lies with both (1) the structure of the health care system and (2) the family structure. Pratt found that when families had wide associations with organizations, engaged in common activities, and used community resources, they used health care services more appropriately. Also, personal health practices were enhanced when husbands were actively involved in internal family affairs, including matters concerning the health care system. She identified certain basic problems with the structure of the medical care system that made it difficult for families to carry out their health care functions.

1. The health care system is organized predominantly around the interests and needs of health care providers rather than consumers. This is operationalized by the preponderant control physicians have over their clients, hospitals, standard fees charged, and so forth. Professional autonomy is highly valued, resulting in inadequate review and control over the members of professional organizations.
2. The hospital is organized bureaucratically, resulting in specialization of functions, rigidity of structure and roles, and depersonalization.

In order for families to become a primary and effective health resource, they must become more involved in the health care team and the total therapeutic process. This implies an equalitarian relationship with health care providers in which both parties can openly express and negotiate in term of their particular needs and interests. Pratt (1976) explains:

> Families cannot become highly responsible about their health care duties if the professionals exclude them from participating in medical management. Nor can families provide good care for sickness at home unless provisions are made for the delivery of health services in the home. (p. 171)

Such a partnership role is needed whether preventive health practices or curative and rehabilitative health needs are under consideration. People must be treated as responsible adults, not passive children, if professionals wish them to assume self-responsibility.

Not only must the family be in partnership with health care providers in directing and implementing its own health care, but clients should also be the ultimate decision makers and managers of those health issues affecting their welfare and lives. In order for clients to engage in effective self-care, they must have the knowledge and skills needed to provide good health care. This means that families need access to the primary sources of health information. Thus professionals must be willing to extend their role to include health education directed toward family self-care.

Most families appear to recognize the need to assume strong management of their own health care. However, both professionals and the health care industry—hospitals, pharmaceutical companies, supply companies, and the health insurance industry—discourage it. Data from Pratt's study revealed that families who were most effective in obtaining appropriate medical services and who practiced a wellness life style on their own were the families referred to as "energized" families. These families assertively sought and verified information, made discriminating decisions, and negotiated aggressively with the health care system, rather than passively accepting and complying (Pratt, 1976, 1982).

HEALTH CARE PRACTICES

Promotion of health practices within the family is a basic goal of family nursing. It becomes critical to gain information regarding the family's health practices to assist the family in health promotion and maintenance.

How well is a family performing the necessary health practices to protect and foster healthy growth and development? One often-used indication of the family's level of functioning is the overall level of health of its family members. This is often inferred by gathering information as to the incidence of disease per member in a specific period of time, realizing, of course, that the ages of individuals and their environment play major roles in the genesis and incidence of disease. Large families and families with young children, for example, have a greater incidence of disease per family. Troubled, problematic families are found to have less resistance to disease and thus have higher rates of disease than families that are functioning well.

In addition to looking at the overall health and illness patterns of family members, the presence or the absence of overt health practices are fruitful assessment areas, providing relevant areas for client education. (See Chapter 2 also.) Four primary areas of health practices will be explored in this section:

1. *Life-style practices*—diet, sleep, and rest patterns, exercise and recreation, drug habits, and self-care.
2. *Environmental practices*—cleanliness and safety practices.
3. *Medically based preventive practices*—general physical examinations and more specifically, vision and hearing examinations, and immunizations.
4. *Dental health practices*.

Life-style Practices

There are hundreds of thousands of Americans who die prematurely each year of diseases caused primarily by unhealthy life-styles. These unnecessary mortalities result from heart disease, cancer, accidents, hypertension, cirrhosis of the liver, suicide, homicide, and diabetes. Cigarette smoking is the chief preventable cause of death in our society. Although the number of smokers has decreased (from 32 percent in 1985 to 29 percent in 1988; (U.S. DHHS, 1989c), smoking is directly responsible for some 390,000 deaths each year in the United States, or more than one out of every six deaths. Cigarette smoking is a major cause of cerebrovascular disease and is associated with lung cancer and uterine cervical cancer (U.S. DHHS, 1989a). Health care, insurance, and lost productivity due to the use of tobacco products cost the United States $52 billion annually (U.S. DHHS, 1990a).

Alcohol, another life-style hazard, is used by more Americans than any other drug, including cigarette tobacco. According to national data, alcohol use declined from 1985 to 1988 (U.S. DHHS, 1989c). Nevertheless an estimated 10.5 million U.S. adults exhibit some symptoms of alcoholism; an additional 7.2 million abuse alcohol but do not show symptoms of dependence. Nearly one-half of all deaths from motor vehicle crashes are alcohol related. It is estimated that 25 percent of all hospitalized persons have alcohol-related problems. The economic cost of alcohol abuse was estimated at $136.3 billion in 1990 (U.S. DHHS, 1990b). Excessive alcohol drinking increases the risk of coronary heart disease, hypertension, stroke, chronic liver disease, some forms of cancer of the oral pharynx, neurological diseases, osteoporosis, nutritional deficiencies, and many other disorders. Even moderate drinking carries some risk in circumstances that require neuromotor coordination and judgment (eg, driving vehicles, working around machinery, and piloting airplanes or boats). Approximately 10 percent of those who consume alcohol in the United States are alcoholics (National Research Council, 1989). Alcohol consumption during pregnancy can damage the fetus, cause low infant birth weight, and lead to fetal alcohol syndrome.

Obesity from overeating and/or reduced physical activity is another example of the results of an unhealthy life-style. Weight gain in adult life is associated with a greater risk of cardiovascular disease, noninsulin-dependent diabetes mellitus, hypertension, gallbladder disease, and endometrial cancer (National Research

Council, 1989). Specific risk factors often discovered in overweight adults during routine health assessments, such as high blood pressure, elevated serum cholesterol, and elevated serum glucose, can be modified by weight reduction.

What we must realize, and this is supported by a myriad of articles and statistics, is that our aggregate health status is not related in any important way to either our health care system or to the medical care provided. When differences among populations and their health status are examined at a specific point in time, socioeconomic, cultural, and environmental factors, plus life-style variation, are found to be much more important than differences in the quantity and quality of health care (LaLonde, 1974; Wildavsky, 1977). Fuchs (1974), in his provocative book, *Who Shall Live?*, makes the role that sociocultural, environmental, and life-style play in health blatantly clear through a comparison of the states of Utah and Nevada in terms of their populations and health status:

> [These] contiguous states . . . enjoy the same levels of income and medical care and are alike in many other respects but their levels of health differ enormously. The inhabitants of Utah are among the healthiest individuals in the United States, while the residents of Nevada are at the opposite end of the spectrum. . . What, then, explains these huge differences? . . . The answer almost surely lies in the different life styles of the residents of the two states. (pp. 52–53)

As a number of authors (Ardell, 1982; Blattner, 1981; Fuchs, 1974; Pelletier, 1979; Pender, 1987; Pratt, 1982) have concluded, the greatest potential for improvement of both overall America's and the individual's health status is through life-style improvement. Personal behavior changes are needed in the areas of diet, exercise, smoking, alcohol, and abusive drug consumption, all of which are critically important factors affecting health.

Family Dietary Practices. The importance of nutritional awareness as a wellness strategy was explored in Chapter 2. In this section, specific assessment areas related to dietary practices are discussed.

Encouraging all family members to keep a 3-day food diary is very helpful in assessing both the quality of their family's diet and how it meets individual nutritional needs. Such a record (3 sequential days' intake) is a stronger indication of a family's eating patterns than is the record of only a single day's intake. A 24-hour food history may not truly represent the family's usual eating patterns (Lacey, 1989). Dietary variations that may occur among individual family members during the day should be included in the journal. Active participation by all family members in completing the food record will enhance the discovery of what family members eat, and where their dietary strengths and deficiencies lie. The 3-day nutrition intake record is an excellent base for assisting families to assess their present nutritional status and begin to develop nutritional goals. The family food diary offered in Figure 16–3 may be used as a guide for data collection.

Assessment of the family's food choices should be a collaborative effort between the family and the nurse. Are a variety of foods consumed from the four food groups each day? Specifically, does the diet contain two 8-ounce servings from the dairy group, two 2- to 3-ounce servings from the meats/protein/fish/beans group, four servings from the bread/cereal group (whole grain or enriched), and four servings from the fruit/vegetable group? Are adequate amounts of dark green or deep yellow fruits or vegetables consumed each day to meet vitamin A requirements? Are vitamin-C-rich fresh fruits and dark green leafy vegetables part of the daily diet? Are low-fat dairy products consumed to meet calcium and vitamin D requirements? Other aspects of the family nutrition analysis should include evaluation for the amount and quality of

	Food Served	Quantity	Comments, factors such as place, activity, money
Breakfast			
Snacks (between meals)			
Lunch			
Snacks (between meals)			
Dinner			
Snacks (between meals)			

Figure 16–3
Family dietary diary (record of family dietary intake for 3 days).

dietary fat, intake of cholesterol and saturated fat, patterns of complex carbohydrate and fiber intake, consumption of sugar and artificial sweeteners, sodium use, processed food intake, alcohol consumption, coffee and tea intake, and the use of dietary supplements.

In analyzing a 3-day food record, the family nurse should determine individual variances. Are any individual family members underweight or overweight for their height and age group? What does each person eat (types of food and quantity) in relation to the family's dietary practices. By learning about family food practices, preferences, and individual dietary habits, the nurse and family will gain a holistic picture of family dietary patterns. For instance, is Johnnie's state of obesity and extensive tooth decay due to his eating excessive amounts of sugars and carbohydrates? If so, is this part of the family's customary diet, along with sedentary activities and poor dental hygiene? Or does the family serve well-balanced meals and Johnnie's sweet intake is at school and/or a reflection of other problems?

Food fads, reduction diets, special dietary beliefs, or culturally based food patterns—such as dietary practices based on a traditional Jewish, Mexican, or Italian pattern, or special food practices based on a philosophic or health commitment such as held by many vegetarians—need to be appraised. Understanding the family's value system and beliefs underlying their food practices is also important and serves as a suitable foundation for later work with them on any modification that might be needed.

Because obesity has been repeatedly demonstrated to be one of the key precursors to chronic illness and shortened longevity, assessing the family's caloric intake and comparing this to their actual caloric need becomes germane to practice.

Additional information relevant in assessing family dietary practices includes an awareness of the function of mealtimes for the family and the family's attitude toward food and mealtimes. Does the family eat together (all meals, only dinner, etc.)? Is mealtime (when they are together) a social, pleasurable experience? How are the meals handled when the family does not eat together? When families are more atomistic or individualistic (each family member doing his/her own "thing"), junk foods and a less adequate diet are often found. When family members do not congregate for at least dinner, it makes it difficult for the family to interact and share with each other, because mealtime is often the one opportunity families have to enjoy each other's company and share important and pleasurable experiences, thoughts, and feelings.

Do parents use the giving and withholding of food as reward and punishment? Where this occurs, the child learns to associate food with approval (love) and disapproval (rejection). Pairing food and social needs for love and acceptance is an unhealthy linkage, as counselors treating the obese will attest.

Shopping, Planning, and Preparation Practices. What are the shopping arrangements? Where is food purchased? Does the family plan for the week or several days at a time, or do they operate on a meal-to-meal basis, shopping for each meal or one day at a time? (The latter is certainly an inefficient means in terms of time and money.) What kind of budgetary limitations exist in their food shopping? If need is present, does family use food stamps? Is food storage and refrigeration adequate? What are usual ways in which food is prepared (fried, boiled, eaten cold, variety of means)?

Shopping, Preparation, and Serving Responsibilities. Who is responsible for each of these tasks? Although we generally assume that the mother–wife is responsible, it is sometimes a role shared with spouse and/or older children.

Family Sleep and Rest Practices. Sleep is a necessary function for quality living. It is thought to fulfill several physiological needs, such as energy conservation, restoration, and protection against exhaustion (Kick, 1989). A major factor in determining how much sleep family members require is age. Infants in the first 6 months of life sleep progressively more in the night than in the day, with requirements for 10 to 12 hours of rest nightly and usually two to three daytime naps by the end of the first year. Toddlers will sleep 8 to 12 hours nightly and have one daytime nap. The preschool-age child requires 10 to 12 hours of sleep. The average school-age child requires 9 to 10 hours of rest each night. The need for sleep declines for adolescents to about 7.5 hours daily. Young and middle-age adults require 6 to 8 hours of sleep. Elderly sleep requirements drop to an average of 6.5 hours. An increase in overall health status, improved mental status, and increased longevity has been positively correlated with regular, adequate rest and sleep habits (Baker, 1985).

Every family has patterns for sleeping, even though in some families these patterns may be erratic due to different work or school schedules, illness, or because of caregiving needs as in the family with a new baby. Assessment of the family's sleep should begin with a sleep history. The following assessment questions may be posed:

1. What are the usual sleeping habits of adults and children? Here one wants to know the number of hours of sleep per night. Are these suitable according to individual's age and health status?
2. Are there *regular* sleeping patterns, with regular hours for going to bed and getting up in the morning? Who decides when the children go to sleep?
3. Where do the family members sleep? In separate or shared beds? Are sleeping arrangements crowded or adequate?
4. Do any family members take naps or have any other regular means of resting?

The nurse should assess if any individual family member has trouble sleeping (insomnia) and if so, what specific type of trouble—falling to sleep, or awakening early without being able to resume sleeping. Frequency and severity of the insomnia should be elicited. Often, sleeping difficulties are due to inadequate sleeping arrangements in the home. A simple sleep diary or log individually kept by each family member may provide additional insight into identifying sleep disturbances.

A deficiency in knowledge of family members' sleep requirements, and what makes a good sleep routine, may be found. New parents may be confused about their baby's irregular sleep schedule. Older adults may lack understanding regarding normal sleep requirements and changes that occur with aging. Many families lack a knowledge of the effects that sedatives and other prescribed drugs, over-the-counter drugs, and illicit drugs have on sleep. The nurse should elicit information from the family as to the possible etiologies of any identified sleep pattern disturbances.

Family Exercise and Recreational Activities. Because regular exercise is found to be a pertinent health habit related positively to overall health, longevity, and improved mental outlook (see Chap. 2), the family nurse should include exercise patterns of the family in her appraisal of family health habits. Specific assessment questions suggested are the following:

1. What types of family recreational pursuits (eg, jogging, bicycling, swimming, dancing, tennis) are engaged in? How often?
2. Does everyone participate?
3. Does the family believe regular aerobic exercise and physical fitness are necessary for good health?
4. Do everyday activities involve any exercise?

Family's Therapeutic Drug Habits. As we know, taking medications is a ubiquitous activity of Americans, with over-the-counter drugs most often used (60 to 70 percent of the time). In a society where pills are regarded as a panacea for everything from sexual problems to headaches, it is no wonder that major community health problems exist in this area.

A significant amount of medication use by families is carried on as an alternative to professional care, because generally the health problems being treated are seen as too trivial to seek medical care or as conditions that the family can adequately handle. A national survey discovered that one half of those sampled undertook self-medication for sore throats, coughs, colds, and upset and acid stomachs. Home over-the-counter medication was found not to be limited to gastrointestinal and upper respiratory complaints, but also covered other body system problems, including the central nervous system, urogenital tract, and skin (Roney and Nall, 1966). Home medication is also frequently used as a supplement to professional treatment. Professional treatments are often altered or modified by patients, as seen in the extensive modifications made to diet and insulin regimen by diabetic patients. Prescribed medications, furthermore are often not taken by patients. One study reported a medication rejection rate of 50 percent (Linnett, 1970).

It is important to assess the family's use of over-the-counter and prescription drugs. What drugs do family members take and for what purpose? By identifying drugs commonly used by the family, the assessor can look for possible side effects or harmful interactive effects. Also, drug usage can tell the nurse something about how the family and/or the family members cope with life events and health problems, as well as how they define health and illness.

Some over-the-counter drugs commonly taken by Americans are potentially harmful, or at best unnecessary. The regular use of laxatives is an example. Although most of the fatal medication poisonings are caused by prescribed medications, with barbiturates heading the list, 20 percent are caused by over-the-counter drugs. Of the nonfatal drug poisonings, aspirin is the leading offender, primarily because of its tendency to produce gastrointestinal bleeding.

In homes where young children are present, storage of drugs and other hazardous substances in safe childproof containers and cupboards is imperative, as the incidence of poisoning among children is very high.

One important factor leading to medication poisonings is the tendency of older families to save and reuse medicines years later. Any nurse who has cared for older patients in their homes will attest to the fact that families will hoard medicines prescribed many years ago and that many of these containers do not even contain the name and dosage of the drug. Such medications undergo change over time and, at best, become ineffective. Often families end up using their old medicines to treat a family member who they perceive to be experiencing the same or similar symptoms as the person for whom the drug was originally prescribed. The possible misdiagnosis by the family presents a further hazard.

In assessing the drug use of older family members, as part of a home health agency visit, it is suggested that the nurse find a way to tactfully review the kinds and age of the drugs stored in the house. By doing so the nurse will be able to go over with the family both the new and old medications and their usage, which may influence the family to properly dispose of drugs that are old and/or unmarked.

In considering drug habits, assessment not only of the use of medications, but also the consumption of caffeine, alcohol intake, and smoking is indicated. Smoking and alcohol intake should be assessed in terms of who uses either substance, and how much, when, and under what situations or circumstances. Is the use of tobacco or alcohol by a family member(s) perceived as a problem by that person or other family members? Does the use of alcohol interfere with their capacity to carry out their usual activities? How long has the present use of alcohol continued? What was the pattern of drinking in the past?

In terms of the group that health care professionals need to be most concerned with helping is the teenage population. This is because smoking often begins during these years.

Family's Recreational Drug Habits. Drug abuse involves the regular taking of a deleterious or noxious quantity of any drug over a period of time, prescribed or illicit. The 1988 National Household Survey (U.S. Department of Health and Human Services, 1989d) conducted by the National Institute on Drug Abuse on illicit use of marijuana, cocaine, heroin, hallucinogens, and inhalants, and nonmedical use of psychotherapeutics (sedatives, tranquilizers, stimulants, or analgesics) found 72.4 million Americans age 12 or older (37 percent of the population) had tried marijuana, cocaine, or other illicit drugs at least once in their lifetimes. Thirty-two percent of the reported illegal drug consumption was found among young adults. In 1988 illicit drug use was admitted to by 17 percent of the youth and 29 percent of adults.

Marijuana remains by far the most commonly used illicit drug in the United States. Almost 66 million Americans (32 percent) have tried marijuana at least once in their lives: 4 million youths, 17 million young adults, and over 45 million adults. Of the 21 million people who used marijuana at least once during the survey period, almost one third, or 6.6 million, used the drug once a week or more. Use of marijuana decreased from 18 million (9 percent) in 1985 to 12 million (6 percent) in 1988.

Marijuana has a toxic effect on brain nerve cells. Researchers have found that chronic use of THC, the psychoactive ingredient in marijuana, destroys nerve cells and causes other pathological changes in the brain, possibly placing long-term marijuana users at risk for serious or premature memory disorders as they age. The daily use of 1 to 3 marijuana joints also appears to produce approximately the same lung damage and potential cancer risk as smoking five times as many cigarettes. Additionally, marijuana elevates heart rate, increases blood pressure, and is believed to adversely affect reproductive functioning in women.

A second illicit drug that is widely used is cocaine. Most clinicians estimate that approximately 10 percent of those who initially use cocaine "recreationally" will go on to serious, heavy use. It is one of the most powerfully addictive of the abused drugs, and is available in several forms. Cocaine is usually sniffed or "snorted", being absorbed through the mucous membranes of the nose. It can also be injected, or after chemical conversion to a purified form known as "freebase" or "crack," it can be smoked. Compulsive cocaine use may develop even more rapidly if the substance is smoked rather than ingested intranasally.

Cocaine acts as a strong central nervous system stimulant. Specific physical effects include constricted peripheral blood vessels, dilated pupils, and increased temperature, heart rate, and blood pressure. Cocaine's immediate euphoric effects, which include hyperstimulation, reduced fatigue, and increased mental clarity, last approximately 30 to 60 minutes.

Cocaine use ranges from episodic to addictive. Episodic cocaine use may produce nasal congestion and a runny nose. Some consistent users of cocaine report feelings of restlessness, irritability, and anxiety. A possible consequence of chronic cocaine "snorting" is ulceration of the mucous membrane of the nose. Addictive cocaine use can sufficiently damage the nasal septum to cause it to collapse. Continuing high doses of cocaine can also result in physiological seizures followed by cardiac or respiratory arrest, coma, or death. The number of cocaine users decreased significantly from 5.8 million in 1985 to 2.9 million in 1988 (U. S. DHHS, 1989d).

There are an estimated 1.1 to 1.3 million IV drug abusers in the United States. Experts estimate nearly 500,000 IV drug abusers inject heroin regularly, while thousands of others inject cocaine or amphetamines (U.S. Department of Health and Human Services,

1989d). These individuals are all at increased risk for AIDS. Since January 1, 1989 data from the National Institute on Drug Abuse indicates that 30 percent of all AIDS cases involve IV drug abuse. Minorities are overrepresented among IV drug users. Among heterosexual IV drug abusers, a disproportionate number (80 percent) of persons with AIDS are blacks and Latinos.

Methamphetamine, also known as "crank," "meth," or "speed," once associated with blue-collar workers and biker gangs, now is gaining increased popularity among college students and young professionals. A frightening form of methamphetamine is a newcomer called ice. Produced in rock-like form, ice is smoked. The drug enters the body faster and its effects are longer lasting when compared to cocaine. Also called crystal meth, it is often odorless, colorless, and tasteless.

Hallucinogens such as LSD, PCP, mescaline, and peyote continue to be a significant problem in the United States. Chronic users of these drugs report memory loss, speech difficulties, depression, and weight loss. When given psychomotor tests, PCP users tend to have lost their fine motor skills and short-term memory. Mood disorders occur.

During the 1988 to 1989 survey (Turner, 1990) it was found that the use of inhalants, and the nonmedical use of psychotherapeutic drugs such as sedatives, tranquilizers, stimulants, and analgesics, decreased to less than 2 percent of the population, being slightly higher for females than males.

The family exercises a profound influence on the onset and continuity of patterns of substance abuse by family members and provides a context for communication of knowledge, skills, and attitudes about substance abuse. Positive social reinforcement (modeling by parents or esteemed family members of substance abuse behavior patterns) may play a major social influence in contributing to youth drug use (Baumrind, 1985). At the other end of the continuum, families may highly discourage substance abuse and openly communicate that illicit drug use is contradictory to family values. Those family members who do become severely drug dependent most often need specialized treatment to become healthy again. A wide range of treatment is available through public and private entities. Recovery treatment centers that incorporate the family into their plan of care more holistically and effectively treat the substance abuser.

Family's Self-care Practices. When assessing a family, a determination is needed of both the family's ability to provide self-care and its motivation and actual competence in handling health matters. For a family to be responsible for its own self-care, it needs to have an understanding of its own health status and/or health problems and the steps needed to improve or maintain its health (Johnson, 1984). Self-care practices involve not only preventive practices, diagnosis, and home treatment of common and minor ambulatory health problems, but also all the procedures and treatments prescribed for the care of illness of a family member, such as giving medications, using special appliances, changing dressings, and carrying out special exercises and diets.

How adequately is the family able to handle the responsibilities of these therapies? Estimates from the literature report that 75 to 85 percent of all health care is provided by self or family, with self-care being the predominant illness response in the older population (Hickey, 1988). These percentages hold for both populations who have and do not have access to professional health services (Levin et al., 1976). There are no firm data demonstrating that lay-initiated self-care is any less effective than professional care (which is about 35 percent effective), or less dangerous (which involves 20 percent iatrogenic ill effects and 4 to 11 percent complications from nosocomial infections) (Levin, 1977). The authors Elliott-Binns (1973) in Britain and Pederson (1976) in Denmark found that 90 percent of self-care procedures taken prior to professional intervention were appropriate and helpful.

An assessment of the family's self-care abilities, focusing on the family's knowledge, motivation, and motor skill strength or coordination necessary to carry out the physical tasks of care, provides the foundation for evaluating the need for nursing intervention. In identifying the family's strengths, resources, and potentials, the nurse should not overlook the possible stressful effects of caregiving on the family unit. Families that assume the major health care responsibility for members who are frail or suffering severe health problems may experience high levels of physical and emotional strain. Financial burdens may also contribute to a family's level of strain.

Studies have shown that female caregivers tend to exhibit higher levels of stress than males. Adult daughter caregivers especially have been found to experience greater familial conflict and household disruption, particularly when married with dependent children (Bass and Noelker, 1987; Cantor, 1983).

Environmental Practices

Environmental practices consist of habits or patterns that positively or negatively affect the family's or its members' health status. For instance, is the family regularly exposed to smoke, herbicides, asbestos, or other harmful substances? Noise pollution may also be harmful, as well as water pollution and radiation exposure.

More and more evidence demonstrates the adverse effects of long-term, low-level exposure to noise and to chemicals in our air, water, and food.

There are a number of dangerous or potentially dangerous substances commonly found in and around homes and offices. A body of scientific knowledge suggests that indoor contaminates especially may present a widespread pollution threat. Concentrations of some airborne pollutants have been found to be as high as 100 times greater indoors than outdoors (U.S. Environmental Protection Agency, 1988). It has been suggested that a wide variety of organic compounds from common household products may contribute to the threat of indoor pollution. According to the Environmental Protection Agency, benzene, a known human carcinogen, has been found in far higher concentrations indoors than outdoors. Benzene is emitted indoors by synthetic fibers, plastics, some cleaning solutions, and tobacco smoke. Commonly used household products such as air fresheners, shoe polish, paints, cleaners, mothballs, and dry-cleaned clothing contain low levels of chemicals that are known animal carcinogens. Cleaning solutions and powders containing chemicals that are toxic, abrasive, or caustic to eyes and mucous membranes are labeled by most manufacturers with warnings about potential dangers. Families should be encouraged to store such substances properly and out of reach of young children.

Noxious byproducts of cigarette, pipe, and cigar smoking such as carbon monoxide and nitrogen dioxide may predispose household occupants, especially children, to pneumonia, other respiratory ailments, and cancer. Formaldehyde, widely used in newer building materials and furnishings, can cause eye, nose, and throat irritation, coughing, skin rashes, headaches, dizziness, nausea, vomiting, and nosebleeds. Products sold to kill household pests may leave pesticide residues, with many of these chemicals having never been tested to determine their health effects. Lead, which adversely affects children's intellectual and emotional growth, can be found in older plumbing and in household dust as old paint deteriorates or is chipped away. Asbestos, found in cement and older insulating materials, can lead to lung cancer or asbestosis, a chronic lung disease. Colorless and odorless radon gas discharged from uranium-bearing rocks and soil beneath homes invades houses through cracks in the foundation. After smoking, radon exposure is estimated to be the nation's leading cause of lung cancer (U.S. Environmental Protection Agency, 1988).

EPA researchers have estimated that indoor pollution, including second-hand tobacco smoke, may account for up to 11,400 deaths each year. Radon exposures may result in anywhere from 3,000 to 20,000 additional deaths. Both urban dwellers and rural residents have tested positive for indoor chemical contamination. A pamphlet, "Inside Story: A Guide to Indoor Pollution," is available from the EPA Information Center, PM-211B, 401 M Street SW, Washington, DC 20460.

The family's hygiene and cleanliness practices may also be considered as environmental practices. Although cleanliness is not "next to Godliness," there are several general health habits that reduce the possibility of infection and its spread.

1. Washing hands before meals and after toileting.
2. Using separate towels. When an infectious skin condition such as scabies or impetigo is present, sharing towels can be an infection route.
3. Drinking from separate cups and glasses that are clean. In families with several children and an overworked and overwhelmed mother, sharing of baby bottles and cups is commonly seen.
4. Bathing and cleanliness. Although this is certainly needed, most health care workers have been found to be overly critical of families that they serve in terms of degree of family cleanliness. We need to carefully differentiate between family hygiene practices that are, in fact, deleterious to health and those that are contrary to our own habits and customs but are *not* harmful in terms of health.

Safety practices could also be included here, but have already been included in Chapter 9 as part of environmental data.

Medically Based Preventive Measures

Complete annual physical examinations for healthy populations are cost ineffective and a waste of our precious health resources (see Chap. 2 for elaboration of this point). On the other hand, a selective preventive-oriented physical examination on a regular periodic basis is cost effective and able to screen for some of the major health hazards.

Annual health assessments (physical examination, history, and diagnostic tests) tailored to the client's age, race, and sex are vital and serve several purposes. They provide the necessary information to jointly establish with the client a health maintenance plan. The preventive health assessment identifies risk factors particular to an individual; for example, an adult who smokes and whose father died of heart disease should be counseled about heart risk factors, because a person with that health profile has twice the risk of incurring heart disease as an individual who does not smoke and has no family history of disease. Health assessments can also detect unnoticed or covert signs and symptoms crucial for case finding (early detection and treatment).

Major risk factors are related to heredity, sex, race, and age. For instance, individuals whose families have had heart disease at early ages or diabetes have an increased likelihood of inheriting a predisposition toward those diseases. Thanks to their sex hormones, premenopausal women are less likely to have myocardial infarctions than men of the same age group. Blacks have more than twice the chance of developing hypertension than whites. And generally, the older one gets, the greater the chance of developing a chronic illness.

This does not imply, however, that the above risk factors are inevitable harbingers of future events. In fact, susceptibility to some diseases can actually be reduced if an attempt is made to attenuate risk factors by improving one's life-style and seeking routine, preventive health care.

What should be included in the annual health assessment of the well adult? Again, opinion varies. The minimum should probably be a general history (review of the systems and any present complaints), blood pressure, vital signs, weight, and urinalysis; for women, a pap smear and breast and pelvic examinations are indicated; for men older than 30 to 35 years of age, an electrocardiogram, heart auscultation, rectal examination, and lipid panel (serum cholesterol and triglycerides) should be performed. Middle-aged men should also have a protoscopy or sigmoidoscopy of the rectum done for detection of cancerous polyps, and blacks should be tested for sickle-cell anemia.

What are the family's feelings about having a "physical" when they are well? Past practices of the family may be a gauge to their feelings; nevertheless, a lack of periodic well-care may also be a function of inaccessibility to, ignorance about, and/or costs of such services, so that in order to ascertain the reasons behind not receiving health examinations, more direct questions may be warranted.

Race, and level of income and education, contribute to class differences in health care service utilization. Minority populations and those with lower levels of income and education utilize health care services less frequently. Nonwhite populations spend fewer days in the hospital, see a physician less often, and are more likely to be treated in a hospital outpatient department than in a physician's office (U.S. DHHS, 1988). For such groups, poor experiences with the health care system are likely to lead to low rates of service utilization for health examinations and treatments.

One contributing factor explaining differences in utilization patterns of medical services is the lack of health care insurance coverage for all families. Approximately two thirds of the U.S. population is covered by employment-related coverage, either individually or through groups sponsored by those other than employers. A total of 74.5 percent of the population is privately insured. Ten percent of the population receives coverage from publicly funded programs such as Medicare and Medicaid, according to data obtained from survey findings conducted by the National Center for Health Services Research. An estimated 15.5 percent of the population, or 37 million Americans, remain without private insurance or public coverage to help pay medical needs (U.S. DHHS, 1989b).

Nearly half of the uninsured population under age 65 is composed of working adults and their dependents. This group represents the largest number of uninsured. Uninsured workers are typically part-time or self-employed, work for small establishments, earn low hourly wages at or near the minimum wage, and work in industries characterized by seasonal or less technical employment such as agriculture, construction, manufacturing, and sales. Other populations especially vulnerable for being uninsured include children, unmarried young adults, older women, lower middle income groups, Latinos, blacks, and families without a working adult living at or near the poverty line (U.S. DHHS, 1989b).

Vision and Hearing Examinations. Health assessments should be supplemented by vision and hearing examinations. This is particularly important, because glaucoma and hearing loss can be detected and can usually be treated effectively or prevented.

Children should have periodic vision and hearing examinations done as part of their well-baby and preschool care. During the school years children are periodically given Snellen tests, a rough screen for common vision problems.

Adults who wear glasses need an eye examination annually, unless visual changes are noted sooner. For others, every other year is adequate. The eye examination should include tonometry testing for detection of glaucoma, which is recommended on a yearly basis for all adults over 40 years of age.

If families do not know of an eye specialist to call, the nurse will need to review with the family the difference in training and focus of an optician, optometrist, and ophthalmologist. If while eliciting a family medical history, the nurse finds a history of glaucoma in the family, he or she should stress an annual eye examination even more vigorously, as there is now an overwhelming evidence of a higher incidence of glaucoma among siblings and offspring of patients with the disease than among the rest of the population (Perkins, 1973).

Because hearing difficulties can lead to serious behavioral and learning problems in school, children should be routinely given an audiometric test during the early school years. Primary care practitioners should also complete rough screening for hearing during well-child care visits.

Although asymptomatic adults may not need annual audiometric testing, if hearing difficulties are noted or an individual is at high risk, testing is indicated. Progressive hearing loss can occur from exposure to certain types of noise. If a client is exposed to a high level of noise at work or home, the nurse should inquire into his or her use of ear protectors and hearing examinations. Hearing loss can also occur with age, due to vascular insufficiency of the cochlea. Smokers have greater hearing loss than nonsmokers, as smoking reduces the blood supply by vasospasm induced by nicotine, by atherosclerotic narrowing of the vessels, and by formation of thrombi in the vessels (Diekelmann, 1977).

Immunization Status. The one most important and specific measure against preventive disease is that of immunization. At least 75 to 80 percent of susceptible children must be immunized to effectively protect a community from preventable communicable diseases (Garner, 1978). Hence promotion of immunization services is a vital and integral part of family health care.

The Department of Health and Human Services instituted a national campaign in 1977 to improve and maintain the immunization levels of children in America (Paskert, 1983). By mid-1985, through legislative regulation of immunization requirements for school attendance, a 96 percent overall immunization level has been achieved in the school-aged population (U.S. DHHS, 1985). The current need is to focus on preschool and infant populations, in which the immunization level is approximately 75 percent to 80 percent (U.S. DHHS, 1987).

For infants and children the need for being adequately protected against tetanus, diphtheria, pertussis (whooping cough), polio, mumps, rubella (German measles), and rubeola (measles) is crucial. Smallpox vaccinations are no longer advised, as the risk of untoward reactions to the vaccine are now greater than the risk of contracting the disease. Flu vaccines and tuberculin skin tests are also recommended for certain age groups and under certain situations. (The conditions and age of the person and the community incidence and exposure risk are important variables here.) Booster shots of diphtheria and tetanus are recommended for adults every 7 to 10 years, because both of these diseases are serious and endemic in the United States today.

When completing an assessment of the immunization status of family members, the types of immunizations received, dates, and any adverse reactions to immunization should be recorded.

Dental Health Care Practices

Dental health practices are vital in maintaining good teeth throughout an individual's life span. The prevalence of dental ill health is great, especially among the poor of our country.

Dental health care includes both preventive care and curative health practices. In order to maintain high-level dental health, a combination of personal habits or practices, as well as preventive care by dentist and/or dental hygienist, should be carried out. The four basic elements for dental health maintenance are:

1. Regular preventive dental services, including dental examination, x-rays, cleaning, education, and for children topical fluoride treatments when indicated.
2. Use of fluoridated water, or if unavailable, prescription for daily oral fluoride liquid or tablets for children.
3. Regular brushing and flossing of teeth after meals.
4. Reduced amounts of certain types of fermentable carbohydrates in the diet. All fermentable carbohydrates have the potential of contributing to the development of dental caries by supplying the raw materials necessary for bacteria in the mouth to produce tooth-decaying acid. Fermentable carbohydrates include sugars, such as found in fruits, honey, and sweets; and cooked starches such as found in bread and potatoes (Loe, 1988).

A survey conducted by the National Institute of Dental Research (NIDR) found that an estimated one half of the nation's school children aged 5 to 17 have no tooth decay at all. This represents a 36 percent reduction in caries from NIDR studies conducted at the beginning of the 1980s (Loe, 1988).

Dental experts suggest factors that contribute toward the improvement in children's dental health may include the widespread use of fluoride, the increased application of sealants, improvement in personal oral hygiene, the receipt of regular professional dental care, and the rise in awareness of the effects of eating habits on the teeth (Loe, 1988).

Fluoride, which can be found in the drinking water supply in some communities, or which is prescribed by dentists as an oral supplement, is recognized as the most effective agent available to protect teeth from decay, preventing nearly two thirds of caries in children. Less helpful but still effective are the various means of applying fluoride topically, including the application of fluoride solutions by many dentists, or the self-administration of fluoride rinses or gels by the patient (American Dental Association, 1988).

Dental caries result from the interaction of several processes, primarily the amount and type of carbohydrates in the diet, the amount of plaque buildup, and resistance of the teeth. Consumption of foods and beverages high in sugar content contribute toward harmful bacteria producing acid for at least 20 minutes after eating. Snacking should be kept to a minimum and confined to foods that do not promote decay—nuts, popcorn, raw fruits, vegetables, and sugar-free drinks. Professional dental care and practicing good daily oral hygiene (brushing and flossing) can control harmful bacteria by removing plaque. Learning how to brush teeth properly to remove plaque is one of the best investments a person can make in preserving his or her own dental health. It is especially important to remove plaque thoroughly from the teeth before bedtime. During sleep less saliva is secreted, and therefore, bacterial acids are diluted less at night (Kandzari and Howard, 1981).

For American adults, periodontal disease continues to be a major dental problem and is the chief cause of tooth loss. Gum disease is thought to affect at least three out of four adults and may strike 95 percent of the population at some time (Kandzari and Howard, 1981; Loe, 1988). Gum disease can be slowed down or prevented by careful attention to brushing, flossing, and regular professional dental care.

The family nurse, in teaching families dental health and hygiene, may wish to check the mouths of some of the children or adults for plaque build-up or bring some disclosing solution that they can use to detect plaque themselves. Teeth should be brushed after meals, and the sooner the better, to prevent sugars from remaining in the mouth. The object of brushing is to remove plaque and food particles from the teeth, which is done by effective friction of the toothbrush (a soft-bristled one) against the surface of the teeth. It is important to use dental floss once a day to supplement brushing, because some surfaces of the teeth and teeth–gum junctions are inaccessible by brushing alone.

Families (both children and adults) need thorough demonstrations of an effective method for brushing teeth. There are several acceptable ways to brush one's teeth; newer methods are much more effective than the older vertical (from gum line or down) method taught in the past. Regular, after-meal brushing and flossing teeth is considered a vital aspect in the prevention of dental caries, gum disease, and periodontal disease.

Treatment of dental problems has not been mentioned except in passing, but is also of vital import. Although prevention has been stressed, early detection and treatment of dental and gum problems will certainly keep more serious problems from developing. Malposition problems—over- and underbites, causing unequal exertion of pressure on teeth—are targets for early detection in children. Orthodontia may be needed to correct these problems, which if untreated could later cause periodontal disease and speech problems, as well as result in cosmetic ill effects.

FAMILY HEALTH HISTORY

This area is significant for several reasons. First, family histories will often identify familial risk factors. Second, the family's experience with certain diseases might possibly have resulted in fears, myths, or misconceptions about these illnesses, and the health worker should be sensitive to these. Third, through eliciting a family medical history, the assessor will learn more about both families of orientation and thus gain a better understanding of the family's past.

The family medical history consists of an identification of past and present environmentally and genetically related diseases of the family of orientation—going back to maternal and paternal grandparents and including aunts and uncles and their children. Besides ascertaining the general health status of all these individuals, the family-centered health worker should specifically inquire about the presence of the following diseases, because people often forget important familial diseases:

1. Environmentally related diseases (to which family members might be or have been exposed).
   a. Psychosocial problems: mental illness and obesity.
   b. Infectious diseases: typhoid fever, tuberculosis, venereal disease, hepatitis, diarrheas (dysenteries), and skin diseases (scabies, lice, impetigo).
2. Genetically linked diseases: epilepsy, diabetes, cystic fibrosis, mental retardation, sickle-cell anemia, kidney disease, hypertension, heart disease, cancer, leukemia, vision and hearing defects, hemophilia, and allergies, including asthma.

Including family history information on the family genogram (see Fig. 8–2) is a useful way of recording this information. The family genogram should include the age of members, whether the individual is living or deceased, the cause of death, level of general health, and presence of chronic disease.

Family Health Records

Families often change physicians, are seen at several agencies or by different specialists for different diseases, and with passing years, and memories fade. All these factors underscore the need for families to keep records of the year-by-year medical events of each of the family members.

Educating families about the importance of maintaining family medical records is an important health education area for assisting families to become responsible for their health care. The data the family maintains will aid the family when new doctors are visited and may also obviate the need for redundant expensive and time-consuming laboratory and diagnostic tests. Moreover, information given in the record may assist a family in obtaining faster and more accurate diagnoses.

When there are young children in the family or adult members, especially oldsters, who have several illnesses and are seeing more than one physician concurrently, it is especially critical to have medical record information. For children, immunization records are important; for adults, diagnostic and laboratory tests, diagnoses, medications taken, and any adverse reactions to them should be carefully recorded.

The following broad areas of health information need to be included:

- Family medical history (see previous section).
- Maternity record.
- Children's heights and weights.
- Adults' weight records.
- Childhood diseases (of children).
- Accident records.
- Major surgeries, illnesses, and hospitalizations.
- Immunization records.
- Allergies.
- Corrective devices (glasses, hearing aids, dental plates, and special shoes are examples).
- Blood groups and Rh factors.
- Blood pressure; and other laboratory tests performed.

FAMILY HEALTH CARE FUNCTION: APPLYING THE FAMILY NURSING PROCESS

☐ ASSESSMENT QUESTIONS

The following areas and questions are germane to assessing the family's health care function.

1. *Family's health belief's, values, and behaviors.* What value does the family assign health? Health promotion? Prevention? Is there consistency between family health values as stated and their health actions? What health-promoting activities does the family engage in regularly? Are these behaviors characteristic of all family members, or are patterns of health-promoting behavior highly variable throughout the family system? What are the family's health goals?
2. *Family's definition of health–illness and its level of knowledge.* How does the family define health and illness for each family member? What clues provide this impression, and who decides? Can the family observe and report significant symptoms and changes? What are the family members' source of health information? How is health knowledge transmitted to family members? How does the family assess its level of health knowledge?
3. *Family's perceived health status and illness susceptibility.* How does the family assess its present health status? What present health problems are identified by the family? To what serious health problems do family members perceive themselves vulnerable? What are the family's perceptions of how much control over health they have by taking appropriate health actions?
4. *Family dietary practices.* Does the family know food sources from the basic four food groups? Is the family diet adequate? (A 3-day food history

record of family eating patterns is recommended). Who is responsible for the planning, shopping, and preparation of meals? How are the foods prepared? Mostly fried, broiled, baked, microwaved, or served raw? What is the number of meals consumed per day? Are there budgeting limitations? Food stamps usage? What is the adequacy of storage and refrigeration? Does mealtime serve a particular function for the family? What is the family's attitude toward food and mealtimes? What are the family's snack habits?

5. *Sleep and rest habits.* What are the usual sleeping habits of family members? Are family members meeting their sleep requirements which are appropriate to their age and health status? Are regular hours established for sleeping? Do family members take regular naps or have other means of resting during the day? Who decides when children go to sleep? Where do family members sleep?
6. *Exercise and recreation.* Are family members aware that active recreation and regular aerobic exercise are necessary for good health? What types of recreational and physical activities do family members engage in regularly? Are these activity patterns representative of all family members or only certain members? Do usual daily work activities allow for exercise?
7. *Family drug habits.* What is the family's use of alcohol, tobacco, coffee, cola, or tea (caffeine and theobromine are stimulants)? Do family members take drugs for recreational purposes? How long has (have) family member(s) been using alcohol or other recreational drugs? Is the use of tobacco, alcohol, prescribed or illicit drugs by family members perceived as a problem? Does the use of alcohol or other drugs interfere with the capacity to carry out usual activities? Do family members regularly use over-the-counter or prescription drugs? Does the family save drugs over a long period of time and reuse? Are drugs properly labeled and in a safe place away from young children?
8. *Family's role in self-care practices.* What does the family do to improve its health status? What does the family do to prevent illness/disease? Who is (are) the health leader(s) in the family? Who makes the health decisions in the family? What does the family do to care for health problems and illnesses in the home? How competent is the family in self-care relative to recognition of signs and symptoms, diagnosis, and home treatment of common, simple health problems? What are the family's values, attitudes, and beliefs regarding home care?
9. *Environmental practices.* How exposed are family members to environmental hazards found in the soil, air, and water? Are family members subjected to high levels of noise on a regular basis? Do family members smoke or are they exposed to smoke while on the job or at home? Do family members use pesticides, cleaning solutions, glues, solvents, heavy metals, or poisons within the home? What are the family's hygiene and cleanliness practices?
10. *Medically based preventive measures.* What are the family's feelings about having physicals when well? When were the last eye and hearing examinations? What is the immunization status of the family?
11. *Dental health practices.* Do family members use fluoridated water, or is a daily fluoride supplement prescribed for the children? What are the family's oral hygiene habits in regard to brushing and flossing after meals? What are the family's patterns of simple sugar and starch intake? Do family members receive regular preventive professional dental care including education, periodic x-rays, cleaning, repair, and for children topical or oral fluoride?
12. *Family health history.* What is the overall health of family members of

origin and marriage (grandparents, parents, aunts, uncles, cousins, siblings, and offspring) over three generations? Is there in the past or present a history of genetic or familial diseases—diabetes, heart disease, high blood pressure, stroke, cancer, gout, kidney disease, thyroid disease, asthma and other allergic states, blood diseases, or any other familial diseases. Is there a family history of emotional problems or suicide? Are there any present or past environmentally related family diseases?

13. *Health services received.* From what health care practitioner and/or health care agency do the family members receive care? Does this provider or agency see all members of the family and take care of all their health needs?
14. *Feelings and perceptions regarding health services.* What are the family's feelings about the kinds of health services available to it in the community? What are the family's feelings and perceptions regarding the health services it receives? Is the family comfortable, satisfied, and confident with the care received from its health care providers? Does the family have any past experience with family health nursing services? What are the family's attitudes and expectations of the role of the nurse?
15. *Emergency health services.* Does the agency or physician the family receives care from have an emergency service? Are medical services by current health care providers available if an emergency occurs? If emergency services are not available, does the family know where the closest available (according to their eligibility) emergency services are for both the children and the adult members of the family? Does the family know how to call for an ambulance and for paramedic services? Does the family have an emergency health plan?
16. *Source of payment.* How will the family pay for services it receives or might receive? Does the family have a private health insurance plan, Medicare, or Medicaid, or must the family pay for services in full or partially? Does the family receive any free services (or know about those available)? What effect does the cost of health care have on the family's utilization of health services? If the family has health insurance (private, Medicare, and/or Medicaid), is the family informed about what services are covered, such as preventive services, special medical equipment, home visits, and so forth?
17. *Logistics of receiving care.* How far away are health care facilities from the family's home? What modes of transportation does the family use to get to them? If the family must depend on public transportation, what problems exist in regards to hours of service and travel time to health care facilities?

FAMILY NURSING DIAGNOSES AND PLANNING

In terms of the types of family nursing diagnoses that are often found in the area of the family's health care function, the number of possibilities are large. Certainly family nursing diagnoses that lead to health-promotional or educational strategies are appropriate here, because knowledge deficits of family members are commonly observed. These knowledge deficits are seen in the various areas discussed in this chapter, such as dietary practices, rest and sleep patterns, exercise practices, drug and alcohol use, life-style practices, and use of health care services.

North American Nursing Diagnosis Association (NANDA) family nursing diagnoses that are behaviorally oriented and deal with health care practice modifications are:

- Altered health maintenance
- Potential altered health maintenance
- Health-seeking behaviors (Carpenito, 1989).

"Health maintenance" family nursing diagnoses identify health care practice areas where the family or sets of family members demonstrate actual or potential inadequate health practices. Specific examples here are in the areas of ineffective or inadequate dental care practices, dietary practices, preventive health care practices, and inadequate family planning. Family health-promotional diagnoses may be subsumed under "health-seeking behaviors," as explained by Carpenito (1989). The definitions of these two broad NANDA nursing diagnoses, made applicable to families and family members, are:

- *Altered health maintenance* (may be potential or actual): "The state in which an individual or group [family or family members] experiences or is at risk of experiencing a disruption in health because of an unhealthy life-style or lack of knowledge to manage a condition" (Carpenito, 1989, p. 382).
- *Health-seeking behaviors:* Extended to the family this diagnoses pertains to a state in which a family or family members "in stable health actively seek ways to alter personal health habits and/or the environment in order to move toward a higher level of wellness" (Carpenito, 1989, p. 408).

Family nurses are challenged to assist the family unit in identifying areas of health risk, in establishing relevant health goals, and in planning for life-style changes that will continue as an ongoing family commitment. For health-promotion planning to be effective, it must be compatible with the family's cultural beliefs and practices. Awareness of the family's cultural interpretation of health, illness, and health care is essential prior to embarking on specific goal-oriented interventions. In addition, family goals should be recorded and prioritized. Major sources of stress, along with any recent or current family developmental or situational transitions, also requires consideration prior to intervention. Collaboration of the entire family in expressing concerns, setting health goals, and planning for life-style modifications, should increase the effectiveness of the nursing interventions.

FAMILY NURSING INTERVENTIONS: GUIDELINES FOR LIFE-STYLE MODIFICATION

Working with families to plan life-style modifications so that health goals can be met, is an important role for the family nurse. Pender (1987) describes useful approaches that may be considered in initiating and supporting family behavior alterations. Specific strategies that nurses may apply in initiating family life-style changes include self-confrontation, cognitive restructuring, modeling, operant conditioning, and stimulus control.

The first technique, self-confrontation, is based on the assumption that clients make changes when they recognize incompatibilities within their own beliefs, values, and behaviors, or between their own behaviors and those of individuals they hold in esteem and wish to emulate. Once this comparison occurs and contradiction is experienced, the client is more likely to change values, attitudes, and behaviors to achieve greater consistency with the self-concept. The nurse, in reviewing family life-style, can provide feedback to families by suggesting areas of inconsistencies between family beliefs or values and current behavior patterns. Contradictions that are of most concern to the family should be the focus for intervention. An example of this can be found in a family that highly values good nutrition as an essential ingredient in maintaining health, and believes its diet is well balanced. Yet family members admit to regularly consuming "fast foods" for lunch during the week. A family confronted with this inconsistency between its beliefs and dietary patterns may then be more motivated to change their behavior.

The cognitive restructuring method of behavior adjustment, which was originally described by Ellis and Grieger (1977), is also known by the term "rational-emotive therapy." The premise behind this approach is that the manner in which the family evaluates a specific situation determines its emotional reaction to the situation. Irrational or illogical self-statements may be generated by unsatisfactory past experiences, with the client skeptical of achieving behavior changes.

Goldfried and Sobocinski (1975) have outlined specific steps for applying cognitive restructuring strategies to improve emotional outlook and foster feelings of success. The nurse utilizing this approach should counsel families to recognize the irrationality in certain beliefs, as in the example where all of a family's members are overweight and firmly convinced that "none of us will ever be thin; we have always been heavy." Cognitive restructuring as an intervention promotes the acquisition of rational positive self-statements and contributes toward clients feeling an increased sense of personal control.

Modeling is a common strategy used in behavior therapy. It is based on the premise that a person will learn through observation, beginning with early childhood and continuing through to adulthood. Modeling is especially helpful when clients are uncertain as to which behavior is necessary to achieve a specific goal. Clients should identify with their models in order for this technique to be effective, with client and nurse working together to select suitable models. The nurse is in a powerful position to positively influence family health by being a role model of healthful living. He or she does this by demonstrating skills that the family seeks to learn, providing needed health education, and expressing encouragement to promote desired family behavior. The technique of modeling may also be used in community organized exercise classes, and in mutual self-help groups such as Weight Watchers or Alcoholics Anonymous. Self-help groups function by offering a setting for role modeling and mutual support (Roth, 1989).

Operant conditioning, based on the principle that behavior is determined by its consequences, can also be an effective behavior modification strategy. Desirable behavior is reinforced to increase the probability that the behavior will be repeated. Positive reinforcers, or rewards, are more effective motivators of behavior change than negative reinforcers or punishments. Nurses applying this intervention strategy should work with families to choose behavior to be changed. Schedules should be developed of how to gradually move toward selected target health-generating behavior, and reinforcement contingencies should be set up. In order to attain family goals, a nurse–family contract with designated rewards for desired behavior may be entered into, so as to provide responsibility guidelines for all family members. Contracting can be enjoyable for the entire family, with family members serving as an important source of motivation for each other. Pender (1987) suggests that operant conditioning works best if the behavior to be reinforced is countable, so that reinforcement may be used correctly. Books that provide information on operant conditioning especially for nurses are *Behavior Modification: A Significant Method in Nursing Practice* (LeBow, 1973) and *Behavior Modification and the Nursing Process* (Berni and Fordyce, 1977).

In stimulus control, attention is directed toward changing the antecedents rather than the consequences of behavior as in operant conditions (Pender, 1987). This method of behavior control suggests that by changing events that precede undesirable behavior it is possible to decrease or eliminate such action, and increase target behavior. Stimulus control concentrates on arranging environmental cues to promote only the desired behavior. Both the Health Belief Model and Pender's Health Promotion Model agree that cues are important factors in promoting health behavior change. Nurses should work with families to accomplish stimulus control by accurately identifying under what conditions desirable behavior occurs more frequently, and under what circumstances undesirable behavior is prompted. Nurses should offer instruction on how to develop sensitivity to appropriate cues, and counsel families on ways to facilitate opportunities for encountering those that are appropriate. Behavioral cues may be taken from a variety of sources. Examples of possible sources include contact with health care professionals, significant others, the communication media, or visual stimuli from the environment such as viewing others participating in the target activity. In addition to environmental cues, nurses can further influence desired action by encouraging families to develop a positive set of internal cues such as "feeling good" or an increased sense of self-esteem. External cues, such as having a family member or friend invite you to an aerobic exercise class, can be combined with internal cues, such as remembering feeling more energetic after exercise sessions. Multiple cues potentiate each other.

Nurses and other health care professionals can assist families to attain a healthier life-style. Specific life-style modification strategies have been suggested as possible nursing interventions in supporting families to increase health-promoting activities and attain family health goals. Continual evaluation of progress toward change in family life-style should be monitored by both the nurse and the family.

□ STUDY QUESTIONS

1. Which of the following are major ways that the family carries out its health care functions? (Select all appropriate answers.)
   a. Family provides preventive health care to its members at home.
   b. Family provides the major share of sick care to its members.
   c. Family pays for most health services received (directly or indirectly).
   d. Family has prime responsibility for initiating and coordinating health services.
   e. Family decides when and where to hospitalize its members.

2. List three primary factors that influence a family's conceptualizations of health and illness and whether they seek health care services.

3. Name the three basic orientations used to define health and illness (according to Baumann). Keeping in mind the two groups studied, correlate the orientation(s) each group identified more frequently.

4. Describe what Koos' central research findings were.

5. Fill in the missing components in this representation of the health belief model (original model).

Health belief model (original):

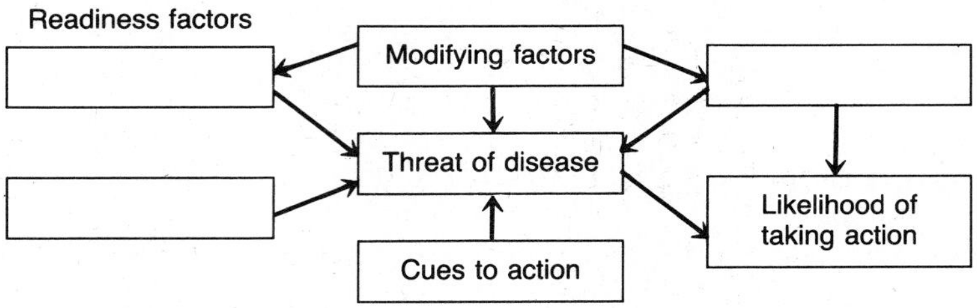

6. Recall the cognitive–perceptual factors suggested as influencing the likelihood of engaging in health-promoting behaviors in Pender's model. What other modifying factors are thought to contribute in activating health-promotion behaviors?

7. Pratt found that on the whole most American families were not adequately performing their vital health care function. On what basis did she conclude this? What are two basic reasons for this inadequacy?

8. In America, our overall health status is most closely related to (choose two):
   a. The quality and quantity of health services we receive.
   b. Our health care system.
   c. Socioeconomic, cultural, and educational factors.
   d. Personal health practices (life-styles).

9. List four assessment areas to cover when appraising a family's dietary practices.

10. The following is a list of several areas that should be assessed under family's sleep and rest practices: number of hours usually slept each night by family members, who takes regular naps during day or what other rest techniques do family members use, and where family members sleep. What important area(s) has (have) been omitted?

11. Formulate three basic questions to ask a family in relation to its exercise and recreational practices.

12. Which of the following substances constitute drugs that need to be assessed by the family completing a family health assessment? (Select all appropriate answers.)
    a. Coffee, tea, cola, and cocoa.

b. Alcohol.
c. Aspirin.
d. Tobacco.
e. Recreational drugs such as marijuana and cocaine.

13. An appraisal of self-care practices involves an assessment of:
a. Preventive and diagnostic practices.
b. Home treatment practices, including home care of sick or disabled members.
c. Determination of the family's ability to provide self-care.
d. (fill in) ______________________________.

14. In regards to health insurance and health care services utilization, what trends are found among those with lower levels of income and education?
a. They visit their physician's office more often.
b. They utilize health care services more frequently.
c. They are more likely to seek health care in hospital outpatient departments.
d. They are vulnerable because of being without health insurance.

15. Indoor pollution was a major area covered under environmental practices. Identify at least two general areas of health advice related to the family's exposure to common indoor contaminants.

16. Name four salient general health education areas for families to learn about concerning dental health.

17. Which of the following measures are generally recommended for plaque control? (Select all appropriate answers.)
a. After-meal toothbrushing.
b. Reduction in dietary sucrose.
c. Daily flossing of teeth.
d. Use of an antiseptic mouthwash twice a day.

18. A family medical history consists basically of two parts. First, information would be elicited about each family member (going back to maternal and paternal grandparents) and his or her present and past health status. What would be the second area of assessment?

CHAPTER SEVENTEEN

Family Coping Strategies and Processes

Learning Objectives

1. Describe the importance of family coping strategies and processes.
2. Present evidence of how adequately families are coping.
3. Define and differentiate the meanings of these terms and concepts: stressor, stress, adaptation, coping, defense mechanisms, and crisis.
4. Identify four broad sources of family stressors.
5. Explain what coping tasks are appropriate for each of the three time phases of stress.
6. Explain the findings of Holmes and Rahe relative to the impact of stressors on individuals.
7. Compare and contrast the Social Readjustment Scale of Holmes and Rahe with the balancing of forces diagram.
8. Trace the sequence of events that occur during a family crisis.
9. Recall several of the important findings from Pearlin and Schooler's study of normative coping tactics.
10. Identify three major variables involved in the development of crisis or successful resolution of the problem (noncrisis), according to Hill's family stress theory.
11. Discuss how Hill's family stress theory has been extended.
12. Briefly describe four functional coping strategies used by families and four dysfunctional adaptive strategies utilized by families.
13. Differentiate whether specific adaptive strategies are functional, dysfunctional, or both (could be either healthy or unhealthy).
14. Identify the two basic purposes of social support systems.
15. Utilizing a family case example:
    a. Assess the family in terms of family coping processes and strategies.
    b. Identify one family nursing diagnosis in the area of family coping.
    c. Propose two family nursing interventions appropriate for resolving or ameliorating the problem.

Families constantly face the need to modify their perceptions and lives. The stimulus for this change comes from within and without. The normal, continually evolving developmental needs of all the family members, in addition to the presence of unexpected situations involving family members, make up the inner demands for change. The external stimuli for change come from the changing society as it interacts with the family during the family's life cycle. General systems theory and family developmental theory both stress the inevitability and ubiquity of family change. Continual demands force the family to adapt—in order for the family to survive, continue, and grow. Family coping processes and strategies are essential for making this possible. A family's perceptions and handling of its problems through use of various coping strategies are crucial to the family's success in dealing with the demands placed on it.

Most important, moreover, family coping processes and strategies serve as vital processes or mechanisms through which the family functions are made possible. Without effective family coping, the affective, socialization, economic, and health care functions cannot be adequately achieved. Hence family coping processes and strategies constitute the underlying processes that enable the family to enact its necessary family functions.

Assessing family coping patterns and resources will provide the foundation for assisting families in their adaptation and in their attainment of a higher level of wellness. Achieving a higher level of wellness is the goal or the *raison d'être* of family nursing practice. Strengthening and encouraging adequate adaptive responses and capacities, as well as reducing the actual and potential stressors from within and outside the family, are part of this broad and encompassing goal. Whether the family is essentially healthy or dysfunctional (at one or the other pole within the health–illness continuum), the family health nurse is still dealing with the same issue: assisting families to help themselves achieve a higher level of functioning or wellness within the context of their particular aims, aspirations, and abilities.

How Well Are Families Coping: The General State of Family Health Today

Families have both great strengths and pervasive weaknesses, as the results of different studies and social indicators make clear. In 1975 authors Yankelovitch, Skelley, and White summarized their findings from 2194 interviews with 1247 families selected by national probability sampling method. They concluded: "What does emerge as heartening news in the present study is a picture of the great strengths and adaptive capabilities of the American family—the flexibility, sturdiness, and vitality of the family" (p. 13).

On the other hand, from community mental health literature, we are reminded of the pervasiveness of mental illness in the community—a sign of the failure of families to cope. The two classic studies of the prevalence on mental disorders in North America attest to this situation (Bloom, 1977). Conducted in the 1950s and 1960s, these studies were based on community surveys of the prevalence of mental disorders rather than on the number of psychiatric patients known to treatment agencies. One study was called the Mid-Manhattan study and involved a sample of 1660 men and women between the ages of 20 and 59 in an area of Manhattan, New York. The second is referred to as the Stirling County study. This survey study consisted of 1000 people in a rural area of Nova Scotia. While the studies differed somewhat in how they defined mental illness, their estimates of the extent of mental illness in the general population were staggering. In the Stirling Country study, it was concluded that at least half of all the adults were currently suffering from some form of psychiatric disturbance. In the Mid-Manhattan study, which used a narrower definition of mental illness, investigators found nearly one-quarter of the respondents to be significantly psychiatrically impaired.

What are some of the major stressors leading to a greater prevalence of mental health problems? Poverty and marital disruption have both been linked with increased rates of mental illness. Families most exposed to hardship are also the least equipped to deal with these stressors (Pearlin and Schooler, 1978). Moreover, of all the social stressors studied relative to their correlation with mental illness, none has been more consistently and powerfully associated with mental illness—using criteria such as psychiatric hospitalizations, suicides, and homicides—than has marital disruption (Bloom, 1977). Marital disruption—divorce, desertion, or death of spouse—affects an enormous number of people yearly, and in many of these cases it can be assumed that a primary underlying problem was the existence of inadequate family coping patterns.

How healthy or unhealthy the American family is judged ultimately depends on the criteria selected to document the family's state of health. If we look at some of the broad social indicators such as proportion of families living at or below the poverty level, proportion of families on welfare, proportion of families without health insurance, infant mortality rate, illiteracy rate, proportion of high school dropouts, and so forth, we would say the American family's health status has taken a downward turn beginning about 1980.

BASIC CONCEPTS AND DEFINITIONS

All of the concepts and terms defined below, with the exception of family coping, are well established and their meanings fairly well agreed on. In defining family coping, definitions of coping as applied to the individual have been adapted to the family.

Stressors refer to the initiating or the precipitating agents that activate the stress process (Chrisman and Fowler, 1980). The precipitating agents that activate stress in the family are life events or occurrences of sufficient magnitude to bring about change in the family system (Hill, 1949). Family stressors can be interpersonal (inside or outside of the family), environmental, economic, or sociocultural events or experiences. Perceptions color the nature and gravity of possible family stressors, because families react not only to the presence of actual stressors, but also to events as they perceive or interpret them. The family's perceptions are of paramount importance. It is significant to note that families that are crisis prone consistently tend to perceive events in a distorted, subjective manner. Events that healthy families would look at objectively and as a challenge are viewed by crisis-prone families as threatening and overwhelming. In these cases extensive stress is experienced which in turn taxes family adaptive capacities.

Stress is the response or state of tension produced by the stressor(s) or by the actual/perceived demand(s) that remains unmanaged (Antonovsky, 1979; Burr, 1973). It is the tension or strain within a person or social system (individual, family, etc) and is a reaction to a pressure-producing situation (Burgess, 1978). Because stress or tension in a family is so difficult to measure, researchers and practitioners alike often assess the pile-up or magnitude of stressors in a family's life to get an estimate of the amount of stress the family is experiencing (Olson et al, 1983).

Adaptation is a process of adjustment to change. The outcome is an altered state of equilibrium or homeostasis. Adaptation may be positive or negative, resulting in the increase or decrease of a family's state of wellness (Burgess, 1978). For example, seeking help from community agencies may be a very positive move when outside assistance is needed to help a child with learning problems; but the same adaptive strategy may be negative if it becomes the predominant way a family solves its problems, because the family does not learn to utilize its own inner resources.

STRATEGIES FOR ADAPTATION

White (1974) identifies three strategies for individual adaptation: defense mechanisms, coping, and mastery—these making up a whole "tapestry of living." These same concepts can be applied to the family.

Defense mechanisms, according to White, are learned, habitual, or automatic (built-in) ways of responding. They are usually tactics for avoiding the problems the stressor poses and are usually used when no apparent solution is known or accessible to a family. Denial of an important family issue is an example of such a defense mechanism, and would be classified as dysfunctional if this is the *habitual* way in which the family deals with its problems. Because defense mechanisms are largely avoidance behaviors, they are usually dysfunctional responses to problems.

Coping strategies, in contrast to defense mechanisms, are viewed as positive strategies of adaptation. Coping consists of problem-solving efforts of an individual faced with demands highly relevant to his or her welfare, but taxing the person's resources (Lazarus et al, 1974). Pearlin and Schooler (1978) add the notion of presumed effectiveness of coping responses when they define coping as any response (behavioral or perceptual—cognitive) to external life strains that serves to prevent, avoid, or control emotional distress. Simply stated, coping efforts or behaviors are positive, problem-specific, active strategies geared towards resolving a problem. Coping is a term that is limited to actual behaviors or cognitions people employ, not to resources they potentially could use.

Mastery, the most positive adaptation mode, is the end result of using effective coping strategies. In this case, situations would be competently handled as a result of effective, well-practiced coping efforts. Mastery is very closely aligned with family competency. Just as individuals gain self-esteem and feelings of competency, so do families. Competence refers to the possessing of sufficient means to meet the exigencies of a situation or task.

Family Coping

Whereas coping refers to the individual, family coping denotes a family group level of analysis (or an interactional level of analysis). Family coping is defined as positive, problem-appropriate, affective, perceptual, and behavioral responses that families and their subsystems employ to resolve a problem or reduce the stress produced by the problem or event. By shifting from the individual level to a family level of coping, coping becomes much more complex. Because of the difficulty assessing family coping efforts, most family coping studies describe a combination of individual and family coping responses made by family members and the family. Family coping responses or behaviors are the specific actions or cognitions family members employ (McCubbin et al, 1981), while coping patterns and strategies are similar responses that cluster into homogeneous sets. Family and individual coping strategies develop and change over time, in response to the demands or stressors being experienced (Menaghan, 1983).

Family coping responses include both internal and external types of coping strategies. Internal coping resources consist of the ability of the family to pull together to become cohesive and integrated. Family integration entails the control of subsystem components through bonds of unity. Families that deal most effectively with their problems are most often the families that are well integrated—where family members are highly committed to the group and its collective goals. Another internal coping resource is role flexibility—being able to modify family roles as needed (Hall and Weaver, 1974).

Hall and Weaver (1974) also emphasize that family communication patterns are of crucial importance in coping. Communication processes in the family greatly influence the quality of the family life. Moreover, in the last analysis, families must choose to grow and learn from their experiences. An element of choice between a set of alternatives exists, and the choices are usually conscious and voluntary, even though heavily influenced by cultural and personal values and norms. Lewis (1976) noted that optimally functioning families were found to excel in *choosing* growth-generating alternatives. In approaching problems, these families explored various options, and if one alternative did not work well, another was tried and evaluated.

External coping resources deal with the family's use of social support systems. In looking at these external resources, it is obvious that families differ in the extent to which they are able to obtain *compliance* from their environments to meet their needs for information, matter, and services. Often financial resources and knowledge of how to get appropriate help are lacking. The family must also be able to reduce some of the demands being made on it. This is accomplished through regulation of family boundaries. Without adequate ability to secure environmental compliance through the effective regulation of family boundaries and bringing in of needed inputs, the family is more at risk.

Crisis

A crisis results because the family's resources and adaptive strategies are not effectively handling the threatening stressor(s). Hence, a family crisis refers to a disruptive state or period in a family's life when an extremely stressful event or series of events significantly taxes on the family's resources and coping abilities, with no resolution of the problem in sight. The family's usually effective problem-solving skills become useless or diminished during this psychosocial emergency (Kus, 1985). Patterson (1988) conceptualizes a family crisis to be the result of an imbalance between demands and resources or coping efforts (Fig. 17–1).

Crisis is characterized by family instability and disorganization. At this time the family generally feels such discomfort that it perceives a greater need for help than during periods of normalcy, and members are more receptive to suggestions and information (Wallace, 1978).

There are two types of crises families undergo: developmental and situational crises. Developmental or maturational crises are those stemming from the stressor events families experience in the process of the psychosocial growth of members. They are inherent within the stages of the normal life cycle of both the family and its members. Situational crises are events or stresses that are not common or normally expected, such as the death of a child or serious illness of one of the family members.

FAMILY STRESS THEORY

One of the primary tasks of a family nurse is detecting when a family is in crisis (although in actuality families range from functioning well to poorly rather than neatly falling into crisis or noncrisis categories). In assessing a family in trouble, it is important to determine (1) whether or not the family's problem is being adequately managed by the family members, (2) if a crisis state exists, or (3) whether the existing problem is part of a chronic inability to solve problems. Nursing intervention varies substantially in each of these cases. Moreover, in working with a family that is not presently having problems, but has had a history of being crisis prone, a family worker would want to be more tuned-in to this tendency so that early problem recognition and assistance can take place.

Hill's Family Stress Theory

Hill's (1949) classic family stress theory is the most eloquent, parsimonious model that describes that factors producing crisis or noncrisis in families. Based on research Hill conducted on war-induced separation and reunion, he developed a family stress theory called ABCX in which he identified a major set of variables

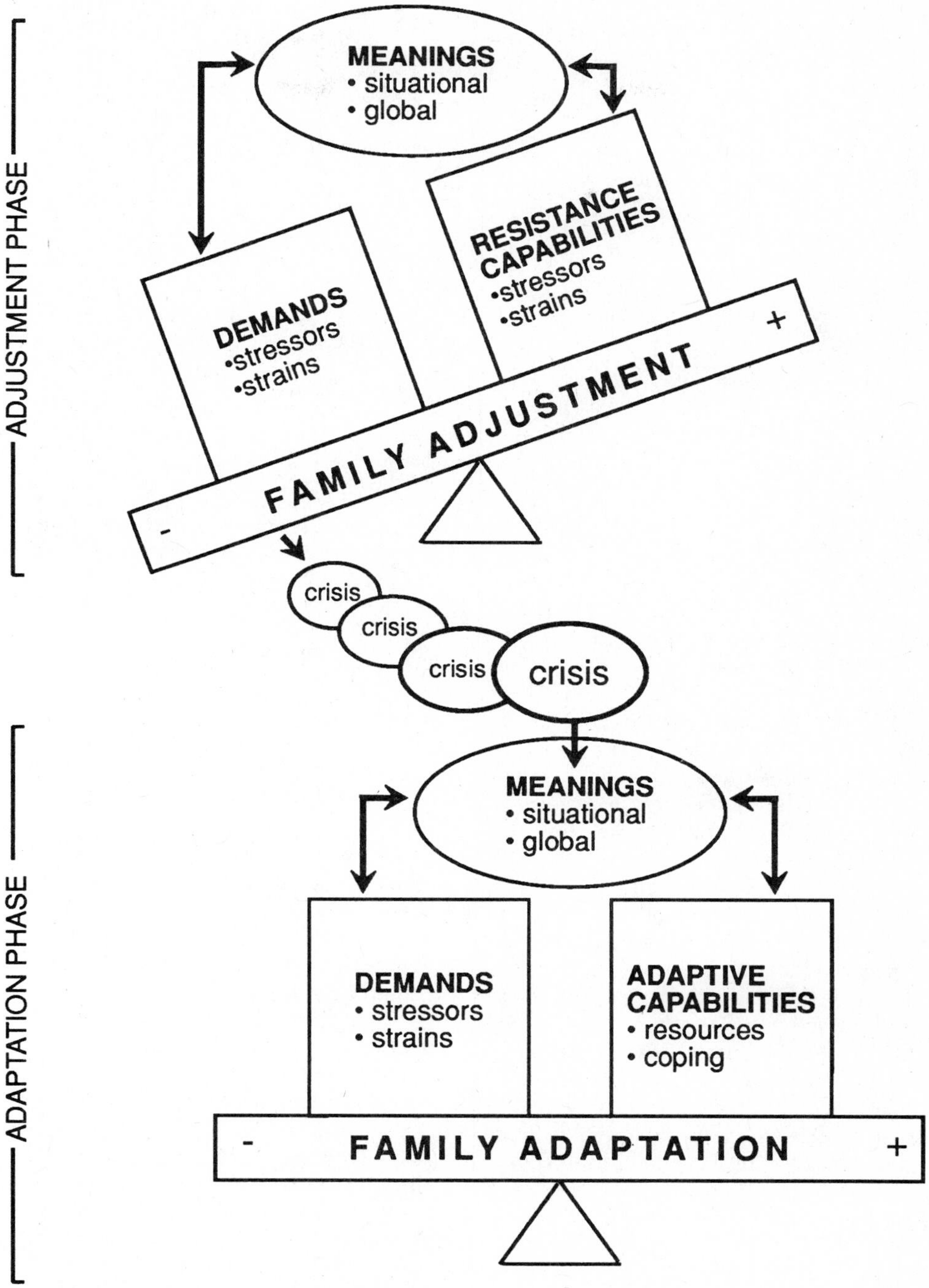

Figure 17–1
The Family Adjustment and Adaptation Response (FAAR) model. (From: Patterson, 1988.)

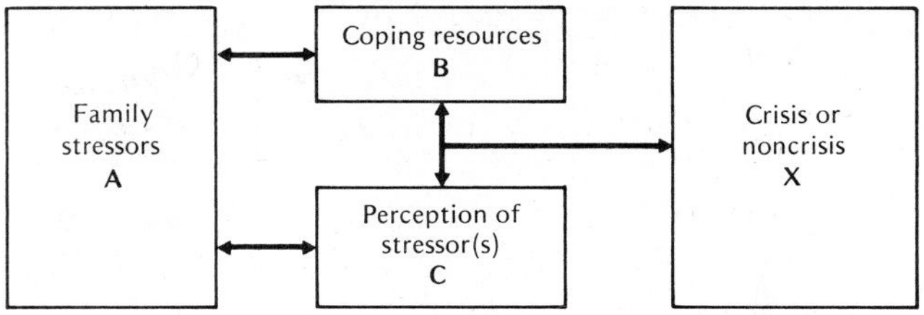

Figure 17–2
Hill's Family Stress Theory (1949). (Adapted from McCubbin and Patterson, 1983b.)

and their relationships that led to family crisis. He also theoretically described a postcrisis "roller coaster" adjustment process families went through. These two parts of his theoretical framework have remained virtually unchanged for the last 40 years. Moreover, this theory has been the basis for many research studies in the family stress and coping area, and has been foundational to the work of Caplan (1964) and other clinicians in generating practice theory and principles in crisis intervention. This framework has two parts. The first is a proposition dealing with the determinants of family crisis:

> A (the event and related hardships) interacting with B (the family's crisis meeting resources) interacting with C (the definition that the family makes of the event) produces X (the crisis). (Hill, 1965, p. 36)

The second part is a more process-oriented statement regarding the course of adjustment following a crisis. Hill (1965) explains that the course of family adjustment following a crisis involves (1) a period of disorganization, (2) an angle of recovery, and (3) reorganization and a new level of organization with respect to family functioning.

Figure 17–2 presents a visual representation of an adaptation of Hill's model. To elaborate further on Hill's model, this model explains what precipitates a crisis in one family and not in another. As seen in Figure 17–2, there are three basic factors involved.

The first is the actual presence of stressors or stressor-events (factor A). The second basic factor influencing the outcome—crisis or noncrisis—in dealing with a stressor is the family's resources and use of coping mechanisms (factor B). Major stressors initially force stereotypic defenses. Later, coping efforts emerge. If the family does not make use of its resources and coping mechanisms from its repertoire of possible responses, the result is the same as if the family did not possess the coping resources. However, the intervention is easier in this case because it is less difficult to assist families to utilize past coping patterns than to help families learn new ways of responding.

Third and most important of the three contributing factors is the family's perception and interpretation of the stressors or stressor-events (factor C). Recall that families that consistently perceive and define events and their situation as threatening and dangerous, rather than challenging will most likely be crisis prone. Functional families are able to see events as understandable and manageable. Hall and Weaver (1974) explain this difference further:

> Successful families have found ways to utilize certain crucial processes to facilitate all the growth-promoting potential in crisis-laden situations. The first of these processes is *cognitive mastery*. . . . A major task is to assist in the development of a cognitive map of what is happening, as a first step in achieving purposeful problem-solving. (p. 5)

Lazarus and co-workers (1974) emphasize the same point by stating that it is the person's or group's cognitive appraisal of the stressor that influences what coping efforts are made as well as the final outcome.

Factor X deals with crisis or noncrisis. Hill (1965) discusses this factor in terms of crisis-proneness in families. Crisis-proneness describes how families handle the B and C factors of the theory. When families are crisis-prone, they tend to experience stressor events (A) with greater frequency and greater severity and define these (C) more frequently as crisis. These types of families are more vulnerable to stressor events because of the meager resources and coping abilities (B) they possess. Also they fail to learn from past crises, leading them to see new stressor events as threatening and crisis provoking.

The X factor tends to be seen by Hill as an "either/or" outcome, although graduations of crisis or noncrisis certainly exist. The disorganizing effects of crisis in the family are seen in family relations and role performance of family members—sexual behavior of the marital couple being a most sensitive index of the presence of crisis (Hill, 1965).

McCubbin and Patterson's Double ABCX Model

The Double ABCX model, developed by McCubbin and Patterson (1983b), extended Hill's ABCX theory. Whereas Hill's theory covered pre-crises variables, McCubbin and Patterson's theory accounts for differences

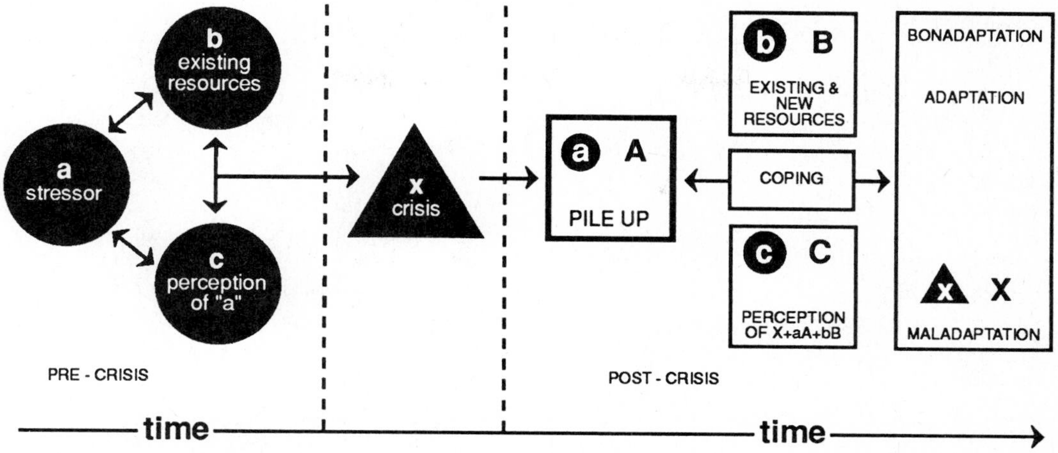

Figure 17–3
The Double ABCX model. (From: McCubbin and Patterson, 1983b.)

in family adaptation in the post-crisis period (Fig. 17–3). Each of the original variables (ABCX) were reexamined and their definitions somewhat modified. Each of the variables in this model is briefly described.

Factor aA, Family Demands: Pile-up. McCubbin and Patterson (1983b) state that rather than just one major stressor, it is the "pile-up of family stressors" that is the important factor in predicting family maladaptation. They point out that because family crises develop and are resolved over a period of time, families are seldom confronted with a single stressor at one point in time. Rather they experience a pile-up of stressors (or demands or changes), particularly in the aftermath of a major stressor such as the diagnosis of cancer in a family member. Davis (1963), in a study of the impact of polio on families, supported the notion that families are not just experiencing one major stressor at a time. He reported that many of the families he observed appeared to be coping with other long-standing problems that tended to merge with those created by the chronic illness stressor.

Five broad types of family stressors and strains contribute to the pile-up. These are (1) the initial stressor and its hardships, (2) normative transitions, (3) prior strains, (4) consequences of family efforts to cope, and (5) ambiguity (both intrafamily and social) (McCubbin and Patterson, 1983b, p. 14).

Factor bB: Family Adaptive Resources. Resources are the family's capabilities to meet the demands the family faces. They consist of family members' personal resources, such as their education, health, and personality characteristics; the family system's internal resources such as flexible roles, shared power, clear communication, and family cohesion; and social support.

Factor cC: Family Definition and Meaning. The definition of this variable is essentially unchanged from Hill's conceptualization of the family's definition of the situation. Positive appraisals of the stressor as well as negative interpretations are included here.

Factor xX: Family Adaptation. Within the Double ABCX model there are three levels of analyses: the individual family member, the family unit, and the community of which the family is a part. Each of these units is described as having both demands and capabilities. "Family adaptation is achieved through reciprocal relationships, where the demands of one of these units are met by the capabilities at another, so as to achieve a balance simultaneously at two primary levels of interaction" between individual and family system and between family system and community (McCubbin and Patterson, 1983b, p. 12).

The concept of family adaptation in the model refers to a continuum of outcomes, ranging from bonadaptation to maladaptation. The Family Adjustment and Adaptation Model shown in Figure 17–1 depicts the idea of balancing of demands and capabilities, which then leads to some level of family adaptation.

Boss' Contextually Based Family Stress Model

Boss (1988), a family researcher, has extended Hill's family stress theory to account for the influence of the family's context. Families do not live in isolation. They are part of a larger context that influences the ABCX variables in Hill's model. Two different contexts in which family stress is mediated are the external and internal context. The family's external context is one the family has no control over. It includes the environment in which the family is embedded, consisting of the constraints of genetics and development, as well as the "time and place" context (history, economics, culture). The family's internal context is made up of three elements that the family has control over and can change. These are the psychological, structural, and philosophical elements. The structural elements are similar to the family structural dimensions in this text, with the exclusion of family values; the psychological context refers to the family's definition of the event/stressor; and the philosophical context refers to the family's values and beliefs. Boss' contextually based model is described as two concentric circles surrounding the ABCX model. The outer circle is the external context, and the inner circle is the internal context.

STRESSORS AND STRESS

Stressors are life events or demands that produce internal stress requiring coping responses. Life stressors, as suggested by a great deal of evidence, are causally associated with both physical and mental illness (Kessler, 1982). The sources of stress, time phases of stress and coping tasks, and the impact of stressors on the family are presented in this section.

Basic Sources of Family Stress

The many changes and stressors a family faces over time may be viewed, as Minuchin (1974) has done, as coming from four basic sources.

Stressful Contact of One Member With Extrafamilial Forces. When one member of the family is stressed by extrafamilial stressors (e.g., loss of job, school problem, legal problem), other family members feel the need to accommodate to his or her changed circumstances. They do this by supporting—the functional way—or attacking the individual—the nonfunctional mode. They may also keep the problem contained within a subsystem, although if the extrafamilial stressor is prolonged and major, its effects "seep" or "ripple" into the other subsystems, thereby affecting the whole family. For example, a father stressed at work comes home and begins criticizing his wife and then redirects his hostility to a child. This reduces the danger to the spouse subsystem, but stresses the child. Or the husband may criticize the wife, who then turns to her daughter for solace and support, thereby creating an unhealthy coalition of mother and daughter against husband.

Stressful Contact of the Whole Family With Extrafamilial Forces. Economic hardships such as poverty and discrimination are two particularly threatening forces straining families today. Family coping mechanisms become overtaxed as family resources are depleted. The family moving to another home, neighborhood, or region of the country is also stressful. Another common stressor immigrant families face is the cultural shock and adjustments that must be made when migrating from one nation and culture to another.

Transitional Stressors. Problems of transition occur in a number of situations, the most common being the developmental changes that the family and family members undergo and the normative changes that occur in family composition. Six of the most frequent transitions in which family nurses become involved are (1) the arrival of a new baby into a family, (2) the emergence of a child into adolescence, (3) the merging of two families through remarriage of single parents, (4) the introduction of an older grandparent into the family due to infirmity or financial reasons, (5) the launching of a young adult from the household, and (6) the loss of a spouse during the last family-cycle stage.

Situational Stressors. This type of stressor is associated with unique, nonnormative, or idiosyncratic problems a family experiences, such as the transitory problems that illness and hospitalization of one of the parents create for the family as a whole. These stressors are unanticipated and may tax a family's coping capacities. For instance, a taxing of coping resources may occur if the illness is serious or prolonged, because this represents a powerful, continuing negative force and creates a need for major change (the redistribution of roles and functions).

Time Phases of Stress and Coping Tasks

When nurses are working with families, they need to be aware of the timing of the stress, as well as the coping tasks family members might use during each of the three periods of stress.

Antestress Period. In the period before actually confronting the stressor (such as the hospitalization of a child), anticipation is usually possible; there is an awareness of impending danger or the perceived threat of the situation. If families or helping persons can identify a future stressor, anticipatory guidance as well as other coping tactics to weaken or reduce the impact of the stressor may be sought or provided. Also, in some situations, moves might be instituted to remove the impending stressor.

The Actual Stress Period. Adaptive strategies during the period of stress usually differ in intensity and kind from those tactics utilized prior to the onset of the stressor and stress. There may be very basic survival, defensive tactics used during this period if the stress in the family is extreme. With tremendous energy expended in dealing with a stressor(s) and stress, many family functions (some which may be crucial to family health) are often temporarily set aside or are inadequately performed until the family has the resources to deal with them again. The most helpful coping responses during stressful periods are often intrafamilial (to be discussed later), and the seeking of spiritual support (Friedman, 1985; Pravikoff, 1985).

Poststress Period. The coping tactics employed following the stress period, termed the posttrauma phase, consist of strategies to return the family to a homeostatic, balanced state. To promote family wellness during this phase, the family needs to pull together, mutually express feelings, and solve their problems (Burgess, 1978) or seek out and utilize familial supports for resolving their stressful situation. A family may also, unfortunately, go through the stressful period, ending up functioning at a lower level of wellness, and thus need professional assistance to help them increase their repertoire of effective coping strategies.

Impact of Stressors

Families daily are bombarded with tension-producing stimuli—some of which are only mildly irritating and hardly noticed, such as traffic noise and poor housing, and some of which are potentially or actually devastating to families, such as marital disruption or the loss of a child (Pearlin and Turner, 1987). Holmes and associates (Holmes and Rahe, 1967) realize the great quantitative and qualitative differences stressors have on individuals, and as early as 1949 began to systematically study the quality and quantity of life changes observed, both desirable and undesirable, which clustered at the time of the onset of an illness. From these data they were able to assign a weight to each of the 43 life events found to be associated with the onset of health problems (Table 17–1).

Other investigations have generated similar lists, all verifying the temporal relationship of high life-change scores preceding illness (Nickolls, 1975). Although these scales were developed for individuals, their applicability to families is significant. Families experi-

TABLE 17–1. SOCIAL READJUSTMENT RATING SCALE OF HOLMES AND RAHE

Rank	Life Event	Value[a]
1	Death of spouse	100
2	Divorce	73
3	Marital separation	65
4	Jail term	63
5	Death of close family member	63
6	Personal injury or illness	53
7	Marriage	50
8	Fired at work	47
9	Marital reconciliation	45
10	Retirement	45
11	Change in health of family member	44
12	Pregnancy	40
13	Sex difficulties	39
14	Gain of new family member	39
15	Business readjustment	39
16	Change in financial state	38
17	Death of a close friend	37
18	Change to different line of work	36
19	Change in number of arguments with spouse	35
20	Mortgage over $10,000	31
21	Foreclosure of mortgage or loan	30
22	Change in responsibilities at work	29
23	Son or daughter leaving home	29
24	Trouble with in-laws	29
25	Outstanding personal achievement	28
26	Wife begins or stops work	26
27	Begin or end school	26
28	Change in living conditions	25
29	Revision of personal habits	24
30	Trouble with boss	23
31	Change in work hours or conditions	20
32	Change in residence	20
33	Change in school	20
34	Change in recreation	19
35	Change in church activities	19
36	Change in social activities	18
37	Mortgage or loan less than $10,000	17
38	Change in sleeping habits	16
39	Change in number of family get-togethers	15
40	Change in eating habits	15
41	Vacation	13
42	Christmas	12
43	Minor violations of the law	11

[a] *Social readjustment rating scale instructions:* Add up value of life crisis units for life events experienced in a two-year period:
Score of 0 to 150—No significant problems.
Score of 150 to 199—Mild life crisis and a 33 percent chance of illness.
Score of 200 to 299–Moderate life crisis and an 80 percent chance of illness.
Score of 300 or over—Major life crisis and an 80 percent chance of illness.
From: Holmes and Rahe (1967).

ence most of these same life crisis events and are also negatively affected by the onslaught of numerous stressors within a short period of time. Extending the work of Holmes and Rahe (1967) and others, McCubbin, Wilson, and Patterson (1981) developed a Family Inventory of Life Events and Changes (FILE) that assesses a family's pile-up of family stressors recently and in the past 3 to 5 years.

It needs to be emphasized that on the Holmes and Rahe scale the three most stressful life events—death of a spouse, divorce, and marital separation—all involve a marital or family disruption. The next five events, in order of stressfulness, include a jail term, death of a close family member, personal injury or illness, marriage, and losing one's job. Again, these events involve the family intimately and affect it powerfully.

Although the work of Holmes and Rahe identified and quantified stressors, epidemiologists have long used a multifactorial model, the epidemiologic triad, based on the interaction of the agent, host, and environment (in contrast to Holmes and Rahe's model, which looks at the "agent" or causative factors only), to explain the state of health, illness, or any point in between on the health–illness continuum. In this chapter, this triadic model has been adapted so that the agent, host, and environmental factors are visualized as weighted forces, both positive and negative, and so that the model applies to the family rather than the individual. These weighted forces are balanced against one another, with the greater forces on either side creating an imbalance toward a higher or lower level of wellness in the family. Using this model, it can be seen that it is not just the magnitude of weighted life events within a specific period of time that causes a greater chance of illness, but that it is the imbalance of stressors compared to assets (with the negative forces offsetting the positive forces because of their greater weight). Moreover, environmental forces, both positive and negative, are considered an inherent facet to be assessed in each of the two sets of forces.

Family problems stem from multiple factors, suggesting how difficult it is to assess families. We have tended to think that in order to eliminate a problem one would need to find a way to eliminate or treat the particular causative factor, rather than view the situation more broadly. By assessing the balance between the stressors (their duration and strength) and the nature and strength of supportive or protective elements, both intrafamilial and extrafamilial, one can either attempt to eliminate or reduce the potency of stressors or to build up and strengthen the family's resources (assets). Figure 17–4 illustrates this "balance" concept and how the family's level of wellness is affected.

Given an assessment of the duration and strength of the family's stressors or current life stressors and other risk factors on the one hand, and of their psychosocial, physical, and environmental assets on the other, it should be easier to anticipate which families are at risk; it may then be possible to reduce or eliminate certain stressors, or conversely to strengthen or add certain assets or resources to modify the balancing of forces in favor of the family's greater health. Furthermore, many of the most stressful life events that cannot be changed may have their impact weakened by preparing the family for the event (anticipatory counseling) or providing reality, present-oriented, short-term counseling such as crisis intervention during the time when the overwhelming stressors are being experienced (Nickolls, 1975).

FAMILY COPING STRATEGIES

The picture of family adaptation to stress emerging from research and theoretical efforts up to about the mid-1970s was that the family was merely a reactor to stress, a "defensive" manager of resources with much tendency towards dysfunction. Fortunately this trend is changing. Many subsequent investigations shifted away from the dysfunctional emphasis to a more positive and broadened interest in the wide array of coping tactics families utilize. With this focus, families tend to be seen as resilient social change agents, innovative and surprisingly effective under stressful conditions (Cleveland, 1980; Venters, 1981).

Normative Coping Responses

Sociologists Pearlin and Schooler (1978) reported an extensive well-conducted study in which they interviewed a sample of 2300 people, ages 18 to 65, representative of the population in the urbanized area of Chicago, to determine the kinds of coping tactics they used and how efficacious these were. Their analysis emphasized the normative coping responses people used in response to life strains in their major social roles (occupational, economic, parental, and marital). This study's significance is that it is one of the few research studies that describe the everyday coping experiences of people. Earlier studies conducted in clinical situations portrayed coping as a highly individualistic defense aroused in very special situations.

As just mentioned, healthy, functional families under stress tend to act in a direction that reduces the stress. Pearlin and Schooler (1978) used this social system characteristic to define the effective coping mechanisms. The coping strategies that led to a reduction in stress in the role being strained were deemed effi-

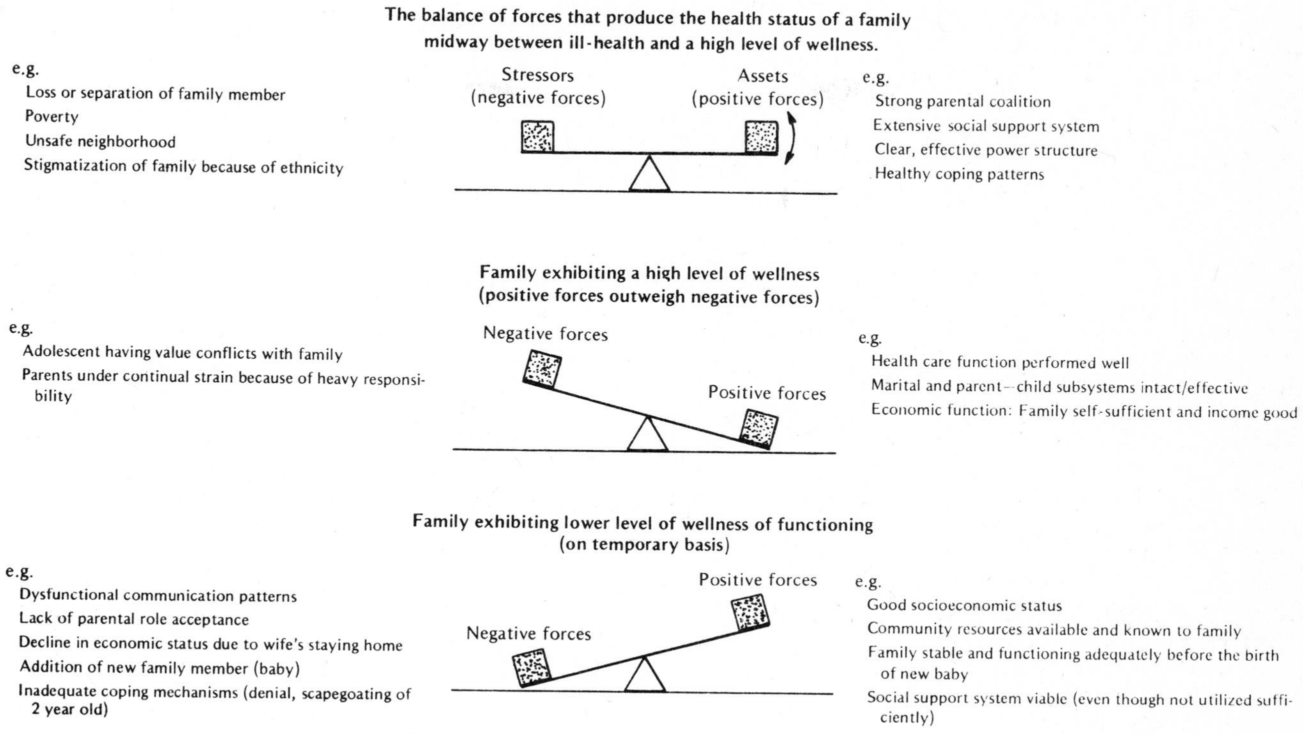

Figure 17–4
The balancing of forces and impact on family health status.

cacious, whereas those responses that did not alleviate or attenuate stress were defined as ineffective.

Pearlin and Schooler (1978) identify three types of coping tactics used extensively by individuals in their social functioning. Each will be described briefly, with a comment as to their effectiveness in reducing stress. Much of this discussion has direct relevance for families and how they cope, because the coping mechanisms used by the adult family members may be taken as representative of those used within sets of family relationships or the family as a whole, assuming that parents set the tone for how the family unit responds.

The first type of coping responses is the type that modifies the stressful situation. This type of coping strategy represents the most direct way to cope with life strains, for it is geared toward altering or eliminating the stressor. Pearlin and Schooler included self-reliance and seeking help from others under this type of coping. In contrast with some of the notions about the inherent helpfulness of social supports, they found that in parental and marital roles, self-reliance was more effective in attenuating stress than was the seeking of help and advice from others. Perhaps those that seek outside help are not the same people as those who successfully receive help. The authors point out that as yet we do not know the conditions under which help from others is effective in modifying stressful situations.

The second type of coping strategy consists of those tactics that function to control the meaning of the problem. "The way an experience is recognized and the meaning that is attached to it determines to a large extent the threat posed by that experience" (Pearlin and Schooler, 1978, p. 6). Thus the same experience may be highly threatening to one family and innocuous to another, depending on family members' cognitive and perceptual evaluation of the event (Lazarus et al, 1974). The following are examples of coping that cognitively neutralize the threats experienced in life: making positive comparisons ("count your blessings," etc); selective ignoring (minimizing the negative elements and maximizing the positive facets); and substitution of rewards (making the most strain-producing experiences the least valued areas of one's life). A substitution of rewards was found to work well in both occupational and economic areas of a person's life. For example, in the economic area where a setback occurred, this usually involved demeaning the importance of money and elevating other aspects of one's life or work such as work hours or fringe benefits. However, in parental and marital roles, this type of coping was not found to be helpful, because one cannot easily relegate one's marriage or children to a less important place on one's list of priorities (Pearlin and Schooler, 1978). The most effective types of coping tactics in both enactment of marital and parental roles were those that entailed involvement (the first-ranked coping tactic), not selective ignoring or manipulating one's values.

The third type of coping tactic includes those mechanisms essentially utilized to help people accommodate to and manage existing stress, rather than deal with the problems or stressor itself. Six coping responses were listed in this category. In marriage, emotional discharge of feelings and controlled reflectiveness were identified, as well as passive forebearance and self-assertion. In parental roles, feelings of potency and helpless resignation were stated as examples. Pearlin and Schooler (1978) discovered that in marriage a reflective probing of problems was more effective than the open and emotional discharge of feelings. In parental areas, the conviction that one has power (potency) to effect change and exert influence over one's children proved to be more helpful in stress management than helpless resignation.

Lastly, the authors point out that use of a variety of coping strategies is usually more effective than having a limited repertoire of coping responses. A single coping tactic, regardless of its effectiveness, cannot possibly be appropriate for the wide range of life strains commonly experienced.

Types of Family Coping Strategies

By including the following strategies as coping strategies, it is assumed that these coping strategies are usually functional—although perhaps the exclusive/predominant or inappropriate use of one could produce dysfunctional family outcomes. Without being specific as to the particular situational and family context, the real functionality of any behavioral pattern cannot be determined.

Family and individual coping efforts and behaviors are problem- or situation-specific. Different circumstances and different problems demand different solutions—that is, employment of different coping responses. However, families do have certain coping styles or propensities, which also influence the particular types of coping efforts the family brings to bear on a problem.

Two broad types of family coping strategies are (1) internal or intrafamilial (within the nuclear family) and (2) external or extrafamilial (outside the nuclear family). Table 17–2 lists both types.

TABLE 17–2. TYPES OF FAMILY COPING STRATEGIES

Internal Family Coping Strategies

1. Family group reliance
2. The use of humor
3. Increased sharing together (maintaining cohesiveness)
4. Controlling the meaning of the problem: cognitive reframing and passive appraisal
5. Joint family problem solving
6. Role flexibility
7. Normalizing

External Family Coping Strategies

1. Seeking information
2. Maintaining active linkages with the community
3. Seeking social support
   - Use of informal social support network
   - Use of formal social systems
   - Use of self-help groups
4. Seeking spiritual support

Internal Family Coping Strategies

Under internal family coping strategies, seven general types of intrafamilial coping strategies are discussed. These are (1) family group-reliance, (2) the use of humor, (3) greater sharing together, (4) controlling the meaning of the problem or reframing, (5) joint problem solving, (6) role flexibility, and (7) normalizing.

Family Group-Reliance. Certain families when under stress will cope by becoming more reliant on their own resources. Families accomplish this by creating greater structure and organization in the home and family. Establishing greater structure is an attempt at greater control over the subsystems and is comparable to the "tighter" regulation of troops in the military under combat conditions. This usually involves tighter scheduling of members' time, more tasks per family member, a more close-knit organization, and a more rigid, prescribed routine. With the closing of family boundaries comes a call for greater family organization and discipline of members, coupled with the expectation that members will be more self-disciplined and conforming. Families utilizing greater control, if successful, also achieve greater integration and cohesiveness.

This type of family coping usually stems from the influence of the traditional Protestant ethic, which values and sees self-control and self-sufficiently as particularly necessary during hardship periods. Concomitant with structuring is a need for members to be "strong" and to learn to conceal feelings and master tension within themselves.

Burgess (1978) points out that this particular coping strategy, involving self-discipline among family members, may be very necessary in stressful situations such as when parents are confronted with a serious accident at home. They must maintain composure and the capacity to problem solve, because they then are responsible for their own lives and those of their children. And, in fact, Pearlin and Schooler (1978) found that self-reliance was an efficacious coping response in the area of enacting one's marital and parental roles. Time management is one particular coping response that follows within this broader coping strategy.

Nonetheless, this strategy can also be dysfunctional if in certain circumstances outside help is needed but not sought. Also if family group-reliance becomes an habitual, pervasive mode of adaptation, the needed flexibility is lost.

Use of Humor. Hott (1977) points out that a sense of humor is an important family asset that contributes to improving the family's attitude toward its problems and health care. Grojahn reiterates this contention further by stating, "Besides maturity, humor implies strength, superiority in face of danger and calamity, victory and triumph over defeat (Wessel, 1975). Humor also is generally acknowledged as a way for individuals and groups to relieve anxiety and tension. Although identified here as functional, if humor is used repeatedly to mask direct emotional expression and cover up and shun problems, its use is obviously dysfunctional.

Greater Sharing Together (Maintaining Family Cohesion). One way of bringing the family closer together and maintaining and managing stress levels and the necessary family morale is by sharing of feelings and thoughts, and engaging in joint family experiences or activities. Greater sharing together produces higher family cohesion, a family attribute that has received wide attention for being a central family attribute (Olson et al, 1979). Redbook editors recognized the significance of families staying close by publishing an interesting article about "Tips for Closer Family Ties" (Lobsenz, 1988). Ten tips are presented on how to help families cope with their problems. Lobsenz recommends: (1) make time together, (2) get to know one another, (3) share problems, (4) make dinnertime a family affair, (5) design a challenging family project, (6) develop rituals, (7) play games together, (8) don't forget a bedtime story, (9) share your work and school lives, and (10) don't let distance come between you.

Perhaps the most crucial sharing together is between the spouses. A confiding relationship, particularly between mates, in which individuals can talk intimately about themselves and their concerns has been shown to be critical for good psychological health in times of stress. The sharing of concerns and feelings is also very advantageous in reducing the family group's tension level. High family cohesiveness is especially helpful when a family has been traumatized, because family members are in much greater need of support (Figley, 1989).

A family's involvement in family rituals that have meaning and value to the family is another way in which the family shares together. Rituals in families are repeated social processes or patterns of interaction that preserve the family identity and give family members a shared definition of the world (Hartman and Laird, 1983). An excellent cultural example of a family ritual is the traditional Jewish custom of sitting shivah—a 7-day period after a funeral in which relatives and close friends visit with the bereaved family and share their thoughts and feelings, providing mutual emotional support and nurturance.

Leisure-time family activities are especially important coping resources to rejuvenate a family's cohesiveness, morale, and satisfaction. The increasing importance of leisure-time activities has been verified in studies of marital satisfaction (Orthner, 1976; Rapoport et al, 1974; West, 1970). Like so many sayings, the adage, "A family that plays together, stays together" contains much truth in it. This coping strategy is ultimately aimed at building greater integration, cohesiveness, and resiliency in the family.

Controlling the Meaning of the Problem by Reframing and Passive Appraisal. One of the primary means Pearlin and Schooler (1978) found to be effective in coping was by use of the mental mechanism—controlling the meaning of the problem, which ameliorates or cognitively neutralizes the threatening stimuli that are experienced in life. As mentioned earlier, the interpretation given to events can make the difference between hyperreacting to a situation (wherein the family experiences great stress); reacting in a realistic way (wherein the situation is seen objectively, appraised accurately); and underreacting (wherein an element of denial may be present and less stress is elicited). Cognitive reframing in the family mental health literature, is the most encouraged way for controlling the meaning of a stressor; "optimistic beliefs" and "positive appraisal" (Folkman et al, 1986) are synonymous terms used. Families that use this coping strategy tend to see the positive facets of life's stress-producing events, as exemplified by the making of positive comparisons ("count your blessings"; "it could have been worse"); selectively ignoring the negative aspects ("I've learned a lot from this negative experience"); and making the stressful events or experiences less important in terms of the family's hierarchy of values (Chesler and Barbarin, 1987; Pearlin and Schooler, 1978).

Reframing is an individual or family perceptual way of coping. Families have shared perceptions or shared subjective realities, and thus will use reframing or hold optimistic beliefs also as a group. In fact, Reiss and Oliveri (1983) state that "the family's shared subjective appraisal of an event is itself a coping process" (p. 65).

Olson and associates (1983) explain that in reframing the family and its members define the stressor event as a challenge that can be overcome. Families tend to use this response not only to minimize problematic circumstances but to prevent potential problems from occurring. Family therapists like Minuchin and Fishman (1981) assist families to reframe their reality. Minuchin and Fishman explain that they first learn of the family's perceptions and interpretations. "The therapist's task then is to convince the family members that reality as they have mapped it can be expanded and modified" (p. 76).

A second way families control the meaning of a stressor(s) is by passive appraisal, sometimes referred also as a passive acceptance. Here families use a collective cognitive coping strategy of viewing the stressor or stressful demand as something that will take care of itself over time and about which there is nothing or little that can be done. As Boss (1988) points out, passive appraisal can be an effective stress-reducing strategy in the short run where in some cases there is nothing that can be done. By passively accepting the situation, a family may more easily tolerate the inevitable or immutable. However, if this strategy is used consistently and over time, its use then inhibits active problem solving and change in families.

Joint Problem Solving. Joint problem solving among family members is a family coping strategy that has been extensively studied via laboratory research methods by a group of family researchers (Straus, 1968; Klein, 1983; Reiss, 1981) and in the natural setting (Chesler and Barbarin, 1987; Figley, 1989). Focusing on the routine and expectable disruptions in family life, researchers have looked at the differences in families' use of joint problem solving. Joint problem solving can be described as a situation where a family jointly is able to discuss a problem at hand, search for a solution governed by logic, and reach a consensus on what to do based upon a fully shared set of cues, perceptions, and suggestions from the various family members. Reiss (1981) calls families that use this type of problem-solving process environment-sensitive families. These types of families see the nature of problems as being "out there" and do not try to make the problem an internal one.

Figley (1989) identified "solution-oriented problem-solving" as being a type of functional coping. Figley explains that families coping with trauma "get stuck" only briefly on who is to blame for the current problems the family is experiencing. The families then move to mobilize their resources to resolve the stress-producing situation.

Role Flexibility. Because of the rapid and pervasive changes in our society and hence in family life, role flexibility, especially among mates, constitute a powerful type of coping strategy. Olson and associates (1979) have defined this capacity as one of the major dimensions of family adaptation. Again, the spousal subsystem's ability to role share and change roles when needed is most important. Switching roles "is highly adaptive externally to the demands of other social institutions and internally to the needs of its own members" (Vincent, 1966, p. 29).

In research on levels of functioning of grieving families, Davies and co-workers (1986) corroborated the importance of role flexibility as a functional coping strategy. They found that the degree to which family roles were flexible or rigid differentiated levels of functioning in their sample of grieving families.

Normalizing. Another functional family coping strategy is the tendency for families to normalize things as much as possible when they are coping with a long-term stressor that tends to disrupt family life and household activities. Multiple authors have used the term "normalizing" to conceptualize how families manage a member's disability (Knafl and Deatrick, 1986). Davis (1963) was the first researcher to use the term "normalization" to describe a family's response to illness or disability. He found that families with children who had polio normalized their situation by minimizing abnormalities in the child's appearance, participating in usual activities, and maintaining ongoing social ties. Darling and Darling (1982) asserted that this coping strategy is the most common mode of adaptation for families with disabled children.

Knafl and Deatrick (1986) analyzed the common categories of behaviors that make up normalization. These were engaging in usual parenting activities, limiting contacts with similarly situated others, making the child appear normal, avoiding potentially embarrassing situations, and controlling information. Keeping "things" normal is also mentioned in several coping studies as a family coping strategy in families with chronically ill children (Friedman, 1985; Schulman, 1976).

External Family Coping Strategies

Although inner coping resources are crucial, most authors writing in this area today also emphasize the necessity for families under stress to bring in or receive greater external information, tangible goods, services, and support—aspects previously discussed in terms of the concept of boundaries in the system's framework. External family coping strategies include seeking information, maintaining active linkages with the broader community, seeking social support, and seeking spiritual support. Most of the discussion in this section describes nuclear family support systems, because social supports are considered a major type of external family coping strategy.

Seeking Information. Families under stress that are more cognitively based respond by seeking knowledge and information concerning the stressor or potential stressor. This acts to increase feelings of having some control over the situation, reduce fear of the unknown, and help the family to appraise the stressor (its meaning) more accurately, in addition to strengthening the family's means of preventing stressors from impinging on it.

Parents who actively cope with parenting by seeking out new information and other resources demonstrate positive results and feelings of coping well with parenting responsibilities (Pearlin and Schooler, 1978). For example, Hoeflin (1954) reports that parents who avail themselves of books and magazines and newspapers to aid them in parenting use significantly more functional child-rearing techniques than parents who do not seek out this type of information. When parents use this activist approach to child rearing, children will also learn to problem solve in active, mastery-oriented ways.

Another research study documenting the use of seeking information as a family coping strategy was by Chesler and Barbarin (1987). In their research on family coping with childhood cancer they found that parents "searched for information" as a means of coping. It helped some parents place their emotional responses in perspective and attenuated some of the uncertainty and fear about their child's prognosis.

Maintaining Active Linkages with the Community. This category differs from coping by using social support systems in that it is a continuing, long-term, and general family coping effort, not one geared to alleviate any one specific stressor. In this case, family members are active participants (as active members or in leadership positions) in clubs, organizations, and community groups. There is extensive use of the society's varied resources and exposure through travel to alternative ways to life (Pratt, 1976).

The rationale for the importance of this linkage as a coping technique is grounded in systems theory, which states that any social system must have a movement of information and activity across its boundaries if it is to perform its functions. Because the family alone cannot serve all its members' and group needs without enrichment from other sources, the initiation and promotion of growth-producing relationships within the neighborhood, town, and wider society is essential (Pratt, 1976). If, however, the family's boundaries are continually open and do not sufficiently allow for family integration and control over input, this strategy then would be dysfunctional.

Seeking Social Support Systems. Seeking social support systems within the family's social network is the major external family coping strategy. In addition to extended families and the whole network of professional services, experts, and bureaucracies, there exists a great reservoir of potential help: kin, friends, neighbors, employers, fellow employees, classmates, teachers, and groups with which a family shares common interests, goals, life-styles, or social identity. Subcultural and reference groups are examples of these types of groups. These groups can also be based on common professional interests, political goals, ethnic identity, or recreational involvements. The family's social networks serve as a third "set of players" for the family wrestling with making suitable arrangements in matters of education, child care, health and welfare services, and so forth (Howell, 1975).

In addition to the discussion in this chapter about seeking family social supports as a type of external family coping strategy, a section within Chapter 8 discusses the concept of social support, social support research findings, and how to assess family social support, using interview questions, the genogram, and the ecomap.

According to Caplan (1974) there are three general sources of social support. These consist of spontaneous, informal networks; organized supports not directed by professional health care workers; and organized efforts by health care professionals. Of these, the informal social network (defined above as the social network) is viewed as the group providing the greatest amount of help in times of need.

The duration and permanency of support systems vary. Some family support systems are long-term or continuous sets of individuals and groups that assist the family in more general life issues such as developmental tasks and situational crisis (eg, a loss of family member). Other support systems may be crisis oriented, dealing with specific issues and are short-term in duration (Hogue, 1977).

A family copes with its problems within its social network; needless to say, it is impossible to survive if one is isolated from outer resources. Every family and person has a unique, special social network that provides important linkages, as well as being critically important to the family's and its members' self-image, sense of belonging, and feeling of group satisfaction (MacElveen, 1978).

Purposes of Social Support Systems. Social networks of support systems have two primary coping purposes: emotional support and direct assistance. First, they provide nurturance and emotional support to family members (Hogue, 1977; MacElveen, 1978). In these types of relationships the nurturing persons or groups care for, support, and emotionally meet some of the psychosocial needs of the family members. Support systems also are concerned with the morale and welfare of the family as a group, and will work to sustain or improve the group's morale and positive motivation. In addition, the family's informal social network provides a family with opportunities for feedback about itself and validation about its expectations and perceptions of individuals and of groups, which, in turn, may improve the family's communication with groups in the community with which it interacts.

Extended families or close friends encourage members to communicate freely about their personal difficulties. The family then shares its problems with this support system and is offered individualized advice and guidance—in keeping with the family's traditions and values. The superiority of extended family and close friends over professionals who do not know the family, in terms of giving help and advice, is often expressed by clients (Friedman, 1985). After all, who knows the family better than these supportive individuals? Can health care professionals have the same keen sense of uniqueness of a particular family that close friends and family have? And who has the greater and more lasting interest in the family's welfare and happiness? The answers to the above speak for the vital nature of social networks.

The second primary purpose support systems achieve is that of task-oriented assistance that extended family, friends, and neighbors often provide. An important element of this assistance is not only telling family members how to find sources of care and assistance in the community, but also giving direct assistance. In our society, usually only close relatives will provide extensive long-term help. Assistance from extended family also takes on the form of direct help, including continuing and intermittent financial aid, shopping, care of children, physical care of old people, performing household tasks, and practical assistance in times of crisis (Caplan, 1974). In times of illness or trouble, this system becomes crucial in assisting families to cope successfully.

The absence of such assistive relationships can generate a sense of vulnerability, especially where use of these assistive relationships, eg, the extended family, is an important culturally derived way of coping. For instance, Friedman (1985) found that the absence of extended family support among Latino versus Anglo families who had a child with cancer was much more disruptive for the family.

Inadequate Use of Social Networks. There is both concern and evidence that many people do not seek needed external help (Pearlin and Schooler, 1978). Several factors inhibit families, especially those in the middle class, from fully utilizing these resources. First, the belief exists that professional services are often best, but because they are very costly and often beyond the family's means, no outside help is sought. Second, while the family is thought of as a place where individuals can let down their defenses and receive and give support and care, some believe that in facing the outside world the family should exhibit independence and self-sufficiency. Despite the fact that family members often yearn to be interdependent, to be supportive of others outside of the family, and to receive support in return, a feeling persists that asking for help or support is a sign of weakness and fallibility. Thus, when a family "fails" to handle its own problems, it "should" be prepared to turn to paid professionals to resolve the problem (Howell, 1975).

Howell (1975) describes closed families as being the mythical standard or the "ideal" family for contemporary life:

> These families provide for their needs either by drawing on their own insular resources or by applying to agencies outside themselves. They are inward-looking units with tight boundaries. . . . For a large proportion of their needs as a group and as individuals, they are expected to be quietly self-sufficient and entirely competent. (p. 72)

In cases of family "failure"—that is, where the family is unable to succeed solely through its own means—professional services are available. The services available to the lower income family or to those who cannot pay full fees, however, are often inadequate or inaccessible. Unfortunately, professionals, rather than encourage self-care and self-control, often rob families of their control over their own problems and, ironically, because of their lack of real understanding and knowledge of the family, may very well provide unsatisfactory solutions (Hogue, 1977).

In contrast with closed families, it has been suggested that open families are able to define their boundaries more loosely and flexibly, according to the needs of members and the group and according to outside demands and requests for help from the social network. Because such boundaries allow for a greater exchange of energy, matter, and information, these families are better able to use the family's informal social network.

A family's use of its social network as a resource for assistance will alter the use of professional services in a more appropriate direction, namely, for those specialized or complex needs that cannot be met by the family's social support system or self-care resources.

Mutual Aid or Self-help Groups. Mutual aid groups have become an increasingly important part of the social support network of many families (Katz and Bender, 1976). Many family members find that they need to share and seek help from others who have the same concerns and needs and share their concerns. Their usual support system does not adequately provide for these needs, some of which are more specialized in nature. As an important coping strategy for these individuals and families, participating in one of these organizations can be seen as part of a search for a supportive and/or assistive system that is sufficiently sharing to mediate communication, guide action, and make personal experiences more bearable (Vickers, 1971).

Individuals and families join mutual aid groups as a coping strategy to meet a wide variety of special needs. Hence self-help groups include a broad gamut of organizations, established with varied purposes and processes. For instance, some self-care groups, such as the Vietnam Veteran's rap groups, are alternative caregiving systems; some such as ostomy clubs are adjuncts to the health care professional's services; some are an expression of democratic, political ideals, such as the National Organization for Women (NOW); and some are vehicles for promoting individual change, such as Recovery and Alcoholics Anonymous.

There is a tremendous growth in urban areas of recovery-oriented self-help groups for family members with addictions (the addicted person and their "codependents"). This rapid growth is evidence of the extent to which addictions (alcohol, drugs, eating) are a problem today, as well as the tendency for families to use self-help groups for coping with this growing problem.

Seeking Spiritual Support. Although most people would think of seeking and relying on spiritual support as being an individual coping response, several studies have reported that family members find it a family way of coping too (Chesler and Barbarin, 1987; Friedman, 1985; Olson et al, 1983). In fact, belief in God and prayer were identified by family members as being either the most important way the family coped with a trying health-related stressor or a very important and frequently employed method in two studies (Friedman, 1985; Pravikoff, 1985). In Pravikoff's study of 28 family members of post-MI patients, the sample was composed of older WASP (White, Anglo-Saxon, Protestants who were middle-class). In Friedman's study (1985) of 55 families with a child with cancer, the families were one half Anglo and one half Latino. Latinos, in comparison to Anglos, relied much more heavily on religion as their most important way of handling their child's cancer. Ethnic differences in family coping with respect to the helpfulness of spiritual supports were quite evident. Olson and associates (1983), in surveying 1200 white middle- and upper-middle-class Lutherans, also found that for coping with everyday life problems, use of religious supports was ranked as very helpful. Spiritual supports have helped families tolerate chronic, long-term strains and contribute to maintaining the family unit. Olson and associates (1983) found that the use of this strategy varies in the family's life cycle stage. For instance, families in their study reported that they used spiritual supports less during the early stages of family life, but used spiritual supports more thereafter.

DYSFUNCTIONAL ADAPTIVE STRATEGIES

Whereas functional families experiencing stress tend to act in a direction that reduces stress, dysfunctional families tend to use habitual defensive strategies that tend not to dissipate the stress or eliminate or attenuate the stressor (White, 1974). Dysfunctional adaptive strategies do temporarily reduce stress, but the stress returns because the underlying stressors are not dealt with. Stress reduction tactics can be functional or dysfunctional. The difference here is that dysfunctional tactics have deleterious effects on family members.

There are various specific dysfunctional strategies families use to attempt to cope with their problem. In most cases these are selected unconsciously, often as responses that their families of origin used in attempting to cope.

As might be expected, the literature dealing with dysfunctional adaptive patterns is much more voluminous than the literature dealing with healthy ways of solving familial problems, this literature having been generated primarily by family and other psychothera-

TABLE 17–3. TYPOLOGY OF DYSFUNCTIONAL FAMILY ADAPTIVE STRATEGIES

I. Denial of problems and exploitation of one or more family members.
   A. Nonphysical, but active overt emotional exploitation: scapegoating, use of threat.
   B. Nonphysical passive emotional exploitation: child neglect.
   C. Both physical and emotional exploitation employed: child abuse, parent abuse, and spousal violence
II. Denial of family problems. Adaptive mechanism impairs family's ability to meet affective function.
   A. Denial seen in family belief system: family myth, use of threat.
   B. Denial maintained through establishment of emotional distancing, certain customs and traditions, triangling, and pseudomutuality.
III. Separation or loss of family member(s). Husband or wife abandonment, institutionalization, divorce, physical absences of family members (alcoholism, physically absent husbands).
IV. Authoritarianism (submission to marked domination).

pists interested in family interaction and process among their troubled clients.

Because no all-encompassing typology or classification of family dysfunctional adaptive strategies exists in the literature, the classification in Table 17–3 was generated to describe major types of family dysfunctional adaptive strategies. It should be noted that each of these dysfunctional family adaptive strategies is used to reduce family stress or tension.

Denial and Overt Exploitation of Family Members

Now that a classification of some of the dysfunctional strategies has been presented, it will be easier to relate the discrete adaptive mechanisms to each other. This section covers the several overt exploitative ways that families reduce tension for the family as a group, but do so at the emotional and/or perhaps physical expense of one or more individual members. Parad and Caplan (1965) explain that emotional exploitation can happen in two basic ways:

> *Passively,* by emotional neglect through concentrating family energies in such a way that the needs of an individual are not attended to, though the details of his own role may not be important in reducing tension; and *actively,* by the *emotional exploitation* of a family member through investing him with a role which does violence to his needs as an individual. (p. 59)

Under this broad category of denial and exploitation, three family dysfunctional patterns will be briefly discussed: family violence, scapegoating, and use of threat.

Family Violence. Family violence is recognized as one of our major public health problems today (Gelles and Strauss, 1988). The professional literature about child abuse and spouse abuse has mushroomed, and there is a concomitant rapid growth of research in this area. Although the basic mechanism of violence (use of physical force by one family member against another) is the same, there are actually five types of family violence: spouse/marital abuse, child abuse (physical and sexual), elder abuse, parent abuse, and violence between siblings. The first two types are more numerous and widely acknowledged than the latter three.

Public awareness of child abuse did not come about until the 1960s when the diagnosis "battered child syndrome" was coined. Family violence as an academic topic of research remained virtually hidden until the early 1970s. Hence, the whole area of family violence and the important underlying family dynamics is relatively new for family health professionals.

It is only recently that a good systematic method of recording reports of child abuse and neglect has been established nationwide, and so even though the number of cases of child abuse appears to be rising rapidly (Fig. 17–5), much of the rise is due to better recordkeeping. Family violence researchers believe that the incidence of family violence has probably not changed much from previous eras, but that the increase is due to greater public and professional awareness and less public tolerance for child abuse, as well as the better recording systems (Strauss et al, 1980).

Extensive research has addressed the factors that are associated with family violence. It is clear that the causes of family violence are multidimensional. As anticipated, those individuals who experienced violent and abusive childhoods are more probable to become abusers. The National Center on Child Abuse and Neglect estimates that 30 percent of individuals who were physically or sexually abused or extremely neglected as children become abusive parents themselves (U.S. DHHS, 1989e). Domestic violence is probably more common in the lower socioeconomic groups, although there is some question about this. It is certainly not confined to any one social class. Most domestic violence is directly related to social stress in families. The violent family is often one that is socially isolated and the existence of personality problems and psychopathology in the family are associated with family violence (Gelles and Maynard, 1987).

One of the main problems in examining family violence data and studies is that the terms "abuse" and "violence" are not conceptually equivalent terms; nor are they consistently defined in the literature. Strauss and associates' (1980) definition of wife and child abuse refers to only those acts of violence that have a high

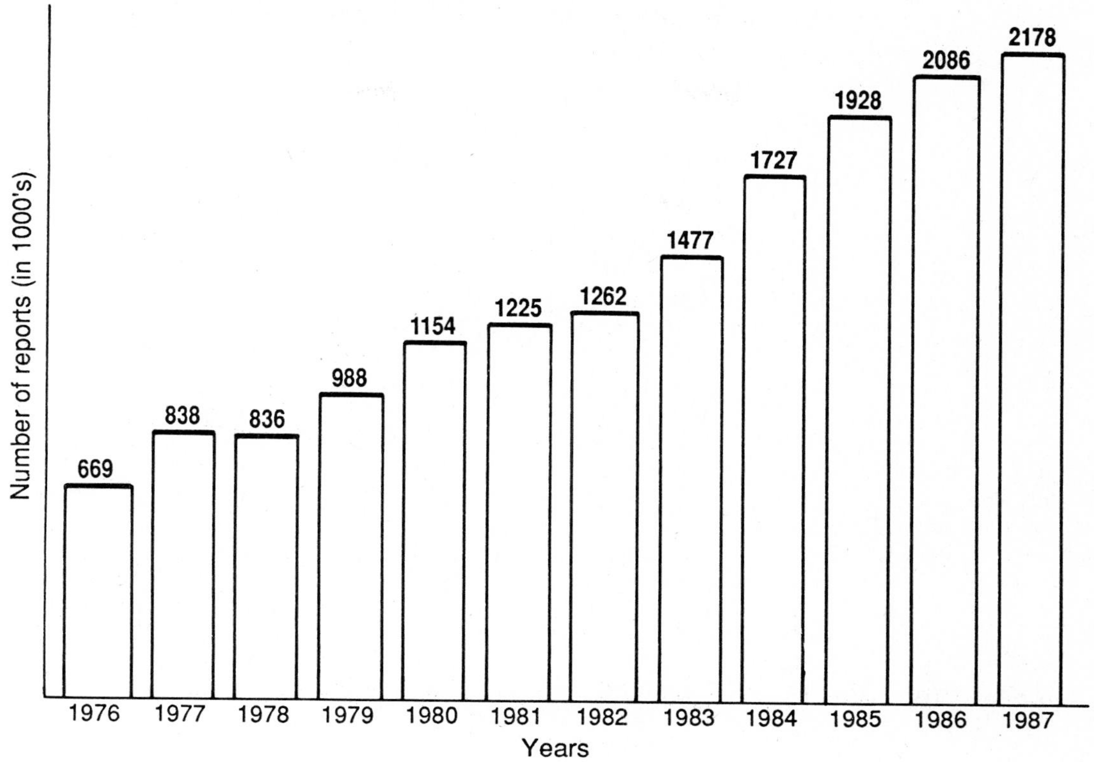

Figure 17–5
National estimates of child abuse and neglect reports, 1976–1987. (From: U.S. Department of Health and Human Services, 1989.)

probability of causing injury to the victim; other authors define family violence as any act of physical aggression regardless of whether it can or does cause injury. Steinmetz (1987) uses a widely referenced definition of family violence, which is that family violence refers to an act carried out by a family member with the intention of, or an act perceived as having the intention of, physically hurting another family member.

Spouse Abuse. Although the use of physical force by one mate against the other (largely husbands against wives) has recently been recognized by the mass media and professionals as a significant social problem (Gelles, 1980), it has been a commonly used tactic for the handling of frustration and stressors throughout our country's history and, as such, has been societally sanctioned.

Estimates of how extensive marital abuse varies. Numerous studies have noted that from 50 to 60 percent of couples report physical violence by a partner at some time during their marriage (Steinmetz, 1987). Strauss and co-workers (1980) in a nationwide survey of 2143 family members found that 16 percent of couples reported some form of violence between spouses during the year of the survey. For about one out of five women, spouse abuse is not an isolated occurrence, but a situation that occurs repeatedly (Steinmetz, 1987).

Strauss (1976) believes that some dynamic is at work in the family that makes the family an arena of physical violence—from slaps to murder. He suspects it is sexism, those beliefs that keep women subordinate, even through force if necessary. Other researchers believe that the power relations (power differential) between men and women and patriarchy in society are primary causes of wife abuse (Gelles, 1987; Pagelow, 1984). In some instances, the marriage license is viewed as legitimizing the husband's right to keep his wife in line, with violence if deemed necessary, despite the fact that similar acts against a person on the street would result in criminal sanctions. However, the legal system presently enforces this "right" to private violence with the doctrine of "spouse immunity" that prohibits a wife from suing her husband for assault and battery in many regions of the country. There is also documentation of widespread refusal of police to interfere in "family fights." This reluctance of police and prosecutors to punish wife-beaters stems from our society's traditional belief that husbands have the right to control their wives (Strauss, 1976).

Extensive research has been done on the factors that are associated with family violence (spousal and child abuse). As anticipated, those individuals who experienced violent and abusive childhoods are more probable to become abusers. Domestic violence is more common in the lower socioeconomic group, although family violence is not confined to that group. Most domestic violence is directly related to social stress in families. And finally, the violent family is often one that is socially isolated (Gelles, 1980).

Contrary to popular thinking, there is no such person as "the battered woman." There are many different types of women who become involved with battering men.

Women who are beaten by their husbands often stay in the marriage with the hope that the husband will change, although statistics indicate he almost never does. Also many battered women lack alternatives (alternate places of live, financial resources). Many of these women remain very passive and are unwilling to run away because they often have come from families where violence was customary, and thus see their predicament as part of "normal" married life. Moreover, some women say that they wanted to keep the family together and had very traditional values about family life. In fact, many wives are unaware that it is illegal for their husband to beat them up. Moreover, many batterers are supermacho types who will not let their wives go out alone, and follow and harass them if they try to run away, leaving the wives with the idea that they will never be able to become free (Benedek, 1978).

Despite the vast numbers of wives who remain in marriages where spousal violence is present, increasingly wives and their children are leaving home. In response to this trend, shelters for battered women are being opened up in communities across the nation. Nurses need to know about these community resources, as well as hot-lines and professional and peer-group counseling services for battered women.

Child Abuse. The family provides an individual's first initiation into uses made of physical force to control and socialize children. Strauss (1976) reports that 93 percent of the parents in one survey in both the United States and England were found to use physical punishment as an important means of reinforcing and sanctioning children's behavior. To these children the message is clear: physical force as a means of imposing one's will on another is effective and is accepted (especially for male children). Boys are encouraged by parents to fight back if they are attacked at school by another child (Strauss, 1976). Moreover, up until recently children were regarded as the possession of their parents—part of a private-ownership view of the family (Daughtery, 1981).

Child abuse is a case in point of the ubiquitousness of physical violence committed by parents against their children to its ugly conclusion. The assaults on children, if complete statistics were available, could turn out to be a more frequent cause of death than such diseases as leukemia, cystic fibrosis, and muscular dystrophy, and may even rank with automobile fatalities. The National Center on Child Abuse and Neglect states that there were almost 2.2 million reports of abused or neglected children nationwide in 1987. This represents an increase of 275 percent since 1976. The increased number of reports of child abuse or neglect between 1976 and 1987 reflects improved recognition, improved statewide reporting, as well as a possibly larger number of affected children (Fig. 17–5). Divorce, alcoholism, drug addiction, mental retardation, emotional illness, unemployment, and financial stressors all play major roles in leading the potentially abusive parent to strike out at a "special child" (Fontana, 1976). According to a 1990 report by the House Ways and Means Committee (Harris, 1991), adult drug use has recently become the predominant characteristic in caseloads of child-protective service agencies in 22 states and the District of Columbia.

In addition to spouse abuse and child abuse, three other groups of abusers that are little talked about are the elder abusers, parent abusers, and sibling abusers. Elder abuse and parent abuse are briefly described here.

Elder Abuse. Elder abuse and neglect, according to a watershed 1985 report by a congressional subcommittee (Larsen, 1989), is a problem that is increasing nationally. In an extensive review of family violence literature, Steinmetz (1987) reported that elder abuse is an area of research that has been virtually ignored until recently. Most of the published articles are personal observations and expert opinion.

The one non-random published study of elder abuse, conducted by Steinmetz (1987), described the study's sample and circumstances under which elderly abuse occurred. Ninety-one percent of her sample were 70 years or older and 85 percent had experienced diminished physical functioning. All elders shared a home with one of their children's family. The abusive techniques used by the caregiving children "ranged from screaming and yelling (30 percent), threatening to send elders to nursing home (8.5 percent), withholding food or medication (17 percent) . . . to physically restraining elder (7.5 percent) and slapping, hitting and shaking (2.5 percent). Overall, 12 percent of the caregivers had used physically abusive acts or the threat of physical violence in an attempt to maintain control" (p. 738).

Families caring for an elderly parent that are experiencing high levels of stress are much more likely to be involved in elder abuse. Also, caregivers who perceive caregiving tasks to be stressful, are more apt to engage in elder abuse (Pagelow, 1984; Steinmetz, 1987).

Parent Abuse. Another form of abuse is between parents and children, where children are old enough to now perpetrate violence against their parents. The children at one point were recipients of violence, and through role modeling learned that the use of violence was a feasible and acceptable mode of expressing anger. In studies that examined this phenomenon, the children were adolescents. In the first national study published (Strauss et al, 1980) of 2143 intact families with adolescent children (10 to 17 years old), 9 percent of the parents reported experiencing at least one attack by one of their children and 3 percent said they had experienced severe violence. In both single- and two-parent families, mothers were more likely to be the victims and sons the perpetrators (Steinmetz, 1987).

In data from a more recent study of parent abuse nationwide (Agnew and Huguley, 1989), the abusing adolescent was more likely to have friends who assaulted their parents; approve of delinquency, including violence; believe that the probability of official sanction for parental assault was low; be weakly attached to parents; and be white.

Scapegoating. Scapegoating is a dysfunctional adaptive mechanism because although it reduces the tension level of the family system and makes the continuance of family homeostasis possible, it does this at the expense of the emotional health of one of its members—the scapegoat or "the identified patient" (McCreery, 1981). The scapegoat's function is to effect a total clearance of the emotional ills that beset the family. This pattern is fairly common in troubled families and can be recognized when a family has achieved unity and cohesiveness while at the same time negatively labeling and stigmatizing one of its members. The identified patient or scapegoat is "selected" to be the focus of its difficulties, thus hiding the real problems within the family (eg, the marital relationship). Thus the deviant within the group may perform a valuable function for the group by channeling group tensions and providing a basis for solidarity" (Bell and Vogel, 1968, p. 412).

How is the scapegoat selected? First, the person must not be someone who has great significance for family survival; thus children are by far the most common choices for being scapegoats. Children are in a relatively powerless position, cannot separate from family, are pliant to behavioral changes, and can adopt the roles parents assign to them. Usually the first child is more vulnerable, because in a faulty marriage further strained by the advent of a child, the stressful marital difficulties are quickly displaced onto the first available and "appropriate" object—the first child. A particular child may also be selected because of his or her age or sex, intelligence, health status, developmental stage, resemblance to another family member with negative attributes, or simple availability. Also, a family member who has already been negatively labeled is particularly vulnerable to scapegoating (Godspeed, 1975; Roberts, 1975).

How does the scapegoating process start and continue? Bell and Vogel (1968) suggest that the family is initially faced with some unresolved tension, often a marital stressor, with the mates having deep-seated fears about their relationship and thus a need to deny the problem's existence. The family's problem is perceived to be insoluble and beyond its coping resources. Because of this, the situation is felt to be a threat or danger to the family's survival and the life goals of its members. Concomitantly, the tension and stress levels rise and throw the family into a state of disequilibrium.

As a result of the increased stress level and precarious family stability, the family attempts to reduce the tension through the exploitation of one or more of its members. Scapegoating reduces family tensions, because tensions, hostilities, and guilt can be directed toward (displaced onto) the identified problem member. Furthermore, the scapegoat begins taking on the assigned roles, which started as negative labeling and later became internalized, that is, into the role of being the scapegoat.

When scapegoating has become an established family adaptive mechanism, family homeostasis is achieved. There is open acknowledgement and labeling of the identified patient or scapegoat. Psychic economy results as group tensions are attenuated by the displacement of anxieties, guilt, and hostility onto an object acceptable to the value system of the family.

Later, when the problem has been further walled off, the individual is reclassified in the family structure as a "problem member," different from all other family members. Although the scapegoat is the victim of hostile projections, because the family is an interactive system, the scapegoat concomitantly works to maintain his or her position as a scapegoat. The parents, to avoid criticism of their treatment of their scapegoated child, define themselves as being victimized by the "problem child" (Vogel and Bell, 1960). Eventually the outside world verifies this differentness by also labeling and stigmatizing the scapegoat. Such labeling maintains the family system's dysfunctionality.

Why would the scapegoat maintain his or her unpleasant role? The answer lies in the self-fulfilling prophesy: a person does what is expected and responds to the reinforcement he or she receives to maintain a certain role. Reinforcement consists of secondary rewards of extra attention, even if negative, and exemption from responsibility.

If the scapegoat leaves the family, is removed by the community, or does not enact the proper role (because of psychiatric treatment), the family will face another homeostatic crisis. At that time the scapegoat may step back into the former role or a new scapegoat may be selected.

In summary, the scapegoating mechanism can be viewed as functional for the family, in that the scapegoat produces family equilibrium on a short-term basis; but it is dysfunctional in the long run for the emotional health of the exploited member and, for that matter, the health of all family members.

Use of Threat. Threat is another dysfunctional coping technique used as a means of keeping the family together at the expense of the emotional health of its members. Smoyak (1969) views threat as a recurrent family dynamic in some troubled families. This technique is employed by the family to produce and maintain connectedness and discourage members' efforts to individuate and achieve separateness. The purpose of doing so is to ensure the survival of the family.

Smoyak (1969) describes the control technique involved in using threat. The initial basis for needing this means of ensuring family survival is that the family system views its surrounding environment as hostile and threatening. The family feels the only way it can survive is to stick together as a closed family system. Family preservation then becomes emphasized over the individual needs of its members, and the family value of connectedness becomes elevated to a place of high importance to maintain the family. Minuchin (1974) refers to these families as "enmeshed" families; Bowen as "undifferentiated" families" (Miller and Winstead-Fry, 1982).

When one or more family members acts in an autonomous, individualistic fashion, the other family members become threatened by the separating individual's impending breach with the family, and thus take action to bring him or her back into the fold. They may do this by themselves threatening to leave the family system, including threats of suicide or self-destructive acts; by threatening social ostracism, forbidding reentry into the family; by threatening an aggressive act against the separating individual; or by threatening emotional rejection—withdrawal of affection and support. These maneuvers, if successful, result in the "deviant" family member retreating from his or her separatist efforts and again conforming to the value of connectedness. Furthermore, once reintegrated, this individual may then take part in sanctioning another member who attempts to individuate.

Forcing deviating members back into the family so that all members espouse connectedness restores the family's equilibrium. However, individuals from such families have severe adjustment problems when they leave the family environment, because they have not learned autonomy, self-directedness, and how to relate effectively with the outside world.

Denial of Family Problems

Denial is a defense mechanism used by family members and the family as a whole. In the short term, family denial is often functional, as it allows the family to "buy time" to protect itself while it gradually accepts a painful event. But in the long term, denial is dysfunctional for a family. There are several denial adaptive mechanisms discussed in this section: family myth, triangling, and pseudomutuality.

The Family Myth. Through the family's belief system, myths can be created about one's family that obscure reality and deny some of the real issues and problems within the group, these problems being perceived as either too painful to be brought out in the open or as unnecessary to discuss because doing so will only make things worse. A family myth refers to a belief that is generated in response to the unfulfilled wishes and expectations of the family, instead of being based on a rational and objective appraisal of the situation (Battiste, 1975). Ferreira (1963) clarifies the concept of family myth as being "a series of fairly well integrated beliefs shared by all family members, concerning each other and their mutual position in the family life, beliefs that go unchallenged by everyone involved, in spite of the reality distortions they may conspicuously imply" (p. 457).

As wish-fulfillment fantasies, family myths are established early in the family cycle to serve as a defense against the limitations that the reality of family life imposes. Family myths thus tend to suspend reality. The more myths a family has, the less realistically a family can judge a situation and the fewer the alternatives they have to draw from. For instance, if a myth exists that the mother needs to be protected and helped, then during times of the father's absence, family's role flexibility is diminished because the mother's ability to function in an instrumental role is stifled by the family myth.

Myths are inner images of the family group, not only the facade that the family holds out to outsiders. Battiste (1975) cites some very good examples of family myths: "We all like to do things together"; "We stay married only because of the children"; "Father is the strong one"; "We're a happy family."

She further explains when to suspect that family myths are operating: "When these inner images a family has of itself seem to not ring true to the outside observer, but when the family clings tenaciously to them, one is probably on the track of a family myth" (p. 101).

As previously mentioned, most family myths begin in the early days of the family, when relationships are being formed and cemented. Family myth formulas for togetherness are sought to promote closeness and set limits on possible untoward interpersonal reactions. Circular, repetitive communication patterns, roles, power, and value characteristics develop based on a myth, which in turn, preserves the family unit (Battiste, 1975).

Occasionally, during a time of family crisis, a family myth will be used as a balancing mechanism. As a means of achieving homeostasis, the myth is called into play when a family experiences stress that threatens to disrupt family functioning. Thus the family myth functions as a defensive mechanism in that it prevents the family from destroying itself by maintaining, and sometimes even increasing, the level of family organization through the establishment of patterns set up as part of the family myth—a myth such as, "When in times of distress, we all help each other" (Peters, 1974).

On the surface, one might say that this "coping" tactic is functional—after all, it provides satisfaction for the family, automatic agreement, a common frame of reference, and stabilizing, reassuring rituals. However, it is a dysfunctional adaptive mechanism because it narrows the vision of reality and the choices or alternatives available. Members react to family issues in a stereotypical, nonindividualized way and become limited in their repertoire of responses used to deal with significant issues and life problems. Thus the growth of the family and its members is stifled because, in the presence of family myths, they will not acquire the feelings of confidence and growth that come from meeting life's problems head-on and confronting life's disappointments with a broad range of possible solutions (Battiste, 1975).

Triangling. Another way of reducing stress either on a short-term or long-term basis within the family is through the use of triangling. This concept was developed by Bowen (1976), a noted family therapist, and applies to the reduction of tension in a dyadic relationship by adding a third member, who then absorbs and diffuses the ongoing tension in the dyadic relationship (Hallen, 1978). In other words, bringing in a third member relieves the emotionality between the original two by shifting the tension to the new dyadic member and making one of the initial partners into an "outsider." The balance of forces within triangles is fluid and may shift either frequently or over long periods of time. In periods of very high stress, a system will triangle in more outsiders, again reducing the stress within the family (Miller and Winstead-Fry, 1982).

For instance, a husband and wife may be involved in an unsatisfactory, argument-laden relationship that results in neither of their needs being met. Triangling in a third person, one of the couple's children, reduces the marital relationship strain. Both mates begin to focus on the child, although one mate usually develops a dyadic relationship with the child and the other mate becomes the third person—the outsider. This process forces the child to take sides: for one parent and against the other. The parent who forms the close relationship with the child tries to fulfill his or her emotional needs through the parent–child relationship, putting new unrealistic demands on this relationship, so that often the newly formed dyad also becomes strained. As a result, the outside parent may again be triangled in, resulting in a shift back to the marital dyad. "If a triangled person remains in this position for a period of time, it is quite possible he/she will develop some physical or emotional problem as an outlet for his/her anxiety" (Francis and Munjas, 1976, p. 38).

Triangling is included here as a dysfunctional coping strategy because it is a commonly used way in which to reduce interpersonal tension within the family without treating the underlying ills of the situation. Although triangling can be looked on as a phenomenon occurring to some extent in all emotionally laden interactions, and especially in dyadic ones under stress, the pervasive use of this stress-reducing mechanism over a long period of time may be considered to be dysfunctional because it does nothing to alleviate the stressor and is injurious to long-term emotional needs of family members.

Pseudomutuality. Pseudomutuality may be classified as a long-term dysfunctional adaptive strategy because it maintains family homeostasis at the expense of meeting the family's affective function—that is, recognizing and responding to the socioemotional needs of its members. The real problem, the inability to foster and maintain intimate, close affective relationships, is covered up by a facade of solidarity and cohesiveness among family members.

Wynne (1958) defines pseudomutuality as "a type of relatedness in which there is a preoccupation of family members with a fitting together into formal roles at the expense of individual identity" (p. 205). As with the use of threat, individual separateness or divergence is forbidden. Individual differentness or divergence is perceived as leading to disruption of the relationship and must therefore be avoided. The use of threat is sometimes used in families displaying pseudomutuality.

These families may desire closeness and intimacy but are afraid of it or are unable to reach one another on a feeling level. Affective communications are almost nil. Each family member strives for relatedness, but feels that other members block his or her efforts at closeness.

To the outside world these families usually present a picture of family solidarity, because their face-saving needs are great. However, they are able to approach this desire only through much formalized or ritualized action, such as giving gifts, celebrating birthdays, holidays, and so forth.

Pseudomutuality is a long-term adaptive strategy used by families. It presents "a stifling structure that constricts autonomy . . . consists of ambiguity, meaninglessness, and emptiness. . . . Individuality poses a great threat, especially with family members who have poor ego structures to begin with" (Silver, 1975, p. 111).

Separation or Loss of Family Member

Another dysfunctional mechanism to reduce tension or stress in the family is for the family members to physically or psychosocially separate from each other. This includes loss of a family member through death or divorce, and psychosocial loss of family member through the member's involvement in an addiction (alcohol, drugs). Only the addicted family is discussed here.

The Addicted Family. Addictions of family members are being understood today as family system problems rather than as individual problems. Steinglass and associates (1987) examined the family system of the alcoholic and clearly demonstrated, in *The Alcoholic Family,* the role that alcohol plays in reducing tension in the family and maintaining homeostasis (albeit it short-lived). Their book charts the developmental course of alcoholism in the family and explains the role that other family members play as co-dependents or enablers of the alcoholic. The 10-year study upon which the book was based challenges many of the commonly held notions about alcoholism and proposes a family systems approach to treating alcoholism.

The role of drugs in families is similar to that of alcohol—only the substance is changed. (It should be noted that many individuals are addicted to more than one drug or to drugs and alcohol.) Certainly the growth in drug addictions has had a tremendous influence on the health care system and treatment modes. In addition to professionally led recovery programs, self-help groups following the 12 steps originally developed to assist alcoholics, are mushrooming nationwide. Many strands of psychosocial theory and practice converge in the current thinking about addiction—family systems theory, chemical dependency theory, child abuse theory, group therapies, and the 12-step self-help programs.

Concerns for family members is evidenced in the literature and in the growth of self-help groups for the "adult child of an alcoholic." Adult children of alcoholics have been profoundly affected by growing up in an alcoholic family, as growing up in these types of families places specific and constant strains on all the family members. As Steinglass and co-workers (1987) showed, the tension/stress level in alcoholic families is like the ocean tides—always changing, with continual ups and downs and maneuvers to keep the system afloat.

Authoritarianism

Submission to marked domination is included in this section as a long-term dysfunctional adaptive strategy, because through the submission of family members to a dominant, ruling figure, usually the husband, family equilibrium is achieved—but again, at the emotional expense of the subordinates and, less obviously, the dominator. Peace and balance may be accomplished on either a short- or long-term basis, but when it is reluctant and forced, anger rages beneath the surface—to be either repressed, with conformity and dependence the outcome, or expressed as depression, somatization, or through acting out behaviors of defiance, antisocial acts, destructiveness, and so on.

Authoritarianism refers to the tendency to give up one's independence due to feelings of powerlessness and dependency and to fuse self with somebody or something outside one's self in order to acquire the power or strength felt lacking. In an authoritarian family, people renounce their own personal integrity and become part of an unhealthy, submissive–dominance symbiosis. The submissive family members are very dependent on the dominant individual. Life as a whole is felt by the submissive members to be something overwhelming, all-powerful, and uncontrollable. Interestingly enough, the dominating member is also dependent on his or her subordinates, because the need for power and control is paramount. Along with having absolute power over the other family members and making them into instruments to be used and exploited, the dominator holds the feeling, "I rule you because I know what's best for you" and "I have done so much for you, now I expect something in return."

As with all the other dysfunctional adaptive strategies, all members in these families suffer. This authoritarian symbiosis curtails efforts of family members to individuate, grow, and become self-directed and independently proficient in life. Moreover, they learn only two ways of relating to people—either as the ruler or the ruled—and with this background they perpetuate these roles in all their other relationships and transmit these interpersonal tendencies to the next generation.

The types of families that fit into this category are those families that do not negotiate on issues, and where the dominant one seeks no input from others before decisions are made. Many families are mildly husband-dominated and function very effectively. It is only when this dominance pattern becomes exaggerated that it becomes a dysfunctional way to adapt to life's stressors.

Cultural patterns must be taken into account when examining whether authoritarianism is an adaptive strategy the family is using. For instance, both Hispanic and Asian families are traditionally patriarchal. However, even in these families marked domination is not salubrious and does not follow the social mores of these cultures.

FAMILY COPING STRATEGIES: APPLYING THE FAMILY NURSING PROCESS

☐ *ASSESSMENT QUESTIONS*

The following questions have been included to assist the assessor in appraising the family coping processes and strategies.

1. What stressors (both long and short-term) are being experienced by the family? Refer to the Social Readjustment Scale of Holmes and Rahe, so that these factors will be identified. Also consider environmental and socioeconomic stressors. Is it possible to estimate the duration and strength of the family stressors? What strengths counterbalance them? Is the family able to handle the usual stresses and strains of daily family life?
2. Is the family able to act based on a realistic and objective appraisal of a stressful situation or event? What is the family's definition of its situation?
3. How does the family react to stressful situations? What coping strategies are being used? What coping strategies has the family employed to deal with what types of problems? Do family members differ in their ways of coping with their present problem? If so, how?
4. Does the family use the following internal coping strategies?
   - Family group-reliance.
   - Use of a sense of humor.
   - Sharing of feelings, thoughts, and activities (maintaining cohesiveness).
   - Controlling the meaning of the problem/reframing.
   - Joint problem solving. What are the problem-solving abilities of various family members? Are they able to articulate their needs and concerns? Can they outline ways of satisfying these needs, arrive at solutions, implement, and evaluate them? (Robischon and Smith, 1977).
   - Role flexibility.
   - Normalizing.
5. Does the family use any of the following external coping strategies?
   - Seeking information.
   - Maintaining linkages with the community (general external involvement).
   - Seeking social support.

Informal support systems (friends, family, neighbors, employers, employees, organizations and groups—self-care or mutual aid groups and other groups with which family members have common interests or goals.
Formal support systems (professional services, both in health and health-related areas).
What support systems fulfill family's needs for support and assistance?
Seeking spiritual supports.
6. In what problem areas or situations has the family, in its dealings over time, achieved mastery?
7. What dysfunctional adaptive strategies has the family used or is the family using? Are there signs of any of the dysfunctionalities listed below? If so, record their presence and how extensively they are used.
Family violence (spouse, child, elder, parent, or sibling abuse).
Scapegoating.
Use of threat.
Child neglect.
Family myth.
Pseudomutuality.
Triangling.
Authoritarianism (marked dominance).

FAMILY NURSING DIAGNOSES

According to the North American Nursing Diagnosis Association (NANDA) classification of nursing diagnoses, there are four nursing diagnoses that specifically cover the focus of family coping processes and strategies. These are:

1. Family coping: Potential for growth
2. Ineffective family coping: Compromised
3. Ineffective family coping: Disabling
4. Potential for violence: (McFarland and McFarlane, 1989).

Other less specific diagnoses—such as knowledge deficit, social isolation, altered health management, and alteration in family processes—could also be used, but they would have to be specified in the defining characteristics and related factors to be sufficiently problem-focused.

The diagnosis of Family coping: Potential for growth, is family-systems-based and is appropriate for situations where the family nurse's goals are to assist families in coping effectively with the family demands/stressors. Families may be successfully adapting at this time, but anticipate certain health stressors and are in need of information to promote health and prevent problems in the future.

The diagnosis of Ineffective family coping: Compromised, is appropriate to use when the family assessment data show that the family is employing adaptive strategies that are ineffective for resolving present stressors and that because of the use of ineffective adaptive strategies, its functioning or adaptation is compromised.

The diagnosis of Ineffective family coping: Disabling, is used "when the behavior of one or more family members incapacitates the family (or individual members) to therapeutically adapt to the existing health challenge" (McFarland and McFarlane, 1989, p. 943). Although the generation and description of this diagnosis was guided by family systems theory, the above definition is ambiguous in terms of how family coping is used. Family coping in this text refers to the coping behaviors or responses made by a subsystem such as parent–child or spousal subsystem or the family as a whole—indicating an interactional level. Hence, the use of this diagnosis for family coping diagnoses should not include individual coping or adaptive responses; the outcome "disabling" would then refer to the family outcome(s).

Although Ineffective family coping: Disabling, can be long or short term, the family is having greater difficulties adapting when this diagnosis is used than when the previous diagnosis is used. Family health and growth are adversely affected here (McFarland and McFarlane, 1989).

In reviewing the diagnosis of Potential for violence, the diagnosis, defining characteristics, and suggested interventions are focused on the potentially violent individual. Using a family-centered approach, each of these areas need to be broadened to incorporate the family system and the family members at risk.

GENERAL FAMILY NURSING INTERVENTIONS

Because of the breadth that this chapter covers, general family nursing interventions are outlined here. Please refer to Chapter 18 for elaboration of the interventions identified in this section. Interventions are based on family assessment data pertaining to family stressors and coping (as outlined in the assessment section), as well as on the family nursing diagnoses.

Assisting Families at Risk to Cope

- Encourage all family members to be involved, especially fathers.
- Support (reinforce) effective coping strategies that families and family members are using to either reduce family tension, control the meaning of stressor(s), or eliminate stressor(s).
- For families that need to learn additional coping strategies, use teaching strategies including role modeling in the four areas listed in Table 17–4. Resources are provided here for stress management, cognitive reframing, life-style alteration, and use of self-help groups and assertiveness training.

For families that are employing ineffective family coping strategies, differentiate between whether the family is chronically dysfunctional (in that case referral for more long-term therapy is indicated) or in acute crisis, but functioning within normal limits until the onset of the stressor(s). In this case, family crisis intervention principles and an empowerment perspective are suggested as guides to family interventions.

1. *Family crisis intervention principles.* Family crisis intervention extends crisis intervention theory by incorporating a family focus. Very briefly, family crisis intervention is a short-term practice model for families experiencing crisis or stress to help them cope with present stressor(s) and future stressor(s). It involves (1) defining the precipitating stressor event and hazardous life events, (2) assessing the family's interpretation of the event(s), (3) assessing the family's resources and methods for coping with stressors, and (4) assessing the family's state of functioning. Based on this model, above, a supportive yet focused problem-solving approach is used to assist the family to mobilize resources (its own and community resources) to resolve the present crisis, and to learn how to prevent and cope with future stressful experiences (Kus, 1985).
2. *Empowering families.* Boss (1988) and Figley (1989), family researchers and clinicians, describe an approach involved with empowering families. Their suggestions extend and enrich the family crisis intervention model. Boss (1988) points out that for families that have been traumatized or victimized, learned helplessness is a common family reaction. If helplessness can be learned, she reasons, then helplessness can be unlearned. Empowerment comes from regaining self-esteem and self-confidence in family members and pride in the family as a team, regaining control over what happens to the family collectively and individually, making sense out of what happened by finding some meaning to the problem(s), and sharing with other family members while actively attempting to prevent the problem or event from recurring. Reassuring families that their reactions to traumatic situations are com-

TABLE 17–4. TEXTBOOK RESOURCES IN STRESS MANAGEMENT, COGNITIVE REFRAMING, LIFE-STYLE ALTERATION, AND USE OF SELF-HELP GROUPS AND ASSERTIVENESS TRAINING

Stress-Management Strategies

Bulechek GM, McCloskey JC, eds. *Nursing Interventions: Treatments for Nursing Diagnoses.* Philadelphia: Saunders; 1985. Chapters on stress management by editors, relaxation training by S. Scandrett and Uecker and music therapy KC Buckwalter, J. Hartsock and J. Gaffney.

Carlson RJ, Newman B, eds. *Issues and Trends in Health.* St Louis: Mosby; 1987. Several chapters on both stress management and exercise.

Lachman VD. *Stress management: A Manual for Nurses.* New York: Grune & Stratton; 1983.

Mealey AR, Richardson H, Dimico G. Family stress management. In: Bomar PJ, ed. *Nurses and Family Health Promotion.* Baltimore: Williams & Wilkins; 1989.

Steiger NJ, Lipson JG. *Self-care Nursing: Theory and Practice.* Bowie, MD: Brady; 1985.

Cognitive Reframing or Reappraisal

Scandrett S. Cognitive reappraisal. In Bulechek and McCloskey (reference above).

Minuchin S, Fishman HC. *Family Therapy Techniques.* Cambridge, MA: Harvard University Press; 1981.

Life-style Alteration

Several chapters in Bulechek and McCloskey (reference above) on various aspects of life-style alteration.

Pender NJ. *Health Promotion in Nursing Practice.* 2nd ed. Norwalk, CT: Appleton & Lange; 1987.

Use of Self-help Groups and Assertiveness Training

Sadler AG. Assertiveness training. In Bulechek and McCloskey (reference above).

Chapter on use of self-help groups. In Steiger and Lipson (reference above).

Trainor MG. Self-help groups as a resource for individual clients and families. In: Clements IW, Roberts FB, *Family Health: A Theoretical Approach to Nursing.* New York: Wiley; 1983.

mon and predictable, thereby "normalizing" their situation, is an effective supportive technique (Figley, 1989).

Figley (1989) implies that empowering families is as much a philosophical attitude toward working with traumatized families, as it is engaging in certain specified activities. When he views and treats dysfunctional families, his approach is tempered by his genuine respect for the natural resourcefulness of families. In the following passage, he explains this perspective:

> I try to empower the family by creating the kind of intervention context that results in the resolution of the traumatizing experience but, just as importantly, that results in the family's giving themselves most of the credit for the accomplishment. Moreover, this approach makes the family feel more confident to face any future traumatic experience equipped with the necessary information, skills, and problem-solving methods. (p. 42).

Protecting Family Members Who Are at Risk for Violence

1. Recognizing and reporting of child abuse.
2. Support and referral for abused spouses, elders, siblings, parents, the abuser, and the family unit.
3. Intra- and Interagency coordination of care to families and family members (Gilliss, et al, 1989).

Referring Families That Exhibit More Complex Family Coping Problems and Dysfunction

Referral and follow-up on ongoing family counseling or therapy; use of family systems approach.

Educating Families About Effective Coping to Promote and Maintain Family Health

Use of teaching strategies to provide family health education in the content areas listed above.

☐ *STUDY QUESTIONS*

1. Family coping is vitally important because (select the best answer):
   a. It is the mechanism through which family functions are made possible.
   b. It provides opportunities for family members to learn.
   c. It leads to problem solving and mastery over family issues and stresses.
   d. It either eliminates stressors or leads to stress-reduction activities.

2. In this chapter, one convincing piece of evidence that shows that many families are experiencing problems in adaptation (family coping) is (select the best answer):
   a. Crisis intervention centers are springing up everywhere.
   b. More money is being pumped into family counseling centers.
   c. The pervasiveness of mental disorders in our communities.
   d. Nursing is increasingly focusing on helping families cope with their health problems.

3. Match the definitions in the right-hand column with the concepts and terms in the left-hand column.

CONCEPTS/TERMS	DEFINITIONS
a. Crisis	1. The end result of functional coping, where repeated successful problem-solving efforts have taken place.
b. Mastery	2. Active, effective adaptive efforts.
c. Defense mechanism	3. The precipitating or initiating events or agents that generate stress.
d. Stressors	4. The general process of adjustment to change.
e. Stress	5. The strain, disequilibrium produced by threat or actual existence of stressors.
f. Adaptation	
g. Coping	

6. Habitual, stereotypic responses to threat or actual presence of stressors.
7. In the presence of the stress and stressors, the family's failure in use of effective adaptive strategies.

4. Minuchin has identified four general sources of family stressors. What are they?

Are the following statements True *or* False?

5. In the antestress period, anticipatory guidance would be contraindicated.

6. Defensive tactics are often necessary adaptive responses during the actual stress period.

7. During the poststress period, coping tactics consist of strategies to return the family to a homeostatic state.

8. In their studies, Holmes and Rahe were able to demonstrate the following relationships (select the best answer):
a. A positive correlation between stressor and stress.
b. A temporal relationship where high life change scores existed prior to the advent of illness.
c. A cause-and-effect relationship between number of life change events and presence of illness.
d. A negative correlation between stress and wellness.

9. The balancing of forces diagram given in Figure 17–4 extends the Holmes and Rahe model in these ways (select all appropriate answers):
a. It includes environmental factors.
b. It is adapted to fit the family system.
c. It takes into account the family's assets and strengths.
d. A higher level of wellness is seen as one type of "imbalance."

10. Pearlin and Schooler conducted a study of normative coping responses and found that in each of the following primary roles certain coping responses were perceived of as more effective by their respondents. Identify an effective coping response for each of the following roles.
a. Occupational and economic role.
b. Marital role.
c. Parental role.

11. Which of the following are two primary variables involved in whether crisis develops or not?
a. Compliance with environment.
b. Perception of event or change.
c. Coping resources.
d. Choice to grow or stagnate.
e. Open or closed communications.

12. Select four functional family coping strategies (two internal coping resources and two external coping strategies) and describe each of these briefly.

13. Select four dysfunctional family adaptive strategies and describe each of these briefly.

Choose the correct answers to the following question.

14. The two prime purposes of social support systems are to:
    a. Provide direct assistance.
    b. Become a family advocate.
    c. Replace professional services.
    d. Provide emotional support.

15. Indicate which of the following are functional (F) or dysfunctional (D) or which could be either (E) depending on the situation.
    a. Family group-reliance.
    b. Scapegoating.
    c. Pseudomutuality.
    d. Sense of humor.
    e. Increased linkage with community.
    f. Spouse violence.
    g. Child neglect.
    h. Triangling.
    i. Social support systems.
    j. Seeking of information.
    k. Role flexibility.
    l. Controlling the meaning of the problem by reframing.

16. Effective coping responses by families usually occur when:
    a. The family has adequate inner and outside resources to draw from.
    b. The crisis-provoking event is interpreted in an objective, realistic manner.
    c. Family bonds and unity exists.
    d. The family has the capacity to shift course and modify roles within the family.

17. The purpose(s) for families utilizing threat as a control mechanism is (are) to:
    a. Maintain authoritarian structure within the family.
    b. Maintain or reinstate connectedness within the family.
    c. Insure the survival of the family group.
    d. Decrease family members' attempts to behave in an autonomous, individualistic manner.

18. In tracing the usual sequence of events that occurs when a family experiences a crisis, or after the family is faced with a stressful event with which it cannot effectively cope, what consequences then follow?

19. Hill's family stress theory has been extended by McCubbin and Patterson as well as by Boss. McCubbin and Patterson extend Hill's theory by (select the correct answers):
    a. Focusing on the postcrisis period of family adaptation.
    b. Modifying the ABCX variables.
    c. Adding coping specifically to the model or theory.
    d. Eliminating the cause–effect aspect of the theory.

Family Case Study*

Read the following family study, then assess the family in the areas of affective functioning and family coping functioning of the family.

Mrs. Ruby Nichols, a 34-year-old obese woman, came to the mental health clinic because, she said, "I just don't know what to do." She was crying hysterically and unable to respond to further questioning. After remaining with her for an hour, the nurse was able to elicit that her 5-year-old foster daughter was being removed from her home per court order. Welfare funds, her only support for herself, her unemployed husband, and their five children, were being terminated in a week, leaving her unable to pay the bills or buy enough food for her family. Although Mrs. Nichols was still tearful and depressed, she was able to be driven home by a community worker.

The following day the nurse made a visit to the Nichols' home. Mrs. Nichols related the following history.

Ruby and John Nichols had been married 15 years. Four children were born of the marriage: Priscilla, 13; Cindy, 10; John Jr., 6; and Lisa, 4. They also had a foster daughter, Ann, age 5. The couple had known each other a year before their marriage in their home town of Smithfield, Louisiana. John was an unskilled laborer, but had always managed to be employed. Ruby had attended business school prior to the marriage and was employed as a bookkeeper until the first child was born. She described her early marriage as fine except for moving so many times, caused by John's "meddling mother." The family would move to get away from his mother, but she would always manage to locate them and appear on the scene. "We were a healthy, happy family and everything was fine as long as John's mother stayed away." Ruby related that this source of conflict between herself and John was resolved each time by a new move on their part. However, she and John never really discussed their mother-in-law problems according to Ruby. Following each new move, Ruby would join clubs and organizations to make new friends and John's work provided a similar opportunity for him. John also spent several evenings a week in the local bar, "shooting the bull" with the boys from work.

The last move was 6 months ago. After 2 months John lost his job and was unable to find another. This resulted in the family receiving welfare, which Ruby and John felt ashamed of, as they had always prided themselves on paying their own bills. Shortly after this, John's mother found the family and moved into town. When she came to visit, a bitter argument ensued regarding John's mother and since then John had been staying away from home and drinking a lot. Moreover, 3 months ago Ruby had abdominal surgery which was followed by complications and a prolonged hospitalization period. During her absence from home, the role of mother was assumed by Priscilla, who managed well with the help from the next door neighbor, Mrs. Law.

Ruby was released from the hospital 3 weeks ago as sufficiently recovered to stay at home. When she got home she perceived that the children had functioned "very well" in her absence; in fact, she felt that they did not need her and even seemed to resent her. John remained away most of the time and was minimally involved in family life during her hospitalization, as well as presently.

A week ago she learned of the court's decision to remove Ann from the home and the termination of welfare funds. Ruby felt herself becoming less and less able to manage and admitted to depression and suicidal thoughts. However, her

* *Adapted with permission from Black (1974).*

concern for her children prevented her from doing anything self-destructive. The next-door-neighbor, Mrs. Law, realizing the gravity of the family's situation, told Ruby to go to the mental health clinic for help.

Subsequent visits to the family revealed that the children were having problems and that Ruby had difficulties relating to their problematic behaviors. It was observed that the children and parents did not discuss these problems or their concerns with each other, and that there was no movement toward sharing their feelings about Ann's leaving, the mother-in-law's disruptive influence, or Ruby's health problems.

Priscilla, age 13, seemed to resent Ruby's return, because it meant the loss of her mothering role. She and her mother have engaged in frequent arguments over the discipline of the younger children, what they should wear, and how they should act. The arguments usually ended with Priscilla leaving the house for long periods of time without telling Ruby where she was. This caused Ruby to worry. Priscilla was not interested in school, her main interest being to grow up as quickly as possible and emulate her mother. She also wanted desperately to be independent and make her own decisions in life. Ruby had "weaned" Priscilla early in terms of her being self-sufficient at home: from age 6 on, Priscilla was caring for her younger siblings and helping her mother out in the home.

Cindy, age 10, seemed unaffected by the situation. She was quite involved with her school activities and Campfire Girls and spent much time in these activities and at her friends' homes. Priscilla and Cindy evidently have a closer sibling relationship than the other siblings do. Cindy tells "all her secrets" to Priscilla when she is upset, worried, or needs someone to talk to.

John Jr., a first grader, was refusing to go to school. Every morning it was now a struggle to get him off to school. He would cry and hang on to his mother. His teacher reported poor school work and lack of attentiveness when he was present.

Lisa, age 4, displayed similar clinging behaviors to that of John Jr. She seemed frightened when mother left the home and was wetting the bed again after having no problems in this area for 2 years. Both John Jr. and Lisa frequently questioned their mother about the recent absence of Ann. They asked if Ann went away because she was "bad."

On the third contact between the family (the parents) and the nurse at the mental health clinic, the nurse asked the parents to describe each child, what he or she was like, and what personal needs or problems they were trying to assist their children with at that time. It was noted that specific information on each child was difficult to obtain. For instance, these general statements were made: "Oh, he (she) is just the average 6-year-old (or whatever age applied)," or "Priscilla's just like all other teenagers, wanting her way all the time," or "I treat all my children the same, regardless." They were able to recognize, though, Priscilla's need to care for her younger siblings and to be independent, but were not open to her staying away from the family very much, or developing a set of friends outside the family with whom she might have frequent social contact.

The mother also recognized that Lisa was very attached to and dependent on her, and needed reassurance that mother would be back when she left home. Additionally, both parents thought Ann's leaving was threatening to the younger children, who might think this might happen to them if they misbehaved. Ruby was trying to spend more time with Lisa to help her with her fears over the mother's separation and Ann's leaving. John showed interest in "comforting" and being involved with Lisa also, since Lisa always responded "in such a cute, loving way to her daddy," according to the mother.

Both parents are able to show affection and warmth to the younger children (John Jr. and Lisa), but do not feel that it is appropriate to be so "physical" when they get older. It was noted that the parents were not physically affectionate to each other and seemed emotionally distant during the interviews. Ruby says that they have never shared their personal concerns with each other much. "It takes another woman to understand my feelings. I used to confide in Priscilla a lot, but since she is upset with me, I haven't been able to talk with her."

20. What short- and long-term stressors are impinging on the family? What strengths counterbalance these stressors?

21. Is the family able to act based on a realistic and objective appraisal of the situation?

22. How does the family react to stressful situations? Both functional and dysfunctional strategies should be described.

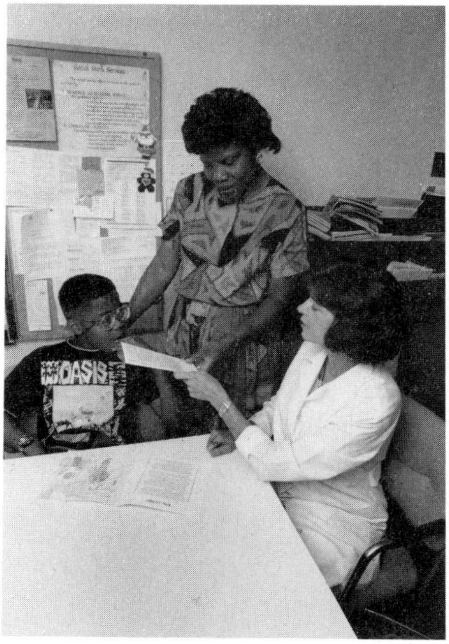

PART IV

General Family Nursing Interventions

Part IV contains only one chapter, a chapter that was added in this third edition and that focuses on the major family nursing interventions that cut across the many possible family nursing diagnoses. Chapter 18 should be referred to when the reader needs more information about one of the six major family interventions: teaching, counseling, contracting, case management, collaboration, and consultation.

CHAPTER EIGHTEEN

Family Nursing Interventions

Learning Objectives

1. Explain how active family participation can be accomplished during the intervention phase of the family nursing process.
2. Relative to the family nursing interventions of teaching, counseling, contracting, case management, and collaboration:
   a. Define and/or explain what the particular intervention strategy entails.
   b. Describe with what types of family nursing diagnoses the intervention strategy would be helpful.
   c. Discuss the limitations of using the intervention strategy.
3. Identify major variables that affect the efficacy of client teaching.
4. Compare the teaching–learning process with the nursing process.
5. Describe the difference between teaching and counseling.
6. Describe the family nurse's role relative to consultation, client advocacy, and coordination.

Upon completion of the planning phase, where goals are formulated, alternative intervention strategies and resources identified, and priorities set, the intervention phase commences. Family nursing intervention is addressed in more general terms in Chapter 3. The present chapter has been added in this third edition to give the reader greater information about major intervention strategies used in family nursing.

In the first and second editions of this book, "direct provision of care" and "case finding/epidemiology" were discussed. These were deleted in this edition, because direct provision of care seems to be individually oriented and case finding/epidemiology seems to be community health oriented. This in no way diminishes their importance. The intervention strategies presented here, however, are those that are applied to the family system or subsystem.

Intervention is a multifaceted process. In working with families, a wide array of interventions are dynamically and flexibly used. Six major family nursing intervention strategies are explored in this chapter: teaching, counseling, contracting, case management, collaboration, and consultation. These strategies cut across many areas of family nursing practice and are applicable with the use of different theories and diagnoses.

Six other types of family nursing interventions are also described, but appear within the chapter where they are most germane. These interventions tend to be more focused on particular aspects of family nursing practice and so are addressed here. The interventions and where they are discussed are as follows:

INTERVENTION	CHAPTER LOCATION
Environmental modification	Chapter 9
Role supplementation and role modeling	Chapter 12
Use of social support and self-help groups	Chapter 8, 17
Family crisis intervention	Chapter 17
Cognitive reappraisal and reframing	Chapter 17
Behavior modification	Chapter 15
Life-style modification	Chapter 16

ACTIVE FAMILY PARTICIPATION

In keeping with the premise that families have the right and responsibility to make their own health decisions, active family participation is an essential approach to be incorporated into each of the subsequent family nursing intervention strategies. Family involvement in the implementation phase often means to engage the family in mutual problem solving, as well as to discuss and decide the best or most feasible approaches to use to accomplish the agreed upon goal(s).

Inclusion of as many family members as possible in planned educational and counseling/supportive sessions is very helpful (Doherty and Campbell, 1988; Drotar, Crawford and Bush, 1984). It allows family members to express themselves and support each other. It also stimulates much-needed group discussion and feedback and assures that all attending members obtain the needed information. One family member may ask novel questions, which then exposes the rest of the participating members to the discussion that follows.

In families with a chronically ill child it often happens that only the mother is involved in managing the child's illness. This most common dysfunctional arrangement leads to the father and healthy siblings feeling "left out" (Drotar et al, 1984), and it progressively distances them from the mother–sick child dyad. It also keeps them from having first-hand information about the health problem and treatment and from having opportunities to discuss problems and support each other.

In caring for a sick family member in the hospital or home, especially if the illness is life threatening, the family members often feel helpless, powerless, and stressed. Wright and Leahey (1987) provide several intervention suggestions aimed at involving the family and reducing its stress. These include teaching caregiving techniques and how to touch and hold the patient without disrupting treatments, as well as encouraging family members to take on particular caregiving roles. Involvements such as these provide the family with a sense of competency (Power and Dell Orto, 1988).

Closely associated with a sense of competency is the notion of empowerment of families. As family nurses, we want to assist families to be empowered so that they may have the knowledge and capability to solve their own health problems, change their own lives, and fulfill their own health goals. Malinski (1987) states that we can empower clients by "recognizing them as equal partners in the health care system and sharing knowledge and skills with them, enabling clients to exercise their autonomy in deciding which options to choose" (p. 28).

TEACHING

A major family nursing intervention is teaching families about health, illness, health and human systems, family dynamics, child rearing, health care treatments, and other related areas. Teaching strategies are processes that facilitate learning. The aim of learning is to support healthy behaviors or to change unhealthy behaviors, albeit alterations of behavior are not always immediate or observable. Steiger and Lipson (1985) enumerate four goals of health teaching (Table 18–1).

Watson (1985) stresses that education provides information to clients, thereby assisting them to cope more effectively with life changes and stressful events. Gaining meaningful information helps family members feel a sense of control and reduce stress. It also enables them to define their own options and problem-solve.

Health teaching today needs to be geared toward assisting the patient and family to engage in self-care and self-responsibility. No longer should health care professionals foster dependency and immaturity. Adult family members need to feel they have the capacity to care for themselves and their family, and the right to sufficient information so that they can make their own decisions. If this philosophy is established

TABLE 18–1. GOALS OF HEALTH TEACHING

1. To provide information so that clients are able to make informed decisions with regard to health and illness.
2. To assist clients to participate effectively in care and cure.
3. To assist clients to adapt to the realities of an illness and its treatment.
4. To assist clients to experience the satisfaction of seeing their own efforts contribute toward improvement of health.

Adapted from Steiger and Lipson (1985).

early in family-nurse relationships, then the traditional superordinate-subordinate positions no longer are appropriate. As health educators, we need to play the role of facilitator and resource person to clients who will decide which options are best for them.

Teaching interventions today often include teaching nursing skills to family caregivers. With the advent of Diagnostic Related Groups (DRGs) and other cost-saving policies by the federal government and other third-party reimbursers, increasing numbers of very sick patients are being sent home. Family-centered home health nurses are assuming much greater responsibility in teaching caregivers how to care for their recovering family members.

Teaching–Learning Process

The teaching–learning process is similar to the nursing process in that both contain the same basic steps: assessment, problem statement (in teaching these are called "learning needs"), goals, implementation, and evaluation.

Assessment. When formally teaching, assessment of the family members' readiness to learn is part of the assessment and is crucial to ascertain before proceeding further. The two types of readiness consist of emotional and experiential readiness. *Emotional readiness* involves the motivation to learn, while *experiential readiness* includes adequacy of background knowledge, mastery of specific skills, and knowledge, attitudes, and values related to learning (Steiger and Lipson, 1985). Readiness is more complex and difficult to assess in a family, because readiness varies among the family members. Adults particularly learn best when they are ready and willing to learn (Knowles, 1973). Watson (1985) contends that more emphasis should be placed on the client's learning process. As part of assessing readiness factors, the family nurse should work within the family's framework to discover family members' perceptions and informational and skill needs.

Problem Identification. Generally speaking, learning needs of families regarding health and illness matters are great, especially when a family member has a serious and complex health problem. Knowledge deficits about family health promotion and all that this entails should, however, not be overlooked as a central focus for teaching.

Among the North American Nursing Diagnosis Association (NANDA) diagnoses that are relevant with respect to teaching interventions, knowledge deficit is probably one of the most germane diagnoses for family nursing. It is a general diagnosis, and so must be further specified in the defining characteristics and contributing factors. Although the NANDA diagnosis is individually oriented it can easily be extended to include the family.

Planning. The establishment of goals or objectives and the ability to measure how well the objectives are met are essential to the teaching–learning process. Short-term and long-term realistic, client-centered goals are often formulated. The simple imparting of information cannot be considered teaching, particularly if there is no evidence that the client has learned or met the objectives of the teaching. Needless to say, for learning to occur, it is crucial that the health educator and client share similar objectives.

Determining the particular teaching strategies to be employed is also part of planning.

Implementation of Teaching Plan. Working with the whole family or sets of relationships within the family makes the actual teaching more complex. Imparting information means that there are probably two different generations to teach and both have different emotional and experiential readiness levels. Teaching the family demands a more flexible, interactive teaching modality. Many times role modeling is used, especially when teaching families how to communicate more clearly and openly.

Teaching in family nursing means much more than the formal, structured imparting of information. It also entails informal teaching—that which goes on in spontaneous client–nurse interactions. It includes modeling, demonstrating, and experiential strategies, which help the family learn new competencies or gain a more positive definition of their situation (called "reframing").

Documentation and Evaluation. Documenting that the teaching has been accomplished, the client's response, and the extent to which the objective(s) have been met—as perceived jointly by nurse and family—completes the teaching–learning process. As with the nursing process, if the goals or objectives were not fully met, then analysis of what barriers to learning existed is in order. With barriers identified, modification of the teaching–learning plan typically follows (Steiger and Lipson, 1985).

Types of Learning

Learning involves acquiring new thoughts and ideas (cognitive learning), attitudes (affective learning), and behaviors (psychomotor skill acquisition) (Bloom, 1956). Recognition is needed of the three kinds of learning when planning teaching interventions, because all three types of learning are important (Lester,

TABLE 18–2. VARIABLES AFFECTING TEACHING EFFECTIVENESS

Client Factors
- Motivation of family members. Motivation is the critical force or drive that activates persons to change.
- Ages of family members.
- Members' psychological state (eg, anxiety, depression level).
- Family members' perception of health problem(s).

Communication Factors
Communication involves the exchange of information between the sender and the receiver. Barriers to communication include those due to:
- Lack of comprehension of subject matter.
- Cultural and language barriers.
- Socioeconomic barriers.
- Inability to communicate clearly with teacher and each other.

Situational Factors
- The environment in which the teaching–learning takes place.
- The timing of the teaching.
- The teaching modalities used.

1986). Moreover, the three types of learning are interdependent. For example, if our attitudes about food and nutrition change, then behavioral changes often follow. Acquiring self-care skills leads to more positive attitudes about self-care.

Variables Affecting Teaching Effectiveness/Learning

There are numerous factors that can positively or negatively influence the efficacy of the teaching intervention. Client and contextual variables that affect teaching effectiveness are listed in Table 18–2.

Informal Teaching: Provision of Information

Where sharing of information occurs in spontaneous encounters between nurse and family members, or information is communicated to family members in an unstructured manner, informal teaching is involved. Doherty and Campbell (1988) detail the skills that health care professionals need when providing ongoing medical information and advice to families. The skills are:

- Regularly and clearly communicating health findings and treatment options to family members.
- Attentively listening to family members' questions and concerns.
- Advising families how to handle the health and rehabilitation needs of the patient. (p. 132)

The type of quality of health information may vary depending on the family members with whom one speaks. Accuracy of information is paramount, however, and who provides what information should be coordinated when nursing and other health care team members are involved.

Providing Information to Families With Critically Ill Members. Clinical practice and family research indicate that in all health care settings families desire more information than they obtain from health care professions. This need for information is heightened when family members are hospitalized and critically ill (Wright and Leahey, 1987). Families want to be regularly informed about their loved one's condition, treatments, and progress. One important strategy suggested (Bozett and Gibbons, 1983) is for the nurse to make regular telephone contact with the family. This strategy has benefits for both the nurse, who now controls the dissemination of information and no longer sees the family as being disruptive and bothersome, and the family, which feels that it does not have to be constantly at the hospital and is less anxious because of the supportive information being regularly provided (Bozett and Gibbons, 1983).

Role Modeling

In addition to informal teaching strategies, role modeling is a powerful modality for teaching family members how to modify their behaviors. This approach is particularly important for pediatric family-centered nurses who serve as important role models when teaching parents; for primary care and community based nurses when they teach positive health behaviors; and for family mental health nurses when they teach family members how to communicate and interact more functionally. "Practice what you preach" is the well-used adage here. "There is nothing less motivating than a health care provider who encourages the client to stop smoking or lose weight yet is overweight and smells of tobacco" (Steiger and Lipson, 1985, p. 15).

Anticipatory Guidance

Anticipatory guidance is an important facet of health teaching. Discussing probable events, feelings, and situations with the family provides for clarification of ideas, reduction of anxiety, and future role change adaptability. Anticipation of and preparation for the coming event will make the event less traumatic for the family and allow family members to better handle the stressor.

An example of the benefits of anticipatory guidance is the success that Lamaze classes enjoy. When labor begins, both parents are fully prepared and usually go through the labor and delivery with excitement and positive feelings. This positive birthing experience gives the parents' positive feedback about their ability to handle future parenting challenges.

In conclusion, teaching interventions are one of the most central types of family nursing interventions. Family health professionals need to keep in mind, however, that knowledge in and of itself does not necessarily lead to needed changes in behavior. As the Health Belief Model describes (Rosenstock, 1974; Pender, 1987), changes in health behaviors are due to multiple factors. A meta-analysis (a synthesis of multiple studies) of patient teaching research demonstrated that patient education outcomes tend to be positive and clearly better than outcomes for patients who had no teaching (Mumford et al, 1982). This meta-analysis also confirmed that in teaching, presentation of knowledge alone is not the most effective option. For instance, approaches that combine information with emotional support to relieve anxiety in one meta-analysis (Mumford et al, 1982) were reported to be superior to the provision of information alone.

COUNSELING

Until recently, counseling has been thought by most nurses to be appropriate only for those in psychiatric–mental health nursing. It is now widely accepted, however, that there are levels of sophistication and complexity in counseling and that family counseling (called family interviewing by Wright and Leahey, 1984) is a core family nursing intervention. Family therapy, an advanced form of counseling, is viewed by this author as well as by the American Nurses' Association Council of Psychiatric-Mental Health Nurses (1982) as requiring advanced education, training, and skills.

Although not called counseling, nursing has long been concerned with nursing's therapeutic interpersonal process (Peplau, 1952). Patterson and Zderad (1976), in their description of humanistic nursing, assert that the crux of nursing is the existence of an authentic dialogue between nurse and patient and that the goal of this dialogue is growth promotion and nurturance of the human potential. Counseling and supportive intervention strategies are congruent with these ideas about nursing's role and goals.

Difference Between Teaching and Counseling

Closely related to teaching, but different, is counseling (Redman and Thomas, 1985). Teaching and counseling have been described as being situated at different ends of a continuum (Fig. 18–1). Applying this perspective,

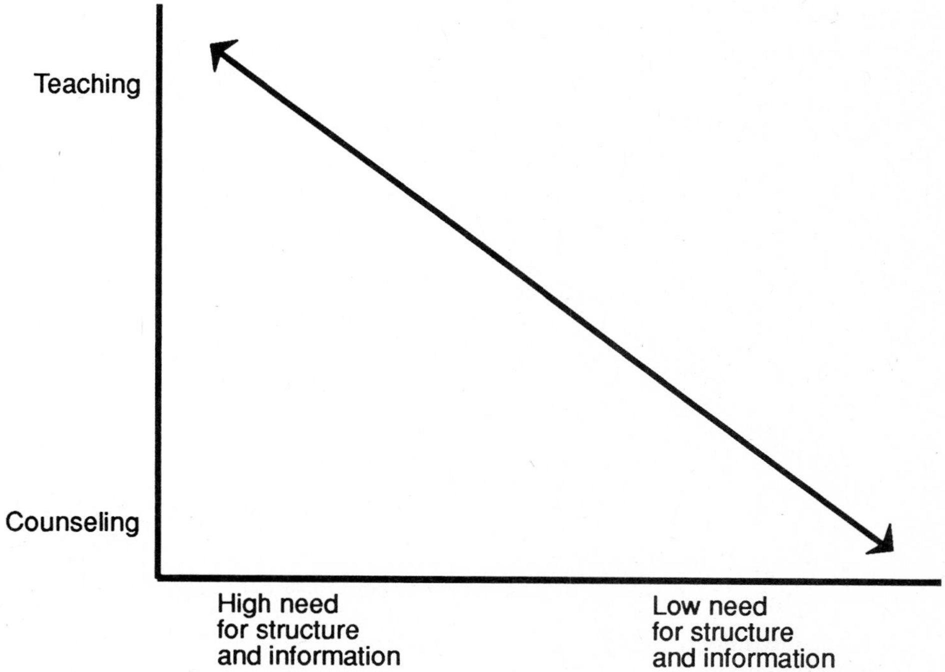

Figure 18–1
Variation in interpersonal intervention approach is influenced by family's need for structure and information.

TABLE 18–3. DIFFERENCES BETWEEN TRADITIONALLY DEFINED TEACHING AND TRADITIONALLY DEFINED COUNSELING

Criteria for Comparison	Teaching	Counseling
Role of nurse	Nurse-directed	Client-directed
Level of family functioning	High dependency (low independence)	Low dependency (high independence)
Type of learning involved	Combination of cognitive, affective, and psychomotor learning	Primarily emotional (affective) and cognitive learning
Goal and modalities used	Nurse-directed	Client-directed
Amount of structure within intervention	High structure	Low structure

teaching is viewed as the mode of choice when working with a family that requires more structure and specific information. Counseling, at the other end of the continuum, is appropriate when working with a family that requires less structure, minimal direction, and more support and encouragement to utilize its own problem-solving skills.

Although this dichotomy makes it sound like the nurse engages either in teaching or counseling, the two strategies can be used almost simultaneously with the same family. The family nurse can teach about the importance of hearing each family member's beliefs and feelings about a particular situation and then in the next breath encourage each member to express his or her own perceptions and feelings. Thus somewhere in the middle of the continuum the nurse uses both strategies flexibly in interactions with families. Table 18–3 presents the major differences between the two intervention strategies.

In this model, teaching is defined in a more traditional sense (structured and instructor-guided), while counseling is defined in a nondirective sense (unstructured and client-guided). The counseling role consists of the family nurse being a facilitator and resource person to the family, leaving the family members to independently make their own decisions. Encouraging the family to explore perceptions and feelings and identify alternatives for coping would be prime goals.

Defining Counseling

Although there are numerous approaches in counseling, all connote an interpersonal intervention process. Banks (1985) offers the following broad definition of counseling:

> Counseling is an interactive helping process between a counselor and a client characterized by the core elements of acceptance, empathy, genuineness, and congruency. This relationship consists of a series of interactions over time in which the counselor, through a variety of active and passive techniques, focuses on the needs, problems, or feelings of the client which have interfered with the client's usual adaptive behavior. (p. 105)

The core elements of counseling, then, are empathy, or the experiencing or sensing of another's feelings and behaviors; acceptance or unconditional positive regard for the client; and congruency or genuineness, being unpretentious and honest in the client–nurse relationship (Rogers, 1951; Truax and Carkhuff, 1967). Underlying these attributes is a respect for others, free of authoritarian judgments and coercive pressure (Banks, 1985), as well as a caring for and about the family.

As with teaching, counseling interventions can be used in addressing many different types of family nursing diagnoses and problems. Of the NANDA diagnoses relevant for family nursing (Table 3–2), counseling is an appropriate type of intervention for all these diagnoses. Family counseling strategies, identified by Doherty and Campbell (1988) as part of their "levels of clinician involvement with families," are summarized in Table 18–4.

Family Counseling of Families in Crisis

Family counseling is often used to help a family deal with a crisis (Hartman and Laird, 1983). One of the nurse's functions here is to increase families' sense of competence, expanding their repertoire of family coping efforts, including aiding the family members in problem solving. Helping families develop their own methods for coming up with solutions to their problems is congruent with a self-care approach to intervention. Moreover, reframing the family members' view of their problem is often used to assist family members to search for alternative behavioral, cognitive, and affective responses to the problem (Hartman and Laird, 1983; Minuchin and Fishman, 1981).

TABLE 18–4. FAMILY COUNSELING STRATEGIES

Feelings and Support Level of Involvement by Family Clinicians

1. Asking the family members questions that elicit their concerns and feelings about health problems and their effects on the family.
2. Empathically listening to their concerns and feelings, normalizing them when appropriate.
3. Supporting family members in their coping efforts.
4. Tailoring health and illness advice to family members' unique needs, concerns, and feelings.
5. Identifying family dysfunction and initiating referral to meet unique needs of family.

Systematic Assessment and Planned Intervention Level of Involvement

1. Engaging family members, even the reluctant ones, in a planned family conference(s).
2. Structuring the family conference so that all participating members have an opportunity and are encouraged to express themselves.
3. Supporting individual members while avoiding forming a coalition with family members.
4. Reframing the family's definition of its problem or situation in a way that makes it seem more positive and manageable.
5. Assisting family members to view their problem(s) as requiring collaborative efforts.
6. Helping the family problem solve and generate alternative mutually acceptable ways to cope with its problem(s).
7. Assisting the family to balance its coping responses in a way that allows for support and cohesiveness and yet does not rob individuals of their autonomy.
8. Identifying family dysfunctions beyond clinician's level of competency and orchestrating referral that educates both family and therapist to the further need for assistance.

Adapted from Doherty and Campbell (1988).

Limitations of and Barriers to Counseling

The barriers to counseling effectiveness are the same as those associated with teaching. Socioeconomic and cultural barriers are particularly troublesome when working with the diverse forms of families nurses serve. Family client motivational problems are also critical barriers to assisting families.

Three additional limitations often curtail what nursing can do in counseling families. First, if the organization for which the family nurse works is not supportive of family nursing counseling interventions (Wright and Leahey, 1984), and hence does not allocate time for this type of intervention or reward the nurse for counseling families, this serves as a major barrier. Second, if the families themselves do not see nurses fulfilling this role, they are often resistant to counseling, unless the nurse can clarify his or her role and gain the participation of the family. A third basic limitation to counseling by family nurses is the reality of today's cost-containment practice mileau. With time and efficiency highly valued to keep costs contained, family counseling activities are often neglected or not feasible.

The decision as to whether to counsel a family is ultimately based upon several primary factors. The first of these is the family's level of functioning, which then implies the intensity or seriousness of the family's problems—or the reverse, the family's health. The family nurse's competence to counsel a particular family is the second consideration. Third, the work context makes a difference. Within the present work environment, is it feasible to counsel the family as needed? If counseling is indicated and mutually agreed upon, then what areas to focus on, who to see, and how long to work with the family are key considerations (Wright and Leahey, 1984).

CONTRACTING

An effective means by which a family-centered nurse can realistically assist individuals and families to engage in self-care is through the use of contracts. Contracting is also an excellent way of involving the family in a collaborative process.

Client contracting has been used in nursing since the 1970s and has been particularly efficacious when working with certain groups of individual clients, such as those with drug and alcohol problems and those who have compliance and pain-control difficulties (Jensen, 1985).

A contract is a working agreement made between two or more people, in this case a family and a nurse. To be timely and relevant, contracts are continuously renegotiable and cover the following areas: goals, length of the contract, client responsibilities (commitments), and health care team members' responsibilities, steps toward meeting the goals, and rewards for meeting goals (Sloan and Schommer, 1975; Steiger and Lipson, 1985). A contract may be written (Table 18–5) or verbal. One of the advantages of making a contract is that at the end of the contract period, progress is evaluated and either a new contract made

TABLE 18–5. BASIC COMPONENTS IN CLIENT CONTRACTING

- Purpose or goals of the contract: short term and/or long term.
- Implementation: activities taken to reach goals and by whom.
- Priorities in terms of goals or activities.
- Reward when goals are met.
- Time parameters: when activities are to be accomplished.
- Reevaluation date to determine progress.
- Cosigners and date: family members and nurse.

or the relationship terminated (Wright and Leahey, 1984).

The philosophy underlying the use of contracts is that of client involvement and the encouragement of self-care and self-responsibility. The contract draws clients in as the chief partners in their health care. Effective use of contract development and implementation is dependent on family involvement. For contracts involving family health problems, it is essential that the contract be made with the responsible and appropriate family members. Otherwise, family system problems cannot be properly addressed.

Nursing Diagnoses and Contracting

According to Jensen (1985), client contracting is particularly appropriate for clients with the following types of nursing diagnoses: noncompliance, knowledge deficit, ineffective coping, alterations in parenting, and self-care deficit diagnoses. Loveland-Cherry (1988 & 1989) encourages family-centered nurses to also use contracting with family health-promotion diagnoses.

Limitations to the Use of Contracting

In client contracting, first and foremost the clients must be actively involved in the development, goal setting, and implementation. Because of this requirement, certain types of clients are automatically not appropriate candidates. Families where the adult members are very dependent, disturbed, cognitively impaired, retarded, or not responsible, are poor candidates because of their inability to help develop and carry out their part of the agreement. Very young children within the family, unless the parent(s) is involved, are also not able to develop or carry through on their commitment.

It is also pointed out in the literature that client contracting takes time and effort, and in contracting the nurse may feel some loss of control, because the majority of the responsibility for implementation shifts to the family client.

In summary, the essential components of this intervention according to the literature (Bulechek and McCloskey, 1985) are identified as (1) active client input into goal setting; and (2) when the goal has been met, the provision of positive reinforcement.

CASE MANAGEMENT

Although nursing case management of families is not directly discussed in the nursing literature, recently nursing case management of the individual client has received substantial attention and interest (ANA Task Force on Case Management, 1988; Baier, 1987; Smith, 1988; Zander, 1988).

Defining Case Management

Case management is seen as both a strategy and a clinical decision-making process. Many definitions of case management appear in the literature. Nevertheless, there is a consensus that the process involves five essential steps: client assessment; planning; linking (referring, coordinating, and advocacy); monitoring; and evaluating (ANA Task Force on Case Management, 1988; Joint Commission for Accreditation of Community Mental Health Service Programs, 1976; Weil et al, 1985). As a process of determining, integrating, and monitoring complex client needs, it seeks to balance quality of care outcomes with efficient use of existing resources. Specific characteristics of case management identified in the literature include (1) its emphasis on active client participation; (2) its holistic orientation; (3) its self-care, self-deterministic orientation; and (4) the coordination and efficient use of a wide range of human services (ANA Task Force on Case Management, 1988; White, 1986).

As can be seen from the above definition, the case-management process and the process used in nursing practice (the nursing process) appear very similar. The crucial difference lies in the breadth and scope of the client assessment (the case management assessment is more comprehensive relative to assessment of psychosocial, environmental, and health-related variables) and the planning and resource identification with clients and members of the service network. This entails greater service coordination (Weil et al, 1985).

Client Advocacy

A major component of case management is client advocacy. An advocate is one who speaks for and on behalf of some other person or group. It is also someone who vindicates or espouses a cause by argument, a defender or intercessor, such as the position of defense attorney assumes. Kosik's (1972) definition relative to client advocacy by nurses extends the above definitions, incorporating a deeper commitment to the client. She explains:

> For me, patient advocacy is seeing that the patient knows what to expect and what is his right to have, and then displaying the willingness and courage to see that our system does not prevent his getting it. The goals of patient advocacy are, first, making a person more independent because he knows the what, why, and how of the system and, second, changing the system to make it more sensitive and relevant by revealing injustices and inadequacies, thereby making complacent continuation of the status quo

> impossible. The nurse may have to make waves. She may have to see that workers and agencies do their jobs and expose the indifference and inhumanity of care givers. (p. 694)

The role of being a client advocate involves informing clients and then supporting them in whatever decision they make. Although a goal of client advocacy is client independence, the advocate may have to accept and perhaps even foster dependency temporarily, for many people, especially the poor, have never had their dependency needs met. And thus we need to start there and assist the person or family to grow.

Community-based family nurses are in a strong position to act as advocates. They are in the community working with families that are often poor and feeling powerless and hopeless. Not only is there a greater need for the community health nurse to assume this role because of client needs, but unless this position is assumed, often one cannot go on to render the other essential services that the family needs. Nurses in hospitals also have an important opportunity to act as family advocates—making sure that families and their members receive needed services and that the services they are receiving are appropriate and of good quality.

Thus the family nurse can be a client advocate in at least two ways: (1) by assisting the client to obtain what he or she is entitled to from the system and (2) by trying to make the system more responsive to client needs in general. Family advocacy can range from calling the welfare department before referring a family, in an effort to pave the way for them, to testifying in court on behalf of a client, calling a meeting with representatives from several agencies to coordinate and improve services to the community, or acting as a political activist working in the political and legislative areas to create needed changes in the health and welfare system for families.

Clark (1984) points out that "advocacy necessitates involvement and commitment. The effective community health nurse cannot be content with the attitude, 'I'd like to help you, but my hands are tied.' Advocacy is not a popular concept" (p. 53), because it often means standing up to other health care and social service professionals and health care agencies for the rights of families. Advocacy also means assisting families to learn how to speak up for themselves—to be their own "best" advocates.

Coordination

The essence of case management is coordination. In fact, case management is often referred to as service coordination, designed to provide multiple services to clients with complex needs within a single locus of control (Seltzer et al, 1989).

The family nurse in community health or primary care is often the key person in the provision of comprehensive, continuous family health care. In addition to the particular functions the nurse is implementing, he or she supports other team members and interprets the nursing objectives and service, as well as coordinates nursing services with the various other services the family is receiving.

Without coordination the client may receive a duplication of some services from different agencies or, even more distressing, a gap in essential areas of need. An illustration of this problem from home health care follows. A rehabilitation clinic patient once remarked to various members of the health care team that she was having difficulty getting out of the bathtub and had no shower facilities to switch to. Each time she mentioned this to the team members they noted her response, but no one made any suggestions of what to do. A social worker, sanitarian, homemaker-home health aid, and visiting nurse were all visiting the family concurrently. In this type of situation it is the nurse's responsibility to make sure that collaboration is taking place and coordinated efforts are being achieved. With a greater number of more acutely and seriously ill patients discharged early from hospital to home and followed by multiservice home health agencies, the nurse's role as case manager or coordinator of services is being expanded. Hospice home care programs are examples of programs where the nurse plays a vital coordination function.

Promoting continuity of care for long-term chronically ill patients and their families is a particularly great need. Discharge planning and implementation is one example of continuity of care. The nurse must make continuing efforts to improve referral systems between the various health care and welfare agencies in the community, and must be willing to share information with referring agencies, given the client's approval. Referral is a two-way street, and communication must flow in both directions for the system to be functional.

In summary, the family-oriented nurse often functions as a bridge between the family and various services by acquainting the family with available community resources, effecting continuity of care, and coordinating and monitoring the services the client is receiving.

Case Management: For Whom?

Great optimism is expressed about how implementation of case management by nurses improves care. For both acute and community settings, among patients where complex and serious health and social problems exist, case management is looked upon as a cost-effective, comprehensive practice strategy.

Case management first appeared in connection with workmen's compensation and physical rehabilitation in the 1940s (Jellinek, 1988) and later, in the 1970s in the social welfare literature (Grau, 1984). Although public health nursing had been using the term "case management" for many years to describe its services, it was not until the middle and late 1980s that the broad field of nursing rediscovered case management.

The client populations for which case-management strategies have been targeted are the frail elderly (Kemper, 1988; Steinberg and Carter, 1983); the physically disabled/rehabilitation client (Kemp, 1981; Roessler and Bolton, 1978); the chronic mentally ill (Goering et al, 1988); the developmentally disabled; the abuse/neglected child (Weil et al, 1985); and more recently, the AIDS client and clients with other complex chronic and life-threatening illnesses (Fisher, 1987; Martin, 1987). With the impact of DRGs and early discharge, case management has been seen as appropriate for acute care patients (Fisher, 1987; Zander, 1988).

Inasmuch as the real thrust of case management is the initiation of linkages between client and needed resources and coordination and advocacy activities, a case management approach could be appropriate for any type of nursing diagnosis. Nonetheless, a case-management strategy and process is a particularly useful type of intervention for use with family clients diagnosed with serious, long-term, or complex needs. Using NANDA nursing diagnoses, the following family-centered nursing diagnoses appear most germane: ineffective family coping, particularly those related to domestic abuse and child abuse or neglect; diversional activity deficit of family; alterations in family processes; grieving; health maintenance; alterations and impaired health maintenance; alterations in parenting; and potential for violence.

Case-Management Studies

The majority of early research investigations of the case-management model were within the context of rehabilitation (Goering et al, 1988). The most extensive evaluation studies of case management, however, were conducted to evaluate "channeling" demonstration projects. Ten projects were funded by the U.S. Department of Health and Human Services in 1980 to evaluate community-based approaches to long-term care for the aged as an alternative and preventive service to institutionalization (Evashwick et al, 1985). Comprehensive case-management services were provided within various types of community-based health, mental health, and social services agencies. The "channeling" case-management services were shown to reduce informal caregiving, increase services to clients, reduce the number of unmet needs of clients, and increase clients' life satisfaction. The results regarding its cost efficiency were less clear, however (Hughes, 1985; Kemper, 1988).

Case Management in Community Health

Within the community health, particularly the home health context, nurses are generally viewed as case managers (Dickinson et al, 1988; Martin, 1987; Wahlstedt and Blaser, 1986). For example, Dickinson and associates (1988) maintain that case management is a primary role of community health and home care nurses, explaining that they help establish and coordinate the many health care, social, fiscal, and environmental services needed for clients and their families.

Limitations and Barriers to Nursing Case Management

There are three primary limitations or barriers to using a case-management approach in family nursing. The first of these is the reimbursement policies that exist in health care. Nurses, except for those in specialized positions where case management is identified as one of their functions, are not paid for providing case management to individuals, let alone to families. Completing a more comprehensive assessment, actively involving the family, and linking, coordinating, and monitoring services takes time. Adequate funding must be available for case management services to be effectively provided.

Second, nurses are not sufficiently educated to function as case managers using the broadened definition of case management described above. "Few basic nursing education programs today, regardless of their level of preparation, provide nurses with the knowledge and skills to function efficiently as case managers" (ANA Task Force on Case Management, 1988, p. 8). Nursing programs typically do not emphasize the assessment of social, economic, and environmental areas, or the initiating linkages and coordinating services to families. For instance, referral for assistance with financial problems resulting from health care expenditures involves the family health professional being knowledgeable about available services and programs, agency referral procedures, and how best to refer the family.

Special programs that teach case-management skills to nurses have been recently developed and implemented. These programs have been evaluated as increasing nurses' documentation of case management services to clients, particularly nurses' patient counseling, education, and health-promotion interventions (Connors, 1988; Winder, 1988).

A third limitation—which is related to the first two barriers—is that health care agencies themselves generally do not see nurses as operating as case managers (social workers are generally seen in this role), or the agencies do not see this broadened responsibility as being within their scope of provided services. In spite of social workers being better educated in some aspects of case management, when clients have complex health problems, nursing case managers often are more appropriate. For instance, this is the current thinking in regard to case management of AIDS clients. The consequences of the disease demand a case manager who is educated in both health and psychosocial/environmental areas.

COLLABORATION

Nursing is only one health service vital to comprehensive health care. As members of a health care team, nurses collaborate and plan comprehensive family-centered care with other team members. Collaboration or collaborative health care refers to care that is provided by several health care professionals who work closely together, in order to offer more comprehensive and integrated care (Glenn, 1987). Collaboration can be considered both as a separate family nurse intervention strategy and as an important strategy used in case management. In both the standards of practice in community health and psychiatric and mental health nursing (ANA Council of Community Health Nurses, 1986; ANA Division on Psychiatric-Mental Health Nursing Practice, 1982), one standard of practice focuses specifically on the nurse's involvement in interdisciplinary collaboration.

The composition of the health team (or health and welfare team) may vary depending on an agency's available resources, the health care professionals' practices, and a family's needs. Doherty (1988), a family therapist, identifies the therapeutic triangle composed of family, family professional, and medical team as being the treatment context within which collaborative health care should take place when families have chronically ill family members.

In a home health agency the team is commonly composed of community health nurse, licensed vocational nurse, homemaker-home health aide, social workers, and physical therapist. The occupational therapist and nutritionist are also often members, or act as consultants to the team. The family physician acts only partially as a team member, because he or she is not present and is often difficult to reach. Many independent health goals need to be formulated by the home health team based on medical information, physician's orders, and client assessments of patient and family. The patient and family themselves are also central members of the team.

In primary health care, the health care team usually involves the physician, nurse practitioner, and clinical nurse. A social worker, nurse's aide/vocational nurse, clinical psychologist, and other physician specialists may also be members of the team.

In the official public health agency, the team may be broader or smaller in size depending on the family's particular health, welfare, and educational needs. The community health nurse working in an official health care agency may be a member of a community-based team working with a young, child-rearing family where the school nurse, teacher, probation officer, caseworker, and psychologist are a part of the team. School nurses routinely function as collaborative members of teams that assess and plan educational programs for the learning-disabled student.

In an acute care setting, physician, nurse, social worker, patient, and family usually make up the team. Family professionals (nurse, social worker, and/or psychologist) need to maintain access and collaboration with the patient's physician, as the disease process and its treatment affect and are affected by the family context.

Collaboration implies a professional, collegial relationship—in which there is mutual respect and egalitarianism and joint decision making (Clark, 1984). An authoritarian type of relationship, where the leadership and direction flow from the physician to nurse to nurse's aide to patient, cannot be considered a team or collaborative relationship. With a hierarchal model (where one person is in charge), communication is not open, direct, or truly two way, and team members' contributions and effective functioning are seriously stifled.

Kindig (1975) points out that the structure of each health care system and the mix of people working on a health care team depend on the needs of the patient population and on the available resources. For the team to function effectively, all members must have a common understanding of their respective roles and responsibilities, as well as the goals of each treatment plan. Moreover, when a health care team continually works together, there is a great need for members to work out the process by which decisions are made, communications channeled, and procedures adopted. If a team runs smoothly, this frees more energy for client care, as less energy will be needed for team maintenance and coping with members' interpersonal problems.

Doherty (1988), speaking about collaboration in primary and secondary care settings, reminds us of the costs of collaboration:

> Collaborating, however, takes effort and accommodation. . . . Physicians must give up some of their unilateral power and psychosocial professionals must give up some of their righteous superiority on the interpersonal dimensions of patient care. (p. 209)

Collaboration: For Whom?

As is mentioned under case management, where individual and family health problems are complex, serious, or long term, interdisciplinary intra-agency or interagency collaboration is indicated. In this way more comprehensive and coordinated health care can be delivered. Other client needs can also be more effectively addressed, such as those dealing with education, environment and housing, mental health, and social areas.

Barriers to Collaborative Health Care

The need for an interdisciplinary process, whereby the efforts and skills of different health care professionals are coordinated, is clear when one adopts the family systems perspective and focuses on ways in which the family both affects and is affected by the health or illness of its members (Glenn, 1987). But as we all are aware, the organization of health care services, especially since cost-containment measures have tightened, is characterized as a biomedical model. Specialist care and fragmentation of services are the norm (Glenn, 1987). Some integrated health care systems are still in place, but the biopsychosocial model, because of economic, political, and social conditions, is presently on the decline. As a result, reimbursement barriers exist, as previously discussed, as well as health care delivery barriers.

Glenn (1987), a family physician and advocate of collaborative health care, writes about the problems in collaboration. The first he addresses is that of power conflicts between health care professionals. "The main conflicts that emerge involve turf and money, authority and power" (p. 160). The most basic issues underlying collaborative health care are economic, however: Who is paying for what and to whom? The way health care dollars are divided is an intrinsic factor that determines health care professionals' roles. Psychosocial aspects of health care receive low priority in terms of reimbursement; and insurance companies generally do not reimburse health agencies for nurses providing family psychosocial care.

CONSULTATION

Consultation is included as a general family nursing intervention because family nurses often serve as consultants to nurses and other professionals in health, welfare, and educational disciplines, and as paraprofessionals when individual and family client information and assistance are needed. Consultation refers to the act of giving professional advice or services. In nursing it usually takes the form of deliberating together about a particular case or client and giving suggestions/information about clients with particular health problems. Or it may entail interviewing a family and providing another assessment of the family and its needs. Lewis and Levy (1982) classify the consultation process into two types. The first type in the above description is an example of indirect consultation, where a case-centered meeting is held and the family is not interviewed by the consultant. The second type of consultation is the latter example, where family members are directly interviewed and a second opinion is given. This particular model is used extensively in medicine.

Family-oriented nurses who function as clinical nurse specialists, school nurses, family counselors, community health nurses, and occupational health nurses include consultation as one important component of their practice. Many family nurses develop special areas of expertise—areas like family and child abuse, family crisis intervention, family health promotion programs, and parenting—and provide assistance to other professionals in these special areas.

☐ *STUDY QUESTIONS*

1. Ways to actively involve families during the implementation phase include (check the appropriate choices):
   a. Asking them questions about how they have solved similar problems in the past.
   b. Advising them to follow prescribed recommendations.

c. Encouraging them to discuss the various options available to them to meet their needs.
d. Bringing all the family members together to discuss what might be done and who could do it.
e. Recognizing that clients often lack the competency to make their own health decisions and, hence, need advice on what decisions to make.

2. Match the specific family interventions (from the left-hand column) with the descriptions of the interventions (in the right-hand column). More than one answer is correct for each intervention.

___ Teaching	a. Role modeling.
___ Case management	b. Involves intra-agency and extraagency linkages.
___ Coordination	c. A working agreement between two or more parties.
___ Advocacy	d. Processes that facilitate learning.
___ Collaboration	e. An interpersonal, interventive process.
___ Consultation	f. Assist families to use their own problem-solving skills and strengths.
___ Contracting	g. Giving professional advice to another helping person.
___ Counseling	h. Speaking for or on behalf of a client.
	i. Working closely with another professional to provide health services.

3. Match the types of limitations/barriers in the right-hand column with the interventions in the left-hand column. More than one limitation/barrier can be associated with each of the interventions.

___ Case management	a. Decreased client motivation to change health behaviors.
___ Teaching	b. Cultural and language barriers between involved parties.
___ Collaboration	c. Families do not see nurses fulfilling this interventive role.
___ Contracting	d. Organization for which nurse works is not supportive of nursing intervention.
___ Counseling	e. Setting for sustained interaction inadequate.
	f. Working relationships are hierarchical or stratified.
	g. Families are leaderless, chaotic, or very dependent.
	h. Inhibiting economic factors (lack of reimbursement, payment for intervention).

Fill in the spaces in the following questions (4–7).

4. Identify three NANDA nursing diagnoses for which teaching would be an appropriate intervention.
a. ____________ b. ____________ c. ____________

5. Identify three NANDA family nursing diagnoses for which counseling would be an appropriate intervention.
a. ____________ b. ____________ c. ____________

6. For what types of families would traditionally defined teaching versus counseling be more appropriate?
____

7. For what type of health problems would family case management be indicated?
____

Are the following statements (8–18) true or false?

8. The steps in the nursing process and the teaching–learning process are the same.

9. In the assessment phase of the teaching–learning process, the sole focus is assessing the learner's readiness to learn.

10. Learning needs are analogous to assessment in the nursing process.

11. Determining the particular teaching strategies to be employed is part of the implementation phase.

12. Contracts can be unwritten or written.

13. Contracts are legal agreements between two sets of individuals.

14. Contracts encourage self-responsibility and self-care.

15. Using contracts greatly aids in the evaluation process.

16. A contract must contain time limitations.

17. A contract is made by the nurse and signed by the patient.

18. A contract spells out goals to be achieved and the respective responsibilities of the involved members.

19. There are many factors that serve to promote or inhibit learning in families. Identify several important inhibiting factors.

20. The nurse is working with a family referred by a physician. Sammy, the 8-month-old son, was recently diagnosed as having leukemia. When the nurse arrives at the home, she discovers that the mother has little knowledge of leukemia, a limited income, and no transportation to medical services. The mother is overprotective and terribly solicitous in her care of her infant son. Identify three appropriate family nursing interventions.

21. The visiting nurse has made her first home visit to an elderly couple. The husband, Mr. Paul, age 80, has severe emphysema and has just been discharged from a local general hospital. The wife is also 80 and has assumed the caretaker role. In completing a nursing assessment, one of the observations

the visiting nurse made is that Mr. Paul is seeing three doctors (a pulmonary specialist, an internist for his "heart condition," and a general practitioner who is a lifelong friend and sees Mr. Paul for immediate problems or "anything else"). His bathroom is filled with prescriptions—new, old, same drugs with different doses, and several drugs that have similar actions—prescribed by the different physicians. The patient, being quite concerned regarding his health, is complying by taking all of these. The wife is confused and finds caring for her bedridden husband alone a real burden. She complains of a continual backache and fatigue. Identify four family nursing interventions.

PART V

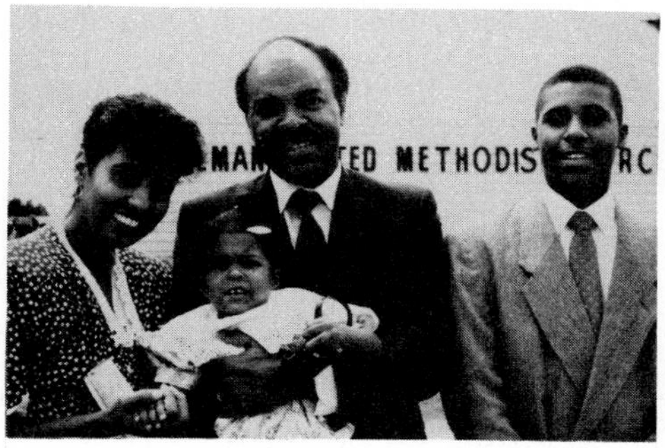

Cultural Differences Among Families

In the last section of this book, a description of families from America's two largest minorities or ethnic groups is presented, in order to show the significance of cultural variation in family life. After a brief overview of each of the two ethnic groups, the Friedman Family Assessment Model (discussed in Chap. 6 and 8–17 and appendix A & B) is used as a framework in describing the family groups. Chapter 8 provides the foundational sociocultural content for these chapters.

CHAPTER NINETEEN

The Mexican-American Family

Learning Objectives

1. Explain the criticism that is made about early writings of social scientists with respect to the Mexican-American family.
2. Discuss why the Mexican-American family has not integrated into the mainstream of American society to the extent that other ethnic groups have.
3. Interpret the meaning of two major family values within the Mexican-American family: familism and the ethic of reciprocity among kin.
4. Describe briefly how the traditional role and power structure of the Mexican-American family is changing.
5. Describe two general socialization patterns among Mexican-American families.
6. Compare American core values with traditional Mexican-American values.
7. Identify the most important structural change occurring in Mexican-American families today.
8. Recognize the functions and primary role of these Mexican folk healers: yerbero, curandero, espiritualisto, and brujo.
9. Recall several common Mexican-American folk illnesses.
10. Identify two central culturally derived family coping patterns of Mexican-Americans and a practice implication emanating from knowledge of culturally derived family coping patterns.
11. Explain three health care practice implications based on Mexican-American culturally patterned beliefs and practices.

THE MEXICAN-AMERICAN OR CHICANO FAMILY*

Family nurse practitioners are increasingly aware of the need for a transcultural and pluralistic perspective in working with diverse ethnic, religious, and cultural groups in American society (Friedman, 1990). There is a demographic imperative, if not a practice imperative, for having a good understanding of the Mexican-American family. The sheer numerical growth of this group in the United States, and the fact that Mexican-American family members tend to have more frequent and serious health problems (Harwood, 1981), provide additional rationale for becoming knowledgeable about the Mexican-American family and its family life patterns.

** The terms Mexican-American and Chicano are used interchangeably throughout this chapter to designate the population of Mexican origin or descent in America.*

Hispanics

Mexican-Americans are the largest ethnic group within the larger Hispanic or Spanish-speaking population within the United States (six out of ten Hispanics are Chicano). People of Spanish origin (Hispanic-Americans) are those people who classified themselves on census documents in one of the specific Spanish/Hispanic categories—Mexican, Puerto Rican, Cuban, South or Central American. Recent census projections report that the Hispanic-American population is rapidly increasing and will after the turn of the century become the largest ethnic minority group in the United States (Vega, 1990).

According to data from the Immigration and Naturalization Service, more than at any time since World War I the United States population increase is driven by immigration, both legal and illegal. Immigrants—7 to 9 million over the 1980 to 1990 decade—are largely from Mexico and Central America, as well as from Asia, South America, and the Caribbean (Barringer, 1990).

The rapid and large growth in the Hispanic-American population is confirmed by U.S. Bureau of the Census data (1983), which estimate that in 1960 there were 3.1 million Hispanic-Americans; in 1970, 9.1 million; and in 1980, 14.6 million. Whereas the white population in the United States increased 9.4 percent from 1970 to 1980, people of Spanish origin increased 61 percent during this same period.

Mexican-Americans comprise over 8 million people in the United States. They are concentrated primarily in the Southwestern United States and are a relatively young population (Barringer, 1990; U.S. Bureau of the Census, 1983).

What specific factors are involved in the tremendous increase of the Hispanic population? The rate of natural increase (births over deaths) among Hispanics is 1.8 percent, one third higher than for blacks. The fertility rate of Chicanos is over 50 percent greater than that of whites (Hayes-Battista, 1990). Also, Hispanic immigration (legal and illegal) is running at the astonishing rate of an estimated one million people per year. Extrapolating from these figures, Hispanics will outnumber blacks within the decade of the 1990s (Fig. 19–1).

Whereas blacks are united by race and a common historic experience of slavery, Hispanic-Americans are united by two powerful forces: their language and their strong adherence to Roman Catholicism. Nevertheless, there are also many factors that divide them into diverse groups. Because of this heterogeneity, only Mexican-Americans—the largest single group of Hispanics—will be addressed in this chapter.

Even among Mexican-Americans, great intra-ethnic variation is present. People of Mexican heritage vary

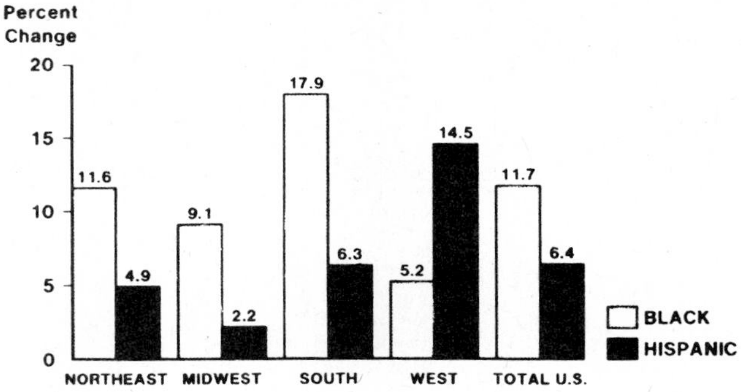

Figure 19–1.
Growth of minorities in the United States, percent change, 1970–1980. (From: U.S. Bureau of the Census, 1980).

by country of origin (United States or Mexico) and self-identification. In addition, socioeconomic, generational, regional, and idiosyncratic factors account for further intragroup diversity (Falicov, 1982).

Generally speaking, first-generation individuals speak Spanish and identify themselves as "Mexicano," whereas second- and third-generation people of Mexican descent speak English and Spanish and usually identify themselves as Mexican or Chicano (Keefe et al, 1978). Another more general term, Latino, is used today to include Mexican-Americans and other Latin American peoples. The term Latino is the preferred term of reference when compared to Hispanic, according to a large survey conducted by the *Los Angeles Times* among the growing Mexican and non-Mexican Latino population in Southern California (Hayes-Battista and Chapa, 1987). In fact, in this survey, most Latinos vigorously rejected the term Hispanic. Latino preserves the flavor of national origin and is culturally and racially neutral. Most Latinos, particularly of the immigrant generation, first describe themselves in relationship to their country of origin before describing themselves as to language, cultural, or race.

The Mexican-American Interface With American Society

Just as slavery provides important keys to understanding the black family, the pattern of labor utilization of Mexicans and Mexican-Americans provides a significant path for understanding the growth and obstacles to the Mexican-American subculture's assimilation into the American cultural mainstream. Historically immigration has been closely tied to Southwestern labor needs. Until recently, job-starved Mexican nationals worked competitively and at lower wage scales than Mexican-Americans either by crossing the border daily, or coming over as *braceros*. (The bracero program, now defunct, permitted Mexican workers to work under contract to the United States when the supply of field workers in this country was evaluated as insufficient) (McLemore and Romo, 1985; Queen and Haberstein, 1974).

According to Queen and Haberstein (1974), Mexican Americans, because of their proximity to Mexico, the fluidity of the border, and the exploitation of the Anglo-dominated agricultural system, have never been able to participate in the usual social processes used by European immigrants to become integrated into and socially mobile within the mainstream of American society.

Chicanos have been, and continue to be, isolated from wider society by religion, language, culture, and social class. Language has served a vital role in maintaining the culture: the Mexican-American family, more than other immigrant families, has continued to speak its native language—Spanish—in the home and community. Social class has also served to isolate Mexican-Americans from the mainstream of the American middle-class society. Quesada and Heller (1977) refer to this alienation as "structural," resulting from class position within society where strong feelings of alienation are coupled with communication problems and enforcement of folkways.

Furthermore, the Anglos' oppressive and discriminatory practices and stereotypic view of the culture have created further problems of social integration. Adding to this situation was the view that many Mexican-Americans held, that the *gringo* is someone from a world alien to their own way of life (Castro, 1978).

Compounding the problem of incompatibility between the larger society and the Mexican-American culture is the ferment being generated by the drastic increases in the population of Spanish-speaking, mostly Mexican, immigrants in many of the areas in the Southwest. The vast influx of Latinos, particularly illegal immigrants, is a prime source of conflict, dissension, and lack of acceptance (Russell and Satterwhite, 1978), because of the social, economic, political, law enforcement, educational, and health impact this rapid population influx has had (Davis et al, 1988).

The type and quality of the interchanges between the family and the external social system significantly affects internal family activities and integration. A major way this occurs is through children's school participation and the father's employment experiences. For instance, the lower- or working-class Mexican-American head of the household has often been unemployed or underemployed in menial positions that constantly erode his self-esteem. He has practically no access to resources that could change his situation, and has had no effective means of making institutions in society respond to his needs. This damaging, limiting process invariably diminishes the internal functioning and role relationships within his family. It has an adverse effect on family leadership and the integration and solidarity of families and their members.

Socioeconomic Considerations

The impact of social class stratification has received sparse attention in the literature about the Mexican-American family, and yet must be taken into account, especially when working with urban Mexican-Americans (Vega et al, 1983). Social class stratification within Mexican-American society reflects the disadvantaged social class status of Mexican-Americans. The proportion of Mexican families in the various social classes does not conform to the American social class distribution of families. Instead, social class distribution is more restricted, reflecting limited social mobility. According to Vega and co-workers (1983), there are four classes in Mexican-American society: the underclass, the low income, the working class, and the middle class.

The underclass are composed of new immigrants who are still in the transition process, while the low-income families are still poor, but have stable unskilled employment and residential stability (Vega et al, 1983).

The largest Latino social class group in most urban areas is the urban working class. Working-class parents have achieved stable employment in skilled or semiskilled occupations and are not economically marginal like the under- and lower-class Latinos.

The middle class is similar to the Anglo-American middle class in that it is a nuclear unit and predominately English speaking. Education is highly stressed and a significant proportion of men are in the skilled trades or in business (Vega, et al, 1983).

Two indicators of Mexican families' precarious status are income and education. The Bureau of the Census (1983) reports that in 1982 it was estimated that the median Hispanic family income was $16,933 per year, in comparison with the median Anglo family income of $23,517 per year. Educationally, the Hispanic is also at a disadvantage when compared to the Anglo; 40.6 percent of all Hispanic adults reported having only an elementary school education (first through eighth grade) in the 1982 intercensus survey (U.S. Bureau of the Census, 1983). A significant factor that lowers the Hispanic's economic status is family size. Hispanics tend to have larger families and more children than non-Hispanics. Hence the ratio of dependence, or the number of persons who rely on the income of the family head, is considerably larger for Hispanics than for non-Hispanics. With larger families and a reduced sal-

There were 31.7 million or 13% persons in the U.S. below the poverty level in 1988.

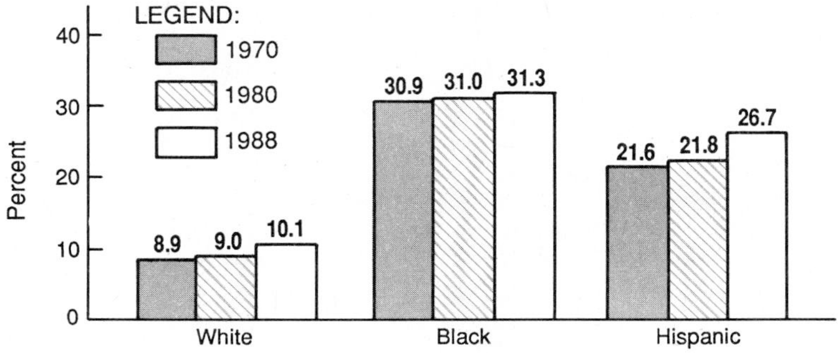

Figure 19–2.
Percent of U.S. population below the poverty line, 1970, 1980, and 1988, by ethnicity. (From: U.S. Bureau of the Census, 1980; 1990.)

ary, 27 percent of all Hispanic families have incomes below the poverty level (Fig. 19–2). Latinos are twice as likely to be poor compared to the general U. S. population (Torres-Gil, 1986).

The Issue of Acculturation

Sociologists have assumed in the past that Mexican-Americans would become acculturated (make the transition from traditional values and behaviors to modern, Western values and modes of behavior) and that social class status was positively associated with modernization, implying that the longer an individual or family is exposed to a dominant culture, the more adoption of the host culture occurs. Although such a formulation has some explanatory value, it fails to delineate which aspects of ethnicity and culture persist over time or the demographic and sociopsychological factors that are likely to affect the acculturation process.

Because of the above shortcomings and the implication inherent within the acculturation notion that the "American" family is the ideal and the "un-American" family less desirable, there is a tendency to move away from acculturation as the sole and central framework for explaining the changes in Mexican-American families. Also, in spite of intergenerational differences, Mexican-American families exhibit a wide range of differences in the extent to which they are acculturated to Anglo society.

Increasing attention is now being devoted to the study of ethnic identity among Chicanos by more objective empirical methods. There is growing recognition that families can be both "modern and ethnic" at the same time (Baca-Zinn, 1981).

There has been tremendous criticism of published literature about the Mexican-American family, especially the early social science literature. Much of the literature is based on opinion and personal observation (Jaramillo and Zapata, 1987). Researchers in their writings failed to recognize and account for the many societal processes (work situation, educational institutions, socioeconomic constraints) affecting the Mexican-American family. In addition, most studies were limited to the lower-class Mexican-American family, and social scientists tended to paint pictures of "black and white" stereotypes of family life and family roles—many times in a pejorative, ethnocentric manner.

Although acculturation has been the primary process used to describe differences between Mexican-American families, we know that this is an uneven process and that some cultural patterns seem to be retained regardless of length or residency in the United States. In the case of the Latino, language is considered to be the best predictor of ethnic identity (Olmedo and Padilla, 1978), and languages spoken a good predictor of acculturation (Sorofman, 1986).

The findings of one study (Keefe et al, 1978) clearly show that even though Mexican-Americans undergo acculturation as evidenced by a decrease in cultural awareness and/or ethnic loyalty, some things do not change. In particular, the importance of the extended family does not wane. In fact, the extended family appears to grow in structure and function when studied across several generations.

THE NORMATIVE FAMILY FORM

Due to the deep commitment to family, more Mexican-American persons live in traditional nuclear families (two parents with children) than white or black persons. According to recent Los Angeles County data, 47.1 percent of Latinos lived in nuclear families while 24.6 percent of whites and 21.8 percent of blacks lived in nuclear two-parent families (Hayes-Battista, 1990).

The idealized and normative Mexican-American family form is the extended family. The extended family living under one roof is not commonly found, however.

Children do not separate from their families of origin psychologically or socially. As children grow up and marry, their families become extensions of the original unit, even though they probably do not live within the same household. The mother's and father's kin are generally of equal importance, with special recognition given to the mother's sisters. Both sets of grandparents are revered. First cousins are especially important secondary kin and are somewhat like sisters and brothers (Queen and Haberstein, 1974). Most social relationships are still based on kinships, and relationships among the extended family are typically closer than in the non-Hispanic family (Keefe, 1984).

The Mexican-American family is typically described as a large and cohesive kin group including both lineal and collateral relatives. Strong and extensive linkages beyond the nuclear family are present, with all relatives having reciprocal rights and duties. In other words, the extended family system, as a concrete manifestation of a familistic orientation, refers to that network of relatives including primary kin (siblings, children, and parents) and secondary kin (aunts, uncles, cousins, nieces, nephews, grandparents).

Godparents (*compadrazgo*) may hold an important place in the family, although the presence and/or role of godparents in Mexican-American families today is more limited (Ramirez and Arce, 1981). *Compadrazgo* refers to the ritual kinship pattern whereby a special linkage is established between two families or two persons by the baptismal ritual. *Compadres* provide coparenthood in time of need but also generate social and interpersonal cohesion, and godparents and godchildren are expected to visit each other and cultivate a close relationship (Queen and Haberstein, 1974).

A well-articulated system of linked nuclear family households exist through which Mexican-American families meet their various life needs. Clearly established patterns of reciprocal help and mutual aid are found between and among extended family members (Miranda, 1977; Vega et al, 1983). This system offers assistance and feelings of security. An example of reciprocity is seen when a poor family becomes too large to support all of its members and, as a result, a child or some of the children are raised by grandparents, uncles, or aunts.

FAMILY STRUCTURE

The descriptions of the Chicano family that follow are culled primarily from fairly recent sources; even then, the reader should particularly keep in mind the possible bias of social class. The reader also needs to keep in mind that cultural norms tend to refer to what ought to be, and that these cultural prescriptions sometimes do not coincide with how things "really" are in families. Because recent research has clarified the wide variation of behavior in Mexican-American families and has dispelled some of our stereotypes of the Chicano family, many of the traditional classic descriptions have been deleted in the third edition of this chapter.

Family Values

Cultures "hang together" on the basis of commonly shared value orientations. For traditional Mexican-Americans, orienting values are present and pervasive, although their actual adherence to these values in family life varies. "An appreciation of their existence and potential impact on family life provides an invaluable perspective for understanding cultural behaviors and expectations" (Vega et al, 1983, p. 199).

Familism. The major theme dominating both the classic and modern portrayal of the Mexican and Mexican-American family is the deep importance of the family to all its members. The set of norms or values related to the importance of the family is referred to as familism. Here "the needs of the family collectivity supercede the needs of each individual family member" (Grebler et al, 1970, p. 369). Heller (1976) states that familism, the opposite of individualism, denotes a set of rights and obligations pertaining to members of a kin network. When strong familistic attitudes prevail, role obligations are seen as mandatory. Familism denotes primacy of one's family (*la familia*) for one's welfare and life (Diaz-Guerrero, 1975).

Mexican-American family values reinforce the system of mutual obligations, support, and reciprocity. Vega and associates (1983) explain other values must be mutually acknowledged in order for mutual support and reciprocity to occur.

> These [values] are mediated by certain values which have received broad attention in the literature: *orgullo* (pride and self-reliance), *dignidad* (dignity), *confianza* (trust and intimacy), and *respecto* (respect). (p. 199)

Table 19–1 compares American and traditional Mexican-American values in some of the major areas of family and personal life. Although clear differences are identified here, again it needs to be stressed that in both American and traditional Mexican-American families heterogeneity abounds and intra-ethnic variation is, indeed, great.

Traditional Mexican-American values, with the exception of familism and a religious orientation, are

TABLE 19–1. AMERICAN AND TRADITIONAL MEXICAN-AMERICAN VALUE DIFFERENCES

Area/Issue	American Central Value Orientation	Traditional Mexican-American Value Orientation
Family	Americans see themselves as individuals first and secondarily as members of families.	Chicanos see themselves as members of families first and as individuals second.
Self versus kin obligations	American culture stresses individuality and independence from family after a certain age. Self-reliance and autonomy are emphasized.	Chicanos believe in ethic of reciprocity within family and kinship group.
Respect and authority structures	Americans value democratic ideals and egalitarianism (to a much greater extent). The elderly do not receive great respect. The authority of the masculine role is gradually diminishing as a result of the societal trend toward egalitarianism.	Greater value on male leadership and respect for and obedience toward the elderly. Authoritarianism is more acceptable.
Progress versus tradition	Americans value progress and change.	Mexican-Americans show more reverence and respect for tradition.
Work	Work and productivity are central, often prominent values of the Anglo culture. Work often becomes a value in itself (more true in the past than today).	Work is seen as a necessity in order to live. Other life experiences—social and emotional experiences—are valued more than work.
Materialism	Materialism is another central American value. Possession of material goods is seen as a sign of success and becomes an end in itself. The cynosures of society as the businessman and financier.	Material objects are viewed as necessities and not as ends in themselves. Social status and prestige are more likely to be derived from an ability to experience things directly and/or through social and family relationships rather than through past successes and accumulation of wealth. Mexican-Americans generally have great reverence for philosophers, poets, musicians, and artists.
Time	"Time is money." Punctuality is equated with goodness and being responsible.	Time is a gift to be enjoyed. The concept of wasting time is not understood. Punctuality is not an important moral value.
Present versus future time orientation	Making plans for the future (planning) is highly valued as a means of getting ahead. Future-oriented.	Enjoyment of the present. Less concern for always living in the future. More present-oriented.
Interpersonal relationships	Americans value openness and directness in communications. (Americans are viewed as being blunt and succinct by Mexican-Americans.) Use of kidding to get messages across more indirectly is acceptable. In interpersonal conflict situations, Americans value "leveling," open dissent, and criticizing each other. Value rational expression of thoughts and not emotional expression as much.	Mexican-Americans value diplomacy and tactfulness, and show concern and respect for others' feelings and dignity. Their manner of expression is more elaborate and indirect. Mexican-Americans value agreement, respect, and courtesy, and are very sensitive to criticism regardless of manner presented. They value being expressive and showing feelings toward another person.
Environmental responses	Americans are less sensitive to the environment and its various forms of stimulation.	Mexican-Americans value greater sensory stimulation within their environments, using a fuller range of senses to experience their environment (vivid colors, expressive music and art, spicy foods).
Relationship to environment	Americans see themselves as mastering the environment.	Chicanos value living in harmony with the environment.
Education	Education highly valued as means to success and way to be productive. Correlated with work and productivity values.	Education is valued but has often been inaccessible, with schools being culturally incongruent with traditional Mexican-American values. Also, many Chicanos are not in tune with success and scientific, individualistic values associated with American education.

Adapted from Murillo (1971).

found among the unacculturated and the poor primarily. Moreover, social class status is a prime determinant of the viability of traditionalism (Moore, 1970).

Martinez (1976) asserts that the poor Chicano family shares many values with other poor families and that these values are actually not so different from those of the middle class. The main difference is that many of the values are ideals or "what should be," rather than what can be. Poor families' "realistic assessment of their capabilities, instead of being received as a healthy and adaptive attitude, has been called fatalism, contentment with their lot, and lack of concern, all implying pathology, differentness, and wrongness. It is this sort of stereotyping that leads people in positions of dominance and control to expect the stereotyped behavior and to plan accordingly" (Martinez, 1976, p. 293).

Value Conflicts. One of the serious problems that occurs as the Mexican-American family interfaces with the larger society is that value conflicts arise. Mexican-American children's socialization experiences (in school and in the *barrio*) often provoke value conflicts between the generations. Many of the primary values of the Mexican-American are incongruent with American core values. This naturally poses significant adaptation problems for Chicano families and individuals. For instance, when Chicano children start school, they soon learn that they and their families are "out of synch" with the wider society.

Vega and co-workers (1983) point out that in low-income areas where Mexican-American families live in *barrios*, the *barrio* also is a powerful socializer.

> The *barrio* has an independent culture and tradition that is neither Mexican alone nor middle class Anglo-American. . . . Often immigrant parents perceive these manifestations as harmless idiosyncracies. However, they may also represent a fundamental affront to values, customs, and decency. (p. 205)

Expectations and sanctions for not conforming to values and social roles within the family are probably more rigidly defined and controlled among Chicanos than Anglos, but nonconformity outside the home is typically not rigidly controlled, as parents perceive limitations on their ability to control the external environment.

Family Roles and Power

The early classic literature about Chicano culture takes cognizance of male dominance in the home. Here, the father is described as unquestionably the head of the family, as well as being "hard, unyielding and strong," exemplifying the traits of *machismo* (Castro, 1978). Family members must show respect for him or he will become angry and may give vent to his wrath by physically striking out. Paz (1973), a noted Mexican author, has described the *macho* or masculine role as incorporating the following elements of arbitrary power: superiority, aggressiveness, insensitivity, and invulnerability. Along with the Chicano male's authoritarian role, he is characterized as providing for his family in the best possible manner he can, priding himself on being the sole provider and being economically self-sufficient.

In this same literature the ideal mother is seen as a soft, nurturing, and self-sacrificing woman, with her traditional and positive role of being in the home, with responsibility to her husband and to her children. In fact, her status and roles are usually defined solely by her marriage and her children.

There has been much criticism over this stereotyping of Mexican-American family roles, both of the conclusions reached and of the theoretical models underlying these past studies. Empirical studies show that patterns of absolute male dominance in conjugal decision making have never been the behavioral norm among Mexicans either in the United States or Mexico (Cromwell and Ruiz, 1979; Grebler et al, 1970; Hawkes and Taylor, 1975). Although the family structure is described as male dominant, the evidence generally suggests the presence of a more egalitarian structure and process, especially when the wife works or the family is not poor (Ybarra, 1982). Moreover, the influence and predominance of *machismo* and the presence of female submissiveness and lack of power are equally controversial generalizations being challenged in Chicano family literature as studies refute the existence of these stereotypes. Chicano scholars on the family argue that there is much diversity within the Chicano family and that many of its present adaptations are due to discrimination and socioeconomic barriers.

Several authors have noted the influence that immigration, urbanization, social mobility, and acculturation have on the Mexican-American family. The Chicano family is being subjected to many of the same societal changes that the Anglo family is facing. The most noteworthy and profound change as noted in recent studies, revolves around the declining primary authority of the male and the greater egalitarianism of spousal roles. The husband's pervasive power has given rise to the wife's feeling a sense of injustice, particularly as she is exposed to American mores and values. Working educated Latino women espouse new aspirations for independence and professional status (Wilkinson, 1987). Large families and the difficulties of finding employment with good wages also compromise the husband–father's ability to provide adequately for the family, which tends to diminish the base for his authority.

Many women, especially the younger ones, are challenging their traditional roles. In the urban areas, the *chicanitas* (adolescent girls) are venturing outside their homes to join social clubs and gangs. *Chicanas* express a need for greater equality in the family and society. Given the increasing occupational opportunities for women and the wish for a higher standard of living, more and more Mexican-American women are working. As a result, traditional male–female roles are changing, among the younger and middle-class couples particularly, and the women of these groups are finding a greater flexibility and choice of options (Miranda, 1977). As with the Anglo families, when women take advantage of educational opportunities and find employment outside the home, their self-image and role expectations change drastically. Education and labor force participation of Latino women are beginning to effect revolutionary changes in the Mexican-American family (Wilkinson, 1987). Hence the Chicano family will face substantial stress due to women's emancipation, generational conflicts, and the decline of the male's patriarchal authority.

Family Communication Patterns

Strong affective communication patterns are characteristic of many Chicano families. There is much warmth and affection shown between mother and children when children are young. In traditional families, respect is shown by children to parents and elders, and females to males of the family.

The Spanish language, being more emotionally-expressive and elaborate than English, shapes the cognitive structure of its speakers. Interpersonal relationships are noted for their tones of respect and hierarchical relationships. As seen in the summary of values, Mexican-Americans value courtesy, respect, maintaining of one's dignity, diplomacy, tactfulness, expressiveness of feelings (emotionality), and agreement. Kidding and open confrontation are not generally sanctioned, because the need to show respect and to "save face" are important.

FAMILY FUNCTIONS

Socialization Patterns

Differences in child rearing and disciplining are notable among Mexican-American families of diverse social classes. Although parental desires for their children may not vary, the ability to realize aspirations does, and hence socialization experiences are clearly varied between social classes (Vega et al, 1983). Nevertheless, in spite of social class differences, children are at the center of family life (Wilkinson, 1987). Also, sex role distinctions through child-rearing practices appear to be reinforced in most Mexican-American families.

Traditionally, the raising of children has been the mother's job, while the father's role has been to work and to form associations with his *compadres* (godparents). However, as with American families generally, this rigid demarcation of roles is rapidly declining. Much more sharing of the child care role is occurring among Chicano couples (Mirandé, 1979).

Mexican-American babies are "wanted, cherished, pampered and thoroughly spoiled." They are regarded as *angelitos*, untouched by evil and sin. Parents and older siblings respond to them in very indulgent, affectionate ways (Queen and Haberstein, 1974).

Socialization strains are common in immigrant Mexican-American families. Among immigrant Hispanic families, researchers have found that children acculturate at a faster rate than adults in the family—a difference that leads to profound intergenerational conflicts. These conflicts are then aggravated by parental attempts to gain control over their children and children rejecting parental efforts (Vega, 1990).

The Health Care Function

Among Mexican-Americans the structure and values of the family are important influencing factors relative to understanding an individual's health attitudes and practices. One can also better understand the shorter longevity and the higher mortality and morbidity rates of Chicanos versus the general American population when the high percentage of this group living at or below the poverty level is taken into account (Angel, 1985).

Health care needs of Mexican-Americans are diverse and depend largely on the specific vulnerabilities and risks associated with social class, environmental, occupational, and life-style patterns. Major health problems and access to health care are concentrated among the poor, the least assimilated, the illegal migrant, and the migrant worker (Angel, 1985).

Health Care Beliefs and Practices. Early studies of health care behavior of Hispanic Americans emphasized the widespread use of folk medicine (Madsen, 1964; Saunders, 1954). Saunders (1954) asserted that Mexican-Americans considered health care as encompassing both scientific and folk cures. Some research on Mexican-Americans shows that folk medicine and beliefs may still persist in rural and urban areas among the lower class (Farge, 1975; Keefe, 1981).

Edgerton and associates (1970) conclude that use of folk healing has all but disappeared in the urban areas of Southern California. In Keefe's (1981) large study of Mexican-Americans in three Southern California communities, there was little indication that *curanderismo* (Mexican traditional folk medical care system) was used. Only 7 percent of the respondents in Keefe's second survey consulted a *curandero* in the last year and one-half of those did so only for a minor medical problem. *Curanderismo* was adhered to most frequently among recent Mexican immigrants who came to the United States after the age of 15, were Spanish-speaking, identified themselves as "Mexicano," and were in the lowest socioeconomic stratum. The respondents who had used *curanderos* believed that folk healers were superior for curing folk illnesses, for curing minor ailments not serious enough to require a doctor's care, and for treating illnesses that physicians could not cure (Keefe, 1981).

Regardless of the degree to which folk medicine is relied upon, there is no empirical evidence indicating that folk medicine and scientific medicine are mutually exclusive systems (Farge, 1975; Kay, 1978; Keefe, 1981; Nall and Speilberg, 1978). Urban Mexican-Americans appear to readily accept modern health care, sometimes supplementing folk medicine with modern medical care or vice versa. Usually there is little incompatibility perceived between the indigenous and the scientific forms of health care.

Traditional Health Beliefs. Most of the Chicano health beliefs are based on assumptions and traditions that have evolved over centuries. In the blending of older European, Spanish-Catholic, and Indian traditions, three basic aspects of Chicano traditional folk health concepts and practices emerge. One aspect is concerned with the specific health beliefs and practices. A second consists of a set of ritualistic acts that are believed to improve health. And lastly, the use of folk practitioners or *curanderos* has evolved (Gonzales, 1976).

Basic to Chicano health beliefs and practices are the health philosophies and ideologies of the culture that circumscribes these beliefs and practices. Dorsey and Jackson (1976) write that the basis for many health beliefs derives from notions about the importance of maintaining equilibrium. Man is viewed holistically, as being in harmony and unity with the natural and supernatural environments. Health is a result of maintenance of this natural state of balance between man and the natural and supernatural worlds. Illness and disease stem from a loss in homeostasis or balance.

Preventive beliefs and rituals are exercised to promote this balance. Prayers, relics, faith, herbs, and spices are all used to ward off disease or to prevent complications of long-term illness. Two examples of the Chicano's concern with maintaining balance are in the consumption of hot and cold foods and in their prenatal health practices. To achieve the necessary balance in the body, foods thought of as "hot" (heavy foods, meats, fatty or spicy foods) are eaten with "cold" foods (vegetables, ice cream), which are considered soothing and fresh to the body. Because pregnancy is seen as a delicate time when imbalances occur easily that can cause great harm to the fetus, the practice of the mother's wearing keys on the night of the lunar eclipse is thought to be protective. Mothers are also urged to maintain good diets, exercise, and take herbs and teas recommended by the *yerbero* (herbalist) or health leader in the family, thus maintaining the delicate balance during the months of pregnancy (Dorsey and Jackson, 1976).

In addition to disease being caused by "imbalances," disease also may be inflicted on an individual as a form of supernatural punishment for wrongdoing (Clark, 1970). Folk illnesses can be caused by a variety of circumstances, although most folk illnesses are believed to be intimately related to faulty social relationships (Herrera and Wagner, 1974; Prattes, 1973).

Some of the specific folk health beliefs, as expressed in form of folk illnesses, are the following. *Mal ojo*, literally translated "bad or evil eye," is believed to be a result of excessive admiration or desire on the part of another. *Mal de susto*, literally translated "illness from fright," is a syndrome believed to be the result of an emotionally traumatic experience. *Empacho* is believed to be caused by food clinging to the wall of the stomach in the form of a ball. *Caida de la mollera* (fallen fontanel) is the one illness that is felt to affect children only and is attributed to a child's being dropped and as the result of a fall. *Mal puesto*, or sorcery, is considered to arise as a consequence of one of three kinds of social relationships: (1) a lover's quarrel, (2) unrequited love, or (3) as a reflection of invidiousness between individuals or nuclear families (Herrera and Wagner, 1974; Prattes, 1973).

Castro (1978) reports that unacculturated Chicano clients see mental illness as a "dreaded affliction." When a person becomes mentally ill, he or she loses the respect of friends and extended family and is viewed as no longer fit to have children or raise a family. The person is socially ostracized and believed to have offended God in some way or be under the influence of a "hex." The mentally ill person's nuclear family feels social disgrace, but continues to love and feel compassion for him or her, in spite of the belief that the individual will never be the same again. Thus for the Mexican-American, mental illness is perhaps one of the most difficult health phenomena with which to cope or for which to seek professional help.

Seeking Health Care. Folk medicine does not treat symptoms of disease conditions alone. Folk medicine views the sick person as a whole psychobiocultural and spiritual being in relationship to the natural and supernatural environments. Whereas Western medicine focuses on epidemiology and pathophysiology, Mexican folk medicine focuses on holistically treating the person.

Typically in the traditional lower-class family, when an individual becomes ill, he or she usually consults the health expert in the family and tries to cure the illness with self-care methods (prayers, diet, household remedies). If this does not relieve the symptoms depending on the type of health problem, he or she may consult a physician, folk practitioner, or sometimes both. Of the folk practitioners, the *yerbero* and then the *curandero* are usually consulted. The types of healing or remedies prescribed are reflective of the healer's perceptions of etiology. In folk medicine, all healing is geared toward restoring the necessary equilibrium or preventing disequilibrium. There are specific household remedies, such as those for being wet and chilled and those for menstruation. Spiritualistic practices are also appropriate for helping with illness considered supernatural in origin. Prayers and ritualistic activities are performed by *espiritualistas,* family, and patient. Herbs are extensively used for treating a multitude of illnesses, some of which have been found scientifically to have great benefit (Dorsey and Jackson, 1976).

Recent studies of Mexican folk health practices demonstrate that Mexican-Americans who use folk medicine do not rely entirely on folk prescriptions for cure, but consider them an important adjunct in expediting solutions to various health problems (Herrera and Wagner, 1974) or as appropriate for folk illnesses.

Folk Healers. Clark (1970), an anthropologist who conducted an extensive ethnographic study of the Mexican-Americans, explains why some Mexican-American people consider folk healers to be vital for meeting their health needs.

> Folk healers are not professionals in the sense that they have formal training in the art of medicine or earn their living by their practice; they are members of the community who are regarded as specialists because they have learned more of the popular medicinal lore of culture than have other barrio people; use language which patients understand and vocabulary familiar to patients; never dictate what must be done, advise the patient what she or he considers appropriate. (p. 207)

There are several levels and types of folk practitioners in most Chicano communities, as described below.

Yerbero(a). The herbalist is an expert in the source, purposes, and derivatives of herbs and spices useful for cure and prevention of disease. As a grower and distributor of herbs, as well as a teacher about their uses, the *yerbero(a)'s* position in the community is one of respect and esteem. Patients will often try family remedies first, herbs from the *yerbero* second, and a visit to the *curandero* and/or physician third (Dorsey and Jackson, 1976).

Curandero(a). The *curandero(a)* is the most respected and specialized folk healer in the Chicano community. The following characteristics of *curanderismo* have been noted: (1) *curanderos* are chosen through divine calling and live in the community; (2) they usually have their practice in their home and their reputation is established by their successes; (3) if respectable, they will not try to cure someone who is incurable, critically ill, or "hexed" (under the influence of a witch or magic); (4) most prescribe prayers, teas, poultices, and herbs; and (5) they do not charge fees, but do accept donations from families (Dorsey and Jackson, 1976; Prattes, 1973).

Espiritualisto(a). This person is a spiritualist who has the ability to analyze dreams and fears, foretell the future, and treat some supernatural and magical diseases (those caused by *brujos*).

Brujo(a). The *brujo(a)* is skilled in the use of magic and witchcraft and can cast spells or hexes on individuals, as well as remove those cast by other magicians. They are honored out of fear rather than admiration (Dorsey and Jackson, 1976).

Access to and Attitudes About Western Health Care. In spite of an increasing reliance on physicians and "scientific health care," especially among second- and third-generation Chicanos, significant barriers to utilization of health care still exist. Access to Western health care has been problematic for many Latinos due to the problems associated with language barriers and lack of health insurance, as well as other cultural differences between Anglos and Latinos. A definite barrier to use of health care services by Mexican-American families is the widespread lack of health insurance benefits. Valdez (1991), in a large study of Latino access to health care, found that 37 percent of Mexican-Americans are not covered for medical care, as compared to 10 percent of Anglos. Another of these barriers is the cultural tradition that "suggests that bad health, though unpleasant, is something that one endures" (Bullough and Bullough, 1982, p. 79). Moreover, when a Mexican-American is in need of medical assistance, he or she is expected to turn to the family first in order to have these needs met. Only when familial resources have been exhausted or under unusual circumstances is it acceptable for the Chicano to seek outside help. These cultural facts are often cited as reasons why it is so difficult for Chicano families and individuals to seek professional help soon enough for their problems (Bullough & Bullough, 1982).

Mexican-Americans generally tend to dread illness and hospitalization more than Anglos do. Perhaps this is due to higher mortality rates or the poorer health the Chicanos experience. Certainly the huge medical expenses the family cannot afford and the estrangement Chicanos often feel when dealing with the health care system contribute to their apprehension of being sick, injured, or hospitalized (Herrera and Wagner, 1974).

Many authors have mentioned that Chicano feelings about health providers and the "scientific" or Western health care systems are usually negative. There are several reasons for this.

1. Health providers use their own medical jargon, which is incomprehensible to Chicano clients.
2. Fee-for-service arrangements between doctors and clients result in feelings of stiffness and mistrust.
3. The Mexican-American feels alienated and lacks confidence in health providers because of the provider's ignorance and arrogance regarding their own traditional beliefs and practices (Farge, 1975; Herrera and Wagner, 1974).
4. Chicanos generally object to clinical, cold, objective attitudes of physicians and nurses and the concept of efficiency, which involves a time orientation valuing speed and results rather than getting to know the patient.

In contrast to the literature that portrays Mexican-Americans as being negative about Anglo health care, Friedman (1985) in a study of 27 Latino families who had a child with cancer, found the parents to be overwhelmingly positive about their health care providers. Not only were parents satisfied with the ongoing care they and their children were receiving, but they also mentioned that doctors, who they saw as "healers," were a prime way that they were able to cope with their child's illnesses.

Family Stress and Coping

Mexican-American families collectively are likely to experience a greater number of major stressors when compared to Anglo families. Certainly poverty, discrimination, cultural conflicts, the immigration experience, social and geographic mobility, and language barriers are primary sources of stress. Substandard housing, inadequate health care and education, and poor employment opportunities are widespread. Immigrant families are identified as a very high risk group in terms of being candidates for family instability and individual health problems (Vega et al, 1983).

Based on the Mexican-American family literature, seeking of social support from the extended family, and of spiritual support, appear to be central culturally derived family coping strategies. This was empirically confirmed in a study by Friedman (1985). Friedman predicted that there would be differences in family coping between Anglo and Latino families. To examine this hypothesis she sampled 28 Anglo and 27 Latino families that had a child with childhood cancer.

Previous studies have empirically demonstrated that the Latino extended family is stronger and more active in providing both instrumental and emotionally supportive assistance than the Anglo family, and thus serves as an important family coping strategy. Moreover, religion, prayer, and reliance on God and saints appear to be more important to Mexican-American than to Anglos, although no comparative studies in this area have been reported. The extent to which Latino families employ fatalism as a passive appraisal type of coping strategy is not entirely clear in the literature, and certainly has been controversial, due to the early anthropological studies that stereotyped all Mexican-Americans as being fatalistic. Yet, Mirowsky and Ross (1984) did find a greater tendency for Latinos to be fatalistic than Anglos, especially among those Latinos with a stronger ethnic heritage.

Friedman's (1985) findings clearly demonstrate that the extended family, especially secondary kin, and religion are significantly more important family coping strategies employed among her sample of Latino families. In fact, Latino parents reported that "God, prayers, and faith" were the most important way Latino families coped with their child's cancer. In terms of the predominant religion among Mexican-American families, 95 percent are Catholic. Mexican Catholicism, it should be noted, varies from American Roman Catholicism. Mexican Catholicism is described as a blend of both Catholicism and Pre-Cortesian Indian beliefs and ideology (Kruszewski et al, 1982). The basic Catholic premise that God governs one's life and ultimately takes it from us, permeates attitudes toward illness.

Anglos, in contrast, reported that spousal support, helpfulness of friends and neighbors, and obtaining medical information are more important family coping strategies. In addition to these apparent ethnic differences, social class of parents also made a difference in family coping patterns. For example, spousal support was reported as a more helpful way of coping by both the middle-class Latinos and Anglos—who generally have more of a companionship type of marriage than lower- or working-class individuals have.

Vega and associates (1986) also studied ethnic differences (Anglo and Latino) in family coping—in the areas of family cohesion and family adaptibility. When comparing families with respect to these two patterns, they found no significant ethnic differences. Both the Latino and Anglo families appeared to be functioning within healthy boundaries in terms of cohesion and adaptability.

One of the major considerations pertaining to culturally derived family coping strategies is the concern about what happens to a family when culturally derived coping strategies are not available. Researchers speculate that the consequences of the Chicano family being heavily reliant on family support (and usually not on support from friends or neighbors) may have adverse effects when the extended family is not present (Keefe et al, 1978; Vega et al, 1983). When Mexican-Americans do not have a local extended family network, they will usually be without other social supports, leaving them less able to cope with stress. Friedman (1985) confirmed the increased vulnerability to stress nuclear families, who were unsupported by extended families, experienced under the prolonged stress of childhood cancer. These families showed much greater familial strains (greater family conflict) and expressions of parental distress.

HEALTH CARE PRACTICE IMPLICATIONS

Based on Chicano culturally patterned beliefs and practices, the following practice implications are suggested.

1. Interactions with Chicanos need to be respectful, friendly, and warm, with sensitivity shown toward the client's feelings (Clark, 1970) and his or her need to maintain dignity. In addition, because the Chicano tends to look on the health care professional as an authority, a structured instructive approach is usually expected and responded to favorably (Nall and Speilberg, 1978).
2. It is well to remember that other family problems may supersede the resolution of health problems. Helping a family tackle their other health-related problems first may leave the way open for the family to engage in solving their primary health concerns.
3. Health workers should not expect a Chicano client to make a medical decision until he or she has a chance to consult with family members. For client compliance, the entire family needs to feel positive about the health decision and feel that the recommended treatment will work. The importance of group responsibility should be recognized. Family health professionals should make an effort to consult with those family members who have authority in the family group. Also, including an older family member, such as the grandmother, in a family discussion is often helpful, because he or she could have substantial influence on what health decisions are made. Meeting with the extended family members to discuss a seriously or chronically ill family member's diagnosis and treatment plan is often an excellent way to operationalize this recommendation.
4. It is best to encourage the whole family or the extended family to adopt a new health program—such as a dietary regimens or obtaining immunizations—rather than encouraging a sole individual to go it alone. People may be more influenced by what other significant family members say and do than by what the health care practitioner thinks.
5. Planning programs to fit Latino cultural patterns and values is an extension of this latter suggestion. Because family involvement and participation works best, planning of family-oriented programs is recommended. Fostering of family group care rather than self-care is another way of stating the above suggestion. Our own cultural bias may be for self-care and individual effort, but for the Latino who values familism, family group care makes more sense.
6. The use of hospitalization for the traditional Mexican-American should be seriously weighed by health care professionals. Integration into Mexican-American culture and its social structure runs counter to the acceptance of health care that involves separation of the patient from his or her family support network. This separation is difficult for the Mexican-American, because the Latino culture and family stress a high degree of psychosocial interdependency (Nall and Speilberg, 1978).
7. Family members including the extended family may want to take an active role in the treatment/rehabilitation of the ill member. It is im-

portant to allow all members of extended family to ask questions and participate in the treatment/rehabilitation as much as possible.

8. When the Mexican-American patient or family believes that Western medicine is more effective in combination with folk medicine for the particular health condition, given that folk remedies are not harmful, support and encouragement of folk remedies in combination with the Western health treatment shows respect and builds trust (Sheppard, 1990).

□ STUDY QUESTIONS

1. Several important factors have adversely influenced the Chicano family's integration into American society, even though some of these same factors may be "positive" for the family. Give three of these factors.

Are the following statements True *or* False?

2. Familism refers to the Mexican-American's propensity to marry early and have a family.

3. In the Chicano family the male and older person have both traditionally held positions of respect.

4. Male dominance in the Chicano family is widespread, the evidence indicating that the father–husband holds absolute power.

5. The institution of having *compadres* among Mexican-American families refers to the custom of having godparents. This custom is, however, declining as a result of acculturation.

6. Which of the following are criticisms that Chicano family scholars and researchers have made about the early writings by social scientists.
   a. They are pejorative.
   b. They tend to describe the Chicano family as homogeneous.
   c. The literature discusses only the middle-class family.
   d. They assume that acculturation will occur uniformly across all facets of family life.
   e. They view the family from a systems, ecological perspective.

7. For each of the following American central values, explain what the corresponding traditional Mexican-American value is:

Area	American Core Value	Tradition Chicano Value
Family	Americans see themselves as an individual first, a family member second.	
Work	Productivity and work are central and prominent values. Work often becomes an end rather than a means to an end.	
Materialism	Possession of material goods is a symbol of success. The greater the accumulation of goods, the greater the prestige.	

(continued)

Area	American Core Value	Tradition Chicano Value
Time and punctuality	"Time is money." Punctuality is a moral value equated with being responsible.	
Interpersonal relationships	American value openness and directness in communication, as well as rationality versus emotional expressiveness.	

Are the following statements True *or* False?

8. The most profound structural change occurring in the Chicano family today is the resurgence of the value of familism.

9. Democratic ideals and verbal facility are taught at a young age in the Chicano family.

10. The ethic of reciprocity in the Latino family has to do with the exchange which takes place between spouses when they role share.

11. Match the description of the folk healer with the type of folk healer.

1. *Yerbero*	a. Herbalist.
2. Conjure doctor	b. Deals with supernatural illnesses.
3. "Granny"	c. Practices witchcraft or magic.
4. *Espiritualisto(a)*	d. Black family's herbalist and midwife.
5. *Brujo(a)*	e. Healer of folk illnesses in the Chicano community.
6. *Curandero(a)*	

12. Fill in the name of each of the following common Mexican folk illnesses from this list of possibilities (mental illness, *empacho, susto, mal ojo, mal puesto, caida de la mollera*).

a. "Bad eye," resulting from excessive admiration or desire on the part of another.
b. Disease given by God or a *brujo* as a hex or punishment on the patient.
c. Affliction caused by food adhering to the stomach wall in the form of a ball.
d. Fallen fontanels (in infants).
e. Sorcery.
f. Illness caused by fright or emotionally traumatizing experience.

13. Based on what is known of Chicano families, and of families in general, identify which of the following practice suggestions would be most appropriate for which group (Chicano family, C; all families, A).

a. Separation of patient from family member(s) should be considered very carefully.
b. Client should not be expected to make a health care decision until he or she has had a chance to consult with the family.
c. It is best to attempt to have the whole family adopt a health promotion or maintenance program.
d. Other family problems may take precedence over health problems, and thus the health worker may have to help the family with its other problems in order for it to be able to resolve health needs.

e. Families need to be spoken to in terms and concepts they understand and suggestions need to appeal to their basic values.
f. An authoritative approach, whereby the health professional conveys expertise and confidence in his/her ability to "heal," is expected.

14. Identify two primary culturally derived family coping strategies of Mexican-Americans. Based on knowledge about culturally derived family coping strategies and an assessment of a Chicano's family's coping responses, state one practice implication.

CHAPTER TWENTY

The Black American Family

Learning Objectives

1. Explain the criticism that is made about the early writings of social scientists with respect to the black American family.
2. Briefly discuss the status of the black American family in the 1990s, relative to social class differences and problems facing the black underclass.
3. Compare the family roles and power structure of black middle-class, working-class, and lower-class families.
4. Broadly describe differences in socialization and marital stability among middle-, working-, and lower-class black families.
5. Identify two traditional folk practitioners in black American communities in the past.
6. Recall two commonly seen responses of black Americans when they initially utilize white health institutions.
7. Explain three health care practice implications based on black family values and coping strategies.

HISTORICAL DEVELOPMENT OF THE BLACK AMERICAN FAMILY

"The family is one of the strongest and most important traditions in the black community" (Franklin, 1988, p. 23). It is unclear as to how much of this tradition is part of the African legacy and how much was developed in the New World.

The development of the contemporary black family is overshadowed by the disastrous legacy of slavery. During the era of slavery, the black family existed only by the consent of the slave owner for the purposes of perpetuating the system and improving his or her economic status. The black family was not autonomous or self-sufficient. Slaves were able to construct a partial family unit when it suited the needs of the slave owners. These units often were mother centered, with the mother–child relationship primary and the husband–wife and father–child relationships tenuous (Rainwater, 1971).

The matrifocal family, which had its inception during slavery, does not exist within black families to any great extent in rural areas today. Blacks in rural areas have been able to maintain two-parent nuclear families to the same extent as similarly situated whites. In agrarian regions, men and women by necessity must function together. In the rural setting, the man has important functions, and it is difficult for women to get along on the farm by themselves. It has been in cities where the black family has disproportionately been headed by women. Here women can earn wages just like a man, and in many cases more easily because of the large number of domestic jobs available. It has also been easier for a mother to receive welfare payments, since she is the bearer and rearer of dependent children (Rainwater, 1971).

DEMOGRAPHIC PATTERNS OF BLACK AMERICANS

Black or African Americans, the largest ethnic group in the United States, comprise approximately 12 percent of the American population, with over 81 percent now living in urban areas (U. S. Bureau the of Census, 1991, April). Two striking developments have occurred within the black population in the United States since the civil rights movement of the 1960s. One is the emergence of an authentic, larger, and economically stronger middle class—better educated, better paid, better housed than for any group of African Americans in the past (Gelman et al, 1988; Hutchinson, 1988). The other development is the emergence and growth of the black underclass (Taylor et al, 1990).

The black middle class grew to about 56 percent of all black wage earners in the 1980s. With a population estimated at 2.5 million, the black underclass is approximately three times larger than it was in the 1970s (Gelman et al, 1988). This group, as discussed in Chapter 8, generates a disproportionate share of the social pathology associated with living in a ghetto—poverty, unemployment, high welfare rates, high crime rates, gang warfare, drugs, dropouts, and teenage pregnancies.

The opportunities of the 1960s and 1970s resulted in the underclass becoming isolated from the more educated and ambitious blacks who took advantage of opportunities to move to more middle-class or integrated neighborhoods and away from the ghettos. For the underclass left behind, the statistics in Table 20–1 bespeak their desperate condition.

TABLE 20–1. SUMMARY OF DEMOGRAPHIC STATISTICS AMONG THE BLACK UNDERCLASS

- In 1985 approximately 55 percent of black families with young children were headed by a single mother. The number of single-parent black families doubled from 1980 to 1987.
- The pregnancy rate among 15- to 19-year-old black girls is more than twice that of white girls in the same age group. Virtually all of these newly created families are poor.
- The black infant mortality rate is twice that of whites.
- Blacks account for one half of all crime, even though they constitute only 11 percent of the U.S. population.
- The rate of unemployment for black youth is more than double that of white youth.
- Black children are three times as likely to live in poverty or in female-headed families.
- The black poverty rate in 1986 was 31 percent of the black population, nearly three times greater than for whites.

Source: Chapman (1988), Edelman (1988), Gelman et al. (1988), Glick (1988a), Meisler and Fulwood (1989).

With the growing proportion of blacks in poverty and the simultaneously rising proportion of blacks at the highest income levels (Malveaux, 1988), a polarity of economic extremes exists within the black community (Levy, 1988). It is important to emphasize this diverse complexion of black families in America. Despite the growing number and worsening status of the black underclass, the majority of black Americans have experienced substantial economic improvements, although certainly more improvement is needed (for instance, the median black income is still only 57 percent of the median white income).

The large and growing number of black teenage pregnancies and resulting single-parent families, which then live in poverty, is a major societal and family health concern. According to some sociologists (Meisler and Fulwood, 1989; Staples, 1985, 1989), the cause of the increased number of black-single-parent families is the shortage of marriageable black males in the underclass. Using data from the Justice Department, Savage (1990) reports that one in four black men in their 20s are in jail or under court control. Further, violence is the number one cause of death (homicides) for black males between 15 and 20 years of age. In fact, black males place at the bottom of nearly every social indicator—highest unemployment, highest infant mortality rate, lowest life expectancy, and poorest educated (Harris, 1990; Savage, 1990). So bad is the black males' situation that the National Association for the Advancement of Colored People (NAACP) calls the black male an "endangered species." Hence, the large number of single-parent families is due, it is reasoned, not to the number of children born to young mothers (the fertility rate has remained about the same for blacks) but to the dearth of black marriages taking place.

Staples, a noted family sociologist, summarizes the problems of the black family as being the same as in the past century. Problems are primarily poverty and racism. Although the future of black middle-class families looks positive, the future of black families in the underclass looks dim. Black men continue to experience widespread problems as noted above, while black women and their roles are in a state of transition—paralleling some changes in American women generally (decreased fertility and greater liberation) (Staples, 1989).

Controversy Over Status of the Black Family

In 1965, Daniel P. Moynihan, who was then Assistant Secretary of Labor, wrote a report that identified the black family with a "tangle of pathology" and deterioration of black society. He concluded that black families were falling apart, basing his conclusions on a myriad of statistical data showing such phenomena as numbers of absent fathers, children on welfare, and juvenile delinquency. This well-known, highly controversial report marked the beginning of the continuing debate and dialogue about the status of the black family, and more importantly, what/who was the victim and the cause. In the last analysis, the real debate centered around who was "to blame" for the multitude of problems besieging black lower-class families. Was it the family itself, the societal treatment of black Americans, or a combination of both external and internal factors. (As we know from other studies, the most potent force for family behavior is external factors, particularly economic constraints.)

Although Moynihan pointed out that the societal treatment of blacks was ultimately to blame, this statement was hidden among the extensive evidence of the black family in trouble. The report also suggested that the black family itself, as a result of its weakening, possessed characteristics inimical to its welfare, as well as to the welfare of its family members and the black community. Moynihan identified the black family's matriarchal structure as a key contributor to the deterioration of the black family. Billingsley and other scholars on the black family disagreed. They saw the black family as a resilient and adaptive system and maintained that black families survived their long journey from Africa to urban America by developing characteristic strength—chiefly a sense of extended family that provides support and nurture during crisis or parental absence (Billingsley, 1968; Williams and Lord, 1978).

In the past decades, controversy over who is to blame for the poor black family's multiple problems has created an atmosphere of defensiveness and not wanting to look squarely at the tremendous problems lower-class and underclass black families are facing. This is now changing. The black community, as well as health and social welfare scholars and practitioners, are closely examining the problems of the poor black family and proposing policy changes and strategies to counter some of the continuing and emergent problems.

One of the significant points of clarification to come from the debate about the status of the black family is that the issues concerning the black family concern the black lower-class family. Notwithstanding the recognition that racism exists against all black Americans, the black middle-class family varies greatly from the lower-class and underclass family. It is similar to its white counterpart in family life-style and does not manifest the extensive strains of the poor black family.

The black family, regardless of social class status, has been repeatedly termed a matriarchal structure, forced into this family form because of the separation of husband and wife during slavery and more recently because of economic realities and welfare restrictions. But according to Billingsley (1968) and Willie (1976), this assertion does not properly account for the total range of black families in our society. First, 78 percent of adult black men and 70 percent of adult women work to support their families. Although still well below the proportion of two-parent white families, 41 percent of black families are two-parent families (Glick, 1988a).

During the last decade significant changes occurred in black families across the nation. The strong family tradition among blacks survived the slave system, discrimination, poverty, and hostile governmental and societial practices and attitudes. Since the 1960s, however, rapid urbanization and especially ghettoization, has had a devastating impact on many blacks who migrated to large cities from rural areas; black males were often unable to find work and governmental policies adversely affected black family strengths (Franklin, 1988). Truncated governmental programs have contributed to the deeper poverty and despair of many black and other ethnic peoples of color. Harriett McAdoo (1988), a black family scholar, asserts that "the need is even greater now to understand the economic situation, cultural patterns and socialization practices of black families" (p. 16).

The black family has adapted to the larger society of which it is a part in various ways, with the common experience of racial discrimination and economic adversity playing very significant roles. Billingsley (1986), a black sociologist, believes that the various structures and functions of black families have resulted largely as adaptive reactions to varying socioeconomic conditions and stressors that threaten black families' survival.

Studying Black Families

As with the Mexican-American family literature, there has been extensive criticism of the writings of social scientists about the black family. Dodson (1988) criticized black family literature as inconsistent, poorly conceptualized, and flawed in terms of research designs. The early black family literature of the 1960s generally saw black families that deviated from mainstream white family life-styles as deviant or pathological. Using the deficit theory (Peters, 1981), the root problem was often believed to reside within black families themselves. Social scientists and the media alike tended to view black families as homogeneous: poor and in trouble. A case of point is a recent analysis of black family articles published in the *Journal of Marriage and the Family* from 1939 to 1987 (Demos, 1990). In these articles sources of distortion were identified. A culture-of-poverty thesis was a prominent focus throughout these years and an obvious source of distortion about the African American family. This focus, encouragingly, has diminished considerably in recent years.

In the last decade or more a number of researchers (Hill, 1970; McAdoo, 1982, 1983; Peters, 1981; Staples, 1985) have looked at black families with a more positive theoretical perspective and also by social class (Billingley, 1968; Coner-Edwards and Spurlock, 1988; McAdoo, 1982). Having this more positive view, black family life is viewed from an ecological, systems perspective "that views Black families as viable, functional, and interacting within mainstream society. . . . This approach assumes that most Black families have developed patterns of behavior and child-rearing attitudes and practices which are appropriate to the values and constraints within their own lives" (Peters, 1981, pp. 73–74).

BLACK AMERICAN FAMILY FORMS AND KINSHIP SYSTEM

Eighty-two percent of all black families were nuclear families in 1985 (Glick, 1988a). Although the female-headed single-parent family is commonly seen (59 percent of all black families were single parent in 1984 according to the U.S. Bureau of the Census [1986]), the modal and ideal black family is the traditional nuclear two-parent family.

One of the distinctive characteristics of black families is the fact that a much higher proportion of black than white family households have extended family members living with them (Hofferth, 1984). Many of the 18 percent of black families that are not nuclear in form consist of groups of relatives such as grandparents and their grandchildren, brothers, sisters, and other relatives excluding parent–child sets living together (Glick, 1988a). Working-class and middle-class black families may have an older relative living in the home providing child care while both spouses work. In the poorer family, the more common pattern is of an older female relative bringing under her wing a younger woman and her children.

Three-generation households typically exist when there is no husband present. Most all married couples have their own apartment or home.

One of the primary cultural patterns noted in the black family literature is the strong reliance on the extended and nuclear family (McAdoo, 1983). Parent–child bonds across the life course are very close (Taylor et al, 1988). Young black couples prefer to live near their families of origin. Strong kinship bonds are also evidenced by the high frequency with which African American families take relatives (especially children under 18) into their households. Black families have developed their own network for the informal adoption of children (Hill and Shackleford, 1986). Babies born out of wedlock are frequently kept in the home; in 1978 fully 90 percent of such black children were reared by parents or relatives, whereas in white families only 33 percent of children born out of wedlock were kept in the home.

Historically the extended family served as a means of pooling meager resources. Today, especially among the poor, financial resources, food, emergency care, and child care are extensively shared among the extended family (Peters and Massey, 1983; Taylor et al, 1988). Child care is often provided by relatives. The grandmother, especially the maternal grandmother, has been the most prominent provider of child care. Today, many of the grandmothers are very young themselves (between 27 and 39). A considerable number of these young grandmothers are feeling resistant to taking on another role—that of grandparenthood—because they still are involved in young adult roles themselves. Role overload has been identified as a problem with "off-timer" young grandmothers (Burton and Bengtson, 1985).

In 1975 the National Urban League reported that one half of all black children between the ages of 3 and 13 whose mothers were working were cared for by relatives. This constitutes a tremendous self-help effort among family, many of whom are already economically strained. Robert Hill of the National Urban League asserts that "the extended family is still one of the most viable institutions for the survival and advancement of black people today" (Williams and Lord, 1978).

FAMILY VALUES AND COPING STRATEGIES

The black family's culturally derived values or ideology is basically conservative; that is, adult members believe in the traditional family structure, in church, hard work, and strong kinship bonds. However, for the poor some of these traditional values have not been realizable, particularly the value of the traditional family structure. It is important to recall here that values are the ideals or "what should be," and the real culture is "what actually is." There is a dissonance between culturally derived family values and the structural conditions in society, particularly for lower-class and underclass blacks. Staples (1985) describes this dissonance as being created because the black male is prevented from fulfilling his normative familial roles, as described earlier. The adaptation of family life that has occurred is seen in the dramatic increase in both households headed by women and out-of-wedlock births. The majority of adult women are not married and living with spouses. Moreover, two out of every three marriages end in divorce (the divorce rate for whites is also high, about 50 percent).

This analysis is presented to emphasize the point that sheer practical necessity often distorts one's values in everyday life and makes family values—what family members say is important—very different from actual behavior. Hence, some coping strategies—that is, how families respond to the demands placed upon them—are more prominently found in the working- and middle-class families, and are discussed in those sections. Those coping strategies that are characteristic of black Americans regardless of social class are addressed here.

The several core coping patterns common to black Americans in the black family literature are:

1. Strong religious commitment and participation.
2. Strong bond with and support from kin and friends.
3. Flexibility in family roles.

The major stressors identified in the literature are racism and oppression—which are felt irrespective of social class—and economic stressors. Included under economic stressors are the stressors of poverty, unemployment/underemployment; housing; and health care (McAdoo, 1983; Staples, 1989). Elaborations on the above coping strategies follow.

Strong Religious Commitment and Participation

A strong commitment to and participation in religion has served as a primary means of coping for both the black individual and family. A religious orientation was a major aspect of the lives of Africans transported here as slaves. During the era of slavery the church played a vital role in helping black Americans cope with the oppression of slavery. It was through the church that blacks learned to use religion as a means to survive (Hill, 1972). Black churches today are descendants of the black church during slavery, where old-time religion and preaching were the mainstay of black family life. Pipes (1988), in studying the old-time religion and preaching, explains that its purpose was to "stir up, to excite the emotions of the audience as a means for their escape from an impossible world" (pp. 55–56).

Today, the black church is still a central institution in black communities. In times of crisis, religion and the church-sponsored social services have been significant supportive elements in revitalizing hope for African Americans (Ho, 1987). The church provides emotional, spiritual, intellectual, and social satisfaction. It is also an important avenue for gaining musical expression and leadership opportunities. Many black families identify elaborate church networks in which their minister and other church "sisters and brothers" are an important informal social network for the family and particularly for the older women members (Boyd, 1982).

Strong Bonds and Support from Kin and Friends

Black families generally have a strong support system composed of kin and friends. As such, this social network represents crucial ways for families to cope. The kin and friendship help–exchange system supplements black families by sharing material, emotional, and social resources (Allen and Stukes, 1982) as well as emergency assistance (Taylor et al, 1988) and care for children, aging parents, and grandparents.

The genesis for strong kinship has been traced back to the traditional African culture (Nobles, 1974). The tradition survived the splitting up of families during slavery and has served to assist the family to deal with the harsh environment in such a way as to ensure survival, security, and self-esteem of its members. Black Americans need support and family involvement, conclude Taylor (1990) and Ellison (1990), who found in research on social support patterns of black Americans that higher levels of familial involvement and subjective family closeness were positively associated with greater family life satisfaction and personal happiness, respectively.

Black "extended families" are not necessarily drawn along "bloodlines" (Hill, 1972). There may be a number of nonkin people who function in important roles in families. It is common practice for long-time friends and neighbors to be brought into the family circle (Carrington, 1978). Nonrelatives were often found to be as influential as relatives, according to one study of black social supports (Manns, 1988). Blacks from lower-class backgrounds were observed to have a greater number of kin and nonkin in their social network than blacks from working- and middle-class backgrounds; the larger network served to offset more adverse life experiences (Manns, 1988).

Family Role Flexibility

Probably the most efficacious family coping strategy in terms of assisting the family to function effectively is the black family's role flexibility and shared decision making (McAdoo, 1988; Peters, 1981). The fluid interchanging of family roles emerged out of economic imperatives of black life (Ho, 1987). In most black families both parents have always had to work outside the home to make ends meet; hence, both parents shared the task of provider, as well as the domestic and child care responsibilities.

Although roles vary considerably between families, sharing of household and child-care tasks between spouses is more common than in white families (McAdoo, H, 1983). Older children in large families become responsible helpers, participating in caring for younger siblings and sometimes working part time to augment the family income. Family teamwork and cooperation are stressed.

FAMILY SOCIALIZATION PATTERNS

Research findings from ecologically oriented and comparative studies represent the most informative and enlightened types of child-rearing studies involving black Americans. In the ecologically oriented studies it is assumed that black families encourage the development of skills, abilities, and behaviors necessary to survive in their environment. In the comparative studies, relevant differences are examined using a relativistic perspective. In general, according to Peters (1988), black families are reported to be strong, functional, and flexible in their socialization practices.

Black Americans provide a home setting that is culturally different from that of white Americans. Children are raised to adjust to the special stress of poverty (in the case of lower-class families) and discrimination, as well as the "ambiguity and marginality of living simultaneously in two worlds—the world of the Black community and the world of mainstream society" (Peters, 1988, p. 233).

Discipline techniques of black parents are reported in some child-rearing research studies to be more direct and physical rather than psychologically oriented (Peters, 1988). Also a high value in individualizing child-rearing practices depending on the child has been observed (Peters, 1988).

A blurring of gender roles was found by some researchers (the stress was on getting the job done rather than matching the job to the child's sex). Parents generally treat children of both sexes the same until early adolescence. At that time sex-based differences in socialization emerge.

There are clear differences in the responsibilities children are given depending on their birth order, with, for example, the oldest child having authority over the child group and the first-born receiving special preparation for a leadership role in the family (Lewis, 1975).

Although child-rearing literature describes mothers' roles in terms of being child centered and in the area of socialization, very little is known about the role of the black father. What has primarily been written has focused on the negative impact of the absent black father (McAdoo JL, 1988b). Where fathers are in the home, researchers have reported sharing of child-care roles and decision making. In comparative studies (comparing white, black, and other ethnic fathers), both black and white fathers are found to be predominantly nurturant, warm, and loving towards their children. Some studies found black fathers to be more restrictive in their expectations and self-reported behaviors towards their children (McAdoo JL, 1988a and b).

Maternal interactive behavior with children and other child-rearing practices are found to differ by social class. As discussed in Chapter 15, socialization practices of parents are molded by what they envision their children as needing to adapt to the world as they see it. Because the worlds of the middle, working, and lower classes are so varied in terms of the skills and behaviors that are adaptive, it stands to reason then that child-rearing patterns would also differ. These differences will be addressed later.

THE HEALTH CARE FUNCTION

A brief review of historic black health practices is instructive for a comprehension of the present-day situation. After slavery and during the reconstruction period in the South, a rise in the use of folk remedies and the midwife or "granny" occurred (Kroska, 1985). As late as 1962 the black midwife was still delivering 42 percent of black babies in the state of Mississippi (Harrison and Harrison, 1971). Their use in the South has been discontinued as a result of legal prohibitions. The use of the conjure doctor, voodoo or hoodoo man, or witch doctor—a practice brought from West Africa—also continued throughout the postemancipation period. Certain diseases were thought to be caused by God or the supernatural, one effect of which was to lead to the fatalism felt by many rural black Americans.

The use of conjure doctors, magical thought patterns, folk practices, and feelings of fatalism are all health attitudes that migrated north with poor black families. Immigrants from Haiti and Jamaica bring traditions of spiritualists, herbalists and voodoo with them also. In some black ghettos today, some lower-class black families continue to use herb doctors, spiritualists, and faith healers. As medical care has become more accessible to black Americans, the use of folk medicine and practitioners has declined considerably. Particularly among the working and the middle classes, only isolated home remedies remain as reminders of the days of "grannies," conjure doctors, and folk health practices.

A considerable proportion of black Americans have

serious problems finding health care. This is partially due to the fact that many poor black Americans do not have health insurance or Medicaid, and many private practitioners refuse to see Medicaid patients. U. S. health statistics provide evidence of the inaccessibility of health care for many black Americans. Edelman (1988) writes that "black children are twice as likely as white children to have no regular source of health care, are more likely to be more seriously ill when they finally do see a doctor, and are five times as likely to have to rely on hospital emergency rooms or outpatient clinics for care" (pp. 286–287). Poor families avoid the expenses of preventive health care, and receive poorer and later prenatal care.

Because many black Americans live in urban, overcrowded ghettos, the health of these individuals is adversely affected. As explained before, the positive correlation between poor general health status and poverty and unsanitary, overcrowded, poor environments, provides evidence of the negative impact of the environment on health (Stokes, 1974).

Folk medicine for a limited number of health problems has remained important in the urban ghettos and in the rural South. Low-income blacks commonly make use of patent medicines and home remedies, secure medical advice from friends, and are reluctant to seek professional health care. Often the poor black person will endure blatant symptoms of ill-health such as unexplained weight loss, abdominal pain, and frequent breathlessness without seeking care. In other words, for families of low socioeconomic status and/or families that feel socially and culturally alienated from available health care, the period of delay is longer. These families will generally exhaust all the home remedies known to kin and friends before feeling forced to turn to health care facilities for help.

Bullough and Bullough (1982) explain that home remedies may have their origins in magical beliefs or have a logical, empirical basis. Two of the more common purely magical actions are putting a knife under the bed of a woman in labor to cut the pain and wearing amulets or charms to ward off disease. Empirical modalities include massage, heat, and tub baths for rheumatoid arthritis, and the application of poultices and the use of herb teas for colds. Older women are the common repository of these folk remedies in today's black families.

New black patients often feel strange, unwelcome, uncomfortable, or mistrustful in white health care facilities (Harrison and Harrison, 1971). "Often there has been so much difficulty working through the system that a patient will come in who assumes she is not going to be treated well" (Monroe, 1989). Monroe asserts that there needs to be an awareness that hostility or avoidance are defensive postures.

SOCIAL CLASS DIFFERENCES

To cope with the enormous sociocultural stresses of daily life—racism, discrimination, and economic isolation—the black family has adapted by developing a variety of family structures, including the patriarchal, egalitarian, and matriarchal forms. The differences in family structure and function can best be understood when one looks at the social class differences. Sociologists Eshleman (1974) and Billingsley (1968) state that the most important variable in understanding the life-style of black families is social class. The impact of socioeconomic status on family structure is seen in the statistics with respect to one- and two-parent families. In black families with incomes below the poverty line, only 20 percent of children live with both parents; while in black families where incomes are above the poverty line, three times more children live with both parents (U.S. Bureau of the Census, 1986).

Black–white family differences are not reducible to simple social class distinctions, however. White middle-class families lack the common identity created by "a sense of peoplehood" (common ethnic identity). Even though lower-class and upper-class black families exhibit dramatic differences in life-styles and family life, they still share a common experience and ethnic identity that makes them feel as "one people," distinct from non-black families, regardless of their social class similarity.

The Black Middle-class Family

In the early 1980s black middle-class and more affluent families comprised about 25 percent of all black families in the United States (Hill, 1981). Levy reported that the more affluent black middle class (those with family incomes over $50,000) increased from 6 to 9 percent from 1979 to 1986, a reflection of the growing number of well-educated black professionals. In recent descriptions of the black middle class, Coner-Edwards and Edwards (1988) identify two categories of families, the "nouveau black middle-class" and the established black middle-class. The first group generally emerged into the middle class from the lower social classes during the window of opportunity of the 1960s and 1970s. The latter category of families includes descendants from middle-class and prominent families. These families appear to have a better sense of belonging than the nouveau black middle-class, who worry about loss of status and stability (Coner-Edwards and Edwards, 1988).

The black middle class is a diverse group, represented by a broad spectrum of income, occupational, and educational levels. For instance, education ranges from completion of high school through postdoctoral education, while occupations include higher-level executives, professors, teachers, small business owners, skilled tradesmen, and technicians.

Families tend to be nuclear in form, generally consisting of husband, wife, and two to three children. Because of their dual employment, cooperative work and team effort of husband and wife are needed. Thus many family tasks such as cooking, cleaning, and shopping are shared, and there is extensive adaptability or flexibility of roles. "Probably the best example of the liberated wife in American society is found in the black middle-class family. Spouses are partners out of economic necessity and have an egalitarian pattern of interaction" (Willie, 1976. p 20). Egalitarian patterns include the sharing of decision making by spouses and more democratic communication patterns. Middle-class black families are more egalitarian than white middle-class families (Willie and Greenblatt, 1978).

The middle-class black family's value system and, consequently, its socialization patterns are largely congruent with those of the dominant culture (Coner-Edwards and Edwards, 1988). Value conflicts emerge as a continual problem, however, because black and white cultures have different value orientations. For the middle-class black there typically is extensive involvement in the nonblack world. This demands that middle-class blacks have the ability to live in two worlds simultaneously (termed being bicultural), managing dual sets of values, expectations, roles, and behaviors.

Racist attitudes and practices are still commonly experienced by black Americans. Because middle-class black parents may not expect, because of discrimination, to get the full benefits for their efforts, they tend to be more protective of their children and act as a buffer between the outer world and the family, to help their children develop their potential while maintaining their self-esteem (McAdoo, 1983).

Social class variability in how black parents rear their children is seen. For instance, middle-class mothers are more vocal with their infants than are lower-class mothers. During later periods of development, middle-class parents are less coercive, restrictive, and arbitrary in their disciplining than lower-class parents. Middle-class parents use more reasoning, support, and communication of democratic approaches and less physical punishment with their children than do lower-class parents (Peterson and Rollins, 1987).

Recent research on the role of black fathers in socialization indicates that middle-income and affluent black fathers look much like their white counterparts in terms of their relationships with their children. John McAdoo (1988b) has noted that when economic status rises within the black family there is an increase in the active participation of black fathers in the socialization of their children. Most middle-class fathers are observed to be warm, nurturant, and loving in their interactions with their children. Some studies also report that black versus white fathers are more restrictive and controlling toward their children (McAdoo, JL, 1988a).

Religion generally has a higher priority for black middle-class than for white middle-class families. Parents tend to be active participants in church affairs, the church serving not only important emotional and spiritual needs but also as a central institution for black social life (Willie, 1976).

Additionally, grandparents, older siblings, or extended family members usually play a more active role in the socialization process than in middle-class white families. It is interesting to note, however, that for upwardly mobile black families, connection with extended family members who have not moved up can be stressful or guilt-producing. A sense of responsibility and an obligation is felt toward those who assisted individuals in moving up or who have not moved up as they have (Coner-Edwards, 1988).

According to several black family scholars (McAdoo, 1983; Peters, 1981; Peters and Massey, 1983), the major stressor in black family life is the psychological and social pressures of racism in the everyday environment. This is termed "mundane extreme environmental stress" in some of the literature (Peters and Massey, 1983). In addition, paralleling large divorce rates in the general U.S. population, marital instability is quite prevalent among the black middle class, posing a stress on all members of the family.

The Black Lower-Middle-Class and Working-Class Family

In the early 1980s working- and lower-middle-class families comprised about 46 percent of all black families (Hill, 1981). Families tend to be nuclear households, but usually have more children (four or more) than do middle-class families. There is also a greater likelihood that a relative or boarder may be part of the household. Many black families from these socioeconomic strata moved to the suburbs in the 1970s and 1980s (Hill, 1981). Again, both parents generally hold jobs. Men tend to work in semiskilled factory, restaurant, or janitorial positions and women are frequently employed at a similar level in community institutions. The parents have often not completed high school, but they desire more education for their own children, and encourage the more motivated children to go to college. Couples usually marry early and begin a family very soon after marriage.

Willie (1976) indicates that the relationship between husband and wife usually takes on an egalitarian character, because cooperation for getting by and survival is a necessity. Hammond and Enoch (1976) confirmed that in their sample of 51 black working-class families, 60 percent of husbands and 57 percent of wives scored their marriage as equalitarian. Because husbands carry out traditional family roles, women generally have more economic control in matters pertaining to the home and children. Additionally, there is a tendency toward some flexibility concerning child-care tasks based on the sex of the child. Lastly, the mother also takes on the social liaison role, primarily with the school and the church.

Respectability is important among black working-class families, with the ownership of one's own home and the good character of one's children being important symbols of the attainment of this value. Of a great significance is one's family. The size of the family may be a source of pride for the parents, as the bearing and rearing of children is considered to be an important responsibility. Working-class parents often make great personal sacrifices for their families, and kinship relationships are strong (Willie, 1976).

Again, religion and the church play a central role in the lives of these families. And the church is often second only to the home as the emotional center of black life (Fellows, 1972).

In regard to child rearing, parents raise their children to assure that they receive the skills and attitudes necessary to survive in the world as the parents perceive it. Thus respectfulness, obedience, conformity to rules, and being "good" are stressed. A strong work ethic exists. During childhood, children are assigned household chores as part of their family responsibility and are encouraged to seek away-from-home jobs for pay when old enough.

Fulfilling the affective functions in the family poses difficulties because of the long hours both parents usually work to provide the necessities of life. Most black working-class families have to give up doing things together as a whole family. Many husbands hold down two jobs, and it is not uncommon for spouses to work different shifts to cover child-care responsibilities. Free time is a premium, but in spite of this, marriage and constancy of family residence are maintained in most families (Willie, 1976).

The Black Lower-Class Family

In the 1980s, the black lower-class family comprised about 31 percent of all black families, a proportion three times that for the white lower class (See Figure 19–2). Poor black families largely live in the urban inner-city poverty areas (Levy, 1988), where social isolation and all the consequences of poverty exist. A chief cause continues to be racial discrimination and economic adversity. Black lower-class families can be divided up into those that represent the working poor and those in the underclass—a group remaining at the bottom of the social ladder and increasingly estranged from mainstream patterns and norms of behavior (Wilson, 1987). The black underclass has increased considerably in size in the last two decades, particularly in the 1980s when fundamental changes occurred in the federal government's response to conditions of poverty (Wilson, 1987). The underclass is described more fully in Chapter 8.

Most married couples have their own households. Poorer black households are much more likely to be single-parent families. It is common to find extended families also, consisting of the grandmother and the mother and her children when no husband is present. Moreover, lower-class black families generally have more children than either the poor white family or the working- or middle-class black family.

In the lower class, desertion and divorce are chief causes for family disruption, although single-parent families are usually not entirely devoid of a male presence. Often the mother will have a boyfriend who visits frequently and acts as companion to the family. Boyfriends and biological fathers often play supportive roles, assisting mothers financially and emotionally (Staples, 1989). If a husband–father is present, he is often unemployed, with the mother on welfare or working in an unskilled job. Even when either spouse is working, the possibility of unemployment is a continual threat.

The primary feature of lower-class black families is their low-income status. Due to the families' impoverished state, they are coerced into making various adaptations, some of which are heavily criticized by the wider society. These adaptations include multigenerational living arrangements and taking in boarders or foster children for pay. Adult heterosexual relationships may involve both marital and parental responsibilities in the absence of marriage. Poor households sometimes forgo conventional morality in order to provide an expedient arrangement for earning sufficient money to live on. "The struggle among poor families is a struggle for existence" (Willie, 1976, pp. 95–98). Movement and instability are great in areas of jobs, residence, and relationships.

Adolescent girls and boys from poor black families tend to have sexual experiences at an early age and have children earlier than their counterparts in the working and middle classes. Premarital pregnancy, though not condoned, is accepted by the family after the fact, as is the belief that, although it may be desirable, it is not necessary to have a man around the house in order to have and raise a family. Many teenage mothers are not marrying today, but raising their children alone, usually with the help of the extended family and friends. Via the process of informal adoption, some young mothers arrange for their children to be raised by kinfolk (Staples, 1989).

Marriage is looked upon ambivalently and in many cases negatively by both sexes, because of the stresses and strains associated with family life (Rainwater, 1971). This ambivalence and negativity has a reality base. Much greater marital instability exists, generally due to economics (unemployment), and, in addition, affectional problems (extramarital relationships) are commonplace.

One of the prevailing myths or stereotypes about the black lower-class family is that it is matriarchal (female-dominated) in structure. There is much convincing evidence that among married couples in the black lower class this is not the case (Cromwell and Cromwell, 1978; Dietrich, 1975; Scanzoni, 1971; Staples, 1976). Dietrich (1975) asserts that matriarchy is not normative in the poor black family. "The study, relying on self-report data from eight samples of black wives in intact nuclear families, reported a predominance of egalitarian decision-making structures in every study population" (Cromwell and Cromwell, 1978, p. 750). Cromwell and Cromwell's (1978) study of lower-class black married couples in Kansas City also suggests that egalitarian decision making predominates.

Because a majority of lower-class black families are female-headed single-parent families, by definition these families are matrifocal. The mother makes most of the necessary decisions and has the greatest sense of responsibility for the family. There is intense loyalty between mothers and grandmothers and their children or grandchildren. Mothers extend every effort to assist their children, even into adulthood; and the grandparents often take on the child-care role and act as prime socializers. Strong loyalty and reciprocity also exists among siblings. The problem here is that when one is in need, all of the siblings are struggling too. Nevertheless, they share their already overcrowded living quarters and often give whatever assistance they can.

The family's values are distinct and different from the wider society's values, thus helping to create the malintegration of this group within and the stigmatization by society of the black lower class. A few selected values will be explained. Fatalism is a common value and one associated with poverty. Black lower-class families learn to hope for little and expect even less. Men and women get sexually involved, but are afraid to trust and commit themselves to each other due to their experience of repeated disappointments. Dependency, rather than self-sufficiency, is an orientation—not really valued, but accepted as a reality and a way to "get by" (eg, it is all right to lean on extended family and on society by receiving welfare). A lack of valuing the achievement and work ethic is apparent, as is the lack of valuing education and future planning. In this regard it must be remembered that family values are reality-based—a reflection of what families can aspire to and expect in life.

Irrespective of social class, kinspeople (grandmothers, aunts, cousins, older siblings) play a more active role in the socialization of black children than is true of white families. In lower-class three-generation maternal households, it is the grandmother who is expected to stay at home with the young children (infants and preschoolers), because the mother has the right to continue outside activities. Some young grandmothers are now resisting this role, however (Burton and Bengtson, 1985).

Rainwater (1971) described the black lower-class family as having little sense of the awesome responsibility of caring for children that the middle-class parent experiences. Although the confinement of being home with infants and preschoolers is also difficult for black mothers and grandmothers, there is not the constant solicitousness that is seen when observing working- and middle-class mothers from various ethnic backgrounds care for their infants.

In single-parent poor homes the maternal household is generally run with a loose organization. Children learn at an early age to fend for themselves, especially if the family is large, with school-agers beginning to shop, cook, go to bed and school on their own, and watch after themselves when mother is gone. Lower-class, three-generation maternal homes are busy with kin and friends coming and going at all times of the day and evening on an unplanned basis. This openness of the home, in part, may be a reflection of the mother's sense of impotence in facing the street system. Although the mother often tries to keep children away from the street when they are young, as they grow older it becomes increasingly futile, and she finally gives up, disengages, and lets the children have their freedom. Black ghetto street life increasingly involves gangs, drugs, criminal activity, and lack of good role models. Poor parents often disengage themselves from their school-age or adolescent son when they feel they are powerless to change the direction of their child's life.

HEALTH CARE PRACTICE IMPLICATIONS

In order to provide more culturally sensitive care, the following practice implications are suggested.

Replacing Stereotypes With Informed Knowledge

Stereotypes about the black American family must be replaced with informed knowledge about cultural differences. Behavior that is not congruent with white middle-class standards should not be prejudged and negatively labeled as deviant or dysfunctional, but evaluated and viewed within the family's cultural and situational context (Mitchell, 1982).

Reevaluating Family Definitions and Use of Social Networks

Family nurses must redefine the family and abandon limiting notions that include only the legally bonded couple or nuclear family in their definition of family (Boyd, 1982). In family assessment and intervention, family nurses should incorporate important people who the family identifies in its social network into the nursing process.

In this regard, because the extended family is usually intact and provides a substantial amount of direct assistance as well as emotional support, this family resource should be considered when working with families. For the older or disabled person, help from extended family is often an invaluable asset that makes the difference between the client having to be placed in a nursing home or cared for in the home. For the family with young children, the assistance of the extended family support system is a central family strength and should be capitalized on in counseling families.

The importance of the role of the older adult woman in the family or grandmother should be especially recognized in working with black families. Parent–child bonds usually exist across the life span and are of critical importance for the provision of assistance (Taylor et al, 1988). Grandmothers are often the repository of both child care expertise and health remedies. They can serve as both a crucial asset and also as a stumbling block if their central role in health matters is not appreciated and they are not brought into important family health decision making.

Assisting With Health-related Family Problems

Poor families, from any cultural group, have survival needs that often supercede the resolution of health problems. Family health workers need to recognize that their role will need to be enlarged in order to assist families with their problems of greater priority. Only after these more pressing problems are resolved can any real energy be given to health needs. Improvement in educational, environmental, social service, and employment opportunities for poor black families is crucial in elevating their health status.

Promotion of Family-centered Health Regimes

In recognition of the powerful influence the family exerts on personal behavior, the whole family should be encouraged to adopt a new health-promotion program, if appropriate, rather than involving only the identified client.

Dealing With Client Discomfort and Mistrust

Health care professionals must be aware of the discomfort and alienation poor black families feel toward white health care facilities. A black family's inactive or nonverbal participation during a first interaction with a health care provider may simply represent the family's initial discomfort or mistrust of the health care provider (Ho, 1987). Interactions need to be warm, sensitive, and respectful of clients' needs, beliefs, and feelings.

With regard to dealing with the black client's initial discomfort and mistrust, some of the ethnic family literature suggests that it is helpful, but not necessary, to have a health care professional be of the same cultural or racial background as the client. Successful assessments and educational and counseling interventions can still be accomplished with black families when the family nurse is of another cultural background and he or she is informed, empathetic, sensitive, and concerned.

☐ STUDY QUESTIONS

1. Which of the following are some of the frequent effects on the black family of slavery, racism, and economic disadvantage (mark true or false after each statement).
   a. The black male's self-esteem is lowered.
   b. The wife becomes submissive to her husband and his primary authority.

c. The self-fulfilling prophecy often occurs in the areas of education and employment.
d. Health-seeking behaviors are exaggerated.
e. A mother-centered family becomes a practical necessity.
f. Traditional husband–wife family roles become rigidly defined.

2. When one examines recent demographic statistics related to the black family, which of the following problems appear to be important? (Select all appropriate answers.)
a. Economic.
b. Parenting and child care.
c. Family planning.
d. Employment.

3. Match the following family attributes with the black family according to social class.

FAMILY ATTRIBUTE	CLASS
a. Respectability is an important value.	1. Middle class
b. Both parents are college-educated and work.	2. Working class
c. Role sharing between husband and wife occurs extensively.	3. Lower class
d. More likely to be single-parent families and/or matrifocal.	4. Underclass
e. A strong achievement orientation is present.	
f. Has the largest family and largest number of relatives living in same household.	
g. Church is a central value and institution.	
h. Egalitarian–autonomic power pattern exists.	
i. Values most incongruent with wider society.	
j. Long-term dependency on public assistance is common.	
k. Families are child centered.	
l. Mothers are more vocal in their interactions with their infants.	
m. Physical punishment is more frequently used.	

4. Black American clients who are new to a health facility often feel uncomfortable initially. What are some of the other feelings or behaviors that have been observed?
a. Overly cooperative
b. Mistrustful
c. Demanding more of a say in their own care
d. Strange and unwelcome
e. Avoidance behaviors

5. Which of the following are criticisms that black family scholars and researchers have made about the early writings on the black family?
a. The authors viewed the black family as being deviant.
b. They tended to describe the black family as homogeneous.
c. The literature was heavily biased in terms of the focus being on the black lower-class family.

d. The writings disregarded the impact of external forces—societal institutions—on the family.
e. Authors viewed the family from a systems, ecological perspective.

6. Two recent striking developments within the black American family are (choose the best answer):
a. The black family has become more assimilated and more egalitarian.
b. The middle class has grown numerically and economically while the underclass has numerically increased but become more economically impoverished.
c. The fertility rate of black women has increased but their marriage rate has decreased.
d. Poor black families have moved into the cities and wealthy blacks have moved into the suburbs.

7. Identify the two traditional folk practitioners used in the past by black families.

8. Briefly describe three family nursing practice implications based upon black family literature.

APPENDIX A

The Friedman Family Assessment Model (Long Form)

The following guidelines represent a collation and abbreviation of the assessment questions/areas that appear at the end of Chapters 6 and 8 to 17, beginning with the assessment of identifying and environmental data, continuing through the assessment of structural and functional dimensions, and concluding with an assessment of family coping. After each broad heading, a footnote alerts the reader as to where the related family theory and further discussion of assessment areas may be found.

The Friedman Family Assessment Model consists of six broad categories:

1. Identifying data
2. Developmental stage and history
3. Environmental data
4. Family structure
5. Family functions
6. Family coping

Each category contains numerous subcategories. Nurses assessing families should decide which subcategories are particularly relevant (after a basic screening type assessment) so that these can be explored in more depth during each family visit/encounter. Not all the subcategory assessment areas may need to be assessed—the depth and breadth of assessment must depend on the family's goals, problems, and resources, as well as the nurse's role in working with the family.

IDENTIFYING DATA

Foundational data that describe the family in basic terms are included in this section.

1. **Family Name**[1]
2. **Address and Phone**[1]
3. **Family Composition**[1]: To gather this information either a table such as Table A–1, or a family genogram (see Fig. 8–2), may be used. To use the table format, after the adult family members, record oldest child first, followed by each succeeding child in order of birth. Include any other related or nonrelated members of household next. If there are extended family members or friends who are considered to be family members, although not living in household, include them also at end of listing. The relationship of each family member to each other, as well as birthdate, birthplace, occupation, and education, should be specified.
4. **Type of Family Form**[1]
5. **Cultural (Ethnic) Background**[2] (including extent of acculturation): In describing this, use the following criteria as guideposts for determining family's cultural and religious orientation.
   - 5.1. Family's or family members' stated ethnic background (self-identified)?
   - 5.2. The family's social network (from the same ethnic group)?
   - 5.3. Family residence (part of an ethnically homogeneous neighborhood)?
   - 5.4. Religious, social, cultural, recreational and/or educational activities (are they within the family's cultural group)?
   - 5.5. Dietary habits and dress (traditional or westernized)?
   - 5.6. Presence of traditional or "modern" family roles and power structure?

TABLE A–1. FAMILY COMPOSITION FORM

Name (Last, First)	Gender	Relationship	Date/Place Of Birth	Occupation	Education
1. (Father)					
2. (Mother)					
3. (Oldest child)					
4.					
5.					
6.					
7.					
8.					

5.7. Home decor (signs of cultural influences)?
5.8. Language(s) spoken in home? Do all family members speak English?
5.9. The portion(s) of the community the family frequents—the family's territorial complex (is it within the ethnic community primarily)?
5.10. The family's use of health care services and practitioners. Does the family visit folk practitioners, engage in traditional folk health practices, or have traditional indigenous health beliefs?
5.11. Country of origin as well as length of time family has lived in the United States (what generation are family members, relative to their immigration status)?

6. **Religious Identification**
   6.1. Do family members differ in their religious beliefs and practices?
   6.2. How actively involved is the family in a particular church, temple, or other religious organization?
   6.3. What religious practices does the family engage in?
   6.4. What religiously based beliefs or values appear central in the family's life?
7. **Social Class Status**[3] (based on occupation, education, and income):
   Economic Status
   Who is (are) the breadwinner(s) in the family?
   Does the family receive any supplementary funds or assistance? If so, from where?
   Does family consider their income to be adequate?
   Social Class Mobility[3]
8. **Family's Recreational or Leisure-Time Activities**[4] Suggested assessment areas pertaining to the family recreational or leisure-time activities include:
   8.1. Identifying the family's activities—what types and how often do these activities occur?
   8.2. Listing the leisure-time activities of family subsystems (spouse subsystem; parent–child subsystems; and sibling subsystems).
   8.3. Exploring the family members' feelings about the family's leisure-time/recreational activities.

DEVELOPMENTAL STAGE AND HISTORY OF FAMILY[5]

9. Family's present developmental stage.
10. The extent to which the family is fulfilling the developmental tasks appropriate for the present developmental stage.
11. The family's history from inception through present day, including developmental history and unique health and health-related events and experiences (divorces, deaths, losses, etc) that happened in the family's life.
12. Both parents' families of origin (what life in family of origin was like; past and present relations with parents of parents).

ENVIRONMENTAL DATA[6]

Environmental data covers the family's universe—from consideration of the smallest area such as aspects of home to the larger community in which the family resides.

13. **Characteristics of Home**[6]
    13.1. Describe the dwelling type (home, apartment, rooming house, etc). Does family own or rent its home?
    13.2. Describe the home's condition (both the interior and exterior of house). House

interior would include number of rooms and types of rooms (living room, bedrooms, etc), their use and how they are furnished. What is the condition and adequacy of furniture? Is there adequate heating, ventilation, and lighting (artificial and daylight)? Are the floors, stairs, railings, and other structures in adequate condition?

13.3. In the kitchen, observe water supply, sanitation, and the adequacy of refrigeration.

13.4. In bathrooms, observe sanitation, water supply, toilet facilities, presence of towels and soap.

13.5. Assess the sleeping arrangements in the house. Are they adequate for family members, considering their age, relationships, and their special needs?

13.6. Observe the home's general state of cleanliness and sanitation. Are there any infestations of vermin (interior especially) and/or sanitation problems due to presence of pets?

13.7. Assess family's subjective feelings about home. Does the family consider its home adequate for its needs?

13.8. Identify the family's territorial unit.

13.9. Evaluate the privacy arrangements and how the family feels about the adequacy of its privacy.

13.10. Evaluate the home's presence or absence of safety hazards.

13.11. Evaluate the adequacy of waste and garbage disposal.

13.12. Assess the family members' overall satisfaction/dissatisfaction with their housing arrangements.

14. **Characteristics of Neighborhood and Larger Community**[6]

14.1. What are the physical characteristics of the immediate neighborhood and the larger community?
Type of neighborhood/community (rural, urban, suburban, intercity).
Types of dwellings (residential, industrial, combined residential and small industry, agrarian) in neighborhood.
Condition of the dwellings and streets (well kept up, deteriorating, dilapidated, being revitalized).
Sanitation of streets, home (cleanliness, trash and garbage collected, etc).
Problems with traffic congestion?
Presence and types of industry in neighborhood (air, noise, or water pollution problems).

14.2. What are the demographic characteristics of the neighborhood and community?
Social class and ethnic characteristics of residents.
Occupations and interests of families.
Density of population.
Recent changes in neighborhood/community demographically.

14.3. What health and other basic services and facilities are available in the neighborhood and community?
Marketing facilities (food, clothing, drug store, etc).
Health agencies (clinics, hospital, emergency facilities).
Social service agencies (welfare, counseling, employment).
Laundromat services for those families in need.
Family's church or temple.

14.4. How accessible are the neighborhood and community schools and what is their condition? Are there busing and integration problems which affect the family?

14.5. Recreational facilities.

14.6. Availability of public transportation. How accessible (in terms of distance, suitability, hours, etc) are these services and facilities to the family?

14.7. What is the incidence of crime in the neighborhood and community? Are there serious safety problems?

15. **Family's Geographic Mobility**[6]

15.1. How long has the family lived in the area?

15.2. What is the family's history of geographic mobility?

15.3. From where did the family move or migrate?

16. **Family's Associations and Transactions with Community**[6]

16.1. *Who* in family uses *what* community services or is known to what agencies?

16.2. How frequently or to what extent do they use these services or facilities?

16.3. What is the family's territorial patterns—communities or areas frequented?

16.4. Is the family aware of community services relevant to its needs, such as transportation?

16.5. How does family feel about groups or

organizations from whom it receives assistance or with whom it relates?

16.6. How does the family view its community?

17. **Family's Social Support System or Network**[7]: Who helps family in time of need for assistance, support, counseling, family activities (babysitting, transportation, etc)?

 17.1. *Informal:* Family's ties with friends, neighbors, relatives (kin), social groups, employers, employees.
 Who are they and what is the nature of their relationship? The family ecomap illustrated in Figure 8–4 is useful for assessing this area as it graphically depicts the family's relationships and interactions with its immediate environment. The family genogram (Fig. 8–2) also provides information on family social support.

 17.2. *Formal:* Family's relationships with helping people from health care and related agencies.

FAMILY STRUCTURE

18. **Communication Patterns**[8]

 18.1. In observing the family as a whole and/or the family's set of relationships, how extensively are functional and dysfunctional communication used?
 Give examples of recurring patterns.
 Are the majority of messages of family members congruent in content and instruction? (Include observations of nonverbal messages.) If not, who manifests incongruency?
 How firmly and clearly do the members state their needs and feelings?
 To what extent do members use clarification and qualification in interacting?
 Do members elicit and respond favorably to feedback or do they generally discourage feedback and exploration of an issue?
 How well do members listen and attend when communicating?
 Do members seek validation from one another?
 To what degree do members use assumptions and judgmental statements in interaction?
 Do members interact in an offensive manner to messages?
 How frequently is disqualification utilized?

 18.2. How are emotional (affective) messages conveyed in the family and within the family subsystems?
 How frequently are these emotional messages conveyed?
 What types of emotions are transmitted within the family subsystems? Are negative, positive, or both types of emotions transmitted?

 18.3. What is the frequency and quality of communication within the communication network and familial sets of relationships?
 Who talks to whom and in what usual manner?
 What is the usual pattern of transmitting important messages? Does an intermediary exist?
 Are messages sent that are appropriate to the developmental age of the members?

 18.4. What types of dysfunctional processes are seen in the family communication patterns?

 18.5. What areas are closed off to discussion that are important issues to the family's wellness or adequate functioning?

 18.6. What are the internal (familial) and external (environmental, socioeconomic, and cultural) influences impinging on the processes and communication patterns?

19. **Power Structure**[9]

 Power Outcomes

 19.1. Who makes what decisions? Who has the last "say" or "who wins?"

 19.2. How important are these decisions or issues to the family?
 More specific questions might include:
 Who budgets, pays bills, decides how money is to be spent?
 Who decides on how to spend an evening or what friends or relatives to visit?
 Who decides on changes in jobs or residence?
 Who disciplines and decides on child's activities?

 Decision-making Process

 19.3. What specific techniques are utilized for making decisions in the family and to what extent are these utilized (eg, consensus; accommodation-bargaining;

compromising or coercion; de facto)? In other words, *how* does the family make its decisions?

Power Bases. The various bases or sources of power are legitimate power/authority and a variation of it, "helpless" power; referent power; expert power or resources power; reward power; coercive power; informational power (direct and indirect); affective power; and tension management power.

19.4. On what bases of power do the family members make their decisions?

Variables Affecting Family Power

19.5. Recognizing the existence of any of the following variables will help the assessor interpret family behavior from which family power can be assessed.
- The family power hierarchy.
- Type of family form.
- Formation of coalition(s).
- Family communication network.
- Social class status.
- Family life cycle stage.
- Cultural and religious background.
- Situational contingencies.
- Person variables (members' ages, gender, self-esteem).
- Spouses' emotional interdependency and commitment to the marriage.

Overall Family System and Subsystem Power

19.6. From your assessment of all the above broad areas, are you able to deduce whether the family power can be characterized as dominated by wife or husband, child, grandmother, etc; egalitarian–syncratic or autonomic; leaderless or chaotic? The family power continuum can be used for a visual presentation of your analysis.

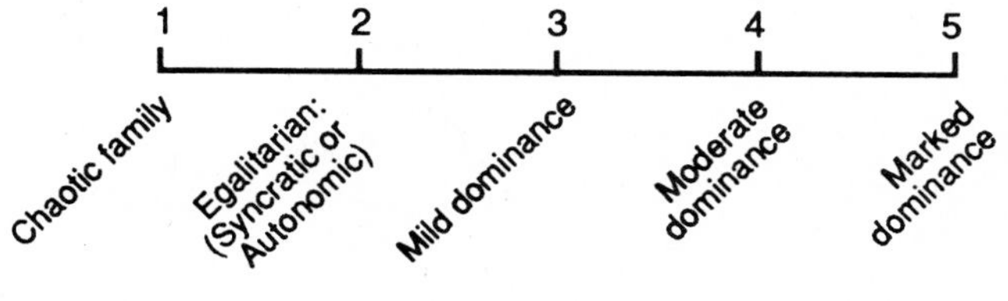

Family Power Continuum: If dominance is found, who is the dominant one?

19.7. To determine the overall power pattern, asking a broad, open-ended question is often illuminating (asking both spouses and children if feasible), examples of which are given below.

Who usually has "last say" about important issues?
Who is really in charge and why (getting at bases for power)?
Who runs the family?
Who wins the important arguments or issues?
Who usually wins out if there is a disagreement?
Who gets his or her way when they disagree?
Are family members satisfied with how decisions are made and with who makes them (ie, the present power structure)?

20. **Role Structure**[10]

Formal Role Structure

20.1. What formal positions and roles do each of the family members fulfill? Describe how each family member carries out his or her formal roles.

20.2. Are these roles acceptable and consistent with family members' expectations? In other words, does role strain or role conflict exist?

20.3. How competently do members perform their respective roles?

20.4. Is there flexibility in roles when needed?

Informal Role Structure

20.5. What informal or covert roles exist in family? Who plays them and how frequently or consistently are they enacted? Are members of the family covertly playing roles different from those which their position in the family demands that they play?

20.6. What purpose does the presence of the identified covert or informal role(s) serve?

20.7. If the informal roles are dysfunctional in the family, who enacted these roles in previous generations?

20.8. What is the impact on the person(s) who play this (these) role(s)?

Analysis of Role Models

20.9. Who were (or are) the models that influenced a family member(s) in his or her early life, who gave him or her the feelings and values about growth, new experiences, roles, communication techniques?

20.10. Who specifically acted as role model for the mates in their roles as parents, and as marital partners, and what were they like?

Variables Affecting Role Structure

20.11. Social class influences: How does social class background influence the formal and informal role structure in the family?

20.12. Cultural influences: How is the family's role structure influenced by the family's cultural and religious background?

20.13. Developmental or life cycle stage influences: Are the present role behaviors of family members developmentally appropriate?

20.14. Situational events: Changes in family member's health status. How have health problems affected family roles? What reallocation of roles/tasks have occurred? How have family members who have assumed new roles adjusted? Any evidence of role stress or role conflicts? How has the family member with the health problem reacted to his or her change or loss of role(s)?

21. **Family Values**[11]

21.1. Use of "compare and contrast" method suggested (with values of either dominant culture, family's reference group—ethnic group with whom they identify—or both).

American Core Values/Family Values

Productivity
Work ethic
Materialism
Individualism
Education
Consumption ethic
Progress and mastery over environment
Future time orientation
Efficiency, orderliness, practicality
Rationality
Democracy, equality, and freedom
"Doing orientation"
Patriarchal authority
The family's interests
The family as a haven
Health

21.2. Is there congruence between the family's values and the family's reference group and/or the wider community?

21.3. Is there congruence between the family's values and the family subsystems' values?

21.4. How important are these identified values to the family?

21.5. Are these values consciously or unconsciously held?

21.6. Are there any value conflicts evident within the family itself?

21.7. How does the family's social class, cultural background, and developmental stage influence its values?

21.8. How do the family's values affect family health status?

FAMILY FUNCTIONS

22. **Affective Function**[12]

Family Need–Response Patterns

22.1. Do family members perceive of the needs of the other individuals in the family?
Are parents (spouses) able to describe their children's and mate's needs and concerns?
How sensitive are family members in picking up cues regarding other's feelings and needs?
Do each of the family members each have someone they can go to within the family to unburden themselves—that is, a confidant?

22.2. Are each member's needs, interests, differentness respected by the other family members?
Does a mutual respect balance exist (do they show mutual respect toward each other)?
How sensitive is the family to each individual's actions and concerns?

22.3. Are the recognized needs of the family members being met by the family, and if so, to what extent? For questions 22.1, 22.2, and 22.3, it is suggested that a list of the family members be included with their needs (as perceived by family members) and the extent to which these needs are being met by the family.

Mutual Nurturance, Closeness, and Identification

22.4. To what extent do family members provide mutual nurturance to each other?
How supportive of each other are they?

22.5. Is a sense of closeness and intimacy present among the sets of relationships within the family?
How well do family members get along with each other?

Do they show affection toward each other?

22.6. Does mutual identification, bonding, or attachment appear to be present? (Empathetic statements, concerns about other's feelings, experiences, and hardships are all indicative.) To answer questions 22.4, 22.5, and 22.6, an attachment diagram is very helpful (see Fig. 14–1).

Separateness and Connectedness

22.7. How does the family deal with the issues of separateness and connectedness?
How does the family help its members want to be together and maintain cohesiveness (connectedness)?
Are opportunities for developing separateness stressed adequately and are they appropriate for the age and needs of each of the family members?

23. **Socialization Function**[13]

23.1. Assess family's child-rearing practices in the following areas.
- Behavior control, including discipline, reward and punishment.
- Autonomy and dependency.
- Giving and receiving of love.
- Training for age-appropriate behavior (social, physical, emotional, language, and intellectual development).

23.2. How adaptive are the family's child-rearing practices for its particular family form and situation?

23.3. Who assumes responsibility for the child-care role or socialization function? Is this function shared? If so, how is this managed?

23.4. How are the children regarded in this family?

23.5. What cultural beliefs influence the family's child-rearing patterns?

23.6. How do social class factors influence child-rearing patterns?

23.7. Is this a family that is at high risk for child-rearing problems? If so, what factors place the family at risk?

23.8. Is the home environment adequate for children's needs to play (appropriate to children's developmental stage)? Are age-appropriate play equipment/toys present?

24. **Health Care Function**[14]

24.1. Family's health beliefs, values, and behaviors:
What value does the family assign health? Health promotion? Prevention?
Is there consistency between family health values as stated and their health actions?
What health-promoting activities does the family engage in regularly?
Are these behaviors characteristic of all family members or are patterns of health-promoting behavior highly variable throughout the family system?
What are the family's health goals?

24.2. Family's definition of health–illness and their level of knowledge:
How does the family define health and illness for each family member? What clues provide this impression, and who decides?
Can the family observe and report significant symptoms and changes?
What are the family members' sources of health information?
How is health knowledge transmitted to family members?
How does the family assess its level of health knowledge?

24.3. Family's perceived health status and illness susceptibility:
How does the family assess its present health status?
What present health problems are identified by the family?
To what serious health problems do family members perceive themselves vulnerable?
What are the family's perceptions of how much control over health they have by taking appropriate health actions?

24.4. Family dietary practices:
Does the family know food sources from the basic four food groups?
Is the family diet adequate? (A 3-day food history record of family eating patterns is recommended).
Who is responsible for the planning, shopping, and preparation of meals?
How are the foods prepared? Mostly fried, broiled, baked, microwaved, or served raw?
What is the number of meals consumed per day?
Are there budgeting limitations? Food stamps usage?
What is the adequacy of storage and refrigeration?

Does mealtime serve a particular function for the family?
What is the family's attitude toward food and mealtimes?
What are the family's snack habits?

24.5. Sleep and rest habits:
What are the usual sleeping habits of family members?
Are family members meeting sleep requirements appropriate to their age and health status?
Are regular hours established for sleeping?
Do family members take regular naps or have other means of resting during the day?
Who decides when children go to sleep?
Where do family members sleep?

24.6. Exercise and recreation:
Are family members aware that active recreation and regular aerobic exercise are necessary for good health?
What types of recreational and physical activities do family members engage in regularly? Are these activity patterns representative of all family members or only certain members?
Do usual daily work activities allow for exercise?

24.7. Family drug habits:
What is the family's use of alcohol, tobacco, coffee, cola, or tea (caffeine and theobromine are stimulants)?
Do family members take drugs for recreational purposes?
How long has (have) family member(s) been using alcohol or other recreational drugs?
Is the use of tobacco, alcohol, prescribed or illicit drugs by family members perceived as a problem? Does the use of alcohol or other drugs interfere with the capacity to carry out usual activities?
Do family members regularly use over-the-counter or prescription drugs? Does the family save drugs over a long period of time and reuse?
Are drugs properly labeled and in a safe place away from young children?

24.8. Family's role in self-care practices:
What does the family do to improve its health status?
What does the family do to prevent illness/disease?
Who is (are) the health leader(s) in the family? Who makes the health decisions in the family?
What does the family do to care for health problems and illnesses in the home?
How competent is the family in self-care relative to recognition of signs and symptoms, diagnosis, and home treatment of common, simple health problems?
What are the family's values, attitudes, and beliefs regarding home care?

24.9. Environmental practices:
How exposed are family members to environmental hazards found in the soil, air, and water?
Are family members subjected to high levels of noise on a regular basis?
Do family members smoke or are they exposed to smoke while on the job or at home?
Do family members use pesticides, cleaning solutions, glues, solvents, heavy metals, or poisons within the home?
What are the family's hygiene and cleanliness practices?

24.10. Medically based preventive measures:
What are the family's feelings about having physicals when well?
When were the last eye and hearing examinations?
What is the immunization status of the family?

24.11. Dental health practices:
Do family members use fluoridated water, or is a daily fluoride supplement prescribed for the children?
What are the family's oral hygiene habits in regard to brushing and flossing after meals?
What are the family's patterns of simple sugar and starch intake?
Do family members receive regular preventive professional dental care including education, periodic x-rays, cleaning, repair, and (for children) topical or oral fluoride?

24.12. Family health history:
What is the overall health of family members of origin and marriage (grandparents, parents, aunts, uncles, cousins, siblings, and offspring) over three gener-

ations? Establish whether there is now or in the past a history of genetic or familial diseases—diabetes, heart disease, high blood pressure, stroke, cancer, gout, kidney disease, thyroid disease, asthma and other allergic states, blood diseases, or any other familial diseases.
Is there a family history of emotional problems or suicide?
Are there any present or past environmentally related family diseases?

24.13. Health care services received:
From what health care practitioner and/or health care agency do the family members receive care?
Does this provider or agency see all members of the family and take care of all their health care needs?

24.14. Feelings and perceptions regarding health care services:
What are the family's feelings about the kinds of health care services available to it in the community?
What are the family's feelings and perceptions regarding the health care services it receives?
Is the family comfortable, satisfied, and confident with the care received from its health care providers?
Does the family have any past experience with family health nursing services? What are the family's attitudes and expectations of the role of the nurse?

24.15. Emergency health services:
Does the agency or physician the family receives care from have an emergency service?
Are medical services by current health providers available if an emergency occurs?
If emergency services are not available, does the family know where the closest available (according to their eligibility) emergency services are for both the children and the adult members of the family?
Does the family know how to call for an ambulance and for paramedic services?
Does the family have an emergency health plan?

24.16. Source of payment:
How will the family pay for services it receives or might receive?
Does the family have a private health insurance plan, Medicare, or Medicaid; or must the family pay for services in full or partially?
Does the family receive any free services (or know about those available to it)?
What effect does the cost of health care have on the family's utilization of health services?
If the family has health insurance (private, Medicare, and/or Medicaid), is the family informed about what services are covered, such as preventive services, special medical equipment, home visits, and so forth?

24.17. Logistics of receiving care:
How far away are health care facilities from the family's home?
What modes of transportation does the family use to get to them?
If the family must depend on public transportation, what problems exist in regard to hours of service and travel time to health care facilities?

FAMILY COPING[15]

25. What stressors (both long- and short-term and socioeconomic and environmental) are being experienced by the family? (Refer to Holmes and Rahe's Social Readjustment Scale.)
Are you able to estimate the duration and strength of the family's stressors?
What strengths counterbalance these stressors?
Is the family able to handle the usual stresses and strains of daily life?
26. Is the family able to act based on a realistic and objective appraisal of the stressful situation?
27. How does the family react to stressful situations (what coping strategies are used)?
What coping strategies has the family employed to deal with what types of problems?
Do family members differ in their ways of coping with their present problem? If so, how?
What are the family's inner coping strategies?
    Family group-reliance.
    Use of humor.
    Sharing of feelings, thoughts, and activities (maintaining cohesiveness).
    Controlling the meaning of the problem/reframing.
    Joint problem solving.

Role flexibility.
Normalizing.
What are the family's external coping strategies?
Seeking of information.
Maintaining linkages with the broader community (general external involvement)?
Informal and formal.
Seeking social support (both formal and informal).
Seeking spiritual support.

28. In what problem areas or situations has the family in its dealings over time achieved mastery?
29. What dysfunctional adaptive strategies has the family used or is the family using? If there are signs of any of the following dysfunctionalities, record their presence and how extensively used:
    - Family violence (spouse, child, elder, parent, or sibling abuse).
    - Child abuse.
    - Scapegoating.
    - Use of threat.
    - Child neglect.
    - Family myth.
    - Pseudomutuality.
    - Triangling.
    - Authoritarianism (submission to marked dominance).

FOOTNOTES

1. Chapter 8.
2. Chapter 8.
3. Chapter 8.
4. Chapter 8.
5. Chapter 6.
6. Chapter 9.
7. Chapters 8 and 17.
8. Chapter 10.
9. Chapter 11.
10. Chapter 12.
11. Chapter 13.
12. Chapter 14.
13. Chapter 15.
14. Chapter 16.
15. Chapter 17.

APPENDIX B

The Friedman Family Assessment Model (Short Form)

The following form is shortened for ease in assessing the O'Shea family (Appendix C) or other families. (Where information is not provided, leave blank or note that a lack of information exists.) If you are not sure what data should be covered in each of the assessment areas below, please refer to Appendix A for the long form, where more detailed questions/areas are presented, or refer to the related chapters where both content and assessment areas are addressed.

Two words of caution are called for before using the following guidelines in completing family assessments. First, not all areas included below will be germane for each of the families visited. The guidelines are comprehensive and allow depth when probing is necessary. The student should not feel that every subarea needs be covered when the broad area of inquiry poses no problems to the family or concern to the health worker. Second, by virtue of the interdependence of the family system, one will find unavoidable redundancy. For the sake of efficiency, the assessor should try not to repeat data, but to refer the reader back to sections where this information has already been described.

IDENTIFYING DATA

1. **Family Name**
2. **Address and Phone**
3. **Family Composition**
   See Table A–1 or Figure 8–2 (family genogram).
4. **Type of Family Form**
5. **Cultural (Ethnic) Background**
6. **Religous Identification**
7. **Social Class Status**
8. **Family's Recreational or Leisure-time Activities**

DEVELOPMENTAL STAGE AND HISTORY OF FAMILY

9. **Family's Present Developmental Stage**
10. **Extent of Developmental Stage Fulfillment**
11. **Nuclear Family History**
12. **History of Family of Origin of Both Parents**

ENVIRONMENTAL DATA

13. **Home Characteristics**
14. **Characteristics of Neighborhood and Larger Community**
15. **Family's Geographic Mobility**
16. **Family's Associations and Transactions With Community**
17. **Family's Social Support Network**
    Ecomap, Figure 8–4 is helpful here.

FAMILY STRUCTURE

18. **Communication Patterns**
    Extent of Functional and Dysfunctional Communication (types of recurring patterns)
    Extent of Affective Messages and How Expressed
    Characteristics of Communication Within Family Subsystems

TABLE B–1. FAMILY COMPOSITION FORM

Name (Last, First)	Gender	Relationship	Date/Place of Birth	Occupation	Education
1. (Father)					
2. (Mother)					
3. (Oldest child)					
4.					
5.					
6.					
7.					
8.					

Types of Dysfunctional Communication Processes Seen in Family
Areas of Closed Communication
Familial and External Variables Affecting Communication

19. **Power Structure**
Power Outcomes
Decision-making Process
Power Bases
Variables Affecting Power
Overall Family Power

20. **Role Structure**
Formal Role Structure
Informal Role Structure
Analysis of Role Models (optional)
Variables Affecting Role Structure

21. **Family Values**
Compare the family to American or family's reference group values and/or identify important family values and their importance (priority) in family.
Congruence Between Family's Values and Values of Family's Subsystems As Well As Family's Reference Group and/or Wider Community
Variables Influencing Family Values
Are these values consciously or unconsciously held by the family?
Presence of value conflicts in family.
Effect of the above values and value conflicts on health status of family.

FAMILY FUNCTIONS

22. **Affective Function**
Family's Need–Response Patterns
Mutual Nurturance, Closeness, and Identification
Family attachment diagram, Figure 14–1 is helpful here.
Separateness and Connectedness

23. **Socialization Function**
Family Child-rearing Practices
Adaptability of Child-rearing Practices for Family Form and Family's Situation
Who Is (Are) Socializing Agent(s) for Child(ren)?
Value of Children in Family
Cultural Beliefs That Influence Family's Child-rearing Patterns
Social Class Influence on Child-Rearing Patterns
Estimation About Whether Family Is at Risk for Child-rearing Problems and If So, Indication of High Risk Factors
Adequacy of Home Environment for Children's Needs to Play

24. **Health Care Function**
Family's Health Beliefs, Values, and Behavior
Family's Definitions of Health-Illness and Their Level of Knowledge
Family's Perceived Health Status and Illness Susceptibility
Family's Dietary Practices
Adequacy of family diet (recommended 24-hour food history record).
Function of mealtimes and attitudes toward food and mealtimes.
Shopping (and its planning) practices.
Person(s) responsible for planning, shopping, and preparation of meals.
Sleeping and Resting Habits
Exercise and Recreation Practices (not covered earlier)
Family's Drug Habits
Family's Role in Self-care Practices
Family's Environmental Practices

Medically Based Preventive Measures (physicals, eye and hearing tests, and immunizations)
Dental Health Practices
Family Health History (both general and specific diseases—environmentally and genetically related)
Health Care Services Received
Feelings and Perceptions Regarding Health Services
Emergency Health Care Services
Dental Health Services
Source of Medical and Dental Payments
Logistics of Receiving Care

FAMILY COPING

25. **Short- and Long-term Familial Stressors**
26. **Family's Ability to Respond, Based on Objective Appraisal of Stress-producing Situations**
27. **Coping Strategies Utilized** (present/past)
    Differences in family members' ways of coping
    Family's inner coping strategies
    Family's external coping strategies
28. **Areas/Situations Where Family Has Achieved Mastery**
29. **Dysfunctional Adaptive Strategies Utilized** (present/past)

APPENDIX C

Case Study of the O'Shea Family*

The O'Shea family was referred to the community health nurse, Ms. Bell, by the county hospital's maternity service for the following reasons. "Mrs. O'Shea has expressed the desire to learn about family planning. She also needs a referral for postpartum and well-baby care." The following information was included in the referral: Mary—age 35; gravida VII, para V, abortions II. Delivered newborn son, Daniel—born 11/3 (5 days ago); birth weight—7 lbs, 2 oz; length—19 inches; hypertension during pregnancy; normal labor and delivery; mother's postpartum status and stay was normal, bonding well with infant.

FIRST HOME VISIT

During Ms. Bell's first home visit, the father and two oldest children were at work and school. From her conversation with the mother and her observations of the home and family members, the following family data were obtained from the nurse's notes. Family: Patrick, father—age 43; Mary, mother—age 35 (looks older, tired and slightly overweight); Joseph, son—age 6; Maureen, daughter—age 5; Betty, daughter—age 4; Richard, son—age 3; and Daniel, son—age 1 week. Pat works as a butcher in his father's small grocery store located in same neighborhood a mile away from home.

The family lives in an older wooden, three-bedroom flat in the Maplewood district—an Irish neighborhood—located 5 miles from a New England city with a population of 300,000. The immediate neighborhood is ethnically and socially homogeneous (working class) and residential, although located very near to a heavily industrialized factory district.

The family's home is rented from a cousin for $600 per month and is sparsely furnished, with a minimum of furniture in each room. The kitchen is clean, containing a small refrigerator and stove. There is one bathroom with toilet and bathtub. The parents have their own room, which they presently share with the newborn (who has a new bassinet the women's group at the parish donated). The girls, Maureen and Betty, have their own bedroom with a double bed, while the boys share the other bedroom, having twin beds and a small chest of drawers. A few area carpets are noted, but few decorations—with the exception of the children's school photos and a photo of the Irish coast on the living room wall and Catholic religious articles in the parent's room and dining room. Curtains matching the tablecloth hung in the dining room, a wedding gift from Mary's mother to them when they were married. A color television set was the centerpiece of the living room. The mother said the home was adequate for their needs, although it was getting smaller with the arrival of another baby.

The outside of the house needed painting but was not cluttered and in fair repair. It was noted, however, that the stairs leading up to the front porch were loose, and there was no railing or lighting. A few children's toys were scattered around the backyard.

Mary was talkative and responsive to questions. When Ms. Bell explained that she had come because of a referral from the county hospital where Mrs. O'Shea had delivered her last baby, Mary was pleased that the nurse had been contacted to visit her. She offered the nurse a cup of coffee as they talked in the living room.

* *Genevieve Monahan revised Appendix C for the third edition.*

NURSE: How are you managing since you have been home from the hospital with your new baby?

MARY: Not too bad, but it sure is harder with five than with four, and being older doesn't help. I just don't have the energy to get up at night and feed Daniel.

NURSE: What kinds of help are you getting?

MARY: My mother came over the first day I was home and Pat's mother came over 2 days ago. They helped by cooking and cleaning up the house a little, and looking after the children. I also have a sister nearby who goes shopping for me sometimes.

NURSE: Anyone else?

MARY: No, that's about it, except for a neighbor and the women from my church, who told me to call if I needed anything. But I wouldn't want to bother them.

NURSE: What about your husband?

MARY: Pat helps a bit with the children, especially with getting them into bed at night. It's hard for him to do much more than that after working all day. Besides, he's pretty conservative and still holds to women being in charge when it comes to taking care of the children. He thinks that if I do need more help it should come from my mother or sister. Pat would usually rather spend his free time playing football or meeting his friends for a beer at the local bar.

NURSE: Is this the way it's been with the other children too—you handling most things by yourself?

MARY: Yes, I'll just have to "offer it up" to the Lord.

NURSE: How have you managed to keep everything going?

MARY: I'm pretty well organized, and I learned quite a bit from my mother about managing a household.

NURSE: Have you found ways to save your energy?

MARY: Mainly it's a question of sleeping when the baby does, letting the other kids watch TV, and not worrying about the housecleaning.

NURSE: Sounds like a good list of priorities. Your health, children, and baby are certainly more important than housework. Is there anything that is important and needs doing that you can't handle?

MARY: Nothing immediately—my family lives here and they help—but I am very worried about getting pregnant again and having more children. I didn't think I would have the need to ask about family planning—I was planning for Richie to be my last. I had two miscarriages since him—1 and 2 years ago—and the doctors told me that I definitely shouldn't have any more children because my blood pressure gets so high. I discussed the problem with our priest, who then spoke to my husband about the rhythm method, but I guess he didn't get the right instructions. Since then, my girlfriends tell me that's not a very good method anyway.

NURSE: So you and your husband have decided not to have more children?

MARY: I'm not sure how Pat feels about it. I told him just yesterday that this was the end of kids for me, and he just looked and listened without a comment—and then just walked into the kitchen and got himself a beer. I can't talk to that man—that's the problem! When he has something on his mind, he sure lets me hear about it. But when I'm talking it's like I'm nagging or like it's not any of his concern.

I think he's torn because he knows how hard our lives would be if we have more, but he's a very devout man and really follows the teaching of the church on this. I'm not sure what he'll say in the end.

NURSE: Would you be willing to tell me a bit more about your marriage?

MARY: Well, we were married when I was 28 and he was 36. I guess that's been 7 years. As you can see, babies started coming pretty quickly after that—one a year until now, including the two miscarriages. We both knew each other from the parish and our parents both live in the neighborhood. We both graduated from Catholic high schools in the neighborhood. After high school Pat went to work in his father's grocery store, was in the service for 3 years, and then when his older brother stopped working for his father, Pat got the job of being butcher in the store—been doing that for his father 4 years now. I worked as a clerk in an electronics factory before we got married. I really liked it there and made a lot of friends at the factory.

I started seeing Pat 3 years after I finished high school, and we went together 5½ years before he asked me to marry him. I was afraid I was going to be an old maid like some of my friends were. Sure was a lot easier being single though, but my family and friends were always hinting and pressuring me to "tie the noose around Patrick."

NURSE: Overall, how would you describe your marriage to Pat?

MARY: Hard work a lot of the time. I always feel like I'm really working at getting along and keeping things on an even keel.

NURSE: Has it always been that way? What was it like in the beginning and after the children came?

MARY: (looking at the nurse with a tired, disappointed expression on her face, and sadness in her eyes): I think our marriage started out all wrong—not that it was so different from any of my friends' and cousin' or sisters' marriages—but it was just not like the marriages I read about in the papers and magazines and see on television. I was raised a strict Catholic, in an Irish school and parish. My grandparents came over from Ireland during the depression. Pat's folks also are Irish, and his father came over here as a teenager and worked in construction until he could save enough to buy a small grocery store—the one he has now. We didn't know much about sex except what we heard from our friends. Our parents never mentioned it, and the nuns certainly never brought it up. Things have changed a lot since then. But we were raised in a time when you didn't have relations until your wedding night. I'm ashamed to say this, but I never really liked having sex that much. It hasn't been the way I thought it would be when I was young. Pat seems to enjoy it pretty well, though I'm not sure.

NURSE: Have you ever discussed it with him?

MARY: Not really. Every time I try I get mortified and then worry that I would hurt his feelings if I told him. Besides, what good would it do?

NURSE: Do you ever talk to your sisters, mother, or friends about it?

MARY: Only my sister and one girlfriend, and they both have the same frustrations. My sister tells me that there are books you can read to make sex more pleasurable—but it seems unnatural to make a study of it like that. Besides, one of the first things I ever learned about it was from my friend's mother, who said it was something you just put up with in marriage.

We used to go out to the movies or friends' homes together—and talk more. But, after the children came we grew apart. Don't misunderstand me, we wanted the children and were happy to see them born, but somehow the demands in raising them caused problems between us. Now we don't talk much, except about the children and money problems—we're always just barely making it through the month. Pat spends more and more time with the boys. You know, going to football, baseball, and basketball games or spending time at the bar. And when he's home, he's really not home. I can't get him to do anything around the house. When I ask him to do something he looks at me as if I'm imposing on him and I'm making his life difficult. When I try to talk to him about problems, he'll say: "Don't bother me with that now. Can't you see that I'm tired. I'll do something about it tomorrow." And tomorrow never comes.

NURSE: I appreciate your sharing so much about your concerns and experience with Pat and the children. You mentioned feeling a little overwhelmed since Daniel's birth and worried about finances. You told me that you've decided that you don't want any more children, and it sounds like you wish that your relationship with Pat was closer, like when you were first married. I would like to offer my support and information, and to work together with you to look at options you have for your concerns.

Ms. Bell then outlined ways that she could help Mary, and asked Mary which problem bothered her most. She then asked permission to make another home visit to meet the rest of the family.

The first visit also consisted of discussing the newborn, Daniel, and Mary's physical health status. Ms. Bell planned to return in a week with information for her on clinic services for the baby and on family planning and postpartum care and follow-up.

SECOND HOME VISIT

During the second home visit 1 week later, the nurse came at 3:30 P.M. when the children were home from school and the father would be there for part of visit (after he returned from work at 4:00 P.M.). After discussing Mary's and Daniel's health and giving Mary appointments for the baby clinic and Mary's postpartum examination at the local health center, the nurse spoke briefly about family planning and asked Mary if she felt that this could be discussed with her husband. Mary agreed, although she did not seem sure about how her husband would react to a woman talking to him about such an intimate subject. However, when Ms. Bell suggested that this might be a way to help both of them talk more directly about this delicate subject, she seemed to reconsider her previous hesitancy and said she thought it would be a good idea.

Before talking with the parents about family planning, Ms. Bell asked them for a brief health history of each of the children and was able to observe and elicit data related to parent–child relationships, parenting roles, and child rearing. She noted that Mary was very warm and cuddly with newborn Daniel. Mary held him close, handled him gently, and appeared relaxed and confident in his care and sensitive to his basic needs. Pat, in contrast, looked proudly at Daniel, but did not hold him, and according to Mary did not get involved in his physical care (nor did he with any of the other children when they were babies).

Both mother and father were warm and Mary physically quite affectionate with Richard, age 3. She seemed quite indulgent with him, letting him "have his way" and giving him a lot of freedom to run around and play.

With the older children—Betty, 4, Maureen, 5; and Joseph, 6—there was not the same permissiveness as observed with Richard. Mary said, "They are older and so need to be more responsible." All three older children were fairly quiet around the nurse. They spoke when spoken to, but otherwise talked quietly with each other or listened. Joseph is the mother's favorite, but both parents say he is too serious and has problems handling himself sometimes, becoming bossy and wanting to take over. Betty is the father's favorite, "since she is petite, very sweet, and looks like Pat's mother."

The parents believe in children behaving and showing respect for their elders and carrying out their responsibilities, even if at these ages they are not expected to do much. The father spanks the children with the palm of his hand on their buttocks if they misbehave. He explained by saying, "None of these newfangled ideas about disciplining for us." It was noticed that children were asked to do several things—pick up the toys from the floor and help their mother.

Both Maureen and Betty acted immediately, while Joseph ignored and then refused until his father yelled at him. No positive reinforcement followed when the children did obey. Maureen and Betty seemed pleased to have a new baby brother, while Richard was jealous of the baby and has been more demanding since the baby's arrival. The parents understand, though, that he feels displaced and jealous and that he needs more parental attention during this time. Joseph states he does not like the new baby.

When asked about each of the children and what they were like, the mother led the conversation although the father chimed in about Joseph and Betty. The descriptions are given in Table C–1. Ms. Bell asked Mary to have the children play in another room and then raised the issue of family planning.

NURSE: Mary, would you be willing to share with Pat our discussion about family planning?

MARY: Yes. Like I tried to tell you Pat, I'm at the end of my rope. I don't want to get pregnant again and I want to look into some kind of family planning method.

NURSE: Pat, I'd like to know how you feel about this.

PAT: I was a little surprised she would bring this up with you, but since she did, I guess we can talk about it. I have felt that my wife is taking things in her own hands—complaining all the time about her life and seeing her job as such a burden. My mother had seven children, and I never heard her complain. It would be very difficult for us if we had another baby—but I can't see any way around it. If the good Lord wants her to have more, then I think she'll just have to accept them and manage with what we have.

TABLE C–1. THE O'SHEA PARENTS' DESCRIPTIONS OF THEIR CHILDREN

	Mother's Description	Father's Description
Joseph, age 6½	He's a bright, independent child. Joseph is the leader of the children at home and school and likes to take over. I try to give him some responsibilities for caring for his sisters and brothers, but have to watch that he doesn't get too bossy. I'm able to talk to Joseph more than the other children. He's a sensitive child and listens to me. I know I'm a little protective of him, but that's just because we're so close to each other.	Joseph is always arguing and wanting his own way. My wife spoils him. He's going to grow up thinking he'll be the President by the time he's 35. He needs to be put in his place by my wife.
Maureen, age 5	Maureen is a helpful child who likes to help me. She is an easy child to raise. She's quiet, likes to play alone and doesn't cause any trouble. Maureen follows her brother Joseph all the time when they play together.	She's great fun.
Betty, age 4	Betty knows how to get people to like her. She's a "people pleaser"—can act cute and sweet when it is in her favor. She needs special watching, however, as she can pull the wool over one's eyes very quickly with her sweet and cunning ways.	The father acts disgusted with his wife's statement and responds by saying: "That's not true. She is a sweet, affectionate little sweetheart. You're just jealous because we have a special relationship."
Richard, age 3	He's always into everything! Very active and inquisitve. I try to let him have a lot of freedom to run around in the house, otherwise he gets so bottled up that he shouts, screams, and makes the rest of us miserable.	He's at the age where we really have to keep an eye on him.

NURSE: Does that mean that religiously you're against any form of family planning?

PAT: Well not exactly. I know that Catholics are not all of the same mind on this issue and that many of them do things to prevent pregnancy. I won't say that my mind is completely closed, but that I have serious questions about it. We tried that rhythm method, but it didn't seem to work.

NURSE: Mary, would you like to say something about this?

MARY: Well, I just can't go on like this. Something has got to be done. You ought to stay home some day, Pat, and just see what raising this many kids is like.

PAT: But our mothers found a way to do it. . . .

MARY: Yes, but things are so much more expensive now, and they never had a choice, but I do. I would like to find out more about what is available and really look into family planning methods.

NURSE: Pat, what's the benefit you see in having more children? Your wife feels it's hard for her to manage now and that further pregnancies are dangerous for her.

PAT: I didn't say I wanted any more. I just said that she's pretty lucky and she doesn't know it. I suppose our family is big enough, but we can't depend on "Russian roulette," I mean the rhythm method, to solve our problem.

NURSE: Do you understand the problem your wife has in having more children now? I mean the hypertension during pregnancy, which has grown worse with each succeeding pregnancy?

PAT: Not really. (Nurse explains the problem and how pregnancy makes problem worse.)

Ms. Bell then asks the spouses if they have discussed their problem or family planning methods with their priest and family doctor, and then suggest that they do this together, because neither priest nor doctor has been approached to discuss the problem. She gives a basic overview of family planning methods that are available, including natural family planning, and gives them a booklet on family planning for more information. Ms. Bell acknowledges their progress in discussing a sensitive subject and encourages them to request further information as needed. She then asks permission to make a follow-up visit.

THIRD HOME VISIT

As the spouses speak to each other and with the nurse, the nurse makes the following observations regarding Pat and the couple's relationship.

Pat seems easygoing, verbal, and quite a conversationalist—as long as he controls the flow. He likes to be the center of attention and loses interest if Mary is talking, in this case, jumping in to refocus attention on himself. He expresses an interest in getting some help for his wife from his mother, but feels that helping himself is "not his job." He says that Mary and his mother don't get along too well together, however, there being too much competition between the two of them. According to Mary, Pat's mother caused tremendous tension during their engagement and early years of marriage. She had bitter arguments with her husband about his mother, but as the mother-in-law finally began to accept the reality of her son's marriage, their problems subsided.

In terms of the marital relationship, there appeared to be no expression of love or affection either physically or verbally. Their relationship was characterized by a lack of empathy or two-way communication between them. One received the impression that Mary was there to meet the needs of her husband, but that he had no similar responsibility to her. Pat expected her to serve him, care for the home and children, and manage with the limited funds he alloted her weekly for groceries and other home and child expenses.

While Pat was present, Mary took little part in the discussions, except when asked direct questions. She acted very self-effacing and subservient in his presence, except when she voiced the opinion that he should spend time with the children to see what it was really like.

Pat did communicate to the children that they should have respect for Mary—because she was their mother. However, in his own communications with her, he did not express much respect. Most communications were in the form of commands, with few requests or room for feedback from his wife. When Mary spoke to him, he seemed to tune her out. Most of the time he halfheartedly agreed that she was right and that he would follow through on such matters as on making appointments with the priest and the doctor, but would not do so.

The children and parents were quite talkative concerning the recent Thanksgiving holiday and other happy events. With pleasant subjects all of the family contributed verbally to family conversations. Unpleasant subjects or angry statements were cut off, such as Joseph's reaction to the new baby, or minimized, such as the mother's feelings of being burdened by too many children. It was also noted that the children spoke directly to their mother, but only indirectly with their father. If they had a request, they would ask their mother to ask their father for permission.

When asked what activities the family engaged in together, Mary reported that family visiting is their most popular and frequent activity. "Movies and eating out are beyond our reach. I like taking the kids to the park, but Patrick doesn't like coming. I go to Mass regularly and so does Pat. We don't travel much—our close relatives live in town and we can't afford traveling much on Pat's salary. Pat's car isn't very dependable. Groceries, clothing and the usual household items we buy at the shopping center. It's about a half-mile from here."

In terms of friendships, Mary states that she has a few old high school friends she still sees occasionally and that Pat sees his friends at sports events or the local bar. But Pat and Mary have no couple friends with whom they engage in social activities.

Ms. Bell asked the couple how they liked the community. Both the parents related that this was the only community and neighborhood they had ever lived in and said, "We like it here. We know where everything is. All of the storekeepers and neighbors are old friends and acquaintances." The family, having lived in the community for many years, was familiar with the community agencies, health centers, and private doctors in town. Up until recently, they used a nearby hospital for children's emergency care; and a family doctor, a general practitioner, for all the health care that they needed, such as maternity and pediatric care. But the parents did not go in for checkups (Pat never had as far as Mary knew), although Mary did have a physical with each pregnancy. Children are only seen when they are sick, with the exception of well-baby care at the health center when they were infants and for immunizations after infancy.

Two months ago, Pat received group medical insurance through his father's store (the father just arranged for it), so their choice of health care was expanded. The family doctor is an older physician whom the family has seen for years. His charges are very low, but Mary feels he is getting too old to keep up with all he needs to know. She used the county hospital to deliver Daniel, because they were not covered by medical insurance at that time and could not raise the money for a private hospital. Now they will have to pay the county back in small payments until their bill is taken care of.

With their expanded health insurance benefits Mary and Pat asked for information regarding regular health care services they might be eligible for. After a bit of prodding from Mary, Pat asked how he might get a physical exam. He also expressed concern about his slow, but steady weight gain, or "gut" since he stopped playing sports.

Dental care for the family has been close to nonexistent. It is obtained at a private neighborhood dental clinic. The mother took Joseph in once when he complained of a toothache. One of his baby teeth had to be filled. The other children have not been seen. Pat and Mary go in when they have problems, and brush their teeth twice a day after meals. Mary is teaching Joseph to brush his teeth now, too.

When Ms. Bell did a nutritional survey of the family, she found that their diet consisted of a lot of starches, mainly potatoes and breads primarily at every meal. Their diet was basically American, with certain Irish specialities included—stews and boiled dinners. The family made little use of fruit or fruit juices, except for bananas, apples when in season, and canned peaches—and occasionally apple or orange juice. One vegetable, in addition to potatoes, was usually eaten with the evening meal, and casseroles, stews, and processed food such as frozen dinners, pizza, chicken pies, and macaroni and cheese were frequently served for dinner. Salads were infrequently eaten; soups were served about every other night, especially in the colder months. The weights of the children were within normal limits, but both parents were 10 to 20 percent overweight (visually) for their height. There were no food allergies among any of the family members, according to their mother.

Their diet for yesterday (excluding Daniel) was:

Breakfast	Cold cereal and whole milk
	Toast—1 to 2 pieces for Joseph, Mary, and Pat
	Coffee—2 cups (parents)
Snacks	Crackers for children (3 to 4 apiece) and milk
	Coffee—mother
Lunch	Soup (tomato)
	Dish of mashed potatoes and butter

	Canned peaches
	Milk
	(Husband and Joseph not home)
Snacks	None
Dinner	Stew with meat (1/2 lb), carrots, potatoes, and celery
	White cake
	Milk—children
	Coffee—wife
	Beer—husband

Because having adequate money for food was mentioned as a monthly concern. Mary was asked whether she received food stamps. When she said she did not, information on the program was provided. The nurse also learned that the family had very little left over each month and that 2 years ago Pat borrowed $2000 from his father to buy a used car (without Mary's knowledge) and still had not been able to pay his father back.

With Ms. Bell's encouragement Mary discussed with Pat her desire to work part time to increase the family income. She mentioned that her mother and sister both offered to take care of the children so that she could do so. They agreed that along with family planning this would be an area for further discussion.

The family associates with several organizations in the community: the parish church and school primarily. The family can walk to both, because they are only five blocks away. The health department, the family doctor, and the family dental clinic are also visited. In addition, the bars Pat frequents, the stores they shop in, and Pat's father's grocery store are all community places and people with whom friendly ties exist. Mary makes all the contacts with church, school, dentist, and doctors. The family's relationships with church, teachers, doctor, health center, dentists, and emergency room seem to have been good. There is public transportation available when family needs it, but Mary drives Pat to work on days that she needs the car, because taking the children with her on the bus is not easy.

Stemming from Mary's extensive experience in raising children and taking them to doctors, she seems to have a good, basic understanding of how to handle common minor illness and injuries. She also is able to explain what to do when more serious injuries occur or symptoms appear. She uses over-the-counter medicines such as aspirin, Tylenol, first-aid medications, Sudafed, and milk of magnesia carefully and correctly and keeps medicines in a safe place out of the reach of the children.

Neither she nor her husband watch their diet or weight or engage in regular exercise. Although she was never active (except doing housework), Pat was very active in sports until recently. For relaxation she watches TV and thinks her husband uses TV and socializing at the bar as ways of relaxing.

When the initial family assessment was completed Ms. Bell discussed her findings with Mary to determine which of the problems posed the greatest threat to family stability. Ms. Bell also asked Mary to identify which problems she felt were most amenable to change and could be worked on by the entire family.

Appendix D presents a family assessment and family care plan for this family.

APPENDIX D

Family Nursing Process Example: The O'Shea Family*

1. **Family Name:** O'Shea.
2. **Address:** Maplewood district, New England city.
3. **Family Composition:** See Table D–1.
4. **Type of Family Form:** Two parent, intact nuclear.
5. **Cultural (Ethnic) Background:** The family is Irish-American and to a large extent unacculturated (Shannon, 1963; Connery, 1968). This conclusion derives from Mary's clearly stated ethnic and religious preferences; the fact that family's social network is from the same ethnic/religious group; the family has resided in same ethnically homogeneous neighborhood for life; visits to extended family and church activities seem to be central activities; family roles and power structure are in keeping with traditional structures within Irish families; home decor is lacking of much visual art and the presence of religious objects is indicative of family's culture and religious orientation; and family stays primarily within ethnic neighborhood.
6. **Religious Identification:** Family actively involved in Catholic religious practices and belief system: attends Mass regularly, consults priest on matters of importance, belief in family and children stressed.
7. **Social Class Status:** Father is sole breadwinner. *Economic status:* Family sees its income as marginal; nevertheless, it is steady. Based on the father's occupation, income (estimated only), and education of parents, family is part of working class.
   Social mobility: The parents of the O'Sheas were poor, and thus Pat feels he, Mary, and the children are more fortunate. In fact, however, the family's history does not indicate much, if any, upward mobility. Actually, with more children the standard of living within their own nuclear family has probably declined.
8. **Family's Recreational or Leisure-time Activities:** Whole family visits extended families together (their most frequent family activity). Mother takes children to park to play. No travel, movies, or eating out because of finances and car's poor condition. Mary and Pat do not go out as couple by themselves or with friends.
9. **Family's Present Developmental Stage:** Family is in the stage of a family with school-aged children.
10. **Extent to Which Family Is Fulfilling Family Developmental Tasks:**
    Family appears to be meeting the family members needs for adequate housing, space, privacy and safety.
    Mother is adequately socializing children (see point 23, socialization function).
    Mother feeling strained in attempting to integrate new child member into family due to her role overload.
    Maintenance of satisfactory parent–child relationships, but decline in satisfaction by wife in marital relationship.
11. **Family's History:** Parents both lived in same

* *Genevieve Monahan revised Appendix D in the third edition.*

TABLE D–1. O'SHEA FAMILY COMPOSITION

Name	Gender	Relationship	Age	Place of Birth	Occupation	Education
O'Shea, Patrick	M	Father	43 years	Maplewood district	Butcher	High school graduate
O'Shea, Mary	F	Mother	35	Same	Housewife	High school graduate
O'Shea, Joseph	M	Son	$6^1/_2$	Same	Student	In first grade
O'Shea, Maureen	F	Daughter	5	Same	Student	In kindergarten
O'Shea, Betty	F	Daughter	4	Same	—	—
O'Shea, Richard	M	Son	3	Same	—	—
O'Shea, Daniel	M	Son	5-day-old infant	Same	—	—

neighborhood and went to same church. Went together $5^1/_2$ years before marriage. During engagement and early years of marriage, sex was an uncomfortable area and later awkward and unsatisfying, reported the wife. Wife feels this has created a lack of closeness between them. Both parents expected children and wanted them, with the exception of the last, which Mary did not want but now accepts warmly.

12. **Parents' Families of Origin:** Father's family: Father came over from Ireland as teenager. Worked for construction companies and saved his money until he could buy the grocery store he now has. Raised family in same neighborhood in a strict Catholic fashion. Mother's family: Her grandparents came over from Ireland during the depression for economic reasons. Raised as Catholic in same neighborhood as family now resides. Both Mary's and Pat's families were mentioned as being poor while they were growing up. No mention of what life with their respective families of origin was like.
13. **Home Characteristics:** Three-bedroom, older wooden house rented from cousin for $600 per month. Outside of house: fair condition, needs paint, loose stairs, and no outside lighting or railing present. Inside of house: minimally furnished. Living room has a color TV. Dining room has lace curtains and tablecloth, a wedding present from Mary's mother. Parents have own bedroom, presently shared with newborn who has a bassinet. The boys have one bedroom, while the girls share the other. Adequate sleeping arrangements in home. Minimal decorations, but several Catholic religious objects and photos of the children were noted. Kitchen contains small refrigerator and stove. One bathroom with toilet and bathtub. Common towels used. Mary considers the house just adequate for their needs now, but becoming more crowded because of the new baby. Safety hazards: outside loose stairs, no railings or outside light.
14. **Characteristics of Neighborhood and Larger Community:** Neighborhood (Maplewood district) is residential and composed of Irish working-class families. Neighborhood is near industrial area and 5 miles from center of city of 300,000 located in New England. Family likes closeness and familiarity of neighborhood, though worried about influx of members of minority groups nearby and rise in crime in the past several years. Family uses nearby shopping center (half mile away) for most of its shopping needs. Family's church and church school located five blocks away. Public transportation available, but Mary has access to husband's car when needed.
15. **Family's Geographic Mobility:** Family members have lived in the same community and neighborhood for all their lives.
16. **Family's Associations and Transactions With Community:** The family is known in parish church and school. Parents go to mass regularly and seem to have close trusting relationship with Father O'Neal. Women's group at church donated bassinet for new baby. Mother acts as liaison with school. Family also relates to the family doctor (although Mary wants to change physicians), family dental clinic, and children's hospital emergency room. In addition to receiving community health nursing visits, mother has taken children to well-baby clinic and for immunizations at the local health department. Family seems to stay primarily within its neighborhood.
    Family not aware of food stamp program (which was explained to Mary).
17. **Family's Social Support Network**
    Informal Systems
    Family, especially parents on both sides and mother's sister, seem to be quite helpful. Pat's

father employs son in his grocery store as butcher and loaned him $2000 for purchase of a car. Pat's mother helped with housework and children when Mary came home from hospital. (Although relations with wife were conflictual during early days of marriage, they are improved but still competitive, according to Pat.) Mary's mother also helped with house and children after Mary returned from hospital and Mary's sister went shopping for her. In addition to her sister, Mary has neighbors she talks to sometimes about her problems. And Pat has his buddies at the tavern that he relates to frequently (the degree of their support is unknown, however).

Formal Systems

Family has ties with priest, doctor, community health nurse, and teachers.

FAMILY STRUCTURE

18. Communication Patterns

Extent of Functional and Dysfunctional Communication (types of recurring patterns): Dysfunctional communication used between husband and wife.

a. Husband gives commands and makes requests without giving opportunity for feedback
b. Wife voices problems and husband minimizes them (does not validate or accept that her problems are real).
c. Wife voices concerns or asks husband's assistance, but he tunes her out, walks away, belittles her, or agrees with her and says he'll follow through, but does not (incongruency). Thus, Pat does not listen to Mary when she is communicating her needs to him.
d. Mary, in turn, does not express herself in some intimate areas due to cultural values and, possibly, fear of rejection. She probably does not directly express her needs in many areas.
e. Neither partner states needs and feelings clearly, except in case of Mary's expressed desire to curtail pregnancies.
f. Rules underlying communication patterns include the following: (1) don't question the status quo and tradition; (2) things are the way they are and complaining won't help or change things (powerless, fatalistic outlook); (3) closedness—husband doesn't want wife becoming exposed to any outside influences.

Extent of Affective Messages and How Expressed: Affective messages are not expressed openly (or privately according to Mary) between spouses. Mary is warm and affectively responsive to Daniel and Richard. She is also verbally warm and close to son Joseph. Father is verbally (and physically?) affectionate to daughter Betty. Pleasant emotions are more openly expressed, whereas negative emotions (anger, unpleasant events) are inhibited. Evidently, family rules exist that prohibit expression of these latter emotions.

Characteristics of Family Communication Network: Children make requests of father through mother. Little direct involvement and communication between father and children (except Betty–father relationship). Quality of communication between spouses poor and limited in scope (mainly regarding children and money problems) and quality (see dysfunctional patterns). Interactions are distant and unsatisfying to wife.

Areas of Closed Communications: Between spouses: inner feelings and perceptions, especially sexual feelings and thoughts.

Familial and External Variables Affecting Communication: Cultural variables are important for this family. Men and women live in different worlds in traditional Irish culture. Roles and worlds are separate, and sexes never learn to communicate adequately with each other. Nor is expression of affection or warmth toward spouse seen as acceptable in public. Sex is riddled with guilt and ignorance, making it difficult for some Irish couples to generate and retain close affective bonds. Socioeconomic stressors (marginal incomes and economic hardships) make family role enactment, housing, and fulfilling of family functions more onerous.

19. Power Structure

Power Outcomes

Husband decides major purchases (car, for example).

Wife is delegated (or relegated) sole roles of housekeeper and child rearer, and allotted a certain portion of paycheck to cover home and family expenses.

Husband in charge of distribution of funds.

Husband in charge of calling priest and doctor to initiate appointment with them.

Decision-Making Process: Husband uses his formal position of dominance to influence family decisions. Process used is accommodation. He seemed to be compromising with wife, under pressure of community health nurse when he agreed to discuss family planning health problems with priest and doctor and attempt to come up with an effective plan to prevent further pregnancies; but because he has not followed through in making appointments, one can question his sincerity in this case. May use de facto process in these cases; by doing nothing he has made the decision.

Power Bases: Father–husband maintains legitimate power or authority, granted to him culturally by virtue of his position in family. Mother has referent power (position of mother is exalted in the Catholic Church), which is more salient in her relationships with her children that it is in her relationship with her husband. Both parents have reward and coercive power over children, and husband has reward/coercive power over his wife, although no description of his using this is evident.

Variables Affecting Family Power Characteristics: Wife's position as go-between in family communication network and as implementer of family decisions should give her increased power; there is no evidence that it is being exercised, however.

Interpersonal Resources: The wife's hesitancy and fear to speak out more often and confront husband reduces what power she does/could have.

Social class/cultural and life cycle factors: Marital expectations that are commonly found in working class predominate. These same marital and family role and power expectations are characteristic of traditional Irish family life. Life cycle of family reduces wife's power and increases husband's power, because wife is burdened with day-to-day household and child-care responsibilities and has no time or energy to exercise whatever influence/power she has.

Overall Family Power

Moderate dominance seen (father dominant), with some dissatisfaction of this situation expressed by wife.

Overall family power:

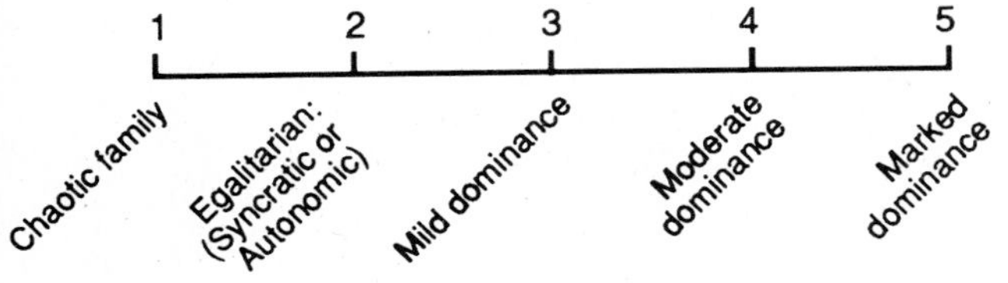

20. Role Structure

Formal Role Structure

Pat: Father and husband. He acts as sole provider for family, and is leader of family. Does not see his position as involving a companionship, recreational, or therapeutic role, however, and only occasionally does he help with the child-care role (when he feels like it). Marital roles enacted, although constricted, appear consistent with his expectations of marital roles.

Mary: Mother and wife. She acts as the homemaker (not shared), involving cooking, shopping, and cleaning home; enacts the child-care role (not shared to any real extent); the recreational role (taking children to park to play). No therapeutic role or companion role enacted in marriage. Sexual role inadequate. Wife has expressed disappointment that the therapeutic role is not present and that the sexual role is unsatisfying (distant communications, no enjoyment in sexual relationship). Wife appears to have some expectations of Pat that are more consistent with American middle-class ideas of marriage, although she seems also resigned to the fact that Pat's traditional expectations of both of their positions in the family are fairly stable and not likely to be changed. She enacts the roles needed to complement husband's role expectations of her, while at the same time trying to limit her family roles in future to some extent by having no more children. Mary definitely shows some role strain in trying to handle child care and all the other mother–wife roles by herself, as well as the possibility that she might return to part-time work.

Joseph: Older son and brother to siblings.

Maureen: Older daughter and sister to siblings.

Betty: Younger daughter and sister to siblings.

Richard: Younger son and brother to siblings.

Daniel: Youngest (baby) son and brother to siblings.

Informal Role Structure

Pat: Leader; distant one (does not get involved in family life); unconcerned one (does wife see him in this way or is this the way she expects husbands to act?)

Mary: Subservient one; go-between role (between children and their father); martyr?

Joseph: Leader of the children, mother's favorite and perhaps confidant, because mother cannot confide in and share affectively with husband. Serious one.

Maureen: Cooperative, compliant one. Follower.

Betty: Sweet one. "People-pleaser" role. Mother perceives her to play cute, manipulative role, whereas father defends her sweetness as being genuine and not manipulative. Father's favorite. Mary is perhaps threatened by husband's affections toward Betty.
Richard: Active one (with explosive temper if exploration and freedom are restricted).
Daniel: No comments by parents.
Variables Affecting Role Structure:
Social class influences: Working-class families are likely to be more traditional in terms of marital roles. Being Irish-American and fairly unacculturated affects family roles. Traditional Catholic background reinforces patriarchal family structure. The family developmental stage and presence of five small children makes wife dependent on husband as sole breadwinner, which further increases his dominance and her dependency.

21. **Family's Values:** In comparing the O'Sheas' values with American and traditional Irish and Irish-American values, the O'Sheas' values are definitely much more in keeping with the traditional Irish values and the working-class values of today. Productivity and success are not primary values. Pat has worked for his father since graduation from high school, except for time he was in the Armed Services. Mary worked in an electronics factory after graduation and until the first child was born. The work ethic and materialism do not seem central in family's life. The family does not value individualism, but familism and the ethic of reciprocity (assisting one's family and church) is salient, as is the value of doing one's duty and playing expected family roles (conformity). Education is not highly valued, nor is progress, change, and mastery; conservatism and fatalistic thinking assume greater importance. No long-term plans were expressed, except Mary's ardent plans to prevent further pregnancies and desire to return to part-time employment. Equality and individual freedom are not inferred to be important values either. The "doing orientation" does not fit this family. Time is not carefully allotted and used. Much of Pat's time outside of work is spent in recreational pursuits (spectator sports and social drinking with friends). Health care and practices are not of prime importance to family.

There appears to be a conflict in values, to some degree, between Mr. and Mrs. O'Shea. Mary obviously feels caught between the values of American society and those of traditional Irish culture that govern family roles, power relationships, and communication. She is trying—not very effectively—to assert herself with her husband, demonstrating the value of egalitarianism, individualism and progress. Pat retains the old traditional values, as stated above. This directly affects the health status of the family, by creating strain in the marital relationship.

22. **Affective Function**
Family Need–Response Patterns
Pat: For the most part, he does not make any of his socioemotional needs known to his wife or children; therefore, they are presumably not adequately met in family. (Perhaps his needs are met through work and socializing with friends at sports events and tavern). He does, however, make his needs for affection and warmth known to daughter Betty, who responds in a sweet, affectionate manner toward him.
Mary: Expressed problem of not being able to talk to husband and of not feeling emotionally close to him. He does not respond to her needs to communicate and does not empathize with her feelings regarding the responsibilities she assumes. Her son Joseph meets some of her socioemotional needs, because she feels she can talk to him, whereas Pat is not available to meet her needs.
Joseph (age 6½): Has need to handle things, lead, and be assertive. His mother gives him this opportunity, Pat feels his son's behavior is inappropriate and feels he should be put in his place. The younger children follow him. Becomes rebellious or bossy when his needs to be assertive are frustrated.
Maureen (age 5): Expresses need to cooperate with and help her mother; emulates mother's behavior and roles. Mary gives her the opportunity to fulfill these needs.
Betty (age 4): Expresses need to please people and be liked. Mother sees this as a way to "get her way" (a form of manipulation). Father sees this need as genuine, and she is his favorite. He responds to Betty's sweetness, reinforcing her behavior and needs to please.
Richard (age 3): Richard has a need to explore and be autonomous. Mary realizes this and responds by letting him run around the house and explore. Also has need for extra attention because of arrival of new baby, which parents understand and are responding to.
Daniel (age 1 to 3 weeks): Needs to trust and have his basic physiological and affectional

needs met. These are being fulfilled ably by the mother.

Mutual Nurturance, Closeness, and Identification: Adequate between mother and Joseph, Maureen, Richard, and Daniel.

Maybe attenuated between Mary and Betty, because Mary may feel threatened by her husband's favoritism and diversion of affections to Betty.

Adequate between father and Betty and father and Richard (?). Remainder of father's relationships with children are distant, and father is relatively uninvolved.

Inadequate between Mary and Pat. Mutual identification involving closeness and nurturance are weak, hence spousal bonds are weak also. She expresses need for greater closeness, whereas he does not express these needs.

Separateness and Connectedness: Not discussed here to any extent. It will become an issue with Joseph soon, because he is assertive, has leadership qualities and needs, and will increasingly wish to individuate. At present conformity and connectedness are valued much more highly than separateness.

23. Socialization Function

Family Child-rearing Practices: Observations limited. Pat advocated old-fashioned child rearing, not "new-fangled" methods. Believes in punishment, respect, and obedience. However, he has a minimal role in implementation, so that Mary may undermine some of his wishes regarding child rearing. From their behavior the children show they have been taught that "children should be seen but not heard" when adults are talking. Mary is very warm and physically affectionate, permissive, and tolerant when children are younger, but when they become preschoolers (age 4 up), she and Pat expect more self-restraint, self-discipline, respect, and obedience. Also could be seen that boys are allowed to be more assertive and aggressive than the girls of family (sex-linked socialization practices are evident).

Adaptibility of Child-rearing Practices for Family's Situation: They appear adaptive in that children are being raised to live in the world as the parents see and experience it. This involves the need to be respectful, obedient, and conforming, and for boys and girls to know their appropriate sex roles and behavior.

Who Is the Socializing Agent? The mother predominantly, but father's influence also present, albeit more indirect. School teachers and priest, in addition to kin, are also socializing agents in children's lives and will become increasingly important as the children age.

Value of Children: They were wanted and accepted. Children appear to be highly valued. Children are highly cherished in the Catholic religion and Irish-American families. Being a mother is the central role for Mary; however she now feels the "burden" of having so many children to care for.

24. Health Care Function

Family's Health Beliefs, Values, and Behaviors: Preventive care for children (except for immunizations) is not given; mother did receive physicals with each pregnancy, hence her health maintenance behaviors are more consistent than her husband's. Pat expressed concern about his steady weight gain and "gut" since he stopped playing sports.

Family's Definition of Health–Illness and Level of Knowledge: By taking children and herself to a physician or clinic when they are not visibly ill means that she acknowledges that health is more than just being able to function or a state of feeling well. Wife is health leader and decides when children are ill and in need of health services. Mother has good basic understanding of how to handle common minor illnesses and injuries. She also knows what to do when more serious injuries occur or symptoms appear.

Family Members' Perceived Health Status: Unknown.

Family Dietary Practices: Adequacy of family diet: From data regarding the family the information was inserted into a food history record (Table D–2) to the extent possible.

Caloric Intake: Adequate, although husband and wife are a little overweight (children's weights are within normal limits). Data obtained via visual inspection only. Cultural food assessment: Stews and boiled dinners prepared. Extensive use of potatoes (the Irish staple); otherwise diet is basically American.

Typicality of 24-hour Diet: This report is typical. Mary said that their diet contains little fruit or fruit juices, except for bananas, apples (in season), and canned peaches—and occasionally apple or orange juice. One cooked vegetable besides potatoes is served at dinner each evening. Soups are eaten three to four times per week; salads are infrequently eaten.

Food Allergies: None noted.

Function of mealtimes and their attitudes toward food and mealtime: Not noted.

TABLE D–2. FAMILY FOOD HISTORY RECORD

Meal	Food Served	Quantity	Individual Differences
Breakfast	Cold cereal	1 bowl	All family ate cereal
	Milk	1/2 cup for cereal	
	Toast, 1 or 2 pieces		Parents only
	Coffee	1 cup	Parents
	Milk	1 cup	Children
Snacks	Crackers	3 or 4 crackers	Children
	Milk	1 glass	
	Coffee	1 cup	Mother
Lunch	Tomato soup	1 bowl	Joseph, Maureen, and father not home
	Mashed potatoes	1/2–1 cup	
	and butter	1 tbsp	
	Canned peaches	1/2 cup	
	Milk	1 cup	
Snacks	None		
Dinner	Stew: containing		All ate stew, but children had smaller servings
	meat	1/4 cup	
	carrots	1/2 cup	
	potatoes	1/2 cup	
	celery	1/4 cup	
	White cake	1 slice	All family
	Milk	1 cup	Children
	Coffee	1 cup	Wife
	Beer	1 cup	Husband
Snacks	Cookies		

Shopping practices and person responsible: Mary goes to nearby shopping center. She has budgetary limitations and just barely gets by each month. She does not use food stamps but is interested in applying to obtain them.

Refrigerator and Stove: Functioning and adequate, though small. Wife is totally responsible for planning, shopping, and preparation of meals.

Sleeping and Rest Practices: Sleeping patterns not noted. Mary stated she used TV for relaxing and that Pat does same, in addition to going over to the bar to socialize and drink for the purposes of relaxation.

Exercise and Recreational Practices: Parents do not have regular exercise program for themselves. It is not mentioned as to whether they believe this is a necessity for health maintenance. Wife gets a moderate amount of exercise doing housework and child-care activities. Husband used to be active in sports but is not presently. He stands at his job (as butcher).

Family's Drug Habits: Husband drinks alcohol (type and amount unknown); socializing at bars is a frequent and central activity for him.

Both parents drink coffee (2 to 3 cups per day noted).

Tobacco is not used.

It is not mentioned whether use of tobacco or alcohol is considered a problem.

Family's use of prescription and over-the-counter drugs:

Use of prescription drugs not noted.

Use of over-the-counter drugs directed by Mary. She uses cold medicines (Sudafed, etc), gastrointestinal medicines (milk of magnesia, etc), first-aid medications, and aspirin correctly and carefully. She also stores medicines in a safe cabinet away from children's reach.

Family's Role in Self-care Practices: See prior comments. Also administers medications carefully and correctly.

Environmental Practices: Environmental hazards are not noted. Family lives close to industrial area, however, where a number of factories are located. No other cleanliness problems noted.

Medically Based Preventive Measures: Children (except when infants) and adults do not have periodic physical examinations.

No information on recency or on vision/hearing examinations or immunization status of family members.
Dental Health Practices: Nutritional: breads and some desserts noted in diet. No candy noted.
Brushing Teeth: Parents brush teeth two times a day after meals. Joseph is being taught to brush teeth. Other children have not started brushing teeth yet.
Use of fluoride: Not mentioned.
No dental check-ups and cleanings. Family visits family dental clinic in neighborhood when dental problems arise. Joseph has had one cavity filled (baby tooth). Parents have been to dentist on a problem basis only. Children other than Joseph have not been seen by a dentist.
Family Health History: No information included.
Health Services Received: Receive pediatric and maternity services from family doctor. Last baby, Daniel, delivered at county hospital because family could not raise necessary funds for private hospital and did not have health insurance at the time. They are now covered by husband's employment, however. Receive well-baby care and immunizations through health department. Pat had never been seen by doctor for physical examinations to Mary's knowledge.
Perceptions/Feelings Regarding Health Care: Family physician (long-time family doctor) is liked, but because family has medical insurance now, Mary would like to switch doctors. Stayed with above physician because his rates were low; but he is old, and Mary is afraid he is not up-to-date in his practice. Mary and Pat asked for information on regular health care services that health insurance covers.
No comments regarding health department services or dental services.
Emergency Health Services: Family uses children's hospital in community when emergency care is needed for children. No mention of where parents go or would go if emergency arose.
Source of Payment: Family has had to assume total expense of medical and dental care up to now. Recently received group health insurance through Pat's father's business (the grocery store). No dental insurance mentioned. Provisions of health insurance not known.
Logistics of Receiving Care: No problems noted. Care has been accessible and mother has car for transportation.

FAMILY COPING

25. Short-term Stressors:

a. Recent addition to family (Daniel), causing need to reallocate resources and relationships in family.
b. Wife's potential to become pregnant again (lack of family planning).
c. Richard's sibling rivalry and acting-out behaviors, although this does not seem to be a serious stressor.
d. Role overload and strain experienced by mother due to the arrival of another baby and heavy household and child-care responsibilities.

Long-term Stressors:

a. Economic: Marginally adequate income ("barely gets by every month") and two outstanding debts to pay off: car and hospital bills. With new baby and inflation, economic problems may increase.
b. Marital: Lack of communication between husband and wife.
c. Role strain of wife (role overload). Mary's role strain appears not to be recognized as burden by Pat and is minimized as a problem within their cultural/religious orientation.
d. Threat of future pregnancies (short- and long-term stressor).
e. Value conflicts between Irish-American subculture and American majority culture.

Strengths That Counterbalance Stressors:
Family has several strong assets that counterbalance to a moderate extent the above family stressors:

a. Husband's steady job (stable provider).
b. Mary's ability and willingness to work and Mary's mother's offer to provide infant care.
c. Permanency of residence. Family knows neighborhood and community, familiar with resources. They like neighborhood's cohesiveness and are well integrated into neighborhood.
d. Social support system of family is moderately strong. Extended family present and assistance available and partially utilized. Also, neighbors and friends were mentioned

as helpful. Church and church school are important resources to family.

e. Health status of family members appears adequate to good with no obvious problems except Mary's hypertension during pregnancies mentioned.

f. Adequate housing and furnishings at present.

g. Adequate health care (except preventive), nutritional practices, and health resources (health services and insurance).

26. **Family's Ability to Base Decisions on Objective Appraisal of Stress-Producing Situation:** Role overload (role strain) experienced by Mary and her expressed need to prevent further pregnancies are the two stress-producing situations occurring during nurse's visits. Mary seems to be able to appraise situations realistically, but Pat denies the significance of her concerns and strains. As a family they have not taken action yet, because Pat was supposed to call the priest and doctor for appointments but has neglected to do so. As a family, parents have not worked together to appraise problems objectively and solve them.

27. **Family's Reaction to Stressors: Functional Coping Strategies Utilized (Present and Past):** The family uses their social support system of extended family and church primarily to assist them in time of need. Inner coping resources are not mentioned as means for dealing with stressors. The family is able to meet the usual stresses and strains of daily life, largely through the efforts of Mary, who is the central figure in the family. Mary and Pat, albeit more reluctantly, are seeking information about health care services.

28. **Problem Areas Over Which the Family Has Achieved Mastery:** This is unclear, but no major areas are identified.

29. **Dysfunctional Adaptive Strategies Utilized (Past and Present):** First, the family does not use its inner resources adequately to deal with stressors. There is no "pulling together," increased cohesiveness, or sharing of feelings and thoughts, during periods of greater demand. Pat goes his own way rather than pitching in as part of the family team. The more overt dysfunctional coping mechanism that can be identified is that of authoritarianism, coupled with an element of neglect. Interestingly enough, this pattern is an exaggeration of the traditional Irish or Irish-American pattern. The stance may be taken that Pat uses his position of dominance too extensively, however, because through his authoritarianism and neglect (his minimal involvement with family life) he stifles the growth and quality of their marital relationship, as well as reduces the quality of his relationship with his children (except with Betty). Mild dominance, where feelings and input are solicited and received from family members, especially the wife, is not detrimental, but the pattern observed in this case study affects the family unit, its subsystems, and the individual family members adversely (Table D–3).

SEE TABLE 10–3 FOR FAMILY NURSING DIAGNOSES AND PLAN OF CARE.

OTHER FAMILY NURSING DIAGNOSES GENERATED FROM O'SHEA ASSESSMENT

- Father–child relationships weak (except for Betty).
- Nutritional deficiencies: Insufficient use of vegetables and fruits, especially ones containing vitamin C; lack of sufficient iron in diet.
- Inadequate dental hygiene and care: Brushing for Maureen and Betty; examinations for whole family.
- Lack of exercise program for the spouses.
- Home safety hazards: No lighting or railings on outside steps. Stair boards loose.

FURTHER ASSESSMENT DATA NEEDED

- Perceived health status of family members.
- Health insurance benefits.
- Family's knowledge regarding how to locate another family physician.
- Family's knowledge of accessible emergency rooms for adults.
- Eye/hearing examinations and immunization status of family members.
- Family medical history.
- Roles: role models of parents.
- Environmental exposure to pollutants from industrial area nearby.
- Spouses' feelings about their sexual relationship and attitudes about counseling.
- Husband's drinking pattern and consumption of alcohol.

TABLE D–3. FAMILY NURSING CARE PLAN AND FURTHER ASSESSMENT NEEDED

Family Nursing Diagnoses Including Contributing Factors	Signs and Symptoms (Identifying Characteristics)	Further Assessment Data Needed	Goals	Interventions	Evaluation
1. Altered marital and parental role performance (role strain/overload) related to arrival of another baby, heavy child-care responsibilities, and inadequate family coping patterns.	No companion role present (couple does not do things together).	Do spouses wish to do leisure time activities together?	*Short-term*: Spouses will be able to discuss their relationship and whether they need to strengthen certain aspects of marriage. *Long-term*: Spousal relationship (subsystem) will be strengthened by enlarging number of roles involved in marital positions (companion, therapeutic, and perhaps sexual) and by improving communications.	Discuss with the couple the stress and role strain they are experiencing with the arrival of the new baby. Help them redefine or reframe the problem as a family problem, not a mother–wife problem. Encourage them to share their concerns about their growing responsibilities and the financial strain. Encourage greater use of existing support system (eg, grandmothers and aunt) to have more leisure time together. Assist the couple to explore options for leisure time that would be satisfying for both of them. Open up discussion with couple about Mary's interest in obtaining part-time job and support her efforts to obtain information. Assist couple to discuss and clarify their roles, expectations of each other, their communications with each other, to open up avenues for modification of their roles/communication to create more functional patterns. Assist couple to identify internal coping mechanisms (eg, humor) or joint problem solving that could be utilized to reduce stressors. Discuss with Pat his willingness to take on some responsibilities with child care and child rearing if Mary returns to part-time work. Support exploration of child care resources/options	To be completed after intervention. Would look at goals to determine to what degree these have been achieved.
Variables Cultural and religious values and norms regarding marital roles and adult roles for women and men. Life cycle of family: high demands being placed on both parents at this stage of family's life. Socioeconomic position: marginal income, limited education, constricted world.	Therapeutic role inadequate. Husband does not listen to wife's concerns. Lack of communication except for money and some of children's problems. Sexual roles unsatisfying.	Does husband feel there is a problem with communication? Does husband feel that sexual roles are problem and an area for improvement? Would wife feel that this is an area she would be too embarrassed to have discussed?			

TABLE D–3. (*Continued*)

Family Nursing Diagnoses Including Contributing Factors	Signs and Symptoms (Identifying Characteristics)	Further Assessment Data Needed	Goals	Interventions	Evaluation
				(aunt or children's grandmother). Explore the couple's perceived need and interest in marital counseling and in receiving information on marital and sexual relationships. Initiate referral(s) if need and interest are present.	
Life cycle of family: high demands being placed on both parents at this stage of family's life. Socioeconomic position: marginal income, limited education, constricted world.	Mates do not "pull together" (become cohesive and reliant on own resources during periods of high demand on family).	Assess couple's, especially husband's, willingness and readiness to explore ways of strengthening marital relationship.		Suggest they discuss family/marriage with priest. See if couple can obtain new, enlightened information and guidance on family planning and marriage. Socioeconomic: Refer to food stamp program.	
2. Alteration in health maintenance: Ineffective family planning.	Wife's hypertension during pregnancies and potential harm to health from subsequent pregnancy.	How do family's priest and physician feel about family planning for couple? What is couple's relationship with physician and priest? Are they the most appropriate resources to refer couple to?	*Short-term*: Couple will be able to accurately describe the types of family planning methods available and acceptable to them (within their cultural/religious belief system).	Help couple explore feelings regarding limiting family, effects of having additional children on family Assist couple to problem solve in making and carrying out decision in this area (resources, who will follow up with contacting them, etc).	To be completed after interventions. Would look at goals to determine to what degree goals have been achieved.
Variables History of high fertility, pregnancies every year. History of hypertension during pregnancies. Cultural/religious in-	Mother does not want more children—strain on herself, budget, housing, etc. Family-planning methods inade-		Couple will be able to explore their thoughts and feelings about having no more children. Husband will understand wife's con-	Refer family to health and religious resources (if needed) as part of problem-solving process. Follow-through with spouses after they have met with physician and priest to dis-	

(*continued*)

TABLE D–3. (*Continued*)

Family Nursing Diagnoses Including Contributing Factors	Signs and Symptoms (Identifying Characteristics)	Further Assessment Data Needed	Goals	Interventions	Evaluation
fluences on family planning. Weak spousal relationship (lack of spousal communication).	quate (not a problem at present, but will be soon). Husband is not sufficiently empathetic with wife's concerns regarding having no more children and passively accepts unplanned pregnancies.		cerns and see problem as a family problem. *Long-term*: Couple will successfully use family planning method(s) to prevent further pregnancies.	cuss any questions, thoughts, or areas where further information is needed, making sure they have sufficient knowledge about family planning methods that were recommended.	
3. Health-seeking behaviors (expressed desire for improvement in preventive health care behavior).	Preventive health services are accessible and family has new health insurance benefits.	What benefits are included under new health insurance policy?	*Short term*: Couple will be able to identify preventive health care services under their new health insurance policy	Review with couple their health insurance policy and determine preventive health care benefits.	To be completed after intervention. Would look at goals to determine to what degree these have been achieved.
	None of the family has had regular preventive dental or medical examinations	Knowledge of age-appropriate preventive health care practices. Immunization status of children.	*Long term*: Family will make full and regular use of all medical and dental benefits eligible for under health insurance benefits. All family members will receive preventive medical examinations allowed by health insurance policy.	Explain the importance of preventive medical and dental examinations. Refer to low-cost community services for care not covered by insurance policy (eg, dental).	

TABLE D–3. (*Continued*)

Family Nursing Diagnoses Including Contributing Factors	Signs and Symptoms (Identifying Characteristics)	Further Assessment Data Needed	Goals	Interventions	Evaluation
			Short-term: Spouses All family members will receive dental checkup and cleaning.		
			Will perform other age-appropriate preventive health behavior (eg, immunizations, safety, stress management, and self-examinations)	Review preventive health care practices that would be beneficial for family group as well as for each member of the family. To expand and reinforce knowledcge, provide health education materials regarding age appropriate preventive health care practices. Refer family members, as needed, to community resources for preventive health behavior modification (eg, health education programs and self-help groups).	
	Parents are both overweight with no regular exercise program.	What kind of physical exercise would couple be willing to participate in? Level of physical activity of children.	Parents will initiate a regular exercise program.	Support husband's concern about need to exercise and positive efforts couple makes to get information or start exercise program.	
	Diet—more fat in diet than recommended. Insufficient fruits and vegetables.	Willingness to alter diet.	Family will alter diet to reduce fat and increase fruits and vegetables.	Compliment parents on the positive aspects of their family diet and encourage them to increase positive dietary patterns. Encourage parents' efforts to improve diet.	
	Husband's use of alcohol by report of wife.	Extent of husband's alcohol use.			

APPENDIX E

Chapter Study Answers

☐ CHAPTER 1 STUDY ANSWERS

1. c, d.
2. d.
3. a, b, and c.
4. b and c.
5. a, b, and c.
6. a and b.
7. *Prevention of illness and risk reduction stage.* Family reinforces health provisions and preventive measures.
8. *Family illness appraisal and symptom experience stage.* Family defines meaning of symptoms/illness.
9. *Care-seeking stage.* Family persuades individual to seek care.
10. *The family's contact with health system stage.* Family is the primary health referral agent (to whom, and when).
11. *Acute response of patient and family stage.* Family defines appropriate activity (roles) of patient during this stage; illness impact on family and often produces crisis in serious, life-threatening situations.
12. *Adaptation to illness and recovery stage.* Family either supports or hinders patient's recovery pattern. Nature of health problem also affects the family's adaptation.

13. a, c, and d.

14. Whereas health refers to the individual's state of functioning (ie, the extent to which an individual functions as an integrated whole person, maximizing his or her potential within his or her environment), family health refers to the adequacy of functioning of the family as a unit or system. Beyond this difference, many finer distinctions exist, such as the use of different indicators used to measure family health and health.

15. Variant family form refers to all family arrangements that deviate from the traditional nuclear family in which the husband/father is the breadwinner, the wife/mother is the homemaker, and children are present in the home.

16. Examples of traditional variant family forms are nuclear dyads (childless couples), single-parent families, single adults living alone, and extended three-generation families.

17. Examples of nontraditional variant family forms are commune families, unmarried parent and child families, unmarried couple and child families, cohabiting couples, and gay/lesbian families.

18. Role conflicts/role overload, role changes, and poverty.

19. Aging population; increase in women's employment; high divorce and remarriage rates, decrease in household/family size (fertility control, postponement of marriage and childbearing are factors creating the decreased size of household/family); increase in births to older mothers.

20. a, b, and c.

21. e. (Factors b and d are also associated with single-parent families and unmarried teenage mothers).

☐ CHAPTER 2 STUDY ANSWERS

1. b.

2. The ordering of priorities is different. The community health nurse is committed to providing services to families to help resolve major *community health* problems in addition to services designed to meet unique health needs of family. The family nurse in other settings/specialties prioritizes the family's particular health needs.

3. b, c, and d.

4. b.

5. a.

6. a.

7. b.

8. c.

9. b.

10. c.

11. a.

12. a.

13. c, d, e, and f; d and e.

14. 1. Recognition of need to change priorities in health care—from crisis-oriented acute care (often the end result of self-destructive life patterns and environmental hazards) to causative factors of major chronic illnesses (life-style and environmental improvements).
2. Growing costs of present health care system with little cost effectiveness.
3. Demystification and discontentment with primary health care.
4. Life-style changes and increased educational levels (a better informed middle class).
5. Problems with accessibility and availability of primary care health services.

15. 1. "Integrated functioning."
2. Continually striving to grow and "maximizing potential" (dynamic state).
3. "Within person's environment." Showing importance of our interaction with the environment.

16. 1. Self-responsibility, self-accountability, and self-care.
2. Nutritional awareness—nutritional patterns that promote health and personal enjoyment.
3. Stress management—learning how to handle stress (keeping it at healthy level).
4. Physical fitness—maintaining a regular exercise program so that physiological and psychological benefits are attained.
5. Environmental sensitivity—to be aware of environmental surroundings and their effects, modifying the physical, social, and personal environments, again, so that positive benefits to health and happiness are accrued.

(See chapter text for a more thorough discussion of these dimensions.)

17. The health-hazard appraisal tool lists basic identifying data on an individual (name, age, race, sex, and occupation) and the rank and nature of the major health problems (causing death) for persons of that age and sex. Prognostic criteria for each of these major health problems are also identified adjacent to problem. The tool then asks for information about client relative to each of these criteria and has space next to client data for treatment advised to reduce risks.

18. Dorothea Orem.

19. Whereas health refers to the individual's state of functioning (ie, the extent to which an individual functions as an integrated whole person, maximizing his or her potential within his or her environment), family health refers to the adequacy of functioning of the family as a unit or system. Beyond this difference, many finer distinctions exist, such as the use of different indicators used to measure family health and health.

20. If family nurses can help families incorporate family health-promotion strategies or incorporate a wellness life-style, most of our health problems will be alleviated or forestalled. Health promotion is much more cost-effective than illness care.

21. b.

☐ CHAPTER 3 STUDY ANSWERS

1. b.

2.
a. 1.
b. 5.
c. 6.
d. 3.
e. 2 and/or 4.
f. 5.
g. 5
h. 2.
i. 5.
j. 4.
k. 7.
l. 4.

3. c.

4. b.

5. a and b.

6. a, b, and c.

7. b or c.

8. e.

9. d and e.

10. Any three:
a. Review written records.
b. Discuss the family with other health care team members who know the family well.
c. Gather whatever information, teaching supplies, and assessment and intervention equipment needed or anticipated.
d. Call family on phone to set up visit if possible.

11. One advantage to using this method of diagnosing is that the symptoms and etiologic factors lead to more comprehensive setting of goals and approaches.

12. All choices (a–e) are correct.

13. All phases, since the family and its members are the crucial, central focus of our services and must be involved in all phases in order for each phase to be accomplished.

14. a. Apathy.
b. Any of the following: difference in value system, difference in perception of problem due to ignorance or fear, and sense of futility about available resources.

15. a. Indecision.
b. Family fears/unexpected concerns.

16. c.

17. d and e.

18. Interview data, observational data, responses from questionnaires, checklists, and agency written records.

19. The theoretical model used; the nature of the diagnosis and goals; the level of the functioning of the family; the family's resources; and family interests and decisions.

20. Freeman's classification.

21. Freeman's classification is nursing action oriented and community health nursing based, while Wright and Leahey classify according to whether the actions are directed toward the family's thoughts/perceptions, feelings, or behaviors. The classification is family and psychosocially oriented.

22. a. l.
b. l.
c. s.
d. s.
e. s.
f. n.

☐ CHAPTER 4 STUDY ANSWERS

1. a. 3.
b. 4.
c. 2 and 6.
d. 5.
e. 7.

2. Its internal dynamics or the interaction between the family members.

3. Role structure, power structure (decision-making processes), and communication patterns. Family stress and coping, status relations, and socialization problems are also correct.

4.

a. 3.	e. 2.
b. 4.	f. 2.
c. 2.	g. 2.
d. 2.	h. 1.

5. a. Nursing theories: specify a nursing focus and suggest nursing actions (what areas to assess and with what emphasis, delineation of goals, and intervention).
b. Family therapy theories: superior in providing clinical application (assessment and intervention) in family mental health settings.
c. Family social science theories: provide full description of family relationships (inner dynamics and external interactions) and family behavior.
d. A theoretical framework provides the mechanism by which we can organize our observations, focus our inquiries, and communicate our findings. A practice theory also guides clinical practice.

6. d.

7. a. 3.
b. 3.
c. 3.
d. 1.
e. 3.

□ CHAPTER 5 STUDY ANSWERS

1. c.

2. Both internal family dynamics (structure) and other internal dimensions (functions and subsystems). The systems interface with other systems and suprasystems, such as reference groups and wider society, which are also assessed.

3. b.

4. a.

5. d.

6. a. 1.
   b. 2.
   c. 1.
   d. 2.

7. *Affective function:* Not being adequately fulfilled for all family members. Minimal data on children, although mother seems quite involved and enjoys her children. Mother is feeling unfulfilled emotionally in her relationship with her husband. No concrete data on husband's feelings, although it appears he has withdrawn from the family affectively.
   Health care Function: Food: mother cooks and provides nutritional meals, although excessive carbohydrates; shelter: adequate home provided; clothing: family adequately dressed; health care: children appear in good health. Would need to assess further this area, as it is inadequately described.
   Reproductive function: Family has seven children. All living with the family.
   Socialization: Emma's central family concern is child rearing; father participates minimally in disciplining and guidance. Family actively fulfills this function via the mother. Social placement: Society will identify family as members of working class.
   Economic function: Father employed and provides family with basic necessities for independent living.

□ CHAPTER 6 STUDY ANSWERS

1. Any three:
   a. A family is seen as a long-lived *small group* that changes *over time.*
   b. Families go through *life cycle stages.*
   c. *During each life cycle stage certain developmental tasks* are germane to a family's functioning.
   d. In families there is *high family member interdependency.*
   e. Family developmental tasks *are derived from* a combination of individual developmental tasks of each family member and the common family functions.
   f. The developmental approach describes *commonalities* in family experiences through time.

2. b.

3. All responses are correct (a–f).

4. c.

5. a, b, d, e, g, and h.

6. b.

7. a, d, and e.

8. a.

9.

FAMILY LIFE CYCLE STAGE	DEFINITION OF PHASE	HEALTH CONCERNS OR NEEDS
I. Married couple	Couple without children	1. Generating satisfying marriage (communications, sexual counseling). 2. Family planning. 3. Prenatal care.
II. Childbearing	Birth of the firstborn until oldest child is 30 months old.	1. Postpartum care, family planning. 2. Sibling rivalry. 3. Infant supervision and education (also family interactions—parental, marital).
III. Preschool age	Oldest child is 30 months to 5–6 years old (when child starts school).	1. Preschooler's accidents and infectious illnesses. 2. Adequate child care facilities. 3. Marital relationship problems.
IV. School age	Oldest child is 6–13 years old.	1. Marital relationship problems. 2. Learning problems of children. 3. Child-rearing practices.
V. Teenage	Oldest child is 13–20 years old.	1. Communication problems (parent–teenager). 2. Discipline and power struggles (parent–teenager).
VI. Families launching young adults	Firstborn through youngest child leave home.	1. Parent–child communication problems. 2. General health promotion. 3. Care of and assistance to aging parents.
VII. Middle-aged parent	Empty nest (no children home) to retirement.	1. Care of and assistance to aging parents. 2. Emergence of chronic illness–need for wellness life-style.

FAMILY LIFE CYCLE STAGE	DEFINITION OF PHASE	HEALTH CONCERNS OR NEEDS
		3. Grandparent role.
VIII. Aging family	Retirement to death of both spouses.	1. Declining health status. 2. Retirement. 3. Death of spouse.

10.

LIFE CYCLE STAGE	DEVELOPMENTAL TASK(S) OF PARENT
I. Stage of marriage	1. None.
II. Childbearing stage	1. Parents learn cues baby expresses in making needs known. 2. Learning to accept child's growth and development (toddler).
III. Preschool age	1. Learning to separate from child.
IV. School age	1. Learning to separate from child continues.
V. Teenage	1. Learning to accept rejection without deserting the child. 2. Learning to build a new life for themselves (marital couple).
VI. Families launching young adults	1. Learning to build a new life for themselves (marital couple) continues.
VII. Middle-aged parents	1. Learning to build a new life for themselves (marital couple) continues.
VIII. Aging family	1. None.

11. d.

12. Emancipation, generation gap, and youth culture.

13. The American family is tremendously affected by the developmental tasks of the adolescent. The turmoil and conflicts between parents and teenagers are inevitable as the teenager's assertion of himself or herself and rebellion is part of becoming independent or emancipated.

14. e.

15. d.

16. b.

17. a.

18. f.

19. g.

20. c.

21. h.

22. a, b, and d.

23. Remarriage, because of its disruptive nature, generally impedes the family's movement through and completion of the family developmental tasks for 2 to 3 years after the creation of the new blended (step-parent) family. After the new family is restabilized (with a new structure, roles, rituals, and rules), the family resumes its normal developmental process.

24. The family's present developmental stage, the extent to which the family is fulfilling its family developmental tasks, the family's history from inception to present, and both parents' families of origin.

25. Teaching and counseling modalities.

☐ CHAPTER 7 STUDY ANSWERS

1. True.
2. False.
3. True.
4. False.
5. True.
6. True.
7. a. Focal system = family.
   b. Suprasystem = wider community.
   c. Interacting systems = health care system, educational system, law enforcement system, welfare system.
   d. Subsystems = spouse, parent–child, and sibling subsystems.
8. See energy, matter, and information exchange and process model (Fig. 7–3). Various examples could be applied, such as:

   Input (= *information*): News of risk of inactivity and benefits of exercise program.

   Flow: Spouse subsystem accepts and internalizes this information.

   Output: Spouses begin dance classes weekly for themselves. They also began hiking with their children on weekends (the energy release—their activity—is the output).

   Feedback: The family members feel better (have more energy, vitality, and strength) plus the parents' figures improve; both then become reinforcers of the exercise program.
9. a. 1.
   b. 2.
   c. 1.
   d. 1.
   e. 3.
   f. 3.
   g. 4.
10. f (see introduction to chapter for relevant discussion).
11. a, b, c, d, e, and h.
12. *Significance of family boundaries:* Boundaries allow for the exchange processes. By controlling the flow in and out of the system, they prevent overload or underload of the system. *Significance of family subsystem boundaries:* They prevent loss of integrity of the system and interference with their vital functions.

13. Family boundaries function adaptively by being selectively permeable—that is, actively expanding (opening up) and retracting (closing down) according to need, thus regulating the amounts of input and output.

14. a. 3.
    b. 1, 2, 3.
    c. 1.
    d. 3.
    e. 2.
    f. 2.

15. Four characteristics of a healthy family are: highly organized and differentiated, autonomous subsystems, tolerance and ability to change internally, and continual openness to new information and other input. (Pratt's characteristics of an energized family are also correct.)

16. a. 1, 3, 7, and 8.
    b. 2, 4, 5, and 6.
    c. 9.
    d. None.

17. a. 5.
    b. 2.
    c. 1.
    d. 3 or 4.
    e. 3 or 4.
    f. 6.
    g. 7.

☐ CHAPTER 8 STUDY ANSWERS

1. Gaining an understanding of the cultural background of a family is essential to family health care, because without this knowledge, family values and behavior cannot be understood or accurately interpreted. Culture permeates and circumscribes familial actions. In the absence of being able to assess accurately, the health care professional then is not in a position to work with the family to assist it in resolving health problems.

2. b.

3. All but e.

4. b and c.

5. c.

6.

1. p.	6. c.	
2. d.	7. g.	11. j.
3. f.	8. m.	12. o.
4. e.	9. n.	13. a.
5. h.	10. l.	14. b.

7. b (usually of husband, but increasingly of both spouses in dual-career families).

8. d.

9. All (a–e).

10. b and c.

11. c, d, and e.

12. b and c.

13. Any three: productivity versus "getting by"; education versus less value on education; mastery over environment versus fatalism, powerlessness against environment; future-oriented, long-range planning versus present-oriented, immediate gratification.

14. a.

15. Use of self-help groups and bringing in people from family's social network to be part of the family unit the nurse is working with.

16. c.

17. a. Teaching families how to reduce costs of health care by presenting options. Teaching them about their insurance coverage and community resources for help.
    b. Other services within the health agency, such as the business office or social worker, or community services, such as the Social Security Administration office or the state vocational rehabilitation office.
    c. Teaching about the benefits to the family of having family recreational and other leisure-time activity. Teaching about what types of recreational activity is healthier and more accessible.
    d. Role modeling and behavior modification (contracting).

☐ CHAPTER 9 STUDY ANSWERS

1. Housing is the symbol of status, of achievement, and of social acceptance. It influences the way in which the individual and family perceive themselves and are perceived by others.

2. Crowding, dilapidation, cockroaches or other insect infestation, and high noise level. Also acceptable answers: social isolation, inadequate space (inadequate internal space of home and arrangement of space in home).

3. Acute respiratory infections, certain infectious childhood diseases, and infectious gastrointestinal diseases. Also acceptable: home accidents, infectious and noninfectious skin diseases, and lead poisoning.

4. c.

5. a, b, and c.

6. b.

7. True.

8. True.

9. True.

10. False.

11. False.

12. True.

Identifying Data

13.1. Composition of family:

Name	Sex	Relationship	Date/Place of Birth	Occupation	Education
Juarez, Mr.	M	Husband/father	1953 Mexico	Dishwasher (full-time)	3rd grade (Mexico)
Juarez, Mrs.	F	Wife/mother	1958 Mexico	Janitorial work (part-time)	3rd grade (Mexico)
Juarez, Maria	F	Daughter	1975 Mexico	Student	?
Juarez, Jose	M	Son	1977 Mexico	Student	?
Juarez, Pedro	M	Son	1980 Mexico	Student	?

13.2. Type of family form: nuclear.

13.3. Religious and cultural orientation: Religion—Roman Catholic; attend mass regularly. Cultural—Ethnicity is Mexican. Family is not acculturated to Anglo culture; evidence—stay within small ethnically based neighborhood territorial complex. Language is Spanish. Family has no community associations except for Spanish-speaking Catholic church. Live within Mexican-American neighborhood; friendly with neighbors. Couple has traditional family structure (patriarchal).

13.4. Social class status: Upper-lower social class. Economically independent. Both parents work in unskilled jobs. Father is primary breadwinner. Parents' education limited to third grade. Income very marginal, but work is steady.

13.5. Social class mobility: Have moved upward from state of dire poverty, where basic necessities—food and shelter—were difficult to obtain to upper-lower class, where family not only has adequate food, but has rented house and both parents have jobs. They are still poor, but relative to their past they have moved upward.

13.6. Developmental stage and history of family: Developmental stage: Family with school-age children. José and Pedro appear to have learning problems and parents have not been to school. By parents not relating to school staff, parents are inadequately promoting school attainment, a developmental task within this stage. Parents were neighbors as children and their families encouraged their marriage. Early marriage (husband was 20, wife 15).

They conceived first child 6 months after marriage and felt positive about pregnancy and birth. All of the children were welcomed additions to the family; they were seen as a natural event in family life. Marital relationship—both partners seem content. Family roles are well-delineated along traditional lines.

13.7. Family's support system: Each other (nuclear family members). May have persons at church or neighbors who serve as supports; however, no information available in this area.

13.8. Recreational activities: Very limited. The mother occasionally takes children to the neighborhood park. No books or toys seen.

Environmental Data

14.1. Home: Noted to be "minimally adequate." Two-bedroom, old, small wooden house; no carpeting, paucity of furniture, clean. Have a stove, refrigerator, washing machine, and radio. Heating is adequate (electric wall heating). Only unsafe condition mentioned was screen off electric wall heater. Inadequate lighting may be safety problem. Types of privacy available: Parents share one bedroom. Have privacy. Boys share another bedroom. Maria does not have the privacy she needs nor a place of her own to play. Family may not perceive themselves as being crowded, since former housing was probably much less spacious.

14.2. Neighborhood and community: Neighborhood is low-income Mexican-American district in Los Angeles. Neighborhood is part of wider Los Angeles community (a large metropolitan, heterogeneous city). Geographic mobility: Moved 1 year ago from northern agrarian area in Mexico to the Los Angeles area.

14.3. Associations and transactions with community: No associations in community except children in school and family attends mass at local Spanish-speaking Catholic church.

14.4. Family's perceptions and feelings about the community: "Neighbors have been friendly." Family likes community, although worried about children's friends and high crime rate.

15. Home safety problems: Absence of fan cover; potential problems due to children's age, parents' probable knowledge deficit regarding safety hazards, and poor housing situation.

16. a. Intervention for actual safety problem: Teach family members about danger of fan's cover being absent and suggest that they either place fan in inaccessible place (after turning it on) or that they replace fan.

b. Intervention for potential problem: Teach primary promotion to reduce likelihood of injury or illness due to potential environmental problems. For instance, because of young children in the home, teach about safe storage of medicines and toxic, poisonous substances and where to get emergency care in the neighborhood/community.

☐ CHAPTER 10 STUDY ANSWERS

1. d and h.

2. *Sender.*
   a. Intention or meaning sent through clear and direct channels.
   Receiver. Intended message and received message are consistent, congruent, and match in meaning.

3. a. 2.
   b. 4.
   c. 2, 3.
   d. 5.
   e. 1.

4. c.

5. b.

6. a.

7. True.

8. a. *Content level.* Disinterest expressed in movie.
   Instructional level. Expression of warmth, sexual attraction, and interest.
   b. *Content level.* Statement of love and demand that child play with toy.
   Instructional level. Expression of rejection of child's request for closeness and attention.
   c. *Content and instructional level.* Both consonant: Demand to stop behavior.

9. Redundancy.

10. Positive feedback loops.

Family Case Study

The following interactional vignettes are followed by interpretations in the brackets:

NURSE: (question directed to husband): What activities did the doctor recommend for you to do this week?

SYLVIA: (interceding): I told Herman that he should take it easy because after all this is his second heart attack and the next one will be his last!
[Speaks for other person; tangentialization and "you should" statement.]

MARIAN: Yes, mother's right. He should be taking it easy. Isn't that right? (Looks at mother for agreement.)
[Short-term, issue-oriented coalition; assumption that father shares their same feelings—lack of exploration or validation with the father.]

NURSE: I understand both of your concerns for your husband's and father's welfare. But, Mr. Katz, I want to know your understanding and feelings about what activities and the amount of exercise your doctor wants you to get.
[Nurse refocuses and paraphrases her question by utilizing an "I want" statement.]

HERMAN: Well, my understanding is that I shouldn't do anything that upsets or fatigues me. And up to now I haven't felt like doing anything much.

NURSE (again looking at Herman): What specifically did the doctor say you should do?

Herman looks at his daughter and then wife, and daughter immediately jumps up to get his written directions on exercises and diet guidelines. Nurse reads these guidelines and explains the concept and importance of the recommended progressive exercise program. As this is being carefully explained, Mrs. K. looks over to the kitchen as if she is disinterested and then walks out to begin lunch preparation.

[Silent disagreement by wife. Perhaps this program violates her need to care for her husband, or maybe she feels it might be too much and is quite concerned over his possible future death. Also, culturally there is a tendency for family members in Jewish families to greatly assist their sick family members and this often runs counter to "pushing" a patient to be more self-sufficient.]

As the exercise program continued to be discussed, Herman remarked:

HERMAN: These activities don't use up much of my time and I'm tired of watching TV. I feel restless 'cause I have nothing to do.
[This is a case of incongruent behavior—between what he is now saying and what he has been doing and saying.]

NURSE: But, Herman, I understand that you have been refusing to get out of bed or dress yourself every day. We discussed last week that you could go outside and sit on the front porch, socialize, play cards and quiet table games, but you have not been interested in doing any of these things.
[Nurse points out the incongruency.]

MARIAN: Dad, you're just stubborn and unwilling to do anything the doctor says!
[Insulting, judgmental remark.]

MOTHER (looking over at her daughter): Oh, Marian, you're always attacking your father. He's just scared to death to move too much for fear of hurting his heart again.
[She interprets his behavior for him, but neglects to ask for feedback or even to look at him for his reaction.]

MARIAN: But you don't help him any by cooking him that rich Jewish food and caring for his every need.
[Attacks with new issue, as well as changing issues—failure to focus on one problem until closure is reached.]

MOTHER: Let's drop it.
[Cutoff in communication.]

13. Extensive use of dysfunctional communication (from short vignette). Most dysfunctional recurring patterns entail: (a) speaking for Mr. K. and daughter and mother assuming that they know his thoughts and feelings; (b) not completing one subject or issue; and (c) not asking for feedback from other family members.

14. They do state some of their fears for and feelings about Mr. K., although they do so indirectly. But none of them state their obvious reticence about the medical regimen.

15. Qualification, clarification, or feedback techniques are not shown in this vignette.

16. The family members sometimes listen to each other. When they agree, they show they are listening particularly. Mother walks away when she doesn't want to hear.

17. Judgmental statements or assumptions are made in speaking for Mr. K.; daughter commenting on father's stubbornness and mother's cooking.

18. The values underlying the family's communication include concern over the father and spontaneity of response.

19. Affective are messages communicated, as in Mrs. K.'s concern for her husband (caring response). However, it was indirectly stated.

20. Nurse asks questions of Mr. K. Both the daughter and wife speak to nurse for him and interact among each other. Herman is passive in interaction except for one interaction where he initiated complaint.

21. *Internal variables.* Family role relationships and power structure (roles of husband–father, wife–mother, and daughter). *External variables.* Cultural influence, as described in the vignette. Home environment is an important variable, because nurse does not have the same influence over the situation. Wife and daughter are the dominant ones here.

22. The answer for question 13 could be used for a family nursing diagnosis: Extensive use of dysfunctional communication among family members. Defining characteristics: Mrs. K and daughter speaking for Mr. K and making assumptions that they know his thoughts and feelings (these are dysfunctional sender characteristics). In addition, tangentialization and distraction—jumping to another topic instead of completing discussion on former topic/issue; lack of exploration—messages are sent, but there is a failure for other family members to clarify the meaning of the message or seek further information, such as when Mr. K explained his restlessness, no one asked him to clarify what he meant (these are dysfunctional receiver characteristics). For related factors see answer 21.

23. Two general nursing interventions. Through teaching and counseling strategies assist family to be more functional in the areas described under defining characteristics. Role modeling particularly should be used. Directly involving Mr. K so that he becomes a more active communicator and speaks for himself is vital here. Having the wife and daughter express their own concerns in a more direct and positive manner (so that the daughter doesn't need to blame or attack the mother) is also suggested.

☐ CHAPTER 11 STUDY ANSWERS

1. a and b.

2. a. 1, 4, 5, and 7.
   b. 2 and 3.
   c. 6 and 9.
   d. 8.

3. Limitations of family power studies (any three):
   a. Lack of good correlation between task allocation and decision making and overall dominance patterns in family.
   b. Focusing on outcome of decision making, which family members have difficulty reporting, rather than process, which gives much greater information regarding family interaction and dynamics.
   c. Methodological: interviewing wife, rather than whole family.
   d. Methodological: solely depending on the self-reporting of family member (interviews), rather than combining with actual observations.

4. a. 3 and 4. f. 9.
   b. 5. g. 2.
   c. 7. h. 10.
   d. 6. i. 11.
   e. 1. j. 8.

5. False.

6. False.

7. True.

8. a. *Consensus.* Both parties discuss and mutually decide.
   b. *Accommodation.* One partner "convinces" other to adjust or they both make concessions.
   c. *De facto.* No conscious, overt decision made, "things just happen."

9. Description of how each of the following variables affects family power:
   a. *Family communication network.* The unequal intensity of family relationships influences power, especially the centrality of one or more members in the network of interactions (an intermediary or go-between). People holding these intermediary positions can screen information as they see fit and can use more intimate knowledge of family members' attitudes and opinions to influence them and obtain more control over decisions.
   b. *Situational changes.* A family life change that is nonnormative may cause the allocation of power to be redistributed. For example, if the mother becomes physically handicapped and can no longer carry out her parenting functions she may lose implementation power.
   c. *Cultural differences.* Cultural differences dictate what power arrangements are seen as "right" and acceptable to the family members.
   d. *Coalition formation.* By forming coalitions, the members of the coalition increase their power relative to other family members.
   e. *Social class.* Social class affects family power by setting up family life conditions that influence the resources each spouse brings to their relationship, the role that tradition plays over new "scientific" or contemporary trends, and more generally, the basic conditions under which the family survives.
   f. *Developmental or life cycle changes.* During the life cycle of the family, demands on the family unit vary, and in response to both internal and external demands, power patterns are altered. For example, couples when first married tend to share decisions more than after children arrive because there is usually more emotional involvement at the start of their relationship.

10. d.

11. b.

12. b.

13. b and d.

14. c and d.

15. c.

16. d.

17. All (a–e).

18. a. Who makes what decisions?

Husband–father. Expected to pay bills, carry out home-maintenance work, garden (his degree of involvement and decision making here is in question).

Wife–mother. She initiates and convinces her husband of the "rightness" of her proposals in areas of major decisions. Also assumes responsibility and decision making in areas of child care, household management, and social activities. Both appear to be responsible for deciding their own work.

Joe (oldest son). In charge of child-care activity in absence of mother.

b. What decision-making techniques are utilized?

No strong evidence of consensus used. (They may not have the communication ability to negotiate and discuss alternatives so that consensual decision making can take place.)

Accommodation: Use of bargaining seen in moving to suburbs and in purchase of home and car.

No use of de facto technique noted (wife is probably too task oriented and too much of a planner for this to happen very often).

c. On what basis is family power derived?

Referent power. The children listen to mother, and although it is not clear if this is out of positive identification or authority, they seem to "mind" when she is not there to enforce the rules (which would indicate reward–coercive power).

Reward–coercive power. The stepfather appears forced to use this type of power base, although ineffectively, because he does not have children's respect, they do not recognize his authority, and he seems not to have expert or informational power to use.

Expert and informational power. It appears that Mrs. Simpson is perceived by Mr. Simpson as having some special competencies or resources that he needs, or greater information on which to base decisions, because he seems to concede to her wishes. Perhaps the "principle of less interest" is operating here.

d. What variables affect family power?

Family communication network. Mrs. Simpson definitely is in a central position as go-between or intermediary between her husband and children. This increases her dominance.

Interpersonal skills. Mr. Simpson lacks confidence in his parenting skills, thus decreasing this effectiveness in this area. Mrs. Simpson undermines his parenting by taking over when the children do not listen to him. Also, he may need her more than she needs him. (Could he be seeking leadership, a mothering figure?)

Social class variables. Family is obviously middle class, and even though the wife "takes over," she is dissatisfied in her husband's role performance. This may be an indication of the disparity between her expectations (the cultural norm of a husband being either a leader or sharing responsibility with wife) and her reality, or her feeling that he is incompetent.

Developmental variable. During this cycle of the family's life, there are many tasks to be fulfilled, and thus the strain is seen in Mrs. Simpson's feeling that she has to assume too much responsibility. Usually there is more division of role responsibilities and decision making.

Cultural variable. The role of the step-father is not crystalized in our society, making it unclear as to the extent of legitimate authority Mr. Simpson has over his step-children.

e. Overall family power typology:

Family power continuum:

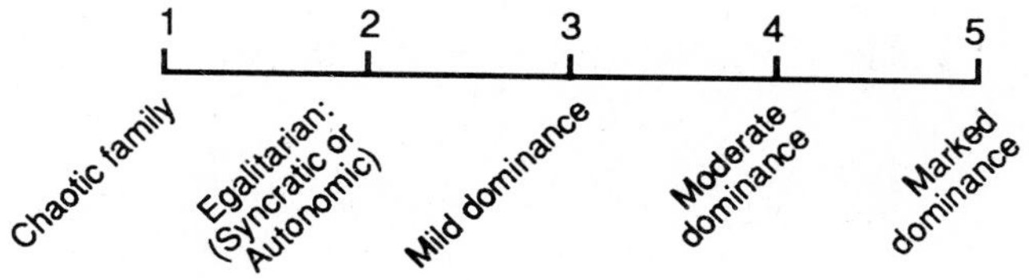

f. Mild to moderate dominance by Mrs. Simpson.

19. Father–child power conflict; marital conflict over lack of exertion of power by step-father in parenting; marital dissatisfaction in area of husband's exercise of parental authority.

20. Counseling of family members, involving exploring their feelings about Mr. Simpson joining of family, his role and authority, and their perceptions of difficulties (goal: development of empathy for each other feelings and concerns). Referral to a marriage and family counseling center may be helpful so that the couple can explore their own marital concerns and how to deal with them.

☐ CHAPTER 12 STUDY ANSWERS

1. a. 4. g. 3.
b. 2. h. 8.
c. 1. i. 9.
d. 12. j. 11.
e. 10. k. 6.
f. 5. l. 7.

2. False.

3. True.

4. False.

5.

Role	Shared Role	Role of Wife–Mother	Role of Husband–Father
Provider	↑	—	√↓
Housekeeper	—	↓	—
Child care	↑	—	—
Recreational	↑	—	—
Kinship	—	√	—
Therapeutic	↑	—	—
Sexual	↑	—	—
Companion	↑	—	—
Health leader	—	√	—

6. d.

7. *Husband:* Feels partial role loss having to share the enacting of provider (breadwinner) role. Necessitates role transitions when he assumes greater (shared) responsibility for child care and perhaps other areas. Usually experiences role changes rather than role conflicts.
Wife: Feels role conflict and strain. Most often still retains the housekeeper role and child-care role (although this is often shared) in addition to working. Her other shared and assumed roles remain also, producing role overload. Commonly feels role strain as a result of role conflict, feeling worried and guilty that she is not spending enough time with children or is hurting husband's pride in being sole provider.

8. *Lower-class Family.* Marital roles: Sexual role less satisfying and diminished in importance, companionship role attenuated, therapeutic role attenuated. Parenting roles: The child-care role is exclusively the mother's domain (and the central role in her life).
Middle-Class Family: Marital roles: Sexual role is shared and more satisfying, companionship and therapeutic roles are strong basis for marriage. Parenting roles: Child-care role shared.

9. a. Integrator (functional).
b. Mediator (functional).
c. Scapegoat.
d. Jester (functional).
e. Child (when formal role is parent).
f. Blocker.
g. The bystander.
h. The placator.
i. The family pioneer (functional).
j. The "great stone face".
k. The pal. (may or may not be functional)
l. Encourager (functional).
m. Harmonizer (may or may not be functional).
n. Initiator-contributor (usually functional).
o. Compromiser (functional).
p. Follower.
q. Dominator.
r. Recognition seeker.
s. Martyr.

10. d.

11. They describe how family members have allocated tasks to fulfill family functions; they disclose the socioemotional needs of family member(s) and the family and whether and how these needs are being met.

12. An individual cannot fully develop because he or she is rewarded only for certain behaviors and thus matures only in these rewarded areas.

13. a. Role overload.
b. Role changes or shifts, which occur if there is remarriage.

14. a. Whether the father (in the case of a step-father family) is a parent or not (parental role confusion).
b. The incompatibility of the wife and mother role. She has divided loyalties (to her children and to her husband), and conflict is seen when being supportive as a wife conflicts with being supportive as a mother.

15. False.

16. True.

17. True.

18. b.

19. c.

20. a.

21. a.

22. c.

23. *Formal role structure of hypothetical family:* The family was characterized by a sharp demarcation of roles (traditional pattern).
Husband–father:
Sole provider—breadwinner role.
Home repairman and gardener role.
Wife–mother:
Child-care role.
Housekeeper role (inside the house).
No roles are shared, nor do they wish to share any roles.
The companionship and therapeutic roles are not present in their marriage.
Sexual roles are not clear, but probably traditional.

24. None present.

25. The Mother feeling role strain and role overload. Marital and parental role conflict and role strain (of marital partners).

26. For role strain: (1) Discuss housekeeper and child care roles with the mother and help her to redefine these roles in terms of what behaviors are necessary to maintain and which behaviors (tasks) can be eliminated or reduced in frequency. (2) Facilitate a discussion between mates of roles that wife–mother has and help her negotiate roles so that there is a more equitable distribution of role responsibilities.
For role conflict: (1) Encourage mother to express her feelings and perceptions about her roles and the incompatibility between the roles she is enacting. (2) Help wife–mother to problem-solve to reduce incompatibilities of present roles and to set priorities.

☐ CHAPTER 13 STUDY ANSWERS

1. a, b, and c.

2. b.

3. b.

4. Four major, recent value changes (any four):
   a. *Individualism.* Greater priority today placed on individual freedom of choice with a concomitant decline in familism.
   b. *Work ethic.* A change from seeing work as an end in itself to a means for obtaining other important aspirations. Decline in belief that hard work will pay off and decline in the intrinsic meaning of work to many individuals.
   c. *Tolerance of diversity.* Studies show that Americans are becoming increasingly tolerant of variation in life-styles and also of ethnic differences. Weakening of the myth of the "melting pot."
   d. *Equality.* Egalitarianism in families and in society is increasing. Women's liberation is probably the strongest force in bringing about this change, but other oppressed groups have also sought and are receiving a fairer share of the resources and more consideration of their rights. These groups include children, the mentally ill, and other stigmatized groups.
   e. *Consumerism.* There has been an increased exploitation of resources and a rise in material indulgence involving the discarding and replacement of goods rather than saving.
   f. *Health and quality of life.* The increasing numbers of middle-class Americans engaging in life-style improvements is evidence of the increased saliency this value has in society.

5. e.

6. a.

7. False.

8. Productivity, materialism, individualism, work ethic, progress, and education.

9. a. Ethnicity, including religious background.
   b. Social class.
   c. Rural versus urban or suburban (geographical location).
   d. Degree of acculturation of dominant cultural values.
   Most important generally: Social class (b).

10. All (a–d).

11. c and d.

12.

AMERICAN CORE VALUES	GARDINER FAMILY VALUES
1. Productivity	1. Probably aspired to being successful—at least get by and be self-sufficient—but were not

12.

AMERICAN CORE VALUES	GARDINER FAMILY VALUES
	able to succeed. (Note wife's frustration and hostility toward husband because of employment problem.)
2. Work ethic	2. Wife appears to be committed to work ethic at home. Husband is not in conformity with this value.
3. Materialism	3. Not present (not realistic for family).
4. Individualism	4. Not evident.
5. Education	5. Not one of the central values for this family. Note lack of educational pursuits by parents and total lack of books at home.
6. Consumption ethic	6. Not present (economically unrealistic)
7. Progress and mastery over environment	7. Progress not implied. Mastery over environment not present. (Again powerless position makes this value unrealistic.)
8. Future orientation	8. Future-time orientation not seen; no planning observed during the time reported.
9. Efficiency, orderliness, and practicality	9. Mrs. G. seemed to place a high value on all these areas.
10. Rationality	10. Value not seen.
11. Democracy, equality, and freedom	11. Democratic functioning not observed in home (authoritarian, wife-dominated power structure).
12. Doing orientation (national character)	12. Wife appeared to be a very active person at home, but her doing was limited to her mother and housekeeper roles.
13. Health	13. Health was not seen as an important (prime) value. Preventive care not sought. Child-care services utilized due to the obvious necessity of receiving treatment for acute problems.
14. Patriarchal authority	14. Not valued (wife-dominated).
15. Family's interests	15. Appeared valued only because no individual interests noted.
16. Family valued as haven	16. This value did not seem to be salient in this family—since warmth, support, acceptance not noted.

13. Practicality, orderliness, cleanliness appear highly valued.

14. Not known.

15. Wife—work oriented; husband—unable to succeed in this area. Value conflict between spouses related to the work ethic. Wife is hard worker and expects husband to be also, and to be the provider for the family.

☐ CHAPTER 14 STUDY ANSWERS

1. a. Provides matrix necessary for individuals to grow and develop into healthy, functional, satisfied people.
   b. This function is central to the formation and continuity of the family unit (without this function being met, the basis for continuing as a family would become tenuous).
   c. No other societal system (institution) is sufficiently involved in fulfilling this task.

   or

   d. Through fulfillment of this function, the family teaches growing individuals how to relate warmly and closely to others.

2. Perception of family members' needs, mutual respect for needs and concerns of family members, and meeting of individual's needs in family.

3. a.

4. All (a–d).

5. a. 4.
   b. 2.
   c. 1.
   d. 1, 2, and 3.
   e. 3.
   f. 1.
   g. 1 and 2.
   h. 4

6. The parental task relative to connectedness and separateness is (1) to provide opportunities for family and children to be together, (2) to have a sense of belonging and familial cohesiveness, and (3) identification so that the children will want to continue to be together and relate as a family. Concomitantly, the parents must provide opportunities for child to progressively have the freedom and autonomy to individuate, become self-directed, competent, and independent outside the family. The family, via parents, must achieve a satisfactory pattern of separateness and connectedness, with both being present and properly emphasized.

7. b and c.

8. Values or priorities (any two):
   a. They are responsive to particular interests and needs of individual family members.
   b. They prize individuality and uniqueness.
   c. They give respect and acceptance to members unconditionally.
   d. Members are encouraged to be independent, creative, and innovative.
   e. Family emphasizes separateness more than most families do.

Family Case Study

Affective Area:

9. To what extent do family members perceive and meet needs of other family members? This involves an analysis of need–response patterns of family.

Family Member	Perceived Need By Parents	Extent Being Met
John (father)	Did not discuss in the vignette.	From study, no evidence that his socioemotional needs are being met; behavioral evidence is that family is not meeting his needs (avoidance behaviors—staying away and drinking excessively).
Ruby (mother)	No family recognition of her feelings of loss and depression or needs (to be able to be good parent) evidenced.	No data implying that family is meeting her needs; in fact, there is evidence that her emotional needs are not being met (physical illness, depression, and suicidal thoughts). Priscilla, her former confidant, is focused on her own needs and is unable to meet Ruby's relational needs.
Priscilla (age 13)	Parents recognize her needs to take on mother role and to be independent.	Since Ruby feels threatened by Priscilla's successful management of the younger siblings while she was gone, she is not able to positively reinforce her parenting efforts now. Neither parent encourages and/or facilitates Priscilla's separating efforts (becoming less involved with the family and more involved with her peer group).
Cindy (age 10)	None expressed.	Obviously, she likes being industrious and involved in projects and social activities outside of the home, which she is able to do. Family is not meeting this need. Her behavior, especially staying away from the home for long periods of time, may be because of the family's inability to meet her socioemotional needs. Priscilla does serve as Cindy's confidant, which provides a vehicle for meeting some of her emotional needs.
John Jr. (age 6)	Only need expressed was that Ann's leaving might threaten younger children and make them feel that if they misbehave, they may be taken away from family.	No evidence that John's socioemotional needs are being met; in fact, there is behavioral evidence (school phobia, clinging to mother, poor school work) that his needs are not being attended to adequately.
Lisa (age 4)	Parents are aware of her problem with separation anxiety and the threatening effect Ann's loss may have.	Both parents evidently spend more time with Lisa, or are planning to give her more attention. She presently has behavioral manifestations of unmet needs; clingingness, frightened when mother leaves, and enuresis, but seems to be the child that is attended to affectively by the parents.

10. *Mutual respect existent?*
There is no direct evidence concerning whether mutual respect exists, but one can infer that there is substantial insensitivity and thus very limited respect accorded to each other's needs, because there is so little perception or recognition of individual needs in the family.

11. *Mutual nurturance provided?*
Again, seems to be limited. It was twice noted that the family members did not share their feelings with each other in the face of present difficulties (this is a primary means of emotional support). Lisa seems to be comforted and nurtured more by the parents than the other family members are. Priscilla also provides nurturance to Cindy.

12. *Closeness and intimacy present among family members?*
There appear to be only three sets of relationships in the family that show these traits: between Cindy and Priscilla, Lisa and Ruby, and Lisa and John. Also, Priscilla and Ruby used to have closer relationship in past. Affectionate feelings, according to the parents, are and should be expressed only to the two younger children. The degree of compatibility is difficult to evaluate from this vignette. No open conflict is described between the children and parents except for the arguments between Priscilla and Ruby. John and Ruby show signs of incompatibility, handling it by withdrawal (John staying away and drinking, and both of them not discussing important issues). Part of lack of spousal discussion of important issues and feelings, however, may be due to social class and cultural role expectations (ie, they do not see this as one of the expected roles in marriage).

13. *Mutual identification and bonding?*
There is evidence that this is present: (1) spouses are staying together (although marital bonds need to be strengthened); (2) Priscilla's emulation of mother's mothering behaviors and role; and (3) separation anxiety of the two younger children when mother leaves.

14. *Issues of separateness and connectedness?*
The information in this area is limited. However, more emphasis is placed on the togetherness aspects with Priscilla and the other children. Parents do not stress individuality and personal growth (which is more of a middle-class phenomenon and luxury).

15. Altered parenting of son John Jr. and Lisa.
Defining characteristics: children clinging to mother, show separation anxiety; John Jr.'s school phobia; the mother is anxious and depressed; the father stays away most of the time.
Related factors: recent hospitalization of the mother; marital strain; children's psychological needs not being recognized or met; poverty; loss of Ann from the family; dysfunctional communication—avoidance of important issues.

16. Teaching: Promoting of open communication and sharing about important issues in family. Hold family conference and discuss what happened to Ann, reasons for her leaving, and that this will not happen to other children. Discuss mother's health problem—asking for members' understanding of both situations and how they feel things are working out now.
Role modeling: Family nurse serves as a role model to family when above

issues are being discussed. Role model open communication, encouraging that each member's opinions, perceptions, and feelings be shared.

☐ CHAPTER 15 STUDY ANSWERS

1. b.

2. Any three:
   a. Language development.
   b. Sociocultural norms and expectations (right and wrong).
   c. Sexual roles.
   d. Individual initiative and creativity.
   e. Acquisition of health concepts, attitudes, and behaviors.

3. b and c.

4. The child-rearing techniques used in a society are culturally patterned, and hence there will be a tendency for families within a particular culture to rear their children similarly. These culturally patterned techniques for child rearing differ from culture to culture, as do the ideas and beliefs about the capabilities and needs of children during their stages of growth and development. Moreover, because socialization patterns differ from one culture to the next, so will personality norms and broad expectations for personal behavior differ.

5. c.

6. a.

7. a. False.
   b. False.
   c. True.

8. a and c.

9. Several important societal changes/issues affecting child rearing (any three):
   a. Day care for children of working mothers and their feelings of guilt about working and dissatisfaction about the facilities available.
   b. The growing number of single-parent families and how well this type of family can fulfill the socialization function.
   c. The growing number of step-parent families and the complex parenting problems this family form faces.
   d. Methods or approaches for assisting families where child abuse or neglect exists.
   e. The emphasis on "unisex" upbringing and its consequences.
   f. Conflicting information from "experts" on how to raise children.

10. a. 4.
   b. 5.
   c. 1.
   d. 2.
   e. 3.

11. Attitudes or beliefs that limit effectiveness include:
   a. Strong beliefs that orderliness, neatness, obedience, degree of restraint or assertiveness, are desirable and should be important to everyone.
   b. Rigid values and beliefs that hold that there is a "right and proper" way to raise children.
   c. Religious convictions suggesting that certain customs and techniques are "good" and others "bad" or "sinful."
   d. The belief that the mother or parents are solely responsible for their children's behavior (blaming the parents).
   e. The attitude that the family's situation is not relevant, or is less significant, whereas what is best for the child is the focus (exclusion of the ecologic unit and the constraints of the family's environment).

12. *Discipline and punishment.* Father administers punishment; uses physical (corporal) means. Parents consider a child's wrongdoing as a reflection of the parents' failure to train their children adequately, and thus they feel threatened and disgraced by their children's misbehavior. The children certainly feel shame for the "loss of face" they have brought to the family. Hence the punishment is more than corporal, because the child being punished also feels the interpersonal sanctions of rejection, disapproval, and withdrawal of acceptance and love.
Rewards. Parents did not express how they reward children, except that Mrs. Chin verbally expressed (in front of children?) that her children, by virtue of their achievements, brought great honor to the family. This may indicate a pattern of verbal praise and acceptance.
Moral training. Family is highly structured and has clear boundaries as to what was right and wrong. This was instilled through careful supervision when the children were young (assumed) and by strict discipline when children were assumed old enough to take on adult behaviors (responsibility, self-sufficiency). When children were young they are given much unconditional love and affection from parents.
Autonomy and dependency. Children were pushed to be autonomous and responsible from school age on; conversely, dependency would not be reinforced positively during these same stages of development.
Initiative and creativity. There was no mention of how parents handled the issues of creativity and taking initiative.
Giving and receiving of love. The mother mentioned the extensive expression of affection to children when they were young, but that from preschool age on (gradually) and especially beginning at school age, children were pushed away from parents' affectively. In fact, parents tried to remove themselves to some extent, so that they could maintain the position of respect vis-à-vis their children.
Training for age-appropriate behaviors. Little is mentioned except that social responsibility (home chores) and school achievement (intellectual development) were stressed and promoted in this family.

13. The child-rearing approach is very adaptive for this family. The parents obviously desire their children to have a better life than they have had. Through their socialization patterns they are training children to be self-sufficient, productive, success-oriented, and independent.

14. The mother may have responsibility for the everyday matters, but the father definitely has ultimate responsibility to administer sanctions for misbehavior and thus ultimate responsibility for socialization. The socialization function is seen as a prime responsibility for this family.

15. There is little data from which to draw conclusions about how children are regarded in this family, but one senses that children are highly valued and are central to the aspirations and life goals of the parents.

16. The family is not acculturated to the dominant American culture. The parents are first-generation Chinese-American; they consider themselves part of the Chinese community, and the values and child-rearing practices they describe are congruent with the traditional values of the Chinese. In describing the Chinese child-rearing practices, Sung (1967) verifies that the Chins' socialization patterns are indeed culturally patterned.

> Discipline is strict and punishment immediate in the Chinese household. . . . The Chinese child is taught that when he does wrong, it is not a personal matter between himself and his conscience; he brings disgrace and shame upon his family and loved one. . . . A Chinese baby may be cuddled and fondled, showered with kisses, and rocked to sleep in his mother's arms, but as the child grows older, the mother withdraws her expression of affection. . . . Chinese parents think they can maintain authority if they are careful to keep a certain distance from their children. . . . The father never tries to be a friend to his son, nor the mother a big sister to her daughter. . . . A parent is the authority that demands obedience, and authority must maintain its dignity (pp. 168–171).

17. *Family nursing diagnosis:* Altered parenting (of Mary by both parents). Defining characteristics: Problem with behavior control (rules and standards change). Mary is allowed to stay home from school when she has a temper tantrum. Mary is disobedient to mother.

- Daughter school phobic.
- Mary hits baby.
- Mother lacks confidence in parenting Mary.
- Father is impatient about problem with Mary.

Related factors

- Father is relatively uninvolved with Mary's care.
- Newborn baby in home.
- Mother is socially isolated (lacks social support) and is unacculturated to American society.
- Mother from Italian family—where familism is a central value of culture—and her family is not here to assist or support her.

Two family nursing intervention strategies:

a. Bring father into child care plan. Both parents together need to sit down with the pediatric nurse practitioner and discuss problems. Father needs to be encouraged to be active in the Mary's child care, even though culturally this was not the traditional role of the father.
b. Set up behavior modification program to eliminate Mary's temper tantrums and refusal to attend school.
c. Teach parents about sibling rivalry—about its causes and ways to reduce rivalry and sibling's regression. Normalize some of Mary's behavior as being commonly seen as a reaction to introducing a new baby (and competitor) into the home.

☐ CHAPTER 16 STUDY ANSWERS

1. All but e. Physicians virtually have total control over when and where to hospitalize their patients.

2. a. Socioeconomic status (also can identify level of knowledge, which is correlated with the educational status and socioeconomic status).
   b. Family's value system or priorities (is also related to socioeconomic status).
   c. Frequency of symptoms of health problem in community (certain prevalent symptoms or problems are accepted as being part of living and thus viewed as inevitable, unavoidable, and "normal").

3.

ORIENTATIONS	GROUPS THAT MENTIONED ORIENTATION MORE FREQUENTLY
a. Feeling-state orientation.	Chronically ill clinic patients (lower socioeconomic group).
b. Performance orientation.	Both groups.
c. Symptom orientation.	Medical student group (younger, presumably well, and of middle- and upper-middle-class background).

4. Koos' study found that as one descends socioeconomic scale, a lack of recognition of and indifference to symptoms of illness increase. Also when these individuals failed to recognize behaviors as indicative of possible disease, they failed to see that medical care was indicated.

5.

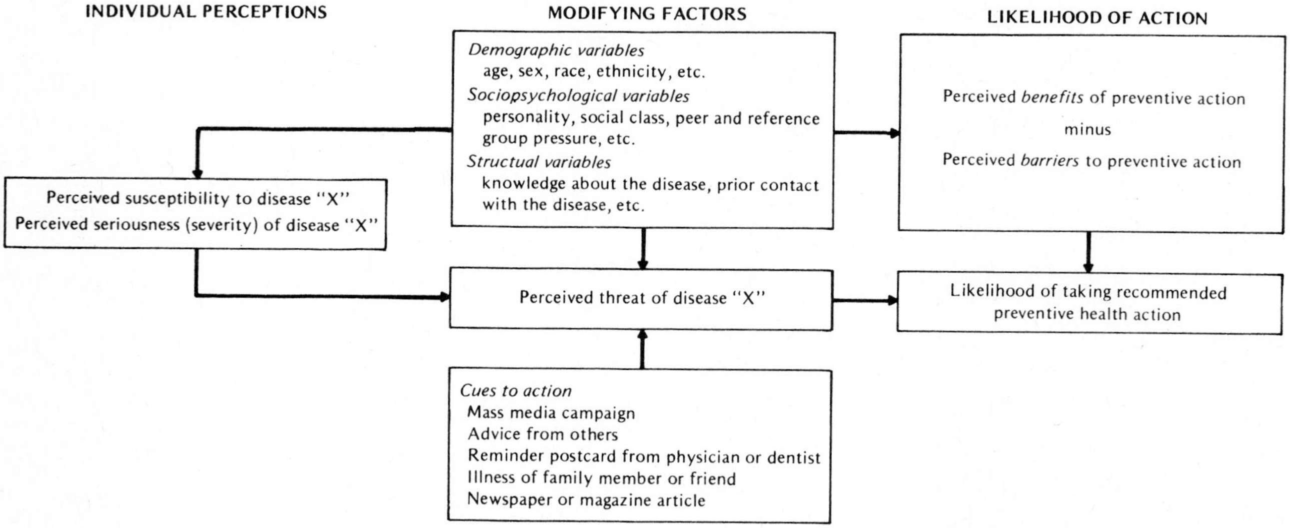

6. Seven cognitive–perceptual factors are identified in the model as the primary motivational mechanisms for engaging in health promoting behavior. They are the importance of health; how health is defined; perceptions of locus-of-control of health; self-efficacy; health status; benefits of health-promoting behaviors; and barriers to health-promoting actions. Modifying factors of demographic and biologic characteristics, interpersonal influences and situational/behavioral factors are proposed as indirectly influencing health behavior patterns. Additionally, internal and external cues may activate health-promoting behaviors.

7. Pratt concluded that American families were generally inadequate in carrying out their health care function based on the following observations:
Many homes are not suitable for maintaining health and controlling infectious disease and accidents (crowdedness, safety hazards, pollution, lack of infectious disease control).
Widespread unhealthful personal and family health practices.
Medication misuse is widespread.
Dependent and/or disabled family members were not cared for or inadequately cared for.
Insufficient or inappropriate use of health services found frequently.
Level of health knowledge inadequate.
Family's self-care practices were not satisfactory.
Reasons for this inadequacy:
Basic structure of the health care system (health care provider dominated; bureaucratic structure).
Family structure itself (family needs to be more widely involved with community and husband–fathers need to be actively involved).

8. c and d.

9. Any four of the following:
   a. Nutritional history (the 3-day family food record).
   b. Observe for variations among family members in terms of quality and quantity of diet. Does visual inspection indicate normal limits for height and weight?
   c. Identify any special family food preferences (culturally, philosophically, or trend-based dietary food patterns).
   d. Psychosocial aspects of mealtimes and eating (food used as a reward or punishment)?
   e. Shopping, planning, food preparation, and serving responsibilities.

10. a. Are there regular times established for children to go to bed and get up? Who decides when children go to sleep?
   b. Do any members of the family have sleeping problems? If so, what kind of problem?

11. a. What types of family recreation involving physical exercise does your family engage in?
   b. How frequently do you as a family go biking, swimming, etc, and does everyone participate?
   c. What effect do you think exercise has on your family's health?

12. All (a–e).

13. The potential for caregiver strain.

14. c and d.

15. a. Always follow the manufacturer's warning on cleaning solutions, powders, or chemically treated materials.
   b. Store toxic, abrasive, or caustic substances properly and out of the reach of young children.
   c. Older buildings should be checked for asbestos and peeling lead paint.
   d. Evaluate the possibility of radon exposure.

16. Four of the following:
- a. Importance of fluoride for increasing resistance of tooth to decay.
- b. Importance of brushing and flossing teeth (and use of an effective method of brushing).
- c. Role of carbohydrates (starches and sugars) in producing dental caries.
- d. Importance of regular dental examination and cleaning of teeth.
- e. Early treatment of dental caries and treatment of major orthodontic problems.

17. a, b, and c.

18. Specific diseases (both genetically based and environmentally related diseases) family members might have had.

☐ CHAPTER 17 STUDY ANSWERS

1. a.

2. c.

3.

a. 7.	e. 5.
b. 1.	f. 4.
c. 6.	g. 2.
d. 3.	

4.
- a. Stressful contact of one member with extrafamilial forces.
- b. Stressful contact of whole family with extrafamilial forces.
- c. Transitional stressors.
- d. Situational stressors.

5. False.

6. True.

7. True.

8. b.

9. b, c, and d.

10.
- a. *Occupational and economic role.* Controlling the meaning of the problem, by minimizing the negative and substitution of other more accessible rewards.
- b. *Marital role.* Self-reliance and involvement (modifying stressful situation) and reflective probing of problems (stress management).
- c. *Parental role.* Self-reliance and involvement (modifying stressful situation) and conviction that one has power to effect change and exert influence (stress management).

11. b and c.

12. *Internal Coping Strategies* (two)

a. *Role flexibility.* Ability of family members to adapt by shifting roles as needed.

b. *Family group-reliance.* The tighter structure and control over subsystems, greater degree of family organization and cohesiveness.

c. *Use of humor.* Improves attitude toward problems and gives some respite and lightness to a stressful situation.

d. *Greater sharing together.* Increasing family efforts to converse about feelings and thoughts, participate in family activities.

e. *Normalizing.* When confronted with a long-term stressor, parents normalize family life to minimize family disruption from stressor.

f. *Controlling the meaning of the problem.* Interpreting or defining a change or event realistically, objectively (where cognitive mastery is involved). Reframing the situation more positively.

g. *Joint problem solving.* The family is able to jointly discuss a problem, search for a solution, and reach a consensus.

External Coping Strategies (two)

a. *Seeking information.* Pertinent information sought to deal with issue/problem at hand.

b. *Maintaining active linkages with broader community.* This is a more general life-style characterization, where family members have open boundaries and continually participate and involve themselves in community organizations and activities.

c. *Seeking social support systems.* Social support systems function to provide support and assistance either more generally or on an as-needed basis. These social support systems are composed of friends, extended family, employers, employees, neighbors, groups (including mutual aid groups), organizations, and professional persons and agencies.

d. *Seeking spiritual supports.* This type of support includes engaging in prayer, rituals, belief in God and attending church/temple together as a family.

13. Dysfunctional family adaptive strategies (any four):

a. *Spouse violence.* In response to pent-up frustrations in marital relationship and hostility of marital partners, one spouse attacks the other.

b. *Child abuse.* Physical violence, usually by one or both parents, against one or more of their children.

c. *Scapegoating.* Selecting one or more family members to be the identified family problem. Negatively labeling and imposing unhealthy exploitative role on to the scapegoat.

d. *Use of threat.* By use of threat or ostracism, expulsion or self-destructive acts, family keeps all its members in conformity. "Separateness" actions by individuals are thus curtailed.

e. *Triangling.* Introduction of a third member into a stressful dyadic relationship when stress level reaches point where stress reduction is sought. This is exploitative of third member and does not confront the problem in the relationship.

f. *The family myth.* Beliefs developed in family about itself which have themes of wish-fulfillment. These tend to hide real problems and limit family's alternatives and problem-solving resources.

g. *Pseudomutuality.* Maintaining pseudo or false closeness. Family members have difficulty in expressing affection and closeness. As a result, they build up all sorts of customs and rituals that structure family members' responses and establish a facade of closeness and solidarity.

h. *Authoritarianism.* This is a long-term adaptive response to deal with feelings of powerlessness and dependency. One member becomes the dominator and the others the subordinates. All "lose" in this type of family structure, because there is no opportunity provided to learn the value of negotiation, discussion, and how to relate effectively with others and yet be autonomous.

14. a and d.

15.

a.	E.	g.	D.
b.	D.	h.	E.
c.	D.	i.	F.
d.	E.	j.	F.
e.	E.	k.	F.
f.	D.	l.	E.

16. all (a–d).

17. b, c, and d.

18. Family functioning continues to decline until either the family seeks or receives assistance and begins to deal effectively with the stressor, or the family reaches a low point in family functioning and then stabilizes at this new, lower level of family function.

19. a, b, and c.

Family Case Study

20. Short-term stressors impinging on the family:
Husband's unemployment.
Being on welfare and then the threat of termination.
Ann's loss (removal from the home).
Ruby's recent ill-health, hospitalization, and convalescence.
Ruby's depression and suicidal thoughts.
Long-term stressors impinging on the family.
The perceived interference of John's mother.
Emotional distance and lack of communication in family and especially within marital relationship.
Continual geographic movement, from one community to the next, so that no stable and sufficient social network is established.
Husband's minimal participation in family life and his excessive and frequent drinking bouts.
Family strengths:
Presence of social support system, although small: receiving help from mental health clinic, Mrs. Law, neighbor.
Ruby's caring for and commitment to children.
Parents' staying together and father's interest in Lisa and his potential of greater participation in family life.
Parents' motivation to find employment, be financially self-sufficient.
Priscilla's interest in and ability for child care.

21. The parents' ability to act based on objective and realistic appraisal of a situation is limited. In terms of the interference of John's mother, they perceived events as problems that they had no control over. They see the problem being John's mother's behavior, rather than a situation in which they need to communicate with each other and John's mother in order to define problems and identify a mutually satisfactory way of handling situation. Data do not reveal their perception of why Ann was removed or why welfare was terminated. Ruby personally distorts the parenting situation, feeling that her children did well without her and did not wish her back.

22. 1. Functional adaptive strategies:
No evidence for the use of some of the internal coping strategies related to family's inner resources such as greater family reliance on themselves, increased sharing of feelings and thoughts, shared activities, and controlling the meaning of the stressors.
Family (Ruby and then family) did seek one support system when problems reached crisis proportions—the mental health clinic. The neighbor, Mrs. Law, has also assisted family. But the family, because of its continual moving, has not developed an adequate social support system.
2. Dysfunctional adaptive strategies:
Use of spousal withdrawal—both spouses do not communicate openly with each other; husband withdraws from family physically and through his drinking.
Use of denial as to the family's real problems. They have seen their major family problem as John's "meddling mother." Use of family myth around this source of conflict was apparent. The family myth, more specifically, has been that "we are a happy family as long as John's mother stays away."

☐ CHAPTER 18 STUDY ANSWERS

1. a, c, and e.

2. Teaching—a, d, and e.
Case management—b and h.
Coordination—b and c.
Advocacy—h.
Collaboration—b, c, e, and i.
Consultation—e and g.
Contracting—c.
Counseling—a, d, e, and f.

3. Case management—b, c, and h.
Teaching—a, b, e, and h.
Collaboration—b, f, and h.
Contracting—a, b, g, and h.
Counseling—a, b, c, e, g, and h.

4. With virtually all NANDA diagnoses, educative interventions could be relevant given clients who are able to understand and learn. Examples (there are many correct answers): (a) knowledge deficit, (b) diversional activity deficit, and (c) health maintenance.

5. a. Ineffective family coping. b. Alterations in family processes. c. Alterations in parenting.

6. Traditionally defined teaching: families with high to moderate dependency. Counseling: families with high to moderate independence.

7. Families with serious, complex and/or long-term health needs. Targeted populations include families with frail elderly, AIDS clients, child abuse, chronically mentally ill, developmental disabled, and physically disabled/rehabilitation patients.

8. True.
9. False.
10. False.
11. False.
12. True.
13. False.
14. True.
15. True.
16. True.
17. False.
18. True.

19. Examples are (a) decreased motivation (denial of learning needs); (b) lack of open communication and/or insufficient exchange of information; and (c) environment is poor for teaching–learning to take place (space, noise problems, interruptions).

20. Teaching, case management (initiating referral), and counseling.

21. Teaching, counseling, case management (service coordination), and collaboration.

☐ CHAPTER 19 STUDY ANSWERS

1. List any three:
   a. Language differences.
   b. Religious differences.
   c. Social class differences (large numbers of peasant agricultural workers and laborers migrated).
   d. American discriminatory and segregation practices.
   e. Mexican-American closeness with Mexico, so that Chicanos can cross back and forth frequently. This consequently strengthens their ties to Mexico and reduces their need to become involved with some of the institutions within the United States.

2. False. (Familism refers to Latinos' deep commitment to their families.)

3. True.

4. False. (Evidence is that the father–husband probably never did hold absolute power, as a normative situation. Although male primary authority is declining, most Mexican-American families are still male dominant.)

5. True.

6. a, b, and d.

7.

Area	Traditional Chicano Values
Family	Chicanos see themselves as members of families first, as individuals second.
Work	Work is seen as a means (a necessity) in order to live. Other life experiences (social and emotional experiences) are valued more than work.
Materialism	Possession of goods and objects are necessary for living, not ends in themselves. Status and prestige are more likely derived from ability to intellectually and emotionally experience things. Social relationships and family are more important than accumulation of wealth.
Time and punctuality	Time is to be enjoyed. Punctuality does not have the moral overtones it does in American society.
Interpersonal relationships	Mexican-Americans value the use of diplomacy and tactfulness. They are concerned about showing respect and are more elaborate, indirect, and emotionally expressive in their communications.

8. False. (The most profound change is the decline of the husband's/father's primary authority and the increase in egalitarianism.)

9. False. (Two major child-rearing patterns are that socialization is distinctly gender role related and that the child-care role is still the mother's responsibility.)

10. False. (The ethic of reciprocity has to do with the system of mutual obligation, support, and assistance within the extended family.)

11. 1. a.
    2. c.
    3. d.
    4. b.
    5. c.
    6. e.

12. a. *Mal ojo.*
    b. Mental illness.
    c. *Empacho.*
    d. *Caida de la mollera.*
    e. *Mal puesto.*
    f. *Susto.*

13. a. c.
    b. c.
    c. a.
    d. a.
    e. a.
    f. c.

14. Family coping strategies: seeking social support from extended family and seeking spiritual support.

15. Practice implications:
   a. If culturally deprived family coping strategies are not being used, explore possible use with family.
   b. Support family's coping strategies.
   c. If family does not have primary culturally patterned coping strategies available and is experiencing frustration because they are not available, attempt to assist family to obtain needed support/assistance. Also the family should be identified as at higher risk for adaptation problems.

☐ CHAPTER 20 STUDY ANSWERS

1. a. True.
   b. False.
   c. True.
   d. False.
   e. True.
   f. False.

2. All (a–d).

3. a. 2.
   b. 1.
   c. 1, 2, and 3.
   d. 3.
   e. 1 and 2.
   f. 3.
   g. 1, 2, and 3.
   h. 1, 2, and 3.
   i. 4.
   j. 4.
   k. 1, 2, and 3.
   l. 1.
   m. 3.

4. b, d, and e.

5. a, b, c, and d.

6. b.

7. Conjure doctors and midwives or grannies.

8. a. Most basic is to abandon stereotypes and be informed and knowledgeable about black families and their cultural background.
   b. Who is in the black family must be identified by the family. Family nurses should incorporate these family members into their assessment and interventions.
   c. Because black families typically have strong bonds between parent and child and with kin and long-time friends, assessment of the characteristics of these important social networks is recommended, as well as assisting families to effectively use these social support resources.
   d. Assisting families with pressing health-related problems first to free them to attend to their health problems.
   e. Promotion of family-centered health regimens and programs.
   f. Realizing the meaning of black clients' initial responses to new health care facilities and/or health providers, and responding in client interactions with empathy, sensitivity, and feelings of concern.

References

Aamodt, A.M. Culture. (1978). In A.L. Clark, (Ed), *Culture, childbearing and health professionals.* Philadelphia: Davis.

Abernathy, W.J. & Schrems, E.L. (1971). *Distance and health services—Issues of utilization and facility choice for demographic strata* (Research Paper No. 19). Palo Alto, CA: Stanford University Graduate School of Business.

Ackerman, N. (1966). *The psychodynamics of family life.* New York: Basic Books.

Adams, B.N. (1971). *The American family.* Chicago: Markham Publishing.

———. (1980). *The family. A sociological interpretation.* Boston: Houghton Mifflin.

Adams, B. & Adams, D. (1990). Child care and the family. In National Council on Family Relations, *2001: Preparing families for the future* (pp. 18–19). Minneapolis, MN: Bolger Publications.

Aday, L.A., Eichhorn, R. (1972). *The utilization of health services: Indices and correlates—A research bibliography* (Publication No (HSM) 73-3003). Washington, DC: Department of Health, Education and Welfare, National Center for Health Services Research and Development.

Agnew, R. & Huguley, S. (1989). Adolescent violence toward parents. *Journal of Marriage and the Family, 51* 3, pp. 699–711.

Ahrons, C.R. (1980, Nov.). Redefining the divorced family. A conceptual framework. *Social Work*, pp. 437–441.

Ahrons, C.R. & Perlmutter, M.S. (1982). The relationship between former spouses: A fundamental subsystem in the remarriage family. In Hansen, J.C. and Messinger, L. (Eds.). *Therapy with remarried families.* Rockville, MD: Aspen.

Ainsworth, M.D. et al. (1966). *Deprivation of maternal care.* New York: Schocken.

Aldous, J. (1974). The making of family roles and family change. *Family Coordinator, 23* (2), 232–237.

———. (1978). *Family careers: Developmental change in families.* New York: John Wiley and Sons.

Allen, W.R., Stukes, S. (1982). Black family lifestyles and the mental health of Black Americans. In F.U. Munoz & R. Ends (Eds.). *Perspectives on minority group mental health* (pp. 45–51). Washington D.C.: University Press of America.

Alpenfels, E.J. (1969). Cancer in situ of the cervix: Cultural clues to reactions. In L.R. Lynch (Ed.). *The cross-cultural approach to health behavior.* Cranbury, NJ: Fairleigh Dickinson University Press.

American Association of Retired Persons. (1990). *A profile of older Americans, 1990.* Washington DC: American Association of Retired Persons.

American Dental Association. (1988). *Seal out decay.* Chicago: ADA Division of Communications.

American Heart Association. (1986). *New dietary guidelines.* Chicago.

American Nurses' Association. (1980). *Social policy statement.* Kansas City: ANA.

American Nurses' Association, Division on Psychiatric-Mental Health Nursing Practice. (1982). *Standards of psychiatric and mental health nursing practice.* Kansas City: ANA.

American Nurses' Association Division on Maternal and Child Health Nursing Practice. (1983). *Standards of maternal and child health nursing practice.* Kansas City: ANA.

American Nurses' Association, Council of Community Health Nurses. (1986). *Standards of community health nursing practice.* Kansas City: ANA.

American Nurses' Association. (1988). *Rehabilitation nursing: Scope of practice.* Kansas City: ANA.

American Nurses' Association Task Force on Case Management. (1988). *Nursing case management.* Kansas City: ANA.

Anderson, E.M. (1964). A continuity of care plan for long-term patients. *American Journal of Public Health, 54*, 308.

Anderson, K.E. (1972). *Introduction to communication theory and practice.* San Jose, CA: Cummings.

Anderson, R., Carter, I. (1974). *Human behavior in the social environment—A social systems approach.* Chicago: Aldine.

Andrews, E. (1974). *The emotionally disturbed family.* New York: Aronson.

Angel, R. (1985). The health of the Mexican origin population. In R. De La Garza, et al. (Eds.). *The Mexican American experience: An interdisciplinary anthology* (pp. 410–426). Austin, TX: University of Texas Press.

Antonovsky, A. (1979). *Health, stress and coping.* San Francisco: Jossey-Bass.

______. (1988). American families in the 1980s. Individualism run amok? *Journal of Family Issues, 8* (4), pp. 422–425.

Araji, S.K. (1977). Husbands' and wives' attitude–behavior congruence of family roles. *Journal of Marriage and the Family, 39* (2), 311–321.

Archer, S. & Fleshman, R. (1975). *Community health nursing.* North Scituate, MA: Duxbury Press.

______. (1985). *Community health nursing* (3rd ed.). North Scituate, MA: Duxbury Press.

Ardell, D. (1982). *Fourteen days to a wellness life-style.* Mill Valley, CA: Whatever Publishers.

Ardell, D. (1977). *High level wellness—An alternative to doctors, drugs and disease.* Emmaus, PA: Rodale Press.

Ardell, D. & Newman, A. (1977). Health promotion—Strategies for planning. *Health Values: Achieving High Level Wellness, 1* (3), 100.

Association for the Care of Children's Health. (1989). Conference Announcement. Washington DC: ACCH.

Atchley, R.C. (1977). *The social forces in later life* (2nd ed.). Belmont, CA: Wadsworth.

Auger, J.R. (1976). *Behavioral systems and nursing.* Englewood Cliffs, NJ: Prentice-Hall.

Austin, R. (1985). Attitudes toward old age: A hierarchical study. *The Gerontologist, 25* (4), 431–434.

Aylmer, R.C. (1988). The launching of the single young adult. In B. Carter and M. McGoldrick (Eds.). *The changing family life cycle* (pp. 191–208). New York: Gardner Press.

Baca-Zinn, M. (1981). Sociological theory in emergent Chicano perspectives. *Pacific Sociological Review, 24* (2), 255–272.

Bahnson, C.B. (1987). The impact of life-threatening illness on the family and the impact of the family on illness: An overview. In M. Leahey and L.M. Wright (Eds.). *Families and life-threatening illness* (pp. 26–44). Springhouse, PA: Springhouse Corporation.

Baier, M. (1987). Case management with the chronically mentally ill. *Journal of Psychosocial Nursing, 25* (6), 17–20.

Baker, T. (1985). Introduction to sleep and sleep disorders. *Medical Clinics of No America, 69,* 1123–1151.

Bandura, A. (1977). *Social learning theory.* Englewood Cliffs, NJ: Prentice-Hall.

Banks, L.J. (1985). Counseling. In G.M. Bulechek & J.C. McCloskey (Eds.). *Nursing interventions: Treatments for nursing diagnoses* (pp. 99–112). Philadelphia: WB Saunders Co.

Baranowski, T. & Nader, P.R. (1985). Family health behavior. In Turk, D.C. & Kerns, R.D. (Eds.), *Health, illness, and families.* New York: John Wiley and Sons.

Barber, B.K. & Thomas, D.L. (1986). Dimensions of fathers' and mothers' supportive behavior: The case for physical affection. *Journal of Marriage and the Family, 48* (4), 783–794.

Barnett, R.C. & Baruch, M. (1987). Determinants of fathers' participation in family work. *Journal of Marriage & Family, 49* (1), 29–40.

Barnett, R. (1986, Nov.). New American Heart Association Guidelines: Reasons of the Heart. *American Health,* 50.

Bass, D. & Noelker, L. (1987). The influence of family caregivers on elder's use of in-home services: An expanded conceptual framework. *Journal of Health and Social Behavior, 28,* 184–196.

Barringer, F. (1990, August 30). Census data show sharp rural losses. *The New York Times,* pp. 1, B12.

Bateson, G. (1958). *Naven,* (2nd ed.). Stanford, CA: Stanford University Press.

______. *Steps to a ecology of the mind.* New York: Ballantine, 1972.

______. (1979). *Mind and nature.* New York: Bantam Books.

Bateson, G., Jackson, D.D., Haley, J. & Weakland, K.J. (1963). A note on the double bind—1962. *Family Process, 2,* 154–161.

Battiste, H.B. (1975). Family myths. In S. Smoyak (Ed.). *The psychiatric nurse as a family therapist.* New York: Wiley.

Baumann, B. (1961). Diversities in conceptions of health and physical fitness. *Journal of Health and Human Behavior, 2* (1), 40.

Baumrind, D. (1978). Parental disciplinary patterns and social competency in children. *Youth and society, 9,* 239–276.

______. (1985). Familial antecedents of adolescent drug use: A developmental perspective. In C. Jones & R. Battjes (Eds.). *Etiology of drug abuse: Implication for prevention.* NIDA Research Monograph. Washington, DC: U.S. Government Printing Office.

Beautrais, A.L., Fergusson, D.M., and Shannon, F.T. (1982). Life events and childhood morbidity: A prospective study. *Pediatrics, 70,* 935–940.

Beavers, W.R. & Hampson, R.B. (1990). *Successful families. Assessment and Intervention.* New York: W.W. Norton & Co.

Beck, D.F. & Jones, M.A. (1973). *Progress on Family Problems.* New York: Family Service Association of America.

Beck, M., et al. (1990, July 16). Trading places. *Newsweek,* pp. 48–54.

Becker, M.H. (1972). The health belief model and personal health behavior. *Health Education Monographs, 2,* 326–327.

______. (1974). *The health belief model and personal health behavior.* Thorofare, NJ: Charles B. Slack.

Bell, R. and Vogel, E.F. (1968). *A modern introduction to the family.* New York: The Free Press.

Bell, R. (1971). *Marriage and family interaction.* Homewood, IL: Dorsey Press.

Belloc, N.B. (1973). The relationship of health practices and mortality. *Preventive Medicine, 2,* 67.

Benedek, E. (1978, December 8). Paper entitled Spousal Abuse, presented at the 1978 Winter Scientific Session of the American Medical Association, Las Vegas, Nevada. Reported by Nelson, H. Abused wives cling to hope, doctors say. *Los Angeles Times*, pp. 1, 18.

Benedict, R. (1938). Continuities and discontinuities in cultural conditioning. *Psychiatry, 1,* 168.

______. (1976). Continuities and discontinuities in cultural conditioning. In P.J. Brink (Ed.). *Transcultural nursing. A book of readings.* Englewood Cliffs, NJ: Prentice-Hall.

Bengtson, V.N. (1985). Diversity in symbolism in grandparental roles. In V. Bengtson and T. Robertson (Eds.). *Grandparenthood* (pp. 11–25). Newbury Park, CA: Sage.

Bengtson, V., Mangen, D., & Landry, P. (1984). Intergenerational linkages. In H. Garms, E.M. Hoerning and A. Schaeffer (Eds.), *Intergenerational relationships.* New York: J. Hogrefe.

Bengtson, V. & Robertson, T. (Eds.). (1985). *Grandparenthood,* Newbury Park, CA: Sage.

Benne, K.D. & Sheats, P. (1948). Functional roles of group members. *Journal of Social Issues, 4* (Spring), 41.

Berardo, F.M. (1988, Dec.). The American family. *Journal of Family Issues, 8* (4), 426–428.

Berkanovic, E. (1976). Behavioral science and prevention. *Preventive Medicine, 5,* 93.

Bernard, J. (1972). *The Future of marriage.* New York: Bantam.

Berne, A.S., Dato, C., Mason, D.J., & Rafferty, M. (1990). A nursing model for addressing the health needs of homeless families. *Image, 22* (1), 8–13.

Berni, R. and Fordyce, W. (1977). *Behavior modification and the nursing process.* St. Louis: CV Mosby.

Berriesi, C.M., Ferraro, K.F. & Hobey, L.L. (1984). Environmental satisfaction, sociability and well-being among urban elderly. *International Journal of Aging and Human Development, 18* (4), 277–284.

Besmer, A. (1967). Economic deprivation and family patterns. In Irelan, L.M. (Ed.). *Low-income life styles.* Washington, DC: United States Department of Health, Education, and Welfare.

Bete, C. (1976). *Don't worry about home accidents.* Greenfield, MA: Channing Bete Co.

Beutler, I.F., Burr, W.R., Bahr, K.S. & Herrin, D.A. (1989). The family realm: Theoretical contributions for understanding its uniqueness. *Journal of Marriage and the Family., 51* (August), 805–816.

Biddle, B.J. & Thomas, E.J. (1966). *Role theory: Concepts and research.* New York: Wiley.

Bild, B.R. & Havighurst, R. (1976). Senior citizens in great cities: The case of Chicago. *Gerontologist, 16* (1), 63.

Billingsley, A. (1968). *Black families in white America.* Englewood Cliffs, NJ: Prentice-Hall.

Blattner, B. (1981). *Holistic nursing.* Englewood Cliffs, NJ: Prentice Hall.

Blank, J.J. & McClmurry, B.J. (1986). An evaluation of consistency in baccalaureate public health nursing education. *Public Health Nursing, 3* (3), 171–182.

Blau, P.M. (1977). *Heterogeneity and inequality: A pragmatic theory of social structure.* New York: The Free Press.

Blieszner, R. & Alley, J.M. (1990). Family caregiving for the elderly: An overview of resources. *Family Relations, 39* (1), 97–102.

Block, F. (1974). *Allocation of time to market and nonmarket work within a family unit.* Unpublished doctoral dissertation, Stanford University.

Blood, R.O. (1969). *Marriage* (2nd ed.). Glencoe, IL: Free Press.

Blood, R.O. & Wolfe, D.M. (1960). *Husbands and wives: The dynamics of married living.* Glencoe, Ill: Free Press.

Bloom, B.S. (1956). *Taxonomy of educational objectives handbook: Cognitive domain.* New York: David McKay.

Bloom, R.L. (1977). *Community mental health. A general introduction.* Monterey, CA: Brooks/Cole.

Blumer, H. (1962). Society as symbolic interaction. In A. Rose (Ed.). *Human behavior and social processes.* Boston: Houghton-Mifflin.

Blumstein, P. & Schwartz, P. (1983). *American couples.* New York: William Morrow.

Bobak, I.M., Jensen, M.D. & Zalar, M.D. (1989). *Maternity and gynecologic care. The nurse and family* (4th Ed.). St. Louis, MO: CV Mosby Co.

Booth, A. & Cowell, J. (1976, Sept.). Crowding and Health. *Journal of Health and Social Behavior, 17,* 218.

Borman, L.D. (1975). *Exploration in self-help and mutual aid.* Evanston, IL: Illinois Center for Urban Affairs.

Boss, P. (1988). *Family stress management.* Newbury Park, CA: Sage.

Bossard, J.H. & Boll, E.S. (1956). *The large family system: An original study in the sociology of family behavior.* Philadelphia: University of Pennsylvania Press.

Bott, E. (1957). *Family and social networks.* London: Tavistock.

Bowdler, J.F. and Barrell, L.M. (1987). Health needs of the homeless. *Public Health Nursing, 4* (3), 135–140.

Bowen, M. (1960). Family concept of schizophrenia. In D.D. Jackson, (Ed.), *Etiology of schizophrenia.* New York: Basic Books.

______. (1976). Theory in the practice of psychotherapy. In P.J. Guerin (Ed.), *Family therapy* (pp. 42–90). New York: Gardiner Press.

Bowen, M. (1978). *Family therapy in clinical practice.* New York: Aronson.

Bower, F.L. (1977). *The process of planning nursing care* (2nd ed.). St. Louis: Mosby.

Bowlby, J. (1966). *Maternal care and mental health.* New York: Schocken.

______. (1977). The making and breaking of affectional bonds. *British Journal of Psychiatry, 133,* 201–210.

Boyd, N. (1982). Family therapy with black families. In E.E. Jones & S.J. Korchin (Eds.), *Minority mental health* (pp. 227–249). New York: Praeger.

Bozett, F.W. and Gibbons, R. (1983). The nursing management of families in the critical care setting. *Critical care update, 10,* 22–27.

Bozett, F.W. (1987). Family nursing and life-threatening illness. In M. Leahey and L.M. Wright (Eds.). *Families and life-threatening illness.* Springhouse, PA: Springhouse Corporation.

Brader, C.J. (1984). *The focus and limits of community health nursing.* Norwalk, CT: Appleton & Lange.

Bradburn, N.M. (1970). *The structure of psychological well-being.* Chicago: Aldine.

Bradt, J.O. (1988). Becoming parents: Families with young children. In B. Carter & M. McGoldrick (Eds.). *The changing family life cycle* (2nd ed.) (pp. 235–254). New York: Gardner Press.

Brazelton, T.B. (1989, February 13). Working parents. *Newsweek,* pps. 66–70.

Brink, P. (1976). *Transcultural Nursing.* Englewood Cliffs, NJ: Prentice-Hall.

Bronfenbrenner, U. (1969). The changing American child—a speculative analysis. In R.L. Coser (ed.), *Life cycle and achievement in America* (pp. 1–20). New York: Harper & Row.

______. (1974). The origins of alienation. *Scientific American, 231,* 53.

______. (1979). *The Ecology of Human Development: Experiments by nature and design.* Cambridge, MA: Harvard University Press.

Bronstein, P. & Cowan, C.P. (1988). *Fatherhood today: Men's changing role in the family.* New York: John Wiley and Sons.

Brothers, J. (1990, June 20). Testing parental philosophies. *The Los Angeles Times,* p. E–4.

Brown, B. (1974). *New mind, new body: Biofeedback, new directions for the mind.* New York: Bantam.

Brown, G.W. & Harris, T. (1978). *Social origins of depression.* New York: The Free Press.

Brown, J.S., Tanner, C.A., and Padrick, K.P. (1984). Nursing's search for scientific knowledge. *Nursing Research, 33* (1), 26–32.

Brown, S.L. (1978). Functions, tasks, and stresses of parenting: Implications for guidance. In: L.E. Arnold (Ed.). *Helping parents help their children.* New York: Brunner/Mazel.

Bruhn, J. & Cordova, F.D. (1978). A developmental approach to learning wellness behavior (Part II). Adolescence to maturity. *Health Values: Achieving High Level Wellness, 2* (1), 20.

Buckley, W. (1967). *Sociology and modern systems theory.* Englewood Cliffs, NJ: Prentice-Hall.

Bulechek, G.M. and McCloskey, J.C. (1985). *Nursing interventions: Treatments for nursing diagnoses.* Philadelphia: WB Saunders.

Bullough, V. & Bullough, B. (1982). *Health care for the other Americans.* E. Norwalk, CT: Appleton & Lange.

Burden, D.S. (1986). Single parents and the work setting: The impact of multiple job and homelife responsibilities. *Family Relations, 35* (1), 37–43.

Burgess, A.W. (1978). *Nursing: Levels of intervention.* Englewood Cliffs, NJ: Prentice-Hall.

Burgess, E.W., Locke, H.J. & Thomas, M.M. (1963). *The family* (3rd. ed.). New York: American Book.

Burr, W.R. (1970). Satisfaction with various aspects of marriage over the life cycle. *Journal of Marriage & Family, 32* (1), 29.

______. (1973). *Theory construction and the sociology of the family.* New York: Wiley.

Burton, L. & Bengtson, V. (1985). Black grandmothers: Issues of timing and continuity of roles. In V.L. Bengtson & J.F. Robertson (Eds.), *Grandparenthood* (pp. 61–78). Newbury Park, CA: Sage.

Bushy, A. (1990). Rural determinants in family health: Considerations for community nurses. *Family and Community Health, 12* (4), 29–38.

Campbell, A., et al. (1976). *The quality of American life.* New York: Russell Sage.

Cantor, M. (1983). Strain among caregivers: A study of experience in the United States. *The Gerontologist, 23,* 597–604.

Cantu, R.C. (1980). *Toward fitness: Guided exercise for those with health problems.* New York: Human Sciences Press.

Caplan, G. (1964). *Principles of preventive psychiatry.* New York: Basic Books.

______. (1974). *Support systems and community mental health.* New York: Behavioral Publications.

______. (1976). The family as a support system. In G. Caplan & M. Killilea (Eds.). *Support systems and mutual help.* New York: Grune & Stratton.

Carey, R. (1989). How values affect the mutual goal setting process with multiproblem families. *Journal of Community Health Nursing, 6* (1), 7–14.

Carlsen, H.J. (1976). The recreational role. In Nye, F.I. (ed). *Role structure and analysis of the family* (Vol. 24). Beverly Hills, California: Sage Publications.

Carpenito, L.J. (1987). *Handbook of nursing diagnoses* (2nd ed.). Philadelphia: JB Lippincott.

______. (1989). *Handbook of nursing diagnosis* (3rd ed.). Philadelphia: Lippincott.

Carrington, R.W. (1978). The Afro-American. In A.L. Clark (Ed.). *Culture, childbearing, and health professionals.* Philadelphia: FA Davis.

Carter, E.A. & McGoldrick, M. (Eds.). (1980). *The family life cycle: A framework for family therapy.* New York: Gardner Press.

______. (Eds.). (1988). *The changing family life cycle: A framework for family therapists* (2nd Ed.). New York: Gardner Press.

Casavantes, E. (1970, Winter). Pride and prejudice: A Mexican American dilemma. *Civil Rights Digest, 3,* 22.

Casey, B.A. (1989). The family as a system. In P.J. Bomar (Ed.). *Nurses and family health promotion* (pp. 37–46). Baltimore: Williams and Wilkins.

Castro, E.M. (1978). The Mexican American: How his culture affects his mental health. In R.A. Martinez (Ed.), *Hispanic culture and health care.* St. Louis: Mosby.

Caudill, W. (1975, April). The individual and his nexus. In L. Nader and T.W. Maretzi (Eds.), *Cultural illness and health.* Washington DC: American Anthropological Association.

Cavan, R.S. (1969). *The American family.* New York: Crowell.

Centers, R., Raven, B.H. & Rodrigues, A. (1971, April). A conjugal power structure. A re-examination. *American Sociology Review, 36,* 245–263.

Chapman, A.B. (1988). Male-female relations. In H.P.

McAdoo (Ed.), *Black families* (2nd ed.). (pp. 190–200), Newbury Park, CA: Sage.

Cherlin, A. & Furstenberg, F.F. (1985). Styles and strategies of grandparenting. In V. Bengtson & J.F. Robertson (Eds.). *Grandparenthood* (pp. 97–116). Beverly Hills, CA: Sage.

———. (1986). *The new American grandparent: A place in the family a life apart*. New York: Basic Books.

Cherry-Loveland, C.J. (1989). Family health promotion and health protection. In P. Bomar (Ed.), *Nurses and health promotion* (pp. 13–25). Baltimore, MD: Williams & Wilkins.

Chesler, M.A. & Barbarin, D.A. (1987). *Childhood cancer and the family*. New York: Brunner/Mazel Publishers.

Chess, S. (1983). Basic adaptation to successful parenting. In V.J. Sasserath (Ed.) *Minimizing high-risk parenting* (pp. 5–11). Skillman, N.J.: Johnson & Johnson Baby Products.

Chilman, C.S. (1966). *Growing up poor* (Publication No. 13). Washington, DC: Department of Health, Education and Welfare, Welfare Administration (U.S. Government Printing Office).

———. (1978, April). Habitat and American families: A social-psychological overview. *Family Coordinator, 27,* 106–109.

———. (1988). Never-married, single, adolescent parents. In C.S. Chilman, E.W. Nunnally, & F.M. Cox, (Eds.). *Variant family forms*. Newbury Park, CA: Sage.

Chin, S. (1985). Can self-care theory be applied to families? In J. Riehl-Sisca (Ed.). *The science and art of self-care* (pp. 56–62). E. Norwalk, CT: Appleton & Lange.

Chrisman, M. & Fowler, M.D. (1980). The system-in-change model for nursing practice. In J. Riedl & C. Roy (Eds.), *Conceptual models for nursing practice* (pp. 74–102). New York: Appleton-Century-Crofts.

Clark, A.L. (1966). Adaptation problems and the expanding family. *Nursing Forum, 5,* 98.

Clark, M. (1970). *Health in the Mexican-American culture: A community study*. Berkeley, CA: University of California Press.

Clark, M.J. (1984). *Community nursing, health care for today and tomorrow*. Reston, VA: Reston Publishing Co.

Clemen, S. (1977). Concepts of culture and value clarification. In S. Clemen, & M. Gregerson, (Eds.), *Family and community health nursing: A workbook*. Ann Arbor, MI: The University of Michigan Media Library.

Clemen-Stone, S., Eigsti, D., & McGuire, S.L. (1987). *Comprehensive family and community health nursing* (2nd ed.). New York: McGraw-Hill.

Clements, I.W., Roberts, F.B. (1983). *Family health. A theoretical approach to nursing care*. New York: John Wiley and Sons.

Cleveland, E. J., & Longaker, W.D. (1972). Neurotic patterns in the family. In G. Handel (Ed.). *The psychosocial interior of the family* (2nd ed.) (pp. 159–185). Chicago: Aldine-Atherton.

Cleveland, M. (1980). Family adaptation to traumatic spinal cord injury: Response to crisis. *Family Relations, 29,* 558–565.

Cline, C.L. (1966, Spring). Five variations in the marriage theme: Types of marriage formation. *Bulletin of Family Development, 3,* 10.

Coddy, B. (1975). The therapist was a gringa. In S. Smoyak, (Ed.). *The psychiatric nurse as a family therapist*. New York: Wiley.

Cogswell, B.E. (1975). Variant family forms and life styles: Rejection of the traditional nuclear family. *The Family Coordinator, 24,* 391–394.

Cohen, S. & Syme, S.L. (1985). Issues in the study of social support. In S. Cohen & L.S. Syme (Eds.), *Social support and health* (pp. 3–20). New York: Academic Press.

Coleman, J.S. (1962). *The Adolescent Society*. Glencoe, IL: Free Press.

Colley, K.D. (1978). Growing up together: The mutual respect balance. In L.E. Arnold (Ed.), *Helping parents help their children*. New York: Brunner/Mazel.

Committee on Public Education. (1973). *The joys and sorrows of parenthood*. New York: Group for the Advancement of Psychiatry.

Conant, L. (1968). The give and take in home visits. In D. Stewart & P. Vincent (Eds.). *Public health nursing* (pp. 51–64). Dubuque, Iowa: William C. Brown.

Coner-Edwards, A.F. (1988). Treatment. In A.F. Coner-Edwards & J.J. Spurlock (Eds.). *Black families in crisis. The middle class* (pp. 213–226). New York: Brunner/Mazel.

Coner-Edwards, A.F., & Edwards, H.E. (1988). Introduction. In A.F. Coner-Edwards & J.H. Spurlock (Eds.). *Black families in crisis. The middle class*. New York: Brunner/Mazel.

Coner-Edwards, A.F. & Spurlock, J.H. (Eds.). (1988). *Black families in crisis. The middle class*. New York: Brunner/Mazel.

Connery, D.S. (1968). *The Irish*. New York: Simon & Schuster.

Connors, H.R. (1988, April). Nurse case management. NAMFE: A three year perspective. *Kansas Nurse,* 8–9.

Cooley, C.H. (1909). *Social organization*. New York: Scribners.

Corrales, R.G. (1975). Power and satisfaction in early marriage. In R.F. Cromwell & D.H. Olson (Eds.). *Power in Families* (pp. 196–215). New York: Sage Publications.

Coser, L.A. (1956). *The Functions of social conflict*. Glencoe, IL: The Free Press.

Cowell, R.T. & Smith, W.M. (Eds.). (1981). *The family in rural society*. Boulder, CO: Westview Press.

Cromwell, R.E. & Olson, D.H. (1975). Introduction. In R.E. Cromwell & D.H. Olson (Eds.). *Power in families* (pp. 2–3). New York: Sage Publications.

Cromwell, R. & Ruiz, R.A. (1979). The myth of macho dominance in decision-making within Mexican and Chicano families *Hispanic Journal of Behavioral Science, 1* (4), 355–373.

Cromwell, V.L. & Cromwell, R.E. (1978, November). Perceived dominance in decision-making and conflict resolution among Anglo, Black and Chicano couples. *Journal of Marriage and the Family, 40,* 749–759.

Cronkite, R.C. (1977). The determinants of spouses: normative preferences for family roles. *Journal of Marriage and the Family, 39,* 575–585.

Crooks, C.E., Iammarino, N.K. and Weinberg, A.D. (1987). The Family's role in health promotion. *Health Values, 11* (2), 7–12.

Crosby, J.F. & Jose, N.L. (1983). Death: Family adjustment to loss. In C.R. Figley & H.I. McCubbin (Eds.). *Stress and the family. Vol. II: Coping with catastrophe* (pp. 76–89). New York: Brunner-Mazel.

Cuber, J.F. & Harroff, P.B. (1966). *The significant Americans: A study of sexual behavior among the affluent.* New York: Appleton-Century-Crofts.

Curran, D. (1983). *Traits of a health family.* Minneapolis: Winston Press.

Daniel, L. (1986). Family assessment. In B.B. Logan and C.E. Dawkins (Eds.). *Family-centered nursing in the community* (pp. 183–208). Menlo Park, CA: Addison-Wesley.

Darling, R. & Darling, J. (1982). *Children who are different: Meeting the challenges of birth defects in society.* St. Louis, MO: CV Mosby Co.

Daughtery, C. (1981). An ecologic perspective of child abuse. In C. Getty & W. Humphreys (Eds.). *Understanding the family* (pp. 298–331). New York: Appleton-Century-Crofts.

Davies, B., Spinetta, J., Martinson, I., McClowry, S. & Kulenkamp, E. (1986). Manifestations of levels of functioning in grieving families. *Journal of Family Issues, 7* (3), 297–313.

Davis, C., Haub, C. & Willette, J.L. (1988). U.S. Hispanics: Changing the face of America. In E. Acosta-Belen & B.R. Sjostrom (Eds.). *The Hispanic experience in the U.S.* (pp. 3–56). New York: Praeger.

Davis, F. (1963). *Passage through crisis: Polio victims and their families.* New York: Bobbs-Merrill.

Davis, K. (1940). The sociology of parent-youth conflict. *American Sociology Review, 5,* 523.

Davis, O.S. (1978). Nursing approach to the postpartum family. In M.L. Moore (Ed.). *Realities in childbearing.* Philadelphia: Saunders.

D'Antonio, W.V. (Ed.). (1983). Family, life, religion, and societal values and structure. In W.V. D'Antonio & J. Aldous (Eds.). *Families and religions.* Beverly Hills, CA: Sage.

D'Antonio, W. V. & Aldous, J. (1983). Introduction. In D'Antonio, W.V., Aldous, J. *Families and religions.* Beverly Hills, California: Sage Publications.

Dell Orto, A.E. (1988). Respite care: A vehicle for hope, the buffer against desperation. In P.W. Power, A.E. Dell Orto, and M.S. Gibbons (Eds.). *Family interventions throughout chronic illness and disability* (pp. 265–284). New York: Springer.

Demos, J. (1970). *A little commonwealth: Family life in Plymouth Colony.* New York: Oxford University Press.

Demos, V. (1990, August). Black family studies in the Journal of Marriage and the Family and the issue of distortion. A trend analysis. *Journal of Marriage and the Family, 52* (3), 603–612.

Deutcher, I. (1964). The quality of post-parental life: Definitions of the situation. *Journal of Marriage & Family, 26,* 52.

Diaz-Guerrero, R. (1975). *Psychology of the Mexican culture and personality.* Austin, TX: University of Texas Press.

Dickinson, D., Clark, C.M.F. & Swaford, M.J.G. (1988). AIDS Nursing Care in the Home. In A. Lewis (Ed.) *Nursing care of persons with AIDS/ARC* (pp. 215–237). Rockville, MD: Aspen.

Diekelmann, N. (1977). *Primary health care of the well adult.* New York: McGraw-Hill.

Dietrich, K.T. (1975). A re-examination of the myth of black matriarchy. *Journal of Marriage and the Family, 37* (2), 367–374.

Dilworth-Anderson, P. & McAdoo, H.P. (1988, July). The study of ethnic minority families: Implications for practitioners and policy makers. *Family Relations, 37* (3), 265–267.

Diosy, L.L. (1956). Socioeconomic status and participation in the poliomyelitis vaccine trial. *American Sociological Review, 21,* 185.

Dodson, J. (1988). Conceptualizations of black families. In H.P. McAdoo (Ed.). *Black families* (2nd ed.) (pp. 77–88). Newbury Park, CA: Sage.

Doherty, W.J. (1988). Implications of chronic illness for family treatment. In C.S. Chilman, E.W. Nunnally and F.M. Cox (Eds.). *Chronic illness and disability* (pp. 193–210). Newbury Park, CA: Sage Publications.

Doherty, W.J. & Baird, M.A. (Eds.). (1987). *Family-centered medical care: A clinical casebook.* New York: Guilford.

Doherty, W.J. & Campbell, T.L. (1988). *Families and health.* Newbury Park, CA: Sage.

Donnelly, E. (1990). Health promotion, families and the diagnostic process. *Family and Community Health, 12,* (4), 12–20.

Dorsey, R.R. & Jackson, J.Q. (1976). Cultural health traditions: The Latino/Chicano perspective. In M. Branch (Ed.). *Providing safe care to ethnic people of color* (pp. 41–79). New York: Appleton-Century-Crofts.

Dougherty, M.C. (1975). A cultural approach to the nurse's role in health planning. In B.E. Spradley (Ed.). *Contemporary community nursing* (pp. 439–445). Boston: Little, Brown.

Douvan, E. & Adelson, J. (1966). *The Adolescent Experience.* New York: Wiley.

Drotar, D., Crawfor, P. & Bush, M. (1984). The family context of childhood chronic illness: Implications for psychosocial intervention. In M.C. Eisenberg, L.C. Sutkin and M.A. Jansen (Eds.). *Chronic illness and disability through the life span. Effects on self and family* (pp. 103–132). New York: Springer.

Duncan, D.F. & Gold, R.S. (May/June, 1986). Reflections: Health promotion. What is it? *Health Values, 10* (3), 47–49.

Dunn, H.L. (1961). *High-Level Wellness.* Arlington, VA: RW Beatty.

Duvall, E.M. (1977). *Marriage and family development* (5th ed.). Philadelphia: Lippincott.

Duvall, E.M. & Miller, B.L. (1985). *Marriage and family development* (6th Ed.). New York: Harper & Row.

Dyer, W. (1973). Working with groups. In A. Reinhardt & M. Quinn, *Family-centered community nursing.* St. Louis: Mosby.

Edelman, C. & Mandle, C.L. (1986). *Health promotion*

throughout the life span. St. Louis, MO: CV Mosby Co.
Edelman, M.W. (1988). An advocacy agenda for black families and children. In H.P. McAdoo (Ed.). *Black families* (2nd ed.) (pp. 286–295). Newbury Park, CA: Sage.
Edgerton, R., Karon, M. & Fernandez, I. (1970). Curanderismo in the metropolis: The diminishing role of folk psychiatry among Los Angeles Mexican Americans. *American Journal of Psychotherapy, 24*, 124–134.
Elder, G. (1974). *Children of the great depression*. Chicago: University of Chicago Press.
Elias, M. (1987, Nov.). Role strained couples. *American Health*, pp. 58–60.
Elkins, C.P. (1984). *Community health nursing-skills and strategies*. Bowie, MD: Robert J. Brady.
Elliott-Binns, D.P. (1973). An analysis of lay medicine. *J. of R. Coll Gen Pract, 23*, 255.
Ellis, A. & Grieger, R. (1977). *Handbook of rational emotive therapy*. New York: Springer.
Ellison, C.G. (1990). Family ties, friendships, and subjective well-being among black Americans. *Journal of Marriage and the Family, 52* (3), 298–310.
Epstein, N.B., Bishop, D.S. & Baldwin, L.M. (1982). McMaster model of family functioning: A view of the normal family. In F. Walsh (Ed.). *Normal family processes* (pp. 115–141). New York: Guilford Press.
Epstein, Y.M. (1981). Crowding and human behavior. *Journal of Social Issues, 37* (1), 126–131.
Erikson, E.H. (1950). *Childhood and society*. New York: Norton.
———. (1959). *Identity and the life cycle. Psychological issues*, Vol. I. New York: International Universities Press.
———. (1963). *Childhood and society* (2nd Ed.). New York: Norton.
Eshleman, J.R. (1974). *The family: An introduction*. Boston: Allyn & Bacon.
Evashwick, C., Nay, J. & Siemon, J.E. (1985). *Case management: Issues for hospitals*. Chicago: Hospital Research and Educational Trust.
Family Service America. (1984). *The state of families, 1984–1985*. New York: Family Service of America.
Fagin, C. (1970). Concluding discussion. In Fagin, C. (Ed.). *Family-centered nursing in community psychiatry*. Philadelphia: Davis.
Falicov, C.T. (1982). Mexican families. In M. McGoldrick, J. Pierce, and J. Giordano (Eds.). *Ethnicity and family therapy*. New York: Guilford Press.
Farge, E.J. (1975). *La Vida Chicano: Health care attitudes and behaviors of Houston Chicanos*. San Francisco: R & E Research Associates.
Fast, I. & Cain, A.C. (1966). The stepparent role: Potential for disturbances in family functioning. *American Journal Orthopsychiatry, 36*, 485.
Fawcett, J. (1984). *Analysis and evaluation of conceptual models of nursing*. Philadelphia: FA Davis.
Feiring, C. & Lewis, C. (1984). Changing characteristics of the U.S. family. In M. Lewis (Ed.). *Beyond the dyad* (pp. 59–89). New York: Plenum Press.
Feldman, F., Scherz, F. (1967). *Family Social Welfare*. New York: Atherton.
Feldman, H. (1961). The development of the husband-wife relationship. Unpublished study supported in part by the National Institute of Mental Health.
———. (1969). Parent and marriage: Myths and realities. Paper read at the Merrill-Palmer Institute Conference on the Family, November 21.
Feldman, F., Scherz, F. (1967). *Family social welfare*. New York: Atherton.
Feldman, J.J. (1976). *The dissemination of health information*. Chicago: Aldine.
Fellows, D.K. (1972). *A mosaic of America's ethnic minorities*. New York: Wiley.
Ferguson, T. (1976). *Medical Self-Care*.
Ferreira, A.J. (1963). Family myth and homeostasis. *Arch Gen Psychiatry, 9*, 457.
Fife, B.L. (1985). A model for predicting the adaptation of families to medical crisis: An analysis of role integration. *Image 17* (4), 108–112.
Filsinger, E.E. (1983). *Marriage and Family Assessment*. Newbury Park, CA: Sage.
Figley, C.R. (1989). *Helping traumatized families*. San Francisco, CA: Jossey-Bass Publishers.
Fine, M.A., Donnelly, B.W. & Voydanoff, P. (1986). Adjustment and satisfaction of parents: A comparison of intact, single parent and stepparent families. *Journal of Fam Issues, 7*, 391–404.
Finley, N.J. (1989). Theories of family labor as applied to gender differences in caregiving for elderly parents. *Journal of Marriage and the Family, 51* (1), 79–86.
Fisher, K. (1987, August). Quality Assurance: Case management. *Quality Review Bulletin*, 287–290.
Fishman, H.C. (1985). Diagnosis and context: An Alexandrian quartet. In R.L. Ziffer (Ed.). *Adjunctive techniques in family therapy*. New York: Grune & Stratton.
Flacks, R. (1971). *Youth and social change*. Chicago: Markham.
Flaskerud, J. (1984, Sept.). Mental health—The culture component. *California Nurse*, 4.
Foley, V.D. (1986). *An introduction to family therapy* (2nd Ed.). Orlando, FL: Grune and Stratton.
Folkman, S., Lazarus, R.S., Dunkel-Schetter, C., De Longis, A. & Gruen, R.J. (1986). The dynamics of a stressful encounter: Cognitive appraisal, coping and encounter-outcomes. *Journal of Personality and Social Psychology, 50*, 992–1003.
Fontana, V.J. (1976). To prevent the abuse of the future. In E. Eldridge and N. Meredith (Eds.). *Environmental issues: Family impact* (pp. 185–189). Minneapolis, MN: Burgess.
Ford, L. (1979). The development of family nursing. In D.P. Hymovich & M.U. Barnard (Eds.). *Family health care*. New York: McGraw-Hill.
Forrest, J. (1981). The family. The focus for health behavior generation. *Health Values: Achieving High Level Wellness, 5* (4), 138–144.
Francis, G.M. & Munjas, B.A. (1976). *Manual of socialpsychologic assessment*. New York: Appleton-Century-Crofts.
Franklin, J.H. (1988). A historical note on black families. In

H.P. McAdoo (Ed.). *Black families* (2nd Ed.) (pp. 23–26). Newbury Park, CA: Sage.

Freeman, R.B. (1970). *Community Health Nursing Practice*. Philadelphia: Saunders.

Friedman, D.B. (1957). Parent development. *California Medicine, 86*, 25.

Friedman, M. (1976). *Assessment of Family Communication Patterns*. Los Angeles, CA: California State University Intercampus Nursing Project.

______. (1985). *Family stress and coping among Anglo and Latino families with childhood cancer*. Unpublished PhD dissertation, University of Southern California.

______. (1986). *Family Nursing: Theory and Assessment* (2nd ed.). Norwalk, CT: Appleton & Lange.

______. (1987). Intervening with families of school-aged children with cancer. In M. Leahey and L.M. Wright (Eds.). *Families and life-threatening illness* (pp. 219–234). Springhouse, PA: Springhouse Publishing Co.

______. (1990). Transcultural family nursing: Application to Latino and Black families. *Journal of Pediatric Nursing, 5* (3), 214–222.

Fuchs, V.R. (1974). *Who shall live? Health, Economics and social choice*. New York: Basic Books.

Fulcomer, D.M. (1977). The family of today. In Clausen, J.P., et al. (Eds.). *Maternity Nursing Today* (2nd ed.). New York: McGraw-Hill.

Furstenberg, F.F. & Nord, C.W. (1985). Parenting apart: Patterns of childrearing after marital disruption. *Journal of Marriage & Family, 47* (4), 893–904.

Galvin, K.M. & Brommel, B.J. (1986). *Family communication: Cohesion and change* (2nd Ed.). Glenview, IL: Scott, Foresman and Co.

Gardner, D., Stewart, N. (1978). Staff involvement with families of patients in critical care units. *Heart and Lung, 1* (1), 105–110.

Garner, M.K. (1978). Our values are showing: Inadequate childhood immunization. *Health Values: Achieving High Level Wellness*, 2 (3), 129.

Geba, B. (1985). *Being at leisure, play at life*. La Mesa, CA: Leisure Science Systems International.

Gebbie, K. (1982). Toward the theory development for nursing diagnoses classification. In M.J. Kim and D.A. Moritz (Eds.). *Classification of nursing diagnoses*. New York: McGraw-Hill.

Gegas, V. (1976). The socialization and child care roles. In F.I. Nye (Ed.). *Role Structure and Analysis of the Family*. Vol. 24. Beverly Hills, CA: Sage.

______. (1979). The influence of social class on socialization. In W.R. Burr, R. Hill, F.I. Nye and I.L. Reiss (Eds.). *Contemporary theories about the family. Vol. I* (pp. 365–404). New York: The Free Press.

Geismar, L.L. & La Sorte, B. (1964). *Understanding the multiproblem family*. New York: Association Press.

Gelcer, E. (1986). Dealing with loss in the family context. *Journal of Family Issues*, 7 (3), 315–335.

Gelles, R.J. (1980). Violence in the family: A review of research on the seventies. *Journal of Marriage and the Family, 42* (4), 873–885.

______. (1987). *The violent home*. Newbury Park, CA: Sage.

Gelles, R.J. & Maynard, P.E. (1987). A structural family systems approach to intervention in cases of family violence. *Family Relations, 36* (3), 270–275.

Gelles, R.J. & Strauss, M.A. (1988). *Intimate Violence*. New York: Simon & Schuster.

Gelman, D. et al. (July 15, 1985). Playing both mother and father. *Newsweek*. pp. 42–50.

Gelman, D. et al. (1988, March 7). Black and white in America. *Newsweek*, pp. 18–23.

Gerson, W.M. (1960). Leisure and marital satisfaction of college married couples. *Marriage and Family Living, 22*, 360–361.

Gilligan, C. (1982). *In a different voice*. Cambridge, MA: Harvard University Press.

Gilliss, C.L. (1989a). Family nursing research, theory, & practice: Our challenges. Presentation at the National Conference on Family Nursing, Sept. 15th: Portland, Oregon.

Gilliss, C.L. (1989b). Why family health care and What is family nursing? In C.L. Gilliss, B.L. Highley, B.M. Roberts, & I.M. Martinson. (Eds.). *Toward a science of family nursing* (pp. 3–8, 64–73). Menlo Park, CA: Addison-Wesley.

Gilliss, C.L., Rose, D.B., Hallburg, J.C. & Martinson, I.M. (1989). The family and chronic illness. In C.L. Gilliss, B.L. Highley, B.M. Roberts, and I.M. Martinson. (Eds.). *Toward a science of family nursing* (pp. 287–299). Menlo Park, CA: Addison-Wesley.

Glasser, P. & Glasser, L. (1970). *Families in crisis*. New York: Harper & Row.

Glenn, M.L. (1987). *Collaborative health care: A family-oriented model*. New York: Praeger.

Glenn, N.D. (Dec., 1988). Continuity versus change, sanguineness versus concern. *Journal of Family Issues, 8* (4), 348–354.

Glick, P.C. (1988). Fifty years of family demography: A record of social change. *Journal of Marriage and Family, 50* (4), 861–873.

______. (1988a). Demographic pictures of black families. In H.P. McAdoo (Ed.). *Black families* (2nd Ed.) (pp. 111–132). Newbury Park, CA: Sage.

______. (1989). The family life cycle and social change. *Family Relations, 38* (2), 123–129.

Godwin, D.D. & Scanzoni, J. (1989). Couple consensus during marital joint decision-making: A context, process, outcome model. *Journal of Marriage and Family, 51* (4), 943–956.

Goeppinger, J. (1982). Changing health behaviors and outcomes through self-care. In J. Lancaster and W. Lancaster (Eds.). *Concepts for advanced nursing practice. The nurse as a change agent*. St. Louis: The C.V. Mosby Co.

Goeppinger, J. & Labuhn, K.T. (1988). Self-health care through risk appraisal and reduction. In M. Stanhope and J. Lancaster, (Eds.). *Community health nursing* (2nd ed.). St. Louis, MO: CV Mosby., pp. 540–553.

Goering, P.N., Wasydlenki, D.A. et al. (1988). What difference does case management make? *Hospital and Community Psychiatry, 39* (3), 272–276.

Goldblum-Graff, D. & Graff, H. (1982). The Neuman model

adapted to family therapy. In B. Neuman (Ed.). *The Neuman systems model. Application to nursing education and practice* (pp. 217–222). New York: Appleton-Century-Crofts.

Goldenberg, I. & Goldenberg, H. (1985). *Family therapy. An overview* (2nd ed.). Monterey, CA: Brooks/Cole Publishing Co.

———. (1990). *Counseling today's families.* Pacific Grove, CA: Brooks/Cole Publishers.

Goldfried, M. & Sobocinski, D. (1975). The effect of irrational beliefs on emotional arousal. *Journal of Consulting and Clinical Psychology, 43,* 504–510.

Goode, W.J. (1959). The sociology of the family: Horizons in family theory. In Merton, R.K., et al. (Eds.). *Sociology today.* New York: Basic Books.

———. (1964). *The family.* Glencoe, IL: The Free Press.

———. (1971). *Introduction to the contemporary American family.* Chicago: Quadrange.

Goodman, E. (1978, June 25). America's war against its children makes monsters of all of us. *Los Angeles Times,* p. 4.

Goodspeed, H.E. (1975). Scapegoating: A process continuing when parents divorce. In S. Smoyak (Ed.). *The psychiatric nurse as a family therapist.* New York: John Wiley and Sons.

Gonzales, E. (1976). The role of Chicano folk beliefs and practices in mental health. In C.A. Hernandez, M.J. Haug, and N.N. Wagner (Eds.). *Chicanos—Social and psychological perspectives.* (2nd ed.). St. Louis, MO: CV Mosby.

Gordan, D. (1991). Medicare's big screening test. *UCLA School of Public Health, 10* (1), 8–10.

Gordon, M. (1976). Nursing diagnoses and the diagnostic process. *American Journal of Nursing, 76,* 1298.

Gordon, M.M. (1964). *Assimilation in American life.* New York: Oxford University Press.

Gordon, M. (1978). *The American family.* New York: Random House.

Gordon, M. (1982). Historical perspective. The national group for classification of nursing diagnoses. In M.J. Kim & D.A. Moritz (Eds.). *Classification of nursing diagnoses.* New York: McGraw-Hill.

———. (1985). *Manual of nursing diagnoses—1984–1985.* New York: McGraw-Hill.

Gorman, G. (1975). New families, new marriages. In S. Smoyak, *The psychiatric nurse as a family therapist.* New York: Wiley and Sons.

Gottlieb, B.H. (1983). *Social support strategies: Guidelines for mental health practice.* Beverly Hills, CA: Sage.

Gottlieb, D. & Ramsey, C. (1964). *The American adolescent.* Homewood, IL: Dorsey Press.

Gottman, J., Notarius, C., Gonso, J. & Markman, H. (1977). *A couples guide to communication.* Champagne, IL: Research Press.

Graedon, T.F. (1985). A transcultural approach to nursing practice. In J.E. Hall & B.R. Weaver. *Distributive nursing practice. Systems approach to community health* (3rd ed.) (pp. 315–331). Philadelphia: Lippincott.

Grau, L. (1984, Nov./Dec.). Case management and the nurse. *Geriatric nursing,* 372–375.

Grebler, L., Moore, J.W., & Guzman, R.C. (1970). *The Mexican-American people: The nation's second largest minority.* New York: The Free Press.

Grotevant, H.D. & Carlson, C.I., (Eds.). (1989). *Family Assessment:* A Guide to Methods and Measures. New York: Guilford.

Gurin, J. (Oct., 1985). Families: A personal way to get unstuck. *American Health,* 39–41.

Gurin, J. and Harris, T.G. (March, 1987). Taking charge: The happy health-confidants. *American Health,* 53–57.

Haber, R. (1987). Friends in family therapy: Use of a neglected resource. *Family Process, 26* (June), 269–281.

Hagestad, G.O. (1988). Demographic change and the life course: Some emerging trends in the family realm. *Family Relations, 37* (4), 405–410.

Hales, D. & Hales, R. (June, 1985). Using the body to mind the mind. *American Health,* pp. 27–32.

Hall, A. & Wellman, B. (1985). Social networks and social support. In S. Cohen & S.L. Syme (Eds.). *Social support and health* (pp. 23–41). New York: Academic Press.

Hall, J., Weaver, B. (1974). Crisis: A conceptual approach to family nursing. In J. Hall & B. Weaver. *Nursing of Families in Crisis* (pp. 3–9). Philadelphia, Lippincott.

Haley, J. (1976). *Problem-solving therapy.* San Francisco, CA: Jossey-Bass.

———. (1980). *Leaving home.* New York: McGraw-Hill.

Hallen, L.L. (1978). Family systems theory in psychiatric intervention. *American Journal of Psychiatry, 74* (3), 463.

Hammond, J. & Enoch, J. (1976). Conjugal power relations among Black working class families. *Journal of Black Studies, 7* (1), 107–127.

Handel, G. (1972). The Psychosocial Interior of the Family (2nd ed.). Chicago: Aldine Atherton.

Hanson, S.M.H. (1987). Family nursing and chronic illness. In L.M. Wright & M. Leahey (Eds.). *Families and chronic illness* (pp. 3–32). Springhouse, PA: Springhouse Corporation.

Hanson, S.M.H. & Bozett, F.H. (Eds.). (1985). *Dimensions of Fatherhood.* Newbury Park, CA: Sage.

———. (1987). Fatherhood and changing family roles. *Family and Community Health, 9* (4), 9–21.

Harburg, E., Erfurt, J.C., Chape, G., Havenstein, L.S. (1973). Socioecological stressor areas and Black-White blood pressure. Detroit. *Journal of Chronic Diseases, 26,* 595–611.

Hardy, M.E. & Conway, M. (1978). *Role theory: Perspectives for health professionals.* New York: Appleton-Century-Crofts.

Hardy, M.E. & Hardy, W.L. (1988). Role stress and role strain. Managing role strain. In M.E. Hardy & M. Conway (Eds.). *Role theory: Perspectives for health professionals* (pp. 159–255). New York: Appleton and Lange.

Hareven, T.K. (1987). Historical analysis of the family. In M.B. Sussman & S.K. Steinmetz (Eds.). *Handbook of marriage and the family* (pp. 37–57). New York: Plenum Press.

Harlow, H. & Harlow, M. (1962, Nov.). Social deprivation in monkeys. *Scientific American,* 54–161.

Harris, L. & Associates (1985). 1985 prevention index/summary report. *Prevention Magazine.*

Harris, L. and Associates. (1983, Oct./Nov.). The prevention index: A report card on the nation's health (Summary report). *Prevention Magazine.*

Harris, L. & Associates. (1975). *The myths and reality of aging in America.* Washington D.C.: National Council on Aging.

Harris, R. (1990, July 10). Blacks: Grim statistics considered threat to race. *Los Angeles Times*, pp. A1, A25.

______. (1991, May 14). A generation of innocents carries drug abuse scars. *Los Angeles Times*, pp. A1, A18 & A19.

Harris, S.E. (1975). Negativity as a major communication pattern in a family. In Smoyak, S. (Ed.). *The psychiatric nurse as a family therapist* (pp. 210–216). New York: Wiley.

Harris, T.G. (1984). From hedonism to health. *American Health, 3* (2), 54–56.

Harris, T. & Gurin, J. (1985, March). The new eighties lifestyle: Look who's getting it all together. *American Health*, 42–47.

Harrison, I.E., & Harrison, D.S. (1971). The Black family experience and health behavior. In C. Crawford (Ed.). *Health and the family* (pp. 175–199). New York: Macmillan.

Hartman, A. (1978). Diagrammatic assessment of family relationships. *Social Casework, 59*, 456–476.

Hartman, A. & Laird, J. (1983). *Family-centered social work practice.* New York: The Free Press.

Hawkins, J. Weisberg, C. & Ray, D. (1980). Spouse differences in communication style. Preference, perception, behavior. *Journal of Marriage and the Family, 42* (3), 585–593.

Harwood, A. (1981). Guidelines for culturally appropriate health care. In A. Harwood (Ed.). *Ethnicity and medical care* (pp. 482–507). Cambridge, MA: Harvard Press.

Hawkes, G.R. & Taylor, M. (1975, Nov.). Power structure in Mexican and Mexican-American farm labor families. *Journal of Marriage and the Family, 37* (4), pp. 807–811.

Haydon, D.F. (1987). The family and health/fitness. *Health Values, 11* (2), 36–39.

Hayes-Battista, D. (1990, April 26). Creating health policy in multi-cultural California. Paper presented at a statewide conference of the California Coalition for the Future of Public Health, Los Angeles, CA.

Hayes-Battista, D. & Chapa, J. (1987). Latino terminology: Conceptual basis for standardized terminology. *American Journal of Public Health, 77* (1), 61–67.

Hayes, M.P. & Stinnett, N. (1971). Life satisfaction of middle-aged husbands and wives. *Journal of Home Economics, 63* (9), 669.

Hazzard, M. An overview of systems theory. (1971). *Nursing Clinics of North America, 6*, 385–393.

Healy, A., Keesee, P.D. & Smith, B.S. (1985). *Early services for children with special needs: Transactions for family support.* Iowa City, IO. Division of developmental Disabilities, University Hospital school, Dept. of Pediatrics.

Heller, P.L. (1976). Familism scale: Revalidation and revision. *Journal of Marriage and the Family, 38* (2), 423–429.

Herbst, P.G. (1954). Conceptual framework for studying the family: Family living regions and pathways, family-living patterns of interaction. In O.A. Oeser & S.B. Hammond (Eds.). *Social structure and Personality in a city.* New York: Macmillan.

Herrera T. & Wagner, N.N. (1974). Behavioral approaches to delivering health services in a Chicano community. In Reinhardt, and M. Quinn (Eds.). *Family-centered community nursing*, St. Louis: CV Mosby.

Hersov, L. (1978, August). British Study Group Presentation. Paper delivered to the Ninth International Congress of the Association of Child Psychiatry and Allied Professions. Melbourne, Australia.

Herzog, E. & Sudia, C.E. Children in fatherless families. (1973). In B.M. Caldwell & M.N. Ricutti (Eds.). *Review of child development research*, Vol. 3, Chicago: University of Chicago Press.

Hickey, T. (1988). Self-care behavior of older adults. *Family and Community Health, 11* (3), 23–32.

Hill, M.S. (1988). Marital stability and spouses' shared time. *Journal of Family Issues, 9* (4), 427–451.

Hill, R. (1949). *Families under stress.* New York: Harper & Row.

______. (1958). Social stresses on the family. *Social Casework, 39*, 142.

______. (1965). *Challenges and resources for family development. Family Mobility in Our Dynamic Society.* Ames, Iowa: Iowa State University.

______. (1970). Interdependence among the generations. *Family development in three generations*, (Chapter 2). Cambridge, MA: Schenkman Publishers.

______. (1986). Life cycle stages for types of single parent families: Of family development theory. *Family Relations, 35* (1), 19–29.

Hill, R.B. (1972). *The strengths of black families.* New York: National Urban League.

______. (1981). *Economic policies and black progress: Myths and realities.* New York: National Urban League.

Hill, R.B. & Shackleford. (1986). The black family revisited. In R. Staples (Ed.). *The black family. Essays and studies* (3rd ed.). (pp. 194–200). Belmont, CA: Wadsworth Publishing Co.

Hill, R. & Hansen, D. (1960). The identification of conceptual frameworks utilized in family study. *Marriage and Family Nursing, 22* (4), 299–311.

Ho, M.K. (1987). *Family therapy with ethnic minorities.* Newbury Park, CA: Sage.

Hobart, C. (1987). Parent-child relations in remarried families. *Journal of Family Issues, 8* (3), 259–277.

Hobbs, D.F. & Cole, S.P. (1976). Transition to parenthood: A decade replication. *Journal of Marriage and the Family, 38* (March), 723–731.

Hoeflin, R. (1954). Child rearing practices and child care resources used by Ohio farm families with pre-school children. *Genetic Psychology Monographs, 84*, 271.

Hoenig, J. & Hamilton, M. (1966). Elderly psychiatric patients and the burden on the household. *Psychiatria et Neurologia, 152*, 281–293.

Hoffer, J. (1989). Family communication. In P. Bomar (Ed.). *Nurses and family health promotion* (pp. 78–89). Baltimore, MD: Williams and Wilkins.

Hofferth, S.L. (1984). Kin networks, race, and family structure. *Journal of Marriage and the Family, 46* (4), 791–806.

———. (1985). Updating children's life course. *Journal of Marriage and the Family, 47*, 93–115.

Hofferth, S.L. & Phillips, D.A. (1987). Child care in the U.S., 1970–1995. *Journal of Marriage and the Family, 49* (3), 559–571.

Hoffman, L.W. (1977, August). Changes in family roles, socialization, and sex differences. *American Psychologist, 32*, 644.

Hogan, M.J., Buchler, C. & Robinson, B. (1984). Single parenting: Transitioning alone. In H.I. McCubbin & C.R. Figley. (Eds.). *Stress and the family, Vol. I: Coping with normative transitions*. New York: Brunner/Mazel.

Hogue, C.G. (1977). Support systems for health promotion. In J. Hall & B. Weaver. *Distributive nursing practice: A systems approach to community health*. Philadelphia: Lippincott.

Holmes, T. (1956). Multidiscipline studies of tuberculosis. In P. Spacer (Ed.). *Personality stress of tuberculosis*. New York: International University Press.

Hollingshead, A.B. (1949). *Elmstown's youth*. New York: Wiley.

———. (1950). Class differences in family stability. *Annuals of the American Academy of Political and Social Science*, 272.

Holman, A.M. (1979). *Finding families*. Beverly Hills, CA: Sage.

———. (1983). *Family assessment: Tools for understanding and intervention*. Beverly Hills, CA: Sage Publications.

Holmes, T.H. & Rahe, R.H. (1967). The social readjustment rating scale. *Journal of Psychosomatic Research, 1*, 213–218.

Homans, G.C. (1958). Social behavior as exchange. *American Journal of Sociology, 63*, 597–606.

Honigman, J.I. (1967). *Personality in culture*. New York: Harper & Row.

Hott, J.R. (1977). Mobilizing family strengths in health maintenance and coping with illness. In A. Reinhardt & M. Quinn (Eds.). *Current practices in family-centered community nursing*. St. Louis, MO: CV Mosby Co.

House, J.S. & Kahn, R.L. (1985). Measures and concepts of social support. In S. Cohen & S.L. Syme (Eds.). *Social support and health* (pp. 83–108). Orlando, FL: Academic Press.

Houseknecht, S.K. (1987). Voluntary childlessness. In M.B. Sussman and S.K. Steinmetz (Eds.). *Handbook of Marriage and the Family*. New York: Plenum Press.

Howell, M.C. (1975). *Helping ourselves: Families and the human network*. Boston: Beacon Press.

Hughes, S.L. (1985). Apples and oranges? A review of evaluations of community-based long-term care. *Health Services Research, 20* (4), 461–488.

Hutchinson, E. (1988, Feb. 28). Black America: Tale of two nations. *Los Angeles Times*, Part IV, pp. 3, 6.

Hutchison, I.W. (1975). The significance of marital status for morale and life satisfaction among low-income elderly. *Journal of Marriage & Family, 35*, 2, 287.

Hymovich, D.P. & Barnard, M.U. (1979). *Family health care*. New York: McGraw-Hill.

Illich, I. (1976). *Medical nemesis, the expropriation of health*. New York: Random House.

Inkeles, A. (1977). Paper presented to American Sociological Association, Washington, DC, in September, 1977. Cited in *Los Angeles Times*, September 20, 1977, Part I, pp. 1, 10.

Irelan, L.M. (1972). *Low income life styles*. US Department of HEW, Social and Rehabilitation Services. Washington DC: U.S. Government Printing Office.

Jackson, D. (Ed.). (1969). *Communication, Marriage, and the Family*. Palo Alto, CA: Science and Behavior Books.

Jackson, D. & Lederer, W. (1969). *Mirages of marriage*. New York: Norton.

Jackson, J. (1966). A conceptual and measurement model for norms and roles. *Pacific Sociological Review, 9*, 35–38.

Jacob, T. & Tennebaum, D.L. (1988). *Family assessment: Rationale, methods, and future directions*. New York: Plenum Press.

Jahoda, M. (1958). *Current concepts of positive mental health. Joint Commission on Mental Illness and Health*. Monograph No 1, New York: Basic Books.

Jaramillo, P.T. & Zapata, J.T. (1987). Roles and alliances within Mexican-American and Anglo families. *Journal of Marriage and Family, 49* (4), 727–735.

Janosik, E.H. & Miller, J.R. (1980). *Family-focused care*. New York: McGraw-Hill.

Jayaratne, S. (1978). Behavioral intervention and family decision-making. *Social Work, 23*, 24.

Jellinek, P.S. (1988, Summer). Case-managing AIDS. *Issues in Science and Technology*, 59–63.

Jensen, D.P. (1985). Patient contracting. In G.M. Bulechek and J.C. McCloskey (Eds.). *Nursing interventions. Treatment for nursing diagnoses* (pp. 92–98). Philadelphia: WB Saunders.

Johnson, C.L. (1975). Authority and power in Japanese-American marriage. In R.E. Cromwell & D.H. Olson (Eds.). *Power in Families* (pp. 182–196). New York: Sage Publications.

Johnson, P.B. (1974). *Social Power and Sex-Role Stereotyping*. Ph.D. Dissertation, University of California, Los Angeles.

Johnson, S.H. (1986). Introduction and Role theory strategies. In S.H. Johnson (Ed.). *Nursing assessment and strategies for the family at risk. High-risk parenting* (2nd ed.) (pp. 1–12 and 388–401). Philadelphia: JB Lippincott.

Johnson, R. (1984). Promoting the health of families in the community. In M. Stanhope & J. Lancaster (Eds.). *Community health nursing* (pp. 330–360). St. Louis: CV Mosby.

Johnston, M. & Sarty, M. (1977). Ethnic differences in sex stereotyping by mothers: Implications for health care. Paper presented to 1977 World Congress on Mental Health, Vancouver, BC, Canada, August, 1977.

Joint Commission on Accreditation of Community Mental Health Service Programs. (1976). *Standards for community mental health centers. Balance service system*. Chicago: Joint Commission of the Accreditation of Hospitals.

Jolly, H. (1975). *Book of child care*. London: Allen and Unwin.

Jones, S.L. (1980). *Family therapy. A comparison of approaches.* Bowie, MD: Robert J. Brady Co.

———. (1986). A reformulation of the interactional approach to family therapy. In A.L. Whall (Ed.). *Family therapy theory for nursing* (pp. 95–126). E. Norwalk, CT: Appleton & Lange.

Jones, S.L. & Dimond, M. (1982). Family theory and family therapy models. Comparative review with implications for nursing practice. *Journal of Psychosocial Nursing and Mental Health Services,* pp. 12–19.

Joos, I.M., Nelson, R., & Lyness, A. (1985). *Man, health, and nursing.* Reston, VA: Reston Publishing Co.

Kagan, J. (1978). The parental love trap. *Psychology Today, 12* (3), 58–59.

Kahn, A.M. (1990). Coping with fear and grieving. In I.M. Lubkin (Ed.). *Chronic illness: impact and intervention* (pp. 179–199). Boston: Jones & Bartlett.

Kalish, R.A. (1975). *Late Adulthood: Perspectives on Human Development.* Monterey, CA: Brooks/Cole.

Kandzari, J.H., & Howard, J.R. (1981). *The well family: A developmental approach to assessment.* Boston: Little, Brown.

Kane, C.F. (1988). Family social support: Toward a conceptual model. *Advanced nursing science, 10* (2), 18–25.

Kane, R.L., Kasteler, J.M., & Gray, R.M. (1976). *The health gap.* New York: Springer.

Kanter, R.M. (1978). Jobs and families: Impact of working roles on life. *Children Today, 7,* 13.

Kantor, D. & Lehr, W. (1975). *Inside the family: Toward a theory of family process.* San Francisco: Jossey-Bass.

Kantrowitz, B. & Wingert, P. Step by Step. *Newsweek* (Special Issue). Winter/Spring, 1990, pp. 24–37.

Kardiner, A. (1945). *The psychological frontiers of society.* New York: Columbia University Press.

Kark, S. (1974). *Epidemiology and community medicine.* New York: Appleton-Century-Crofts.

Katz, A.H. & Bender, E.I. (1976). *The strength within us.* New York: Franklin Watts.

Kay, M.A. (1978). The Mexican American. In A.L. Clark (Ed.). *Culture, childbearing and health professionals.* Philadelphia: Davis.

Keefe, S.E. (1984). Real and ideal extended familism among Mexican Americans and Anglo Americans: On the meaning of "close" family ties. *Human Organization, 43,* 65–70.

Keefe, S.E. (1981). Folk medicine among urban Mexican-Americans: Cultural persistence, change and displacement. *Hispanic Journal of Behavioral Science, 3* (1), 41–48.

Keefe, S.E., Padilla, A.M. & Carlos, M.L. (1978). The Mexican-American extended family as an emotional system. In J.M. Casas and S.E. Keefe (Eds.). *Family and mental health in the Mexican-American community.* Los Angeles: Spanish-speaking Mental Health Research Center, UCLA.

Keeney, B. (1982). What is an epistemology of family therapy? *Family Process, 21,* 153–168.

Kell, D., & Patton, C. (1978). Reaction to induced early retirement. *Gerontologist, 18,* 173–180.

Kelley, T. et al. (1977). What the family physician should know about treating elderly patients. *Geriatrics, 32* (9), 97.

Kelly, J.R. (1978). Family leisure in three communities. *Journal of Leisure Research, 10* (1), 47–60.

Keller, S. (1974). Does the family have a future? In R.L. Coser (Ed.). *The family* (2nd ed.). New York: St. Martins Press.

Kemp, B.J. (1981). The case management model of human service delivery. *Annual Review of Rehabilitation, 2,* 212–238.

Kemper, P. (1988, April). The evaluation of the national long-term demonstration. *Health Services Research, 23* (1), 161–174.

Kendall, J.H. (1974). Maternal behavior one year after early and extended postpartum contact. *Dev Med Neurol, 16,* 172.

Kennedy, G.E. (1989). Involving students in participatory research on fatherhood. A case study. *Family Relations, 38* (4), 363–37.

Kerckhoff, R.K. (1976). Marriage and middle age. *Family Coordinator, 25* (1), 7–10.

Kessler, R.C. (1982). Life events, social supports, and mental health. In W.R. Gove (Ed.). *Deviance and mental illness.* Beverly Hills, CA: Sage.

Kick, I. (1989). Sleep and the family. In P. Bomar (Ed.). *Nurses and family healthy promotion.* Baltimore, MD: Williams & Wilkins.

Kidwell, J., Fischer, L., Dunham, R.M. & Baranowski, M. (1983). Parents and adolescents: Push and pull of change. In H.I. McCubbin & C.R. Figley (Eds.). *Stress and the Family: Coping with Normative Transitions.* New York: Brunner/Mazel.

Kievit, M.B. (1968). Family roles. In Rutgers School of Nursing. *Parent-Child Relationships—Role of the Nurse.* Newark, NJ: Rutgers University.

Kiester, E. (1976, Feb.). Marriage the second time around. New York: *Family Circle,* pp. 2–4.

Killien, M.G. (1985). An environmental approach to nursing practice. In J.E. Hall & B.R. Weaver (Eds.). *Distributive nursing practice: A systems approach to community health* (2nd ed.). (pp. 259–277). Philadelphia: Lippincott.

Kindig, D. (1975). Interdisciplinary education for primary health care team delivery. *Journal of Medical Education, 50,* 102.

King, I. (1981). *A theory for nursing: Systems, concepts, process.* New York: John Wiley and Sons.

———. (1983). King's theory of nursing. In I.W. Clements & J.B. Roberts (Eds.). *Family health: A theoretical approach to nursing care* (pp. 177–187). New York: John Wiley and Sons.

Kingson, E.R., Hirshorn, B.A., & Cornman, J.M. (1986). *Ties that bind. The interdependence of generations.* Washington, DC: Seven Locks Press.

Kirschenbaum, H. (1977). *Advanced value clarification.* La Jolla, CA: University Associates.

Kirschling, J., Gilliss, C. et al. (1989). Persons who describe themselves as family nurses: Why they are, where they practice and what they do. Handout at presentation by the Special Interest Group, Family Nursing Continuing Education Project, Oregon Health Sciences University, at the National Family Nursing Conference, September 1989. Portland.

Kitson, G.C., Babri, F.B., Roach, M.J. & Placidi, K.S. (1989). Adjustment to widowhood and divorce. *Journal of Family Issues, 10* (1), 5–32.

Klaus, M.H. & Kendall, J.H. *Maternal-Infant Bonding.* St. Louis: C.V. Mosby, 1976.

Klein, D.M. (1983). Family problem-solving and family stress. In H.I. McCubbin, M.B. Sussman, & J.M. Patterson (Eds.). *Social stress and the family.* (Special issue) In *Marriage and Family Review, 6* (1/2), 85–112.

Kluckholm, F.R. Dominant and variant value orientations. In P. Brink (Ed.). *Transcultural nursing.* Englewood Cliffs, NJ: Prentice-Hall, 1976, pp. 63–81.

Knafl, K.A. & Deatrick, J.A. (1986). Concept analysis: An analysis of the concept of normalization. *Research in Nursing and Health, 9* (3), 215–222.

Knapp, D.A., Knapp, D.E., & Engle, J. (1966). The public, the pharmacist and self medication. *Journal of the American Pharmacology Association, 56,* 460.

Knowles, M. (1973). *The adult learner: A neglected species* (2nd ed.). Houston, TX: Gulf Publishing Co.

Kobasa, S.O. (Sept., 1984). How much can you survive? *American Health,* pp. 64–78.

Kobrin, F.E. & Goldscheider, G. (1978). *The ethnic factor in family structure and mobility.* Cambridge, Mass: Ballinger.

Kohlberg, L. (1970). Education for justice: A modern statement of the platonic view. Moral Education: Five Lectures. Cambridge, MA: Harvard University.

Kohn, M.L. (1969). Social class and parent-child relationships: An interpretation. In R.L. Coser (Ed.). *Life cycle and achievement in America* (pp. 21–42). New York: Harper Torchbooks.

______. (1977). *Class and conformity. A study of values* (2nd ed.). Chicago: University of Chicago Press.

Komarovsky, M. (1964). *Blue-collar marriage.* New York: Random House.

Koos, E. (1954) *The health of regionville.* New York: Columbia University Press.

Koshi, P.T. (1976). Cultural diversity in the nursing curricula. *Journal of Nursing Education, 15,* 14.

Kosik, S.H. (1972). Patient advocacy or fighting the system. *American Journal of Nursing, 72,* 694.

Kosten, T.R., Jacobs, S.C. & Kasl, S.V. (1985). Terminal illness, bereavement and the family. In D.C. Turk & R.D. Karns (Eds.). *Health, illness and families. A life span perspective* (pp. 311–334), New York: John Wiley and Sons.

Koten, J. (March 9, 1987). A once tightly knit middle class finds itself divided and uncertain. *Wall Street Journal,* Section 2, p. 25.

Kozol, J. (1990). The new untouchables. *Newsweek.* (Special Issue on the 21st Century Family). Winter/Spring, 1990, pp. 48–53.

Kraft, I., Fushello, J., & Herzog, E. (1968). *Prelude to school: An evaluation of an inner-city preschool program.* Washington DC, Children's Bureau Research Reports, No 3.

Kranichfield, M.L. (1987). Rethinking family power. *Journal of Family Issues, 8* (1), 42–56.

Kroeber, A.L. (1948). *Anthropology.* New York: Harcourt, Brace.

Kroska, R.A. (1985). Ethnographic research method. A qualitative example to discover role of granny midwives in health services. In M. Leininger (Ed.). *Qualitative research methods in nursing.* New York: Grune & Stratton.

Kruszewski, A., Anthony, R., Hough, L. & Ornstein-Galicia, J. (1982). *Politics and society in the Southwest.* Boulder, CO: Westview Press.

Kunst-Wilson, W. & Cronenwett, L. (1981). Nursing care for the emerging family: Promoting paternal behavior. *Research in Nursing and Health, 4,* 201–211.

Kus, R.J. (1985). Crisis intervention. In G.M. Bulechek & J.C. McCloskey (Eds.). *Nursing interventions: Treatments for nursing diagnoses* (pp. 277–287). Philadelphia: WB Saunders.

Lacey, K. (1989). Nutrition. In P. Swinford & J. Webster (Eds.). *Promoting wellness: A nurse's handbook.* Rockville, MD: Aspen.

Lachman, V.D. (1983). *Stress management: A manual for nurses.* New York: Grune & Stratton.

LaLonde, M. (1974). *A new perspective on the health of Canadians.* Ottawa: Government of Canada.

Lamb, M.E. (1987). *The father's role: Cross-cultural perspectives.* Hillsdale, NJ: Lawrence Erlbaum Associates.

Lange, S. (1970). Transactional analysis and nursing. In C. Carlson (Ed.). *Behavioral Concepts and Nursing Intervention.* Philadelphia: Lippincott.

Langlie, J.K. (1979). Interrelationships among preventive health behaviors. A test of competing hypotheses. *Public Health Reports, 94,* 216–225.

Langman, L. (1987). Social stratification. In M.B. Sussman & S.K. Steinmetz (Eds.). *Handbook of marriage and the family* (pp. 211–249). New York: Plenum Press.

LaRocca, S. (1978). An introduction to role theory for nurses. *Supervisor Nurse, 9* (12), 41–45.

LaRossa, R. & La Rossa, M.M. (1981). *Transition to parenthood. How infants change families.* Newbury Park, CA: Sage.

Larrabee, E. (1973). Comments to Loretta Ford's research. An ethnic perspective. *Community nursing research: Collaboration and completion,* Denver, CO: Western Institute of Higher Education Commission.

Larsen, D. (1989). Elder abuse. *Los Angeles Times.* February 5, 1989. Part IV, p. 1.

Lasch, C. (1977). *Haven in a heartless world. The family beseiged.* New York: Basic Books.

______. (1979). *The Culture of Narcissism.* New York: W.W. Norton & Co.

Laslett, P. (1979). *The world we have lost* (2nd ed.). New York: Scribners.

Lauver, D. (1980). Recognizing alternatives: A process for client centered health care. *Health Values: Achieving High Level Wellness, 4* (3), 134–138.

Lawton, M.P. (1980). *Environment and aging.* Monterey, CA: Brooks Cole Publishers.

______. (1985). Housing and the living environment of older persons. In R. Binstock and E. Shanas (Eds.). *Handbook of aging and the social sciences* (pp. 450–478). New York: Van Nostrand Reinhold Co.

Lazarus, R., Averill, J.R., & Opton, E.M. (1974). The psychology of coping. Issues in research and assessment. In

G.R. Coelho, D.A. Harburg & J.E. Adams (Eds.). *Coping and adaptation.* New York: Basic Books.
Lazlo, E. (1972). *The systems view of the world.* New York: George Braziller.
Leavell, H., Clark, E.G., Gurney, B., et al. (1965). *Preventive medicine for the doctor in his community: An epidemiologic approach* (3rd. ed.). (pp. 19–28). New York: McGraw-Hill.
Leavitt, M.B. (1982). *Families at risk: Primary prevention in nursing practice.* Boston: Little, Brown.
Leahy, K., Cobb, M., Jones, M. (1977). *Community health nursing* (3rd ed.). New York, McGraw-Hill.
LeBow, M. (1973). *Behavior modification: A significant method in nursing practice.* Englewood Cliffs, NJ: Prentice-Hall.
Lederer, W.J. & Jackson, D.D. (1968). *Mirages of marriage.* New York: W.W. Norton & Co.
Lee, G.R. (1978). Marriage and morale in later life. *Journal of Marriage & Family, 40* (1), 131.
______. (1979). Effects of social networks on the family. In W. Burr, Hill, R., Nye, F.I., & Reiss, I.L. (Eds.). *Contemporary theories about the family,* Vol. I. New York: The Free Press.
Lee, G. & Lancaster, J. (1988). Conceptual models for community health nursing. In M. Stanhope & J. Lancaster (Eds.). *Community health nursing* (2nd ed.). (pp. 131–148). St. Louis, MO: CV Mosby.
Leighton, D., Harding, J.S., Macklin, D.B. et al (1963). *The Character of danger.* New York: Basic Books.
LeMasters, E.E. (1957). Parenthood as crisis. *Marriage and Family Living, 19* (2), 352.
______. (1974). Parents without partners. In A. Skolnick & J.H. Skolnick (Eds.). *Intimacy, family and society.* Boston: Little, Brown.
Leininger, M. (1970). *Nursing and anthropology: Two worlds to blend.* New York: John Wiley.
______. (1974). Transcultural nursing; A promising subfield of study for nurses. In A. Reinhardt & M. Quinn (Eds.). *Family centered community nursing* (pp. 7–44). S. Louis: Mosby.
______. (1976). *Transcultural health care issues and conditions.* Philadelphia: Davis.
Leonard, G. (1976, May 10). The Holistic Health Revolution. Los Angeles, *New West,* p. 43.
LeShan, E.J. (1973). *The wonderful crisis of middle age.* New York: McKay.
Leslie, G.R. (1976). *The family in social context* (3rd ed.). New York: Oxford University Press.
Leslie, G.R. & Korman, S.K. (1989). *The family in social context* (7th ed.). New York: Oxford University Press.
Lester, P.A. (1986). Teaching strategies. In S.H. Johnson. *Nursing assessment and strategies for the family at risk. High-risk parenting* (2nd ed.). (pp. 415–433). Philadelphia: JB Lippincott.
Lesthaeghe, R. (1983, Sept.). A century of demographic and cultural change in Western Europe. *Population and Development Review,* pp. 411–435.
Levin, L.S. (1977). Forces and issues in the revival of interest in self-care: Impetus for reduction in health care. *Issues in self-care (Health Education Monographs), 5* (2), 116.
Levin, L.S., Katz, A. & Holst, E. (1976). *Self-care—Lay initiatives in health.* New York: Prodist Press.
Levin, R.J. & Levin, A. (1975, Sept.). Sexual pleasure. The surprising preferences of 100,000 women. *Redbook,* pp. 51–58.
Levine, E.M. (1988). The realities of day care for children. *Journal of Family Issues, 8* (4), 451–454.
Levy, F. (1988, February 28). Black America: Tale of two nations. *Los Angeles Times,* Park IV, pp. 3 and 6.
Lewis, D. (1975). The black family. Socialization and sex roles. *Phylon, 2,* 221–237.
Lewis, A. & Levy, J.S. (1982). *Psychiatric liaison nursing. The theory and clinical practice.* Reston, VA: Reston Publishing Co.
Lewis, J.I., Beavers, W.R., Gossett, J.T., & Phillips, V.A. (1976). *No single thread: Psychological health in family systems.* New York: Brunner/Mazel.
Lewis, L. (1970). *Planning patient care* (2nd ed.). Dubuque: William C. Brown.
Lewis, O. (1961). *Children of Sanchez.* New York: Random House.
Libman, J. (1988). Growing up too fast. *Los Angeles Times,* August 9, 1988, Part V, p. 1.
Lidz, T. (1963). *The family and human adaptation.* New York: International Universities Press.
Linnett, M. (1970). Prescribing habits in general practice. *Proceedings of the Royal Society of Medicine, 61,* 613–615.
Linton, R. (1945). *The cultural background of personality.* New York: Appleton.
Litman, T.J. (1971). Health care and the family—A three generational study. *Medical Care, 9,* 67.
______. (1974). *Health care and the family: A three generational study.* Washington DC: Division of Community Health Services and Medical Care Administration, US Public Health Service.
______. (1974). The family as a basic unit in health and medical care—A social behavioral overview. *Social Science and Medicine, 8,* 502–506.
Littlefield, V.M. (1977). Emotional considerations for the pregnant family. In J.P. Clausen, M.H. Flook, B. Ford, M.M. Green, & E.S. Popiel. (Eds.). *Maternity nursing today* (2nd ed.). New York: McGraw-Hill.
Litwak, E. (1972). Occupational mobility and extended family cohesion. In I.L. Reiss (Ed.). *Readings on the Family System* (pp. 413–431). New York: Holt, Rinehart & Winston.
Lobsenz, N.M. (1975). *Sex after sixty-five.* Public Affairs Pamphlet, No. 519. New York: Public Affairs Committee.
______. Tips for closer family ties. *Redbook,* May, 1988.
Loe, H. (1988). Americans are smiling at fewer cavities. *Food Insight Reports.* Washington, DC: International Food Information Council.
Lopata, H. (1973). *Widowhood in an American city.* Cambridge, MA: Schenkman Publishing Co.
Love, L. (1970). Process of role change. In C. Carlson (Ed.). *Behavioral concepts and nursing intervention.* Philadelphia: Lippincott.
Loveland-Cherry, C. (1988). Issues in family health promo-

tion. In M. Stanhope, & J. Lancaster (Eds.). *Community health nursing* (2nd ed.). St. Louis, MO: CV Mosby.
———. (1989). Family health promotion and health protection. In P. Bomar (Ed.). *Nurses and family health promotion.* Baltimore, MD: Williams & Wilkins.
Lowenthal, M.F. (1972). Some potentialities of a life-cycle approach to the study of retirement. In F.M. Carp (Ed.). *Retirement.* New York: Behavioral Publications.
MacElveen, P.M. (1978). Social networks. In D.C. Longo & R.A. Williams (Eds.). *Clinical practice in psychosocial nursing: Assessment and intervention.* New York: Appleton-Century-Crofts.
MacKay, D. (1968). The informational analysis of questions and commands. In W. Buckley (Ed.). *Modern systems research for the behavioral scientist.* Chicago: Aldine.
Macklin, E.D. (1988). Nontraditional family forms. In M.B. Sussman & S.K. Steinmetz (Eds.). *Handbook of marriage and the family* (pp. 317–353). New York: Plenum Press.
Maddox, M.A., & Tillery, M. (1988). Elderly image seen by health care professionals. *Journal of Gerontological Nursing, 14* (11), 21–25.
Madsen, W. (1964). *The Mexican-American of South Texas.* New York: Holt-Reinhart & Winston.
Mallinchak, A.A., Wright, D. Older. (1978, March/April). Americans and crime: The scope of victimization. *Aging,* 281–282.
Malinski, V.M. (1987). Nursing science within the science of unitary human beings. In V.M. Malinski (Ed.). *Explorations on Martha Rogers' science of unitary human beings* (pp. 25–32). E. Norwalk, CT: Appleton-Lange.
Malveaux, J. (1988). The economic statuses of black families. In H.P. McAdoo (Ed.). *Black families* (2nd ed.). (pp. 133–147). Newbury Park, CA: Sage.
Mancini, J.A. & Orthner, D.K. (1988). The context and consequences of family change. *Family Relations, 37* (4), 363–366.
Manisoff, M. (1977). Psychosocial and cultural factors in family planning. In J.P. Clausen, M.H. Flook, B. Ford, M.M. Green, & E.S. Popiel. *Maternity nursing today,* (2nd ed.). New York: McGraw-Hill.
Manns, W. (1988). Supportive roles of significant others in black families. In H.P. McAdoo (Ed.). *Black famlies* (2nd ed.). (pp. 270–283). Newbury Park, CA: Sage.
Marmor, J. (Fall, 1988). Access to health care. A growing crisis. *UCLA Public Health.* Los Angeles: UCLA School of Public Health, pp. 1–5.
Martin, J.P. (1987). Sustaining care of persons with AIDS. In J.D. Durham & F.L. Cohen (Eds.). *The person with AIDS: Nursing perspectives* (pp. 161–177). New York: Springer.
Martinez, C. (1976). Community mental health and the Chicano movement. In C.A. Hernandez, M.J. Haug & N.N. Wagner (Eds.). *Chicanos—Social and psychological perspectives,* (2nd ed.). St. Louis: Mosby.
Martinez, E.A. (1988). Child behavior in Mexican American/Chicano families. Maternal teaching and child-rearing practices. *Family Relations, 37* (3), 275–280.
Martinez, R.A. (Ed.). (1978). *Hispanic culture and health care.* St. Louis: Mosby.
Maslow, A. (1954). *Motivation and personality.* New York: Harper & Row.
Matteoli, R. (1974). *The orientation phase of the professional nurse–family relationship.* Los Angeles: Intercampus Nursing Project, California State University, Los Angeles.
Mattessich, P. & Hill, R. (1987). Life cycle and family development. In M.B. Sussman & S.K. Steinmetz (Eds.). *Handbook of marriage and the family* (pp. 437–469). New York: Plenum Press.
Matthews, S.H. & Rosner, T.T. (1988). Shared filial responsibility: The family as the primary caregiver. *Journal of Marriage and the Family, 50* (1), 185–195.
McAdoo, H.P. (1978). Minority families. In J.H. Stevens & M. Mathew (Eds.). *Mother/child; Father/child relationships* (pp. 178–180). Washington, DC: The National Association for the Education of Young Children.
———. (1982). Stress absorbing systems in black families. *Family Relations, 31* (3), 479–488.
———. (1983). Societal stress; The black family. In H.I. McCubbin & C.R. Figley (Eds.). *Stress and the family. Vol. I: Coping with normative transitions* (pp. 178–187). New York: Brunner/Mazel.
———. (Ed.). (1988). *Black families* (2nd ed.). Newbury Park, CA: Sage.
McAdoo, J.L. (1988a). Changing perspectives on the role of the black father. In P. Bronstein & C.P. Cowan (Eds.). *Fatherhood today. Men's changing role in the family* (pp. 79–92). New York: John Wiley and Sons.
———. (1988b). The roles of black fathers in the socialization of black children. In H.P. McAdoo (Ed.). *Black families* (2nd ed.). (pp. 258–268). Newbury Park, CA: Sage.
McClelland, D., Constantine, C.A., Regaldo, D., & Stone, C. (1978, June). Making it to maturity. *Psychology Today,* pp. 45–47.
McClowry, S., Gilliss, C.L. & Martinson, I.M. (1989). The process of grief in the bereaved family. In C.L. Gilliss, B.L. Highley, B.M. Roberts, and I.M. Martinson, (Eds.). *Toward a science of family nursing* (pp. 216–225). Reading, MA: Addison-Wesley.
McCown, D.E., Delamarter, D., Schroeder, B. & Liegler, R. (1989). Family recreation and exercise. In P. Bomar (Ed.). *Nurses and family health promotion* (pp. 216–236). Baltimore, MD: Williams & Wilkins.
McCreery, A. (1981). Scapegoating. A survival phenomenon. In C. Getty and W. Humphreys (Eds.). *Understanding the family* (pp. 479–487). New York: Appleton-Century-Crofts.
McCubbin, H. & Dahl, B. (1985). *Marriage and family: individuals and life cycles.* New York: John Wiley and Sons.
McCubbin, H.I. & Figley, C.R. (Eds.). (1983). *Stress and the family:* Vol. 1. Coping with normative transitions. New York: Brunner/Mazel.
McCubbin, H.I. & McCubbin, M.A. (1988). Typologies of resilient families: Emerging roles of social class and ethnicity. *Family Relations, 37* (July), 247–254.
McCubbin, H.I., McCubbin, M., Nevin, R.S. & Cauble, E. (1981). Coping health inventory for parents (CHIP). In H.I. McCubbin & J.M. Patterson (Eds.). *Systematic assessment of family stress resources and coping.* St. Paul,

MN: Family Social Sciences Department, University of Minnesota.

McCubbin, H.I., and Patterson, M. (1983a). The family stress process: The double ABCX model of adjustment and adaptation. In H.I. McCubbin, M.B. Sussman, and J.M. Patterson (Eds.). *Social stress and the family.* (Special issue) In *Marriage and Family Review, 6* (1/2), 7–27.

McCubbin, H.I. & Patterson, M. (1983b). Family transitions: Adaptation to stress. In H.I. McCubbin & C.R. Figley (Eds.). *Stress and the family: Coping with normative transitions* (pp. 5–25). New York: Brunner/Mazel.

McCubbin, H.I., Wilson, L., & Patterson, J.M. (1981). Family inventory of life events and changes (FILE). In H.I. McCubbin & J.M. Patterson (Eds.). *Systematic assessment of family stress, resources, and coping.* St. Paul, MN: Family Social Sciences Department, University of Minnesota.

McCullough, P.G. & Rutenberg, S.K. (1988). Launching children and moving on. In B. Carter & M. McGoldrick (Eds.). *The changing family life cycle* (pp. 285–308). New York: Gardner Press.

McDonald, G.W. (1980, Nov.). Family power: The assessment of a decade of theory and research, 1970–1979. *Journal of Marriage and the Family, 42* (4), 841–854.

______. (1977). Family power, reflection and direction. *Pacific Sociological Review, 20,* 609–614.

McFarland, A.J. (1988). A nursing reformulation of Bowen's family systems theory. *Archives of Psychiatric Nursing. II* (5), 319–324.

McFarland, G.K. & McFarlane, E.A. (1989). *Nursing diagnosis and intervention.* St. Louis, MO: CV Mosby Co.

McFarlane, J.M. (1986). *The clinical handbook of family nursing.* New York: John Wiley & Sons.

McGoldrick, M. (1988). The joining of families through marriage: The new couple. In B. Carter and M. McGoldrick. *The changing family life cycle* (pp. 209–233). New York: Gardner Press.

McGoldrick, M. & Gerson, R. (1985). *Genograms in family assessment.* New York: W. W. Norton and Co.

McKinley, D. (1964). *Social class and family life.* Glencoe, IL: The Free Press.

McLachlan, J.M. (1958). Cultural factors in health and disease. In E.G. Jaco (Ed.). *Patients, physicians, and illness.* New York: The Free Press.

McLanahan, S. & Booth, K. (1989). Mother-only families: Problems, prospects and politics. *Journal of Marriage and the Family, 51* (3), 557–580.

McLemore, S.D. & Romo, R. (1985). The origins and development of the Mexican-American people. In R.D. De La Garza et al. (Eds.). *The Mexican-American experience: An interdisciplinary anthology.* Austin: University of Texas Press.

McQuade, W. Aikman, A. (1975). *Stress.* New York: Bantam.

Mead, G. (1934). *Mind, self and society.* Chicago: University of Chicago Press.

Mechanic, D. (1964). Influences of mothers on their children's health attitudes and behavior. *Pediatrics, 33,* 445.

Mederer, H. & Hill, R. (1983) Critical transitions over the family life span. Theory and research. *Marriage and Family Review, 6,* (1/2), 39–60.

Meisenhelder, J.B. (1982). Boundaries of personal space. *Image, 14* (1), 16–19.

Meisler, S. & Fulwood, S. (1989, July 17). Number of inner-city single parents on rise. *Los Angeles Times,* p. A 14.

Meissner, M.W. et al. (1975). No exit for wives: Sexual division of labor and the cumulation of the household demands. *Can Rev Sociol Anthropol., 12,* 424.

Meleis, A.I. (1975). Role insufficiency and role supplementation. *Nursing Research, 24* (2), 264.

______. (1985). *Theoretical nursing.* Philadelphia: JB Lippincott.

Meleis, A.I. & Swendsen, L.A. (1978). Role supplementation—an empirical test of a nursing intervention. *Nursing Research, 27* (1), 11.

Melson, G.F. (1983). Family adaptation to environmental demands. In H.I. McCubbin & C.R. Figley (Eds.). *Stress and the family. Vol I: Coping with normative transitions* (pp. 149–162). New York: Brunner/Mazel.

Menaghan, E.G. (1983). Individual coping efforts and family studies. Conceptual and methodological issues. In H.I. McCubbin, M.B. Sussman & J.M. Patterson (Eds.). *Social stress and the family.* (Special issue) In *Marriage and Family Review, 6* (1/2), 113–135.

Mendes, H.A. (1988). Single-parent families: A typology of life-styles. In Wells, J.G. (Ed.). *Current issues in marriage and the family* (4th ed.) (pp. 247–259). New York: Macmillan Co.

Mercer, R.T. (1989). Theoretical perspectives on the family. In C.L. Gilliss, B.L. Highley, B.M. Roberts, & I.M. Martinson (Eds.). *Toward a science of family nursing.* Menlo Park, CA: Addison-Wesley.

Merton, R.K. (1957). *Social theory and social structure.* New York: Free Press.

Messer, A. (1970). *The individual in his family: An adaptational study.* Springfield, IL: Thomas.

Milardo, R.M. (1988). *Families and social networks.* Newbury Park, CA: Sage.

Miller, B. (1990). Gender differences in spouse caregiver strain: Socialization and role explanation. *Journal of Marriage and the Family, 52* (2), 311–321.

Miller, B.G. & J.A. Myers-Wells. (1983). Parenthood: Stresses and coping strategies. In H.I. McCubbin & C.R. Figley (Eds.). *Stress and the family. Vol I. Coping with normative transitions* (pp. 54–73). New York: Brunner/Mazel.

Miller, B.G. & Sollie, D.L. (1980). Normal stresses during the transition to parenthood. *Family Relations, 29* (4), 459–465.

Miller, J.G. (1969). Living systems. Basic concepts. In W. Gray, F. Duhl, & N. Rizzo (Eds.). *General systems theory and psychiatry.* Boston: Little, Brown.

Miller, S.R. & Winstead-Fry, P. (1982). *Family systems theory in nursing practice.* Reston, VA: Reston.

Millington, M.J. & Zieball, C.W. (1986). Financial strategies. In S.H. Johnson (Ed.). *Nursing assessment and strategies for the family at risk. High risk parenting.* (2nd ed.) (pp. 473–487). Philadelphia: JB Lippincott.

Minuchin, S. (1974). *Families and family therapy.* Cambridge, MA: Harvard University Press.

———. (1977). Constituting a therapeutic reality. In T. Buckley et al. (Eds.). *New directions in family therapy* (pp. 3–18). Oceanside, NY: Dabon Science Publications.

Minuchin, S. & Fishman, H.G. (1981). *Family therapy techniques.* Cambridge, MA: Harvard University Press.

Minuchin, S., Rosman, B.L., & Baker, L. (1978). *Psychosomatic families. Anorexia nervosa in context.* Cambridge, MA: Harvard University Press.

Mirandé, A. (1977). The Chicano family: A re-analysis of conflicting views. *Journal of Marriage and the Family, 6* (1), 751–755.

Mirandé, A. (1979, October). A reinterpretation of male dominance in the Chicano family. *The Family Coordinator,* 473–479.

Mirowsky, J. & Ross, C.E. (1984). Mexican culture and its emotional contradictions. *Journal of Health and Social Behavior, 25* (1), 2–13.

Mishel, M.H. (1974). *Patient problems in self-esteem and nursing intervention.* Los Angeles: California State University, Los Angeles, Trident Shop.

Mischke-Berkey, K., Warner, P. & Hanson, S. (1989). Family health assessment and intervention. In P. Bomar (Ed.). *Nursing and family health promotion* (pp. 115–154). Baltimore, MD: Williams & Wilkins.

Mitchell, A.L. (1982). Barriers to therapeutic communication with Black clients. In B.W. Spradley (Ed.). *Readings in community health nursing* (2nd ed.). Boston: Little, Brown.

Mitchell, B.A., Wister, A.V. & Burch, T.K. (1989). The family environment and leaving the parental home. *Journal of Marriage and the Family, 51* (3), 605–613.

Monroe, L.D. (1989, August 19). Culture shock hits health care. *Los Angeles Times,* Part I, pp. 1, 30.

Moore, D. (1983, Jan. 30). America's neglected elderly. *New York Times Magazine,* 30–37.

Moore, J.W. (1970). *Mexican Americans.* Englewood Cliffs, NJ: Prentice-Hall.

Moorek, K., Spain, D. & Bianchi, S. (1984). Working wives and mothers. *Marriage and Family Review, 7* (3/4), 77–98.

Morehead, S.A. (1985). Role supplementation. In G.M. Bulechek, J.C. McCloskey, & M.K. Aydelotte. *Nursing interventions: Treatments for nursing diagnoses* (pp. 152–159). Philadelphia: WB Saunders.

Moynihan, D.P. (1965). *The Negro family: A case for national action.* Washington, DC: U.S. Government Printing Office.

Mueller, D.P. & Cooper, P.W. (1986). Children of single parent families: How they fare as young adults. *Family Relations, 35* (1), 169–176.

Mumford, E., Schlesinger, H.J. & Glass, G.V. (1982). The effects of psychological intervention in recovery from surgery and heart attacks: An analysis of the literature. *American Journal of Public Health, 72,* 141–151.

Murdock, G.P. (1949). *Social structure.* New York: Macmillan.

Murillo, N. (1971). The Mexican-American family. In C.A. Hernandez, M.J. Haug, N.N. Wagner (Eds.). *Chicanos: Social and psychological perspectives* (pp. 97–108). St. Louis, MO: CV Mosby Co.

———. (1976). The Mexican-American family. In C.A. Hernandez, M.J. Haug, & N.N. Wagner (Eds.). *Chicanos: Social and psychological perspectives* (2nd Ed.) (pp. 15–25). St. Louis: Mosby.

Murphy, J.F. (1983). Conflict theory. In I.W. Clements & J.B. Roberts (Eds.). *Family health: A theoretical approach to nursing care* (pp. 123–144). New York: John Wiley and Sons.

Murray, R. & Zentner, J. (1975). *Nursing concepts for health promotion.* Englewood Cliffs, NJ: Prentice-Hall.

Murray, R. & Zentner, J. (1985). *Nursing concepts for health promotion.* (3rd ed.). Englewood Cliffs, NJ: Prentice-Hall.

Naisbitt, J. (1984). *Megatrends.* New York: Warner Communications Co.

Nall, F.C. & J.S. Speilberg. (1978). New York social and cultural factors in the responses of Mexican Americans to medical treatment. In R.A. Martinez (Ed.). *Hispanic culture and health care.* St. Louis: Mosby.

Napier, A.Y. (1988). *The fragile bond.* New York: Harper & Row.

National Center for Health Statistics: *Mortality Reports, 1972–1973.* Washington DC: Govt. Printing Co.

———. 1986. Advance report on final natality statistics, 1984, Vol. 35, No. 4, Supplement, July 18.

National Center for Health Statistics. (1989). *Monthly Vital Statistics Report,* Sept. 26, 1989. Washington DC: U.S. Govt. Printing Office.

National Council for Family Relations. (1989). Facts shared on rural poverty. *NCFR Report,* June, 1989, p. 13.

National Research Council. (1989). *Executive summary, diet and health: Implications for reducing chronic disease risk.* Washington, D.C. National Academy Press.

Nelson, H. & Roark, A. (1985, April 7). Health care crisis: Less for more. *Los Angeles Times,* Part I, p. 1, 24, 25, 27, 28.

Neser, W. (1975). Fragmentation of black families and stroke susceptibility. In B. Kaplan and J. Cassel *Family and health: An epidemiological approach.* Chapel Hill, NC: Institute for Research in Social Science.

Neuman, B. (1982). *The Neuman systems model.* Application to nursing education and practice. Norwalk, CT: Appleton-Century-Crofts.

Nobles, W. (1974). African root and American fruit: The Black family. *Journal of Social and Behavioral Sciences, 20,* 52–64.

Nock, S.L. (1988). The family and hierarchy. *Journal of Marriage and the Family, 50* (4), 957–966.

Norbeck, J.S. & Tilden, V.P. (1983, March). Life stress, social support, and emotional disequilibrium in complications of pregnancy: A prospective, multivariate study. *Journal of Health and Social Behavior,* 1983, *24* (1), 30–46.

Nortan, A.J. & Glick, P.G. (1986). One-parent families: A social and economic profile. *Family Relations, 35* (1), 177–181.

North American Nursing Diagnosis Association. NANDA approved nursing diagnostic categories. (1988). *Nursing Diagnoses Newsletter, 15* (1), 1–3.

Nickolls, K. Life crisis and psychosocial assets: Some clinical implications. In B.H. Kaplan & J.C. Cassell (Eds.). *Family and health: An epidemiological approach*. Chapel Hill, NC: Institute for Research in Social Science.

Nye, F.I. (1974). Emerging and declining roles. *Journal of Marriage and the Family, 36* (2), 238.

______. (1976). Role constructs: Measurement. In I. Nye (Ed.). *Role Structure and Analysis of the Family,* Vol. 24. (pp. 23–28). Beverly Hills, California: Sage.

Nye, F.I. (Ed.). (1976). *Role structure and analysis of the family,* Vol 24. Beverly Hills, CA: Sage.

______. (1979). Choice, exchange, and the family. In W.R. Burr, Hill, R., Nye, F.I., & Reiss, I.L. (Eds.). *Contemporary theories about the family, Vol. II.* (pp. 1–41). New York: The Free Press.

Nye, F.I. & Berardo, F. (1966). *Conceptual frameworks for the study of the family.* New York: Macmillan.

Nye, F.I. & Gegas, V. (1976). The role concept: Review and delineation. In F.I. Nye (Ed.). *Role structure and analysis of the family,* Vol. 24. Beverly Hills, CA: Sage, 1976.

Ogburn, W.F. (1933). The family and its function. *Recent Social trends in the United States.* New York: McGraw-Hill.

Olmedo, E.J. & Padilla, A.M. (1978). Empirical and construct validation of a measure of acculturation for Mexican Americans. *Journal of Social Psychology, 105* (1), 179–187.

Olson, D.H. & Cromwell, R.E. (1975). Methodological issues in family power. In R.E. Cromwell & D.H. Olson (Eds.). *Power in Families* (pp. 142–145). New York: Sage Publications.

Olson, D.H., Cromwell, R.E. & Klein, D.M. (1975). Beyond family power. In R.E. Cromwell & D.H. Olson (Eds.). *Power in Families* (pp. 236–239). New York: Sage Publications.

Olson, D.H., McCubbin, H.I. & Associates. (1983). *Families: What makes them work.* Newbury Park, CA: Sage.

Olson, D.H., Sprenkle, D.H., & Russell, G.S. (1979). Circumplex model of marital and family systems. *Family Process, 18,* (1), 3–28.

Oppenheim, M. (1984, Sept.). The "big four" tests you really need. *American Health,* 80–89.

Orem, D.E. (1980). *Nursing: Concepts and practice* (2nd ed.). New York: McGraw-Hill.

______. (1983). The self-care deficit theory of nursing. A general theory. In A. Clements & F. Roberts (Eds.). *Family health: A theoretical approach to nursing care.* New York: John Wiley and Sons.

Orthner, D.K. (1976). Familia ludens: Reinforcing the leisure component in family life. In E. Eldridge & N. Meredith (Eds.). *Environmental issues: Family impact.* Minneapolis: Burgess.

Osmond, M.W. (1978). Reciprocity: A dynamic model and a method to study family power. *Journal of Marriage and The Family, 40* (1), 51.

Otten, A.L. (Jan. 27, 1989). Extended families: As people live longer, houses become homes to several generations. *Wall Street Journal, CXX* (19), 1.

Otto, H. (1973). A framework for assessing family strengths. In A. Reinhardt & M. Quinn (Eds.). *Family-centered community nursing* (pp. 87–93). St. Louis: Mosby.

Padilla, E.R. (1976). The relationship between psychology and Chicanos: Failures and possibilities. In C.A. Hernandez, M.J. Haug, & N.N. Wagner (Eds.). *Chicanos—Social and psychological perspectives.* (2nd ed.) (pp. 282–290). St. Louis: Mosby.

Pagelow, M.D. (1984). *Family violence.* New York: Praeger.

Pallett, P.J. (1990). A conceptual framework for studying family caregiver burden in Alzheimer's-type dementias. *Image, 22* (1), 52–58.

Papernow, P.L. (1984). The stepparent cycle. An experiential model of stepfamily development. *Family Relations, 33* (3), 355–363.

Parachini, A. (June 9, 1987). New guidelines for physical exams. *Los Angeles Times,* Part V, 1–2.

Parad, H.J. & Caplan, G. (1965). A framework for studying families in crisis. In H.J. Parad (Ed.). *Crisis intervention: Selected readings* (pp. 55–60). New York: Family Service of America.

Parsons, T. (1951). *The Social System.* Glencoe, IL: Free Press.

Parsons, T. & Bales, R.F. (1955). *Family socialization and interaction process.* New York: Free Press.

Parsons, R., Bales, R.F., & Shils, E.A. (1953). *Working papers on the theory of action.* Glencoe, IL: Free Press.

Paskert, C. (1983). Progress and focus on the national childhood immunization program. *Journal of School Health,* August, pp. 357–359.

Pasquali, E.A., Arnold, H.M., De Basio, N., & Alesi, E.G. (1985). *Mental Health Nursing* (2nd ed.). St. Louis: Mosby.

Patterson, J.M. (1988). Chronic illness in children and the impact on families. In C.S. Chilman, E.W. Nunnally, & F.M. Cox (Eds.). *Chronic illness and disability* (pp. 69–107), Newbury Park, CA: Sage.

Patterson, J.M. & Zderad, L. (1976). *Humanistic nursing.* New York: John Wiley and Sons.

Paul, W. & Paul B. (1975). *The marital puzzle.* New York: Norton.

Paz, O. (1973). The sons of La Malenche. In L.I. Duran & H.R. Bernard (Eds.). *Introduction to Chicano studies.* New York: Macmillan.

Pearlin, L. (1983). Role strains and personal stress. In H.B. Kaplan (Ed.). *Psychological stress* (pp. 3–31). New York: Academic Press.

Pearlin, L. & Schooler, C. (1978). The structure of coping. *Journal of Health and Social Behavior, 19* 19–21.

Pearlin, L. & Turner, H.A. (1987). The family as a context of the stress process. In S.V. Kasl & C.L. Cooper. *Stress and health: Issues in research methodology.* New York: John Wiley and Sons.

Peck, J.S. & Manocharian, J.R. (1988). Divorce in the changing family life cycle. In B. Carter & M. McGoldrick. *The changing family life cycle* (pp. 335–369), New York: Gardner Press.

Pederson, P. (1976, August 2). Varighed fra sygdoms begyndelse til henvendelse til prakliserende laege. *Ugekr Laeg, 138,* 32.

Pender, N.J. (1986). Health promotion: Implementing strategies. In B.B. Logan & C.E. Dawkins (Eds.). *Family-*

centered nursing in the community (pp. 296–334). Reading, MA: Addison-Wesley.

Pender, N.J. (1987). *Health promotion in nursing practice.* (2nd ed.). E. Norwalk, CT: Appleton & Lange.

Pelletier, K. (1977). *Mind as healer, mind as slayer.* New York: Dell.

———. (1979). *Holistic medicine.* New York: Delta/Seymour Lawrence.

Peplau, H. (1952). *Interpersonal relations in nursing.* New York: GP Putnams' Sons.

Perkins, E.J. (1973). Screening for ophthalmic conditions. *Practitioner, 211,* 171–177.

Perkins, H.W. & Harris, L.B. (1990). Familial bereavement and health in adult life course perspective. *Journal of Marriage and the Family, 52* (1), 233–241.

Perry, S.E. (1983). Attachment theory. In I.W. Clements & F.B. Roberts (Eds.). *Family health: A theoretical approach to nursing care* (pp. 109–122). New York: Wiley.

Peters, L.R. (1974). Family team or myth. In Hall, J.E., Weaver, B.R. (Eds.). *Nursing of families in crisis* (pp. 226–237). Philadelphia: Lippincott.

Peters, M.F. (1981). "Making it" Black family style: Building on the strengths of Black families. In N. Stinnett, J. De Frain, K. King et al. (Eds.). *Family strengths: Roots of well-being* (pp. 73–91). Lincoln, NB: University of Nebraska Press.

Peters, M.F. & Massey, G. (1983). Mundane extreme environmental stress in family stress theories: The case of Black families in White America. In H.I. McCubbin, M.B. Sussman & J.M. Patterson (Eds.). *Social stress and the family—Marriage and Family Review, 6* (1/2), 193–218.

Peterson, G.W. & Rollins, B.C. (1987). Parent-child socialization. In M.B. Sussman & S.K. Steinmetz (Eds.). *Handbook of marriage and the family* (pp. 471–507). New York: Plenum Press.

Peterson, L.R., Maynard, J.L. (1981, Jan.). Bringing home the bacon doesn't mean I have to cook it too. *Pacific Sociological Review, 24* (1), 87–106.

Piaget, J. (1971). *Science of education and the psychology of the child.* New York: Viking Press.

Pifer, A. & Bronte, L. (1986). Introduction: Squaring the pyramid. In A. Pifer & L. Bronte (Eds.). *Our aging society.* New York: W.W. Norton.

Pilisuk, M. & Parks, S.H. (1983). Social support and family stress. In H.I. McCubbin, M.B. Sussman & J.M. Patterson (Eds.). *Social stress and the family.* (Special issue) In Marriage and Family Review, *6* (1/2), 137–156.

Pipes, W.H. (1988). Old-time religion. Benches can't say amen. In H.P. McAdoo (Ed.). *Black families* (2nd ed.). (pp. 54–76). Newbury Park, CA: Sage.

Pleck, J.H. (1985). *Working wives/working husbands.* Beverly Hills, CA: Sage.

Pollack, D. (1981, April 5). The stepparent. How to put your best foot forward. *Fresno Bee.* Part B1, B4.

Power, P.W. & Dell Orto, A.E. (1988). Approaches to family intervention. In P.W. Power, A.E. Dell Orto & M. Gibbons (Eds.). *Role of the family in the rehabilitation of the physically disabled* (pp. 321–330). Baltimore: University Park Press.

Pratt, L. (1976). *Family structure and effective health behavior. The energized family.* Boston: Houghton-Miffin.

———. (1977). Changes in health care ideology in relation to self-care by families. *Health Education Monograph, 5* (2), 121–122.

———. (1982). Family structure and health work: Coping in the context of social change. In H.I. McCubbin, A.E. Cauble, & J.M. Patterson (Eds.). *Family stress, coping, and social support* (pp. 73–89). Springfield, IL: Charles C. Thomas.

Prattes, O. (1973). Beliefs of the Mexican American family. In D. Hymovich & M.V. Barnard (Eds.). *Family health care* (pp. 131–137). New York: McGraw-Hill.

Pravikoff, D. (1985). Family coping and perception of the situation in families with an actual or suspected myocardial infarction. Unpublished Master's Thesis. Los Angeles: California State University, Los Angeles.

Preto, N.G. (1988). Transformation of the family system in adolescence. In B. Carter & M. McGoldrick (Eds.). *The changing family life cycle* (2nd ed.). (pp. 255–283). New York: Gardner Press.

Price, J.A. (1976). North American Indian families. In C.H. Mindel & R. Haberstein (Eds.). *Families in America: Patterns and variations.* New York: Elsevier.

Prohaska, T.R., Leventhal, E.A., Leventhal, H. et al. (1985). Health practices and illness cognition in young, middle aged and elderly adults. *Journal of Gerontology, 40* (5), 569–578.

Queen, S.A. & Haberstein, R.W. (1974). *The family in various cultures.* Philadelphia: Lippincott.

Quesada, G.M. & Heller, P.L. (1977). Sociocultural barriers to medical care among Mexican Americans in Texas. *Medical Care* (suppl), *15* (5), 93–100.

Rainwater, L. (1971). Crucible of identity: The Negro lower-class family. In J.H. Bracey, A. Meier, & E. Rudwick (Eds.). *Black matriarchy: Myth or reality?* (pp. 76–109). Belmont: CA: Wadsworth.

———. (1972). Fear and house as haven in the lower class. In R. Gutman (Ed.). *People and buildings.* New York: Basic Books.

Ramirez, O. & Arce, C. (1981). The contemporary Chicano family: An empirically-based review. In A. Baron (Ed.). *Explorations in Chicano psychology.* New York: Praeger.

Rapoport, R., Rapoport, R. & Thiessen, V. (1974). Couple symmetry and enjoyment. *Journal of Marriage and the Family, 36* (3), 588–591.

Raths, L.E., Harmin, M. & Simon, S.B. (1978). *Values and teaching: Working with values in the classroom* (2nd ed.). Columbus, OH: Charles E. Merrill.

Rauckhorst, L.M., Stokes, S.A., & Mezey, M.D. (1982). Community and home assessment. In B.W. Spradley (Ed.). *Readings in community health nursing* (2nd ed.). (pp. 154–165). Boston: Little, Brown.

Raush, H., Goodrich, W., & Campbell, J.D. (1963). Adaptation to the first years of marriage. *Psychiatry, 26,* 368–371.

Raven, B.H., Center, R., & Rodrigues, A. (1975). The bases of conjugal power. In R.E. Cromwell & D.H. Olson

(Eds.). *Power in families* (pp. 217–232). New York: Sage Publications.

Rayner, J.F. (1970). Socioeconomic status and factors influencing the dental health practices of mothers. *American Journal of Public Health, 60,* 1250.

Rebelsky, F.G. Infancy in two cultures. (1967). *Psychologie Ned Tydschr Psychol Grensgebieden, 22,* 379.

Redman, B.K. & Thomas, S.A. (1985). Patient teaching. In G.M. Bulechek & J.C. McCloskey (Eds.). *Nursing interventions: Treatments for nursing diagnoses* (pp. 160–172). Philadelphia: W.B. Sauders Co.

Reed, K. (1982). The Neuman systems model: A basis for family psychosocial assessment and intervention. In B. Neuman. *The Neuman systems model. Application to nursing education and practice* (pp. 188–195). New York: Appleton-Century-Crofts.

Reed, P.G. (1986). The developmental conceptual framework: Nursing reformulations and applications for family therapy. In A. Whall (Ed.). *Family therapy theory for nursing: Four approaches* (pp. 69–91). Norwalk, CT: Appleton & Lange.

Reich, C. (1970). *The greening of America.* New York: Bantam.

Reinhardt, A. & Quinn, M. (Eds.). (1973). *Current practices in family-centered community nursing.* St. Louis: Mosby.

Reiss, D. (1981). *The family's construction of reality.* Cambridge, MA: Harvard University Press.

Reiss, D. and Oliveri, M.E. (1983, Spring/Summer). Family stress as community frame. *Marriage and Family Review, 6* (1/2), 61–83.

Reiss, I.L. (1965). The universality of the family: A conceptual analysis. *Journal of Marriage and the Family, 27,* 443.

______. (1976). *Family Systems in America* (2nd ed.). Hinsdale, IL: Dryden Press.

Richardson, W. (1970). Measuring the urban poor's use of physicians: services in response to illness episodes. *Medical Care, 8,* 132.

Rippe, J.M. (1989). For a life long healthy heart: Choose exercise. *Newsweek,* February 13, 1989, pp. S-8 & S-10.

Roack, A.C. (1988). Parenting: Fads, theories change with the years. *Los Angeles Times* (July 24, 1988), pp. A-1 and A 24.

Roberts, R.H. (1975). Perceptual views of family members of the identified patient. In S. Smoyak (Ed.). *The psychiatric nurse as a family therapist* (pp. 156–163). New York: Wiley.

Robiscon, R. & Smith, J.A. (1973). Family assessment. In A.M. Reinhardt & M.D. Quinn (Eds.). *Current practice in family-centered community nursing,* Vol I. St. Louis: Mosby.

Rodgers, R.H. (1973). *Family interaction and transaction: The developmental approach.* Englewood Cliffs, NJ: Prentice-Hall.

Rodman, H. (1965). *Marriage, family and society.* New York: Random House.

Roessler, R. & Bolton, B. (1978). Coordination of human services. In R. Roessler & B. Bolton (Eds.). *Psychological adjustment to disability* (pp. 145–161). Baltimore: University Park Press.

Rokeach, M. (1973). *The nature of human values.* New York: The Free Press.

Rogers, C. (1951). *Client-centered therapy: Implications and theory.* Boston: Houghton Mifflin Co.

Rogers, M.F. (1974). Instrumental and infra-resources: The bases of power. *American Journal of Sociology, 79,* 1423.

Rollins, B.C. & Feldman, H. (1970). Marital satisfaction over the family life cycle. *Journal of Marriage and the Family, 32,* (1), 20–25.

Rollins, B.C. & Thomas, D.L. (1979). Parental support, power and control techniques in the socialization of children. In W.R. Burr, R. Hill, F.I. Nye & I.L. Reiss (Eds.). *Contemporary theories about the family,* Vol. I New York: The Free Press.

Roney, R.G. & Nall, M.L. (1966). *Medication practices in a community: An exploratory study.* Menlo Park, CA: Stanford Research Institute.

Rose, A.M. (1962). *Human behavior and social processes.* Boston: Houghton Mifflin Co.

Rosenstock, I.M. (1974). Historical origins of the health belief model. In M. Becker (Ed.). *The health belief model and personal health behavior* (pp. 1–8). Thorofare, NJ: Charles Slack.

Ross, C.E., Mirowsky, J. & Goldsteen, K. (1990). The impact of the family on health: The decade in review. *Journal of Marriage & the Family, 52* (4), 1059–1078.

Rossi, A.S. as cited in Woodward, K.L. et al. (1978, May 15). Saving the family. *Newsweek,* 67.

Rossi, A.S. (1986). Sex and gender in the aging society. In A. Pifer and L. Bronte (Eds.). *Our aging society* (pp. 111–139). New York: W.W. Norton and Co.

Roth, P. (1989). Family social support. In P.J. Bomar (Ed.). *Nurses and family health promotion* (pp. 90–102). Baltimore, MD: Williams & Wilkins.

Roy C. (1983). Analysis and application of the Roy adaptation model. In I. Clements & F. Roberts (Eds.). *Family health: A theoretical approach to nursing care.* New York: John Wiley and Sons.

Rubin, R. (1967). Attainment of the maternal role. 1. Processes. *Nursing Research, 16,* 237.

______. (1967). Attainment of maternal role. 2. Models and referrants. *Nursing Research, 16,* 342.

Ruesch, H., Barry, W., Hertel, R., Swain, M. (1974). *Communication conflict and marriage.* San Francisco: Jossey-Bass.

Rushing, W. (1968). Individual behavior and suicides. In J.P. Gibbs (Ed.). *Suicide* (pp. 96–121). New York: Harper & Row.

Russell, G. (1977, August 29). The American underclass. *Time Magazine,* 16–19.

Russell, G. & Satterwhite, B. (1978, October 16). It's your turn in the sun. *Time,* p. 48.

Ryan, M.C. & Austin, A.L. (1989). Social supports and social networks in the aged. *Image, 21* (3), 176–179.

Safilios-Rothschild, C. (1976, May). A macro and micro-examination of family power and love: An exchange model. *Journal of Marriage & the Family 38* (2), 355–362.

______. (1976). The dimensions of power distribution in the family. In H. Grunebaum & J. Christ (Eds.). *Contempo-*

rary marriage: Structure, dynamics and therapy. Boston: Little, Brown.

Samuelson, R.J. (October 20, 1986). The discovery of money. *Newsweek*, p. 58.

Santi, L.L. (Nov., 1987). Changes in the structure and size of American households: 1970 to 1985. *Journal of Marriage and the Family, 49* (4), 833–837.

Satir, V. (1967). *Conjoint family therapy.* Palo Alto, CA: Science and Behavior Books.

______. (1972). *Peoplemaking.* Palo Alto, CA: Science and Behavior Books.

______. (1975). Intervention for congruence. In V. Satir, J.S. Stachowiak & H.A. Taschman (Eds.). *Helping families to change.* (pp. 79–104). New York: Jason Aronson.

______. (1983). *Conjoint family therapy* (3rd. ed.). Palo Alto, Calif: Science and Behavior Books.

Saunders, L. (1954). *Cultural differences & medical care: The case of the Spanish-speaking people of the Southwest.* New York: Sage Foundation.

Saunders, L.E. (1969). *Social class and postparental perspective.* Doctoral dissertation, University of Minnesota.

Savage, D.G. (1990, February 27). One in four young black males in jail or in court control, study says. *Los Angeles Times*, p. A 1 and 16.

Scanzoni, J. (1971). *The Black family in modern society.* Boston: Allyn & Bacon.

Scanzoni, J. (1987). Families in the 1990's. *Journal of Family Issues, 8* (4), 394–421.

Scanzoni, J. & Szinovacz, M. (1980). *Family decision-making. A developmental sex role model.* Newbury Park, CA: Sage.

Schonfield, D. (1982). Who is stereotyping whom and why? *The Gerontologist, 22*, 267–272.

Schorr, A.L. (1970). Housing and its effects. In H.M. Proshansky, et al. (Eds.). *Environmental psychology.* New York: Holt, Rinehart, & Winston.

Schraneveldt, J.D. (1973). The interactionist framework in the study of the family. In A. Reinhardt & M. Quinn (Eds.). *Family-centered community nursing.* St. Louis: Mosby.

Schulman, J.L. (1976). *Coping with tragedy: Successfully facing the problem of a seriously ill child.* Chicago: Follett Publishing Co.

Schultz, D.A. (1972). *The changing family.* Englewood Cliffs, NJ: Prentice-Hall.

Schwartz, G. & Merton, D. (1967). The language of adolescents: An anthropological approach to the youth culture. *American Journal of Sociology, 72*, 459.

Schwartz, P. (1987). The family as a changed institution. *Journal of Family Issues, 8* (4), 455–459.

Scotch, N. & Greiger, J. (1962). The epidemiology of rheumatoid arthritis—A review with special attention to social factors. *Journal of Chronic Diseases, 15*, 1037.

Sears, R, Maccoby, E. & Levin, H. (1957). *Patterns of child rearing.* New York: Harper & Row.

Sells, J.W. (1973). *Seven steps to effective communication.* Atlanta: Forum House.

Seltzer, M.M., Litchfield, L.C., Lowy, L. & Levin, R.J. (1989). Families as case managers: A longitudinal study. *Family Relations, 38* (3), 332–336.

Selye, H. (1974). *Stress without distress.* New York: Lippincott.

Sena-Rivera, J. (1980). La familia Hispania as a natural support: Strategies for prevention in mental health. In R. Valle & W. Vega (Eds.). *Hispanic natural support systems: Mental health promotion perspectives.* Berkeley, CA: State of California Department of Mental Health.

Shanas, E. (1980, Feb.). Older people and their families. The new pioneers. *Journal of Marriage and the Family, 42* (1), 9–15.

Shanas, E. et al. (1968). *Old people in three industrial societies.* New York: Atherton.

Shapiro, J. (1989). Stress, depression and support group participation in mothers of developmentally delayed children. *Family Relations, 38* (2), 169–173.

Shapiro, V. (1983). Growing hand in hand: Infants and parents at risk. In V.J. Sasserath & R.A. Hoekelman (Eds.). *Minimizing high-risk parenting.* Skillman, NJ: Johnson & Johnson Baby Products Co.

Shaw, S.M. (1988). Gender differences in the definition and perception of household labor. *Family Relations, 37* (3), 333–337.

Sheppard, H. (1990, February 5). How Hispanic cultural patterns affect caregivers. *The Nurse's Newspaper*, pp. 15–16.

Silver, J. (1975). Solidarity versus pseudomutuality. In S. Smoyak (Ed.). *The psychiatric nurse as a family therapist* (pp. 106–113). New York: Wiley.

Simmel, G. (1955). *Conflict and the web of group affiliations.* Englewood Cliffs, New Jersey: Prentice-Hall.

Skinner, D. (1984). Dual-career families: Strains of sharing. In H.I. McCubbin & C.R. Figley (Eds.). *Stress and the family. Vol I: Coping with normative transitions.* New York: Brunner/Mazel.

Slater, P. (1970, July). Culture in collision. *Psychology Today*, pp. 31–33, 66–68.

Sloan, M., Schommer, B. (1975). The process of contracting in community nursing. In B. Spradley, (Ed.) *Contemporary community nursing* (pp. 221–229). Boston: Little, Brown.

Smelzer, N.J. & Halpern, S. (1978). The historical triangulations of family, economy and education. In J. Demos & S.S. Boocock (Eds.). *Turning points: Historical and sociological essays on the family.* Chicago: The University of Chicago Press.

Smith, G.R. (1988, June 13). Exploiting the public agenda. Advancing new opportunities for public health nursing. Paper presented at American Nurses Foundation, Louisville, KY.

Smith, H. (1985). What research is telling us about family recreation. *Perspectives on family recreation and leisure.* Centennial National Conference American Alliance for Health, Physical Education and Dance (ERIC Document Reproduction Service, No. ED 263-1061.

Smoyak, S. (1969). Threat: A recurring family dynamic. *Perspectives in Psychiatric Care, 7*, 267–268.

______. (1975). Introducing families to family therapy. In S.

Smoyak (Ed.). *The psychiatric nurse as a family therapist.* New York: Wiley.

———. (1977). Introduction: Symposium on parenting. *Nursing Clinics of North America, 12,* 447.

Sobel, E.G. & Robischon, P. (1975). *Family nursing: A study guide.* St. Louis, MO: CV Mosby.

Sorofman, B. (1986). Research in cultural diversity. Defining diversity. *Western Journal of Nursing Research, 8,* 121–123.

Speck, R.V. & Attneave, C. (1973). *Family networks.* New York: Random House.

Spence, W.R. (1989). *Weight control.* Waco, TX: Health EDCO.

Spiegel, J. (1957). The resolution of role conflict within the family. *Psychiatry, 25,* 1.

Spiegel, J. (1971). Cultural strain, family role patterns and intrapsychic conflict. In J. Howells (Ed.). *Theory and practice of family psychiatry.* New York: Brunner/Mazel.

Spinetta, J.J. & Deasy-Spinetta, P. (1981). *Living with childhood cancer.* St. Louis, MO: CV Mosby.

Spitze, G. (1988). Women's employment and family relations: A review. *Journal of Marriage and the Family, 50* (3), 595–618.

———. (1957). The resolution of role conflict within the family. *Psychiatry, 25,* 1.

Spitzer, W. & Brown, B. (1975). Unanswered questions about the periodic health examination. *Annals of Internal Medicine, 83,* 257.

Spock, B. (1974). *Baby and child care* (3rd ed.). New York: Pocket Books.

Sprey, J. (1969). The family as a system in conflict. *Journal of Marriage and the Family, 31* (4), 699–706.

———. (1972). Family power structure: A critical comment. *Journal of Marriage and the Family, 34* (2), 235.

———. (1979). Conflict theory and the study of marriage and the family. In W.R. Burr, R. Hill, F.I. Nye & I.L. Reiss (Eds.). *Contemporary theories about the family, Vol. II* (pp. 130–159). New York: The Free Press.

Sprey, J. & Matthews, S. (1982). Contemporary grandparenthood. A systematic transition. *Annals of the American Academy of Political and Social Science, 464,* 91–103.

Stachowiak, J. (1975). Family structure and intervention strategies. In V. Satir, J. Stachowiak & H.A. Taschman (Eds.). *Helping families to change* (pp. 105–131). New York: Jason Aronson.

Staples, R. (1976). The Black American family. In C.H. Mindel & R.W. Haberstein (Eds.). *Ethnic families in America.* New York: Elsevier.

———. (1985). Changes in black family structure: The conflict between family ideology and structural conditions. *Journal of Marriage and the Family, 47* (4), 1005–1013.

———. (1989). Family life in the 21st century. In C.L. Gilliss, B.L. Highley, B.M. Roberts & I.M. Martinson (Eds.). *Toward a science of family nursing* (pp. 156–170). Menlo Park, CA: Addison-Wesley.

Stea, D. (1965, Autumn). Space, territory, and human movement. *Landscape,* 14.

Steiger, N.J. & Lipson, J.G. (1985). *Self-care nursing: Theory and practice.* Bowie, MD: Brady Communications Co.

———. (1970). Space, territory, and human movements. In Proshansky, H.M. et al. *Environmental psychology* (pp. 37–44). New York: Holt, Rinehart, & Winston.

Steinberg, R.M. & Carter, G.W. (1983). *Case management and the elderly.* Lexington, MA: Lexington Books.

Steinglass, P. (1978). The conceptualization of marriage from a systems theory perspective. In T.J. Paolino & B.S. McCrady (Eds.). *Marriage and marital therapy: Psychoanalytic, behavioral, and systems theory perspectives.* New York: Brunner/Mazel.

Steinglass, P., Bennett, L.A. Wolin, S.J. & Reiss, D. (1987). *The alcoholic family.* New York: Basic Books.

Steinmetz, S.K. (1987). Family violence. Past, present and future. In M.B. Sussman & S.K. Steinmetz (Eds.). *Handbook of marriage and the family* (pp. 725–765). New York: Plenum Press.

Stetz, K., Lewis, J. & Primomo, J. (1986). Family coping strategies and chronic illness in the mother. *Family Relations, 35,* 515–522.

Stinnett, N. (1979). In search of strong families. In N. Stinnett, B. Chesser & J. De Frain (Eds.). *Building family strengths—Blueprints for action.* Lincoln, Nebraska: University of Nebraska Press.

Stokes, L.G. (1974). Delivering health services in a Black community. In A. Reinhardt & M. Quinn (Eds.). *Family-centered community nursing.* St. Louis: Mosby.

Strauss, M.A. (1968). Communication, creativity, and problem-solving ability of middle and working class families in three societies. *American Journal of Sociology, 73,* 417–430.

———. (1976). Marital violence. Paper presented at American Psychological Association Convention, Chicago, 1975. Cited in E. Eldridge & N. Meredith (Eds.). *Environmental issues: Family impact* (pp. 177–178). Minneapolis, MN: Burgess.

Strauss, M.A., Gelles, R.J. & Steinmetz, S.K. (1980). *Behind closed doors: Violence in the American family.* New York: Anchor Press.

Strayhorn, J.M. Jr. (1977). *Talking it out: Guide to effective communication.* Champagne, IL: Research Press.

Strodtbeck, F.L. (1978). Family interaction, values, and achievement. In D.C. McClelland, et al. (Eds.). *Talent and society* (pp. 135–194). New York: Van Nostrand.

Stryker, S. (1964). The interactional and situational approaches. In H.T. Christensen, (Ed.). *Handbook of marriage and the family.* Chicago: Rand McNally.

Suchman, E.A. (1965, Fall). Stages of illness and medical care. *Journal of Health and Human Behavior, 6,* 114–128.

Sung, S.L. (1967). *The story of the Chinese in America.* New York: Collier.

Sussman, M.B. (1974). Family systems in the 1970s: Analysis, policies, and programs. In A. Skolnick, & J.H. Skolnick (Eds.). *Intimacy, family and society* (pp. 579–598). Boston: Little, Brown.

Sussman, M.G. & Slater, S.B. (1963, August 28). Reappraisal of urban kin networks—Empirical evidence. Paper presented at the Annual Meeting of the American Sociological Association, Los Angeles, CA.

Sussman, M.B. et al. (1971). Changing families in a changing society. Forum 14 in Report to the President: White House Conference on Children. Washington DC: Government Printing Office.

Swendsen, L.A. & Meleis, A.I. (1978, March/April). Role supplementation for new parents—a role mastery plan. *American Journal of Maternal-Child Nursing X* (2), 84.

Syme, S., Hyman, M. & Enterline, P. (1964). Some social and cultural factors associated with the occurrence of coronary heart disease. *J Chronic Dis, 17*, 277.

Synder, W.K. (1988). *Sudden infant death syndrome. Self-help support groups. An annotated bibliography* (Fall, 1988). McLean, VA: National Sudden Infant Death Syndrome Clearinghouse.

Szinovacz, M.E. (1987). Family power. In M.B. Sussman & S.K. Steinmetz (Eds.). *Handbook of marriage and the family* (pp. 651–693). New York: Plenum Press.

Tadych, R. (1985). Nursing in multiperson units: The family. In Riehl-Sisca, J. (Ed.). *The science and art of self-care.* pp. 49–55 E. Norwalk CT: Appleton & Lange.

Taylor, C. (1970). In horizontal orbit. New York: Holt, Rinehart & Winston.

Taylor, R.J. (1990). Need for support and family involvement among Black Americans. *Journal of Marriage and the Family, 52* (3), 584–590.

Taylor, R.J., Chatters, C.M. & Mays, V.M. (1988). Parents, children, siblings, in-laws, and non-kin as sources of emergency assistance to Black Americans. *Family Relations, 37* (3), 298–304.

Taylor, R.J., Chatters, C.M. Tucker, M.B., & Lewis, E. (1990). Developments in research on black families: a decade review. *Journal of Marriage and the Family, 52* (4), 993–1014.

Teachman, J.D., Polonko, K.A. & Scanzoni, J. (1987). Demography of the family. In Sussman, M.B. & Steinmetz, S. (Eds.). *Handbook of Marriage and the Family* (pp. 3–36). New York: Plenum Press.

Thomas, W.I. (1923). *The unadjusted girl.* New York: The Social Science Research Council (Later publication in 1967 by New York: Harper & Row).

Tinkham, G., Voorhies, E. (1977). *Community health nursing—Evolution and process.* New York: Appleton-Century-Crofts.

______. (1984). *Community health nursing—Evolution and process* (2nd ed.). New York: Appleton-Century-Crofts.

Toffler, A. (1970). *Future Shock.* New York: Warner Communications.

Toffler, A. (1990). Power shift. Knowledge, wealth, and violence at the edge of the 21st century. *Newsweek,* Oct. 15, 1990, pp. 85–92.

Toman, W. (1961). *Family constellation.* New York: Springer.

Torres-Gil, F. (1986). Hispanics: A special challenge. In A. Pifer & L. Bronte (Eds.). *Our aging society* (pp. 219–242). New York: W.W. Norton and Co.

Toynbee, A.J. (1955, March). We must pay for freedom. *Women's Home Companion,* pp. 52–53.

Trainor, M.G. (1983). Self-help groups as a resource for individual clients and families. In I.W. Clements & F.B. Roberts (Eds.). *Family health: A theoretical approach to nursing care* (pp. 45–56). New York: John Wiley and Sons.

Travelbee, J. (1969). *Intervention in psychiatric nursing.* Philadelphia: FA Davis.

Travis, J. (1976). *Wellness workbook.* Wellness Resource Center, Mill Valley, CA.

Treas, J. & Bengston, V. (1987). The family in later years. In M.B. Sussman & S. Steinmetz (Eds.). *Handbook of marriage and the family* (pp. 625–648). New York: Plenum Press.

Tripp-Reimer, T., Brink, P.J., Saunders, J.M. (1984, March/April). Cultural assessment: Content and process. *Nursing Outlook, 32* (2), 78–82.

Tripp-Reimer, T. & Lauer, G.M. (1987). Ethnicity and families with chronic illness. In L.M. Wright & M. Leahey (Eds.). *Families and chronic illness* (pp. 77–100). Springhouse, PA: Springhouse Corporation.

Troits, P.A. (1982). Conceptual, methodological and theoretical problems in studying social support as a buffer against life stress. *Journal of Health and Social Behavior, 23* (June), 145–159.

Troll, L. (1971). The family of later life: A decade review. *Journal of Marriage and the Family, 33,* 263–275.

Truax, C. & Carkhuff, R. (1967). *Toward effective counseling and psychotherapy.* Chicago: Aldine.

Turk, K.C. & Kerns, R.D. (1985). The family in health and illness. In D.C. Turk & R.D. Kerns (Eds.). *Health, illness and families. A life span perspective* (pp. 1–22). New York: John Wiley and Sons.

Turner, R.H. (1970). *Family interaction.* New York: John Wiley and Sons.

______. (1962). Role taking: Process vs. conformity. In A.M. Rose (Ed.). *Human behavior and social processes* (pp. 20–40). Boston: Houghton-Mifflin.

Turner, V. (1990, Winter). A look at methamphetamine. *People reaching out newsletter.* Youth and Family Center for Substance abuse Counseling and Information.

United Press International. (1990). Tax report says rich gained, poor lost during the 80's. February 6, 1990, *Los Angeles Times,* p. A4.

U.S. Bureau of the Census. (1974, March). Household and family characteristics, *Current population reports,* Series P-20, No 276. Washington DC: Government Printing Office, 2, 4, 13.

______. (1978). *Statistical abstracts of the U.S.* (99th ed.). Washington DC: Government Printing Office.

______. (1980). *Statistical abstracts of the U.S.* (101st ed.). Washington DC: Government Printing Office.

______. (1981). *Statistical abstracts of the U.S.* (102nd ed.). Washington DC: Government Printing Office.

______. (1982). *Statistical abstracts of the U.S.* (103rd ed.). Washington DC: Government Printing Office.

______. (1983). *Statistical abstracts of the U.S.* (104th ed.). Washington DC: U.S. Government Printing Office.

______. (1984). Projections of the population of the United States, by age, sex, and race: 1983–2080. *Current populations reports,* Series No 952, p. 25.

______. (March, 1985). Households, families, marital status and living arrangements. *Current population reports.* Series P-20, No. 402, Washington DC: US Government Printing Office.

______. (1986). Marital status and living arrangements: March 1985. *Current Population Reports.* Series P-20, No. 410, Washington DC: U.S. Government Printing Office.

______. (1988b). *Statistical abstracts of the U.S., 1988.* (108th Ed.). Washington DC: Govt Printing Office.

______. (1989). *Statistical abstracts of the U.S.* (109th Ed.). Washington DC: U.S. Government Printing Office.

______. (1990, Jan.). How we're changing. *Current Population Reports,* Series NO 164, p. 23. Washington DC: U.S. Government Printing Office.

U.S. Bureau of the Census. (1991, February). *Census & You, 26* (2). Washington DC: U.S. Government Printing Office.

U.S. Bureau of the Census. (1991, April). *Census & You, 26* (4). Washington DC: U.S. Government Printing Office.

U.S. Department of Agriculture. (1985). *Dietary guidelines for Americans* (2nd ed.). USDA, Dept. of Health and Human Services.

U.S. Department of Health, Education and Welfare. (1972, June). *Periodontal Disease and Oral Hygiene Among Children.* US Public Health Services, Series 11, No 117.

U.S. Department of Health, Education, and Welfare. (1983, May 30). *Monthly Vital Statistics Report, 23,* 13.

U.S. Department of Health and Human Services, Center for Disease Control. (1985). *Diphtheria, tetanus, and pertussis: Guidelines for vaccine prophylaxis and other preventive measures.* Atlanta, MMWR July 12, pp. 405–426.

U.S. Department of Health and Human Services, Center for Disease Control. (1987). *The 21st immunization conference proceedings.* CDC. Atlanta. June 8–11.

U.S. Department of Health and Human Services. (1988). *Health in the United States.* National Center for Health Statistics. DHHS Pub. No. (PHS) 88-1232.

______. (1989a). *Reducing the health consequences of smoking: 25 years of progress, a report of the Surgeon General.* DHHS Pub. No. (CDC) 89-8411.

______. (1989b). *A profile of uninsured Americans.* National Center for Health Services Research and Health Care Technology Assessment. DHHS Pub. No. (PHS) 89-3443.

______. (1989c). *National household survey on drug abuse. National Institute on Drug Abuse.* DHHS Pub. No (ADM) 89-1636.

______. (1989d). *Highlights of the 1988 national household survey on drug abuse.* National Institutes on Drug Abuse. NIDA Capsules, CAP 20, C-86-13, p. 2.

______. (1989e). *Child health USA '89.* Office of Maternal and Child Health. HRS-M-CH 8915, October, 1989.

______. (1990a). *Smoking and health: A national status report.* Office on Smoking and Health. DHHS Pub. No (CDC) 87-8396.

______. (1990b). *The seventh special report to the U.S. Congress on: Alcohol and health.* Alcohol, Drug Abuse, and Mental Health Administration. Washington, DC: US Gov't Printing Office.

U.S. Environmental Protection Agency. (1988a). *The inside story: A guide to indoor pollution quality.* United States Consumer Product Safety Commission. EPA 400/1-88/004. Wash. DC: U.S. Government Printing Office.

U.S. Public Health Service. (1979). *Healthy people: The surgeon general's report on health promotion and disease prevention.* U.S. DHEW (PHS). #79-55071.

______. (1980). *Promoting health/preventing disease: Objectives for the nation.* USDHEW (PHS).

U.S. Senate Select Committee on Nutrition and Human Needs. (1975). *Nutrition and Health—An Evaluation of Nutritional Surveillance in the U.S.* Washington, D.C.: U.S. Government Printing Office.

U.S. Senate Special Committee on Aging (in conjunction with the American Association of Retired Persons, the Federal Council on Aging and the U.S. Administration on Aging. (1987–1988). *Aging America: Trends and projections.* Washington DC: U.S. Government Printing Office.

Valdez, R. (1991). Latino access to health care. *Health, 10* (1), 3.

Vega, W.A. (1990). Hispanic families in the 1980s: A decade of research. *Journal of Marriage and the Family, 52* (November): 1015–1024.

Vega, W.A., Hough, R.L. & Romero, A. (1983). Family life patterns of Mexican Americans. In A.J. Powell (Ed.). *The psychological development of minority children* (pp. 194–215). New York: Brunner/Mazel.

Vega, W.A. et al. (1986). Cohesion and adaptability in Mexican-American and Anglo families. *Journal of Marriage and the Family, 48* (4), 857–867.

Venters, M.H. (1981). Familial coping with chronic and severe childhood illness: The case of cystic fibrosis. *Social Science and Medicine, 19A,* 189–197.

Ventura, J.N. (1987). The stresses of parenthood reexamined. *Family Relations, 36,* (1), 26–29.

______. (1989). First births to older mothers, 1970–1986. *American Journal of Public Health, 79* (12), 1675–1677.

Vernez, G., Burnam, M.A., McGlynn, E.A., Trude, S. & Mittman, B.S. (1988, February). *Review of California's program for the homeless mentally disabled.* Santa Monica, CA: The Rand Corporation.

Vickers, G. (1971). Institutional and personal roles. *Human Relations, 24* (5), 433.

Vickory, D. & Fries, J. (1981). *Take care of yourself–A consumer's guide to medical care,* Revised Edition, Reading, MA: Addison-Wesley.

Vincent, C. (1966). Familia spongia: The adaptive function. *Marriage and the Family, 28* (1), 29–36.

Vincent, C.E. (1970). Mental health and the family. In P.H. Glasser & L.N. Glasser (Eds.). *Families in Crisis.* New York: Harper and Row.

Vincent, J. & Ransford, H.E. (1980). *Social stratification.* Boston: Allyn & Bacon.

Visher, E.B. & Visher, J.S. (1979). *Stepparent Families: Myths and Realities.* Secaucus, NJ: Citadel.

Visiting Nurse Association of Omaha. (1986). *Client management information system for community health nursing agencies. An implementation manual.* Bethesda, MD: USDHHS, Division of Nursing. Pub # NTIS HRP-0907023. For sale by the National Technical Information Service, 5285 Port Royal Rd., Springfield, VA 22161.

Vogel, E. & Bell, N. (1960). The emotionally disturbed child as a family scapegoat. In N. Bell & E. Vogel (Eds.). *A*

Modern introduction to the family. New York: Free Press.
von Bertalanffy, L. (1950). The theory of open systems in physics and biology. *Science, 111*, 23–29.
———. (1966). General system theory and psychiatry. In S. Arieti (Ed.). *American Handbook of Psychiatry*, Vol. 3, (pp. 705–721). New York: Basic Books.
Von Bertalanffy, L. General system theory: A critical review. (1968). In W. Buckley (Ed.). *Modern Systems Research for the Behavioral Scientist*. Chicago, IL: Aldine.
Voydanoff, P. & Donnelly, B.W. (1988). Economic distress, family coping and quality of family life. In P. Voydanoff and LeMajka, L.C. (Eds.). *Families and economic distress*, (pp. 97–115). Newbury Park, CA: Sage.
Vuchinich, S. (1987). Starting and stopping spontaneous family conflicts. *Journal of Marriage and the Family, 49* (3), 591–601.
Wahlstedt, P. & Blaser, W. (1986). Nurse case management for the frail elderly: A curriculum to prepare nurses for that role. *Home Healthcare Nurse, 4* (2), 30–35.
Walker, A.J. (1990). Gender and families. In National Council on Family Relations. *2001: Preparing families for the future*, (pp. 16–17). Minneapolis: National Council on Family Relations.
Wallace, A.M. (1978). Typology of stressors: A developmental view. In A.W. Burgess (Ed.). *Nursing: Levels of intervention* (pp. 76–108). Englewood Cliffs, NJ: Prentice-Hall.
Waller, W. (1938). *The Family: A Dynamic Interpretation*. New York: Dryden Press.
Wallerstein, J. & Kelly, J.B. (1980). *Surviving the break-up: How children and parents cope with divorce*. New York: Basic Books.
Walters, J. (Ed.). (1976). Fatherhood. (Special issue) In *Family Coordinator, 25*.
Warner, W.L. (1953). *American life*. Chicago: University of Chicago.
Watzlawick, P., Beavin, J.H., & Jackson, D.D. (1967). *Pragmatics of Human Communication*. New York: Norton.
Watson, J. (1985). *Nursing. The philosophy and science of caring*. Denver, CO: Colorado Associated University Press.
Weatherley, R.A. & Cartoof, V.G. (1988). Helping single adolescent parents. In C.S. Chilman, E.W. Nunnally & E.M. Cox (Eds.). *Variant family forms*, (pp. 39–55). Newbury Park, CA: Sage.
Weaver, G.R. (1976). American identity movements: A cross-cultural confrontation. In E. Eldridge & N. Meredith (Eds.). *Environmental issues: Family impact*. Minneapolis: Burgess.
Webster's New Collegiate Dictionary. (1988). Springfield, MA: Merriam.
Weeks, G., Jackson, J. (1982). The power of powerlessness. *The American Journal of Family Therapy*, 44–47.
Weil, M., Karl, J.M. & Associates. (1985). *Case management in human services practice*. San Francisco: Jossey-Bass.
Weiner, N. (1948). *Cybernetics*. New York: Wiley.
Weinert, C. & Long, K.A. (1987). Understanding the health care needs of rural families. *Family Relations, 36* (4), 450–455.
Weiss, R.S. (1988). On the current state of the American family. *Journal of Family Issues, 8* (4), 468–470.
Wessell, M.L. (1975). Use of humor by an immobilized adolescent girl during hospitalization. *Maternal Child Nursing Journal, 4* (1), 35–48.
West, P. & Merriam, L.E. (1969). Camping and cohesiveness: A sociological study of the effect of outdoor recreation on family solidarity. *Minnesota Forestry Research Notes*, 201.
———. (1970). Outdoor recreation and family cohesiveness: A research approach. *Journal of Leisure Res., 2*, 251–259.
Whall, A.L. (1981, Jan.). Nursing theory and the assessment of families. *JPN and Mental Health Services*, 30–36.
———. (1983). Family system theory. Relationship to nursing conceptual models. In J. Fitzpatrick & A. Whall (Eds.). *Conceptual models of nursing: Analysis and application* (pp. 69–93). Bowie, MD: R.J. Brady Co.
———. (1986a). The family as the unit of care in nursing: A historical review. *Public Health Nursing, 3* (4), 240–249.
———. (1986a/b). *Family therapy theory for nursing*. E. Norwalk, CT: Appleton & Lange.
Whall, A.L. & Fawcett, J. (1991). Family therapy development in nursing: State of the science and art. Philadelphia: FA Davis.
White, B.B. (1989). Gender differences in marital communication patterns. *Family Relations, 28* (2), 89–105.
White, L. (1988). Freedom versus constraint. *Journal of Family Issues, 8* (4), 468–470.
White, M. (1986). Case management. In M. Maddox (Ed.). *The encyclopedia of aging*. New York: Springer.
White, R.W. (1974). Strategies of adaptation: An attempt at systematic description. In G.V. Coehlo, D.A. Hamburg & J.E. Adams (Eds.). *Coping and adaptation*. New York: Basic Books.
Whiting, B. (1974). Folk wisdom and child rearing. Merrill-Palmer Quarterly, *20* (1), 9.
Wilberding, J.Z. (1985). Values clarification. In G.M. Bulechek, J.C. McCloskey (Eds.). *Nursing interventions: Treatments for nursing diagnosis* (pp. 173–184). Philadelphia: WB Saunders.
Wildavsky, A. (1977). Doing better and feeling worse: The political pathology of health policy. *Daedalus, 106*, 105.
Wiley, D.J.D. (1989). Family environmental health. In P.J. Bomar (Ed.). *Nurses and family health promotion* (pp. 293–319). Baltimore MD: Williams & Wilkins.
Wilkinson, D. (1987). Ethnicity. In M.B. Sussman & S.K. Steinmetz (Eds.). *Handbook of marriage and the family* (pp. 183–210). New York: Plenum Press.
Williams, D.A. & Lord, M. (1978, May 15). Blacks: Fresh trials. *Newsweek*, pp. 77–78.
Williams, J.I. & Leaman, T. (1973). Family structure and function. In H. Conn & R. Rakel (Eds.). *Family practice*. Philadelphia: Saunders.
Williams, R.M. (1960). *American society: A sociological interpretation* (3rd ed.). New York: Knopf.
Willie, C.V. (1976). *A new look at black families*. Bayside, NY: General Hall, Inc.
Willie, C.V. & Greenblatt, S. (1978). Four classic studies of power relationships in Black families: A review and look to

the future. *Journal of Marriage and the Family, 40*, 691–694.

Wills, T.A. (1985). Supportive functions of interpersonal relationships. In S. Cohen & S.L. Syme (Eds.). *Social support and health* (pp. 61–82). Orlando, FL: Academic Press.

Wilson, M.T. (1988). The family with a school-age child and the family with an adolescent. In B.J. Bradshaw (Ed.). *Nursing of the family in health and illness* (pp. 176–213, 214–255). E. Norwalk, CT: Appleton & Lange.

Wilson, W.J. (1987). *The truly underclass.* Chicago, IL: The University of Chicago Press.

Winder, P.G. (1988, July). Case management by nurses at a county facility. *Quality Review Bulletin*, 215–219.

Winnick, A.J. (1988). The changing distribution of income and wealth in the United States, 1960–1985: An examination of the movement toward two societies, "separate and unequal." In P. Voydanoff and L.C. Majka (Eds.). *Families and economic distress* (pp. 232–260). Newbury Park, CA: Sage.

Woods, N.J., Yates, B.L. & Primomo, J. (1988). Supporting families during chronic illness. *Image, 21* (1), 1989, 46–50.

Woodward, K.L. (1990, Winter/Spring). Young beyond their years. *Newsweek* (Special Issue), pp. 54–60.

Woodward, K.L., Lord, M., Maier, F., Foote, D.M. & Malamud, P. (1978, May 15). Saving the family. *Newsweek*, 67–71.

Wolfe, S. & Badgley, F. (1972). Patients and their families (Part 2 of The family doctor). *Millbank Mem Fund Bull, 50* 73.

World Health Organization. (1974). *Community health nursing report of the WHO expert committee.* Technical Report Series No. 558, Geneva: WHO.

Wright, L.M. & Leahey, M. (1984). *Nurses and families, A guide to family assessment and intervention.* Philadelphia: FA Davis.

______. (1987). Families and life-threatening illness: Assumptions, assessment, and intervention. In M. Leahey and L.M. Wright (Eds.). *Families and life-threatening illness.* (45–58) Springhouse, PA: Springhouse Corp.

______. (1988). Family nursing trends in academic and clinical settings. *Proceedings of the international family nursing conference.* May, 1988. Calgary, Alberta, Canada.

Wynne, L.G. et al. (1958). Pseudomutuality in the family relationships of schizophrenics. *Psychiatry, 21*, 205.

Yankelovich, D. (1975). How students control their drug crisis. *Psychology Today, 9* (5), 39–42.

______. (1981). *New rules.* New York: Bantam Books.

Yankelovich, D. & Gurin, J. (1989, March). The new American dream. *American Health*, pp. 63–67.

Yankelovitch, Skelley, and White, Inc. (1975). *The American family report: A study of the American family and money.* Minneapolis: General Mills.

______. (1979). *Family health in an era of stress. General Mills family report: Report 1978–1979.* Minneapolis: General Mills.

Ybarra, L. (1982, February). When wives work: The impact on the Chicano family. *Journal of Marriage and the Family, 44*, 169–180.

Young, C. (1982). Family systems model. In I.W. Clements, D.M. Buchanan. *Family Therapy, A Nursing Perspective* (pp. 101–109). New York: Wiley.

Yura, H., Walsh, M. (1978). *The nursing process.* New York: Appleton-Century-Crofts.

Zander, K. (1988). Nursing case management: Strategic management of cost and quality outcomes. *Journal of Nursing Administration, 18* (5), 23–30.

Zuk, G.H. (1966). The go-between process in family therapy. *Family Process, 5*, 162.

Index